ILLUSTRATED ESSENTIALS IN ORTHOPEDIC PHYSICAL ASSESSMENT

RONALD C. EVANS, D.C., F.A.C.O., F.I.C.C.
Chiropractic Neuro-Orthopedic Associates;
Chairman of the Iowa Board of Chiropractic Examiners
of the Department of Professional Licensure,
State of Iowa,
Des Moines, Iowa;
Examiner Emeritus
American Board of Chiropractic Orthopedists
of the American Chiropractic Association
Washington, DC

Photography by Miriam C. Dunlap BA, MA

with 643 illustrations

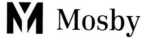

St. Louis Baltimore Boston Chicago London Madrid Philadelphia Sydney Toronto

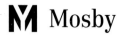

Dedicated to Publishing Excellence

Publisher: George Stamathis
Editor: Martha Sasser
Project Manager: Mark Spann
Production Editor: Amy Wastalu
Layout Artist: Doris Hallas
Manufacturing Supervisor: Theresa Fuchs
Designer: David Zielinski

Printed in the United States of America

Mosby–Year Book, Inc.
11830 Westline Industrial Drive
St. Louis, Missouri 63146

Library of Congress Cataloging in Publication Data

Evans, Ronald C.
    Illustrated essentials in orthopedic physical assessment / Ronald
C. Evans ; photography by Miriam C. Dunlap.
       p.   cm.
    Includes bibliographical references and index.
    ISBN 0-8016-6612-0
    1. Orthopedics--Diagnosis.   2. Physical diagnosis.   3. Physical
orthopedic tests.   4. Joints--Range of motion--Measurement.
I. Title.
    [DNLM: 1. Joint Diseases--diagnosis--atlases.   2. Bone Diseases-
-diagnosis--atlases.   WE 17 E92i 1994]
RD734.E93   1994
617.3--dc20
DNLM/DLC
for Library of Congress
                                                                    93-33257
                                                                    CIP

94 95 96 97 98 CA /MV 9 8 7 6 5 4 3 2

ILLUSTRATED
ESSENTIALS IN
ORTHOPEDIC
PHYSICAL
ASSESSMENT

For Linda, with love and pride—
RCE

Preface

The basic observation of a patient's antalgia and exacerbative movements allows the formulation of the presenting signs and symptoms into a recognizable disease syndrome. The essence of diagnosis is the clinically demonstrable or reproducible signs of disease.

Many physicians associate an aura of mysticism with the ease and speed with which the orthopedic specialist arrives at a diagnosis. It is in fact, the specialist's development of interviewing, observation, and physical testing skills that allows proceeding directly to the heart of the patient's problem.

I have been privileged in private practice to be challenged by myriad orthopedic health problems presented by my patients. I believe that my early and fumbling years were well tolerated by these patients. They may have become well in spite of my efforts. They have remained loyal indeed.

In later years of practice, many of the early patients return with new diseases. These diseases are often much more difficult to diagnose and to treat. My skills as an orthopedic specialist have been honed to a fine edge out of necessity. Some of these patients will not live long enough to give me yet another chance to get it right.

The perspective of the role of the physician in modern medicine has changed. Physicians are no longer viewed as the omnipotent beings they were formerly thought to be. The physician is expected to recognize personal skill limitations and make appropriate consultations and referrals. Patients expect the correct diagnosis the first time around. At the least, they deserve that.

This book is created to relieve the frustration and discomfort for two parties in their quest for wellness. First are the physicians and orthopedic specialists, who labor mightily in pushing, pulling, poking, bending, and twisting patients' body parts as they search for the cause of the suffering. Second are the patients, who have been not-so-gently pushed, pulled, poked, bent, and twisted into inhuman configurations, as they wait furtively for the discovery of the cause of their anguish. I salute both parties for their endurance in seeking the origin of disease.

Each chapter of *Illustrated Essentials in Orthopedic Physical Assessment* has a specific format. The format lends to the quick referencing of tests and maneuvers and cross referencing of associated procedures.

Each chapter introduction addresses the various unique considerations or pathologies of the focal joint. The introductory section contains the index of the tests presented and illustrated in the chapter.

Range of motion for the joint is included. These illustrations depict the expected full ranges of movement for the joint. The discussion further identifies the amount of lost motion that can affect the activities of daily living.

Muscle testing for each joint is also included. This section identifies the musculature that is the prime mover of the joint, the innervation and the action of the muscle.

Each chapter contains testing procedural flow charts. These charts identify the test procedure(s) used to objectify the symptoms of pain, paralysis, weakness, and loss of sensation. The chart provides a plan of examination and selections of tests for the joint.

Each test, maneuver, sign, law, or phenomenon is presented separately. The common usage name for the test, as identified in Stedman's, Dorland's, or Churchill's medical dictionaries, is used as the heading for the test. This name is followed by equally common synonyms and eponyms. Eponyms for certain examinations vary from locale to locale or among institutions within the same area. Such observations are a reflection of the training center's influence. This is especially true where the names of prominent local physicians are frequently used for these examinations. Occasionally the same test is given two or more names, or the name can apply to more than one test or sign. In a problem-oriented situation, eponyms are routinely used in the physical evaluation process. Familiarity with the terms and techniques used in determining regional problems enables the physician and assistant to record and clarify an orthopedic examination.

A *test* is part of the physical examination in which direct contact with the patient is made. It also may be a chemical test, x-ray, or other study. All tests described in his book will relate to the physical examination.

A *sign* is elucidated by a test or a particular maneuver. A sign can be simply a visual observation (for example, antalgia), and it is an indication of the existence of a problem perceived by the examiner.

A *maneuver* is a complex motion or series of movements, used either as a test or treatment. A maneuver is also a method or technique.

A *phenomenon* is any sign or objective symptom or any observable occurrence or fact.

A *law* is a description of a phenomenon that is so thoroughly tested and accepted that it is regarded as a principle governing like phenomena.

For each testing procedure in the book, a general comment is presented about the pathologic condition targeted by the test. This comment is followed by a discussion of how the test is conducted. Each procedure is supported by photo illustrations and legends. Each test is cross referenced with other supportive tests and procedures. An accurate documentation or reporting statement is provided for each test. When possible, a "clinical pearl" identifies the subtle nuances or finesse of the tests that the author has gleaned from empirical practice.

The references are listed for each chapter. This listing is extensive and in some instances reflects older volumes or works than is commonly found in scientific literature today. These older references are the original work of the creators of various tests or procedures in this book. Preserving the books in these reference lists is an attempt to preserve a continuum in the developments of orthopedic investigation.

Finally, about the references used:

"When you steal from one author, it's plagiarism; if you steal from many, it's research."

W. Mizner 1876

"For such kind of borrowing as this, if it be not bettered by the borrower, among good authors is accounted *plagiare.*"

John Milton 1649

Although the various tests and procedures in this book are presented in an anatomical or regional format, the application of the tests are accomplished in a more natural flow of examination procedures. The natural flow of the examination usually moves the patient from the standing position, through sitting, supine, and side-lying positions to the prone position. Appendix B lists the tests found in this book according to the position of the patient.

Acknowledgements

Numerous individuals come to mind for their contributions to this book, and they are indeed too many to list. They are the physicians who attended my lectures and took the time to tell me about or demonstrate for me various orthopedic tests and signs. I am sure that in many instances the uniformed or casual onlookers thought that grown men were wrestling in public. In fact we were exchanging the latest testing procedures. I will always be grateful to these keepers of the empirical body of medicine and science. Without their thirst for knowledge and scientific rationale, this book could not have been written.

More specifically, I must acknowledge three great mentors in chiropractic orthopedics, Dr. Joseph J. Sweere, Dr. Russell G. Hass (deceased) and Dr. Robert N. Solheim (deceased). It was my fortune to be the student of these men of orthopedic science. Their challenges kept me advancing in my fundamental knowledge in orthopedic medicine, and their educational excellence caused me to grow. This book is a product of that growth. Their guidance and vitality have been the breath of life for the entity of orthopedic specialization within the scope of chiropractic practice.

My contemporaries, Dr. James R. Brandt, Dr. Bruce V. Gundersen, Dr. Gregory R. Norton, and Dr. Leonard E. Toon have contributed their time and diligence to the preparation of this text. Without their critical commentaries more errors in preparation would have slipped through my fingers. I am ever indebted to their willingness to participate in this academic exercise.

Two individuals, Mrs. Pamela Schwartz and Mrs. Linda Evans, have been tireless in their efforts to keep up with my revisions of the manuscript. I am sure they thought the stream of changes would never end. I am grateful for their accuracy and speed at typing and proofreading.

The photographer, Miriam C. Dunlap, could not have worked harder to achieve any higher degree of excellence with the illustrations. She pushed the models to exceed their known abilities, squeezing out every detail of movement or position. Her work embodies the constant search for perfection, and her efforts served as a guide for me to create prose equal to the illustrations.

The primary photographic model, Ms. Lisa Bates, demonstrated interminable patience in achieving just the right position or look of a test or procedure. This is matched by her great physical beauty. I am grateful for her stamina and physical pliability.

Two support personnel were very important to the photographic portion of the project. The first is Chef David Larsen, who provided catering and did a wonderful job of feeding our bodies and spirits during the long and arduous shoots. It is no small miracle that the models were the same size at the end of all the shooting sessions as they were at the beginning. The second person is Mr. Rod Slings, who provided the make-up for the photo shoots. A supreme cosmetics supplier, Rod was able to disguise the everyday surface wear and tear on the models. Thanks for making us look good.

Ms. Amy Wastalu, the production editor for this text, is the finest. With cheer and enthusiasm she has redirected my meandering prose into sharp focus. She has persuaded this work to rise above mundane scientific literature to become a useful instrument in the search for relief of patient suffering. I am ever indebted for her pursuit of excellence and for her patience.

Last but not least, I thank Mr. James Shanahan, acquisitions editor for Mosby. Mosby has been wonderful throughout this endeavor and Mr. Shanahan has provided the necessary encouragement at the most difficult times. This book would not exist without his persistence. I look forward to our next collaboration.

Introduction

Solving a patient's health problem can be a demanding exercise of orthopedic medical detection and logical deduction. Each health problem is a new diagnostic jigsaw puzzle for which the pieces must be found and fitted together in a carefully organized manner. Success requires an organized thought process in approaching the patient's problem. There must be a clear plan to follow and a particular aim in each stage of the investigation.

First, it must be determined if a lesion of the musculoskeletal system is present. This determination is accomplished by analysis of the history and physical examination.

Second, the location of the lesion must be determined. Is it possible to locate the lesion at one site, or are multiple sites involved? A system must be developed by the examiner to relate the signs and symptoms to a basic knowledge of musculoskeletal anatomy.

Third, what pathologic conditions are capable of producing the lesions?

Fourth, from careful analysis of the history and examination and by intelligent use of ancillary tests, which of these suspected conditions is most likely to be present?

Each examination or investigation should have a plan for including or excluding a specific member of a "short list" of suspected conditions. It is always the failure to have such an organized plan or approach that makes the diagnosis of orthopedic health problems so artificially difficult. Routine steps must be followed but not blind routine or blunderbuss investigations.

Diagnosis purely by comparison with previous cases is reserved for the physician or orthopedic specialist who is very experienced and remembers the cases very accurately, but this combination is not the norm. The entry level physician or orthopedic specialist will come nearer to diagnostic accuracy by logically progressing through the medical investigation paradigm.

Despite all this, however, the right approach will never be achieved until one misconception is laid to rest. This misconception is that the exact solution of an orthopedic problem does not matter very much and that such a solution will be of academic interest only, with no useful nonsurgical treatment. Such a view is nonsense. It is true that health science is frustrated in treating motor neuron disease; no cure exists for hereditary ataxia, and no reliable method exists to prevent relapses in disseminated sclerosis. Contrary to many beliefs, these diseases occupy only a small part of the orthopedist's time.

Think for a moment of the transformation in the last 30 years in the treatment of cervical spine trauma, intervertebral disc prolapse, carpal tunnel syndrome, and deficiency neuropathies. Think of the influence of physiologic therapeutics in hypersensitivity states and in acute episodes of soft-tissue disease, of the continuing progress of manipulative therapy in certain facets of the migraine headache process, mechanical lower-back disorders, and in trigeminal neuralgia. Consider the advances of chiropractic orthopedics in treating various forms of benign spinal compression.

Finally, the solution of an orthopedic problem takes time. A solution cannot be rushed, and the examiner must never allow the approach to be influenced by the exhortations of optimistic colleagues to "just glance at this case while passing" or to "just run over the musculoskeletal system, it won't take 5 minutes." It will, it always does, and so it should.

Contents

ILLUSTRATED ESSENTIALS IN ORTHOPEDIC PHYSICAL ASSESSMENT

Diagnostic Instrumentation

Some tests and maneuvers that aid in the substantiation of the patient's complaint require instrumentation. Information derived from the objective assessment is part of the data needed to arrive at a diagnosis and analysis. Equally important is the information derived from the subjective history and the impressions derived from diagnostic imaging. At times there may be a need for referral to facilities that may have more diverse or specific diagnostic abilities, such as advanced imaging methods, neurodiagnostic testing, laboratory, or psychologic assessment.

The basic elements of examining the patient include: vital signs, observation and inspection, palpation, neurologic evaluation, range of motion studies, clinical laboratory, orthopedic tests, and diagnostic imaging.

VITAL SIGNS

Vital signs include the brachial blood pressure, peripheral pulse rate, respiration rate, height, weight, and vital capacity. The instruments used in these measurements include the stethoscope, the spirometer, scales, tape measures, and the blood pressure cuff.

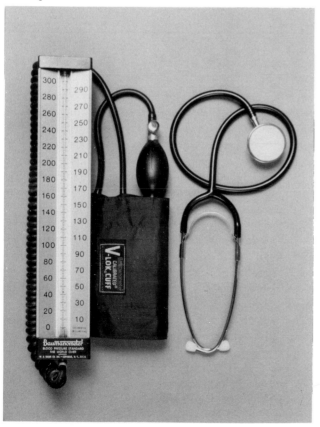

OBSERVATION AND INSPECTION

Observation and inspection of the patient occur anytime during the examination or history interview, especially when the patient is not aware of the observation. The examiner notes the following: (1) posture, for antalgia or deformities; (2) gait, noting if there is a need for assistance; and (3) spinal symmetry, especially noting prominences or elevations, flattenings or depressions, and scoliosis or abnormalities of the anteroposterior curvature. The examiner also determines whether any scars are present, noting location, size, and direction.

PALPATION

This is the process of touching or feeling the patient's body, joints, and any contiguous structures. The purpose of palpation is to locate and substantiate areas of tenderness and abnormal muscle tone. Palpation also allows the physician to identify a localized increase or decrease in superficial temperature and the presence of induration and masses. Palpation can be performed with the fingertips, by percussion (gently tapping with a reflex hammer), with vibration (using a C-128 tuning fork), or with the blunt end of a cotton tip applicator. This examination can be accomplished in the standing, sitting, or prone positions. Effective spinal palpation is also accomplished in the sitting or kneeling Adam's position.

NEUROLOGIC EVALUATION

The neurologic evaluation involves locating the lesion; testing deep tendon, superficial, and pathologic reflexes; testing cranial nerve and brainstem function; measuring of body parts (mensuration); grading muscular strength; and testing the gross sensory modalities.

Cerebral dysfunction is determined during the consultation by noting the patient's mannerisms and orientation in time and space and of body parts. Further evaluation of lesions in the cerebrum require sophisticated imaging systems and electroneurodiagnostic testing.

Cerebellar lesions are associated with repeated cogwheel-type physical actions while the patient's eyes are open. The posterior columns of the spinal cord are the source of the dysfunction when repeated physical actions are smooth and occur while the patient's eyes are open. However, these same actions cannot be repeated with the eyes closed, which

Fig. 1–1, left. Wall-mounted sphygmomanometer and stethoscope. Most significant heart sounds occur in the 200 to 500 Hz frequency range, but human auditory sensitivity is limited below 1000 Hz. Stethoscopes amplify the lower frequencies.

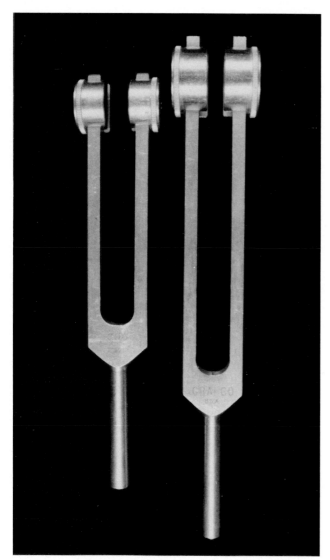

Fig. 1–2 Aluminum alloy tuning forks, available in C-64, C-128, C-256, C-512, C-1024, C-2048, and C-4096 vibrations. The lower frequency tuning forks are the usual choices for bone vibration conduction studies.

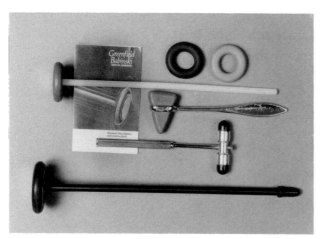

Fig. 1–4 From top to bottom the Greenfield Babinski reflex hammer, Taylor reflex hammer, Buck's neurologic hammer, Babinski reflex hammer.

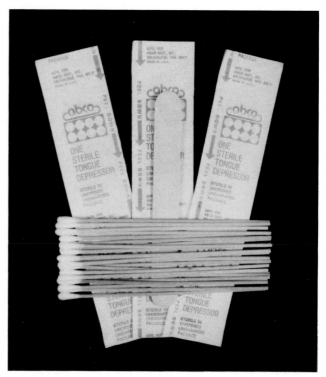

Fig. 1–3 Single-tipped cotton applicators are both economical and versatile and can be used in the following settings: emergency room, examining room, outpatient clinic, and laboratory, and on dressing carts. Sterile tongue depressors are usually made from white birchwood that is 1/16″ thick. These tongue depressors are evenly cut and highly polished for smooth and clean edges, ends, and surfaces.

is known as Romberg's sign. Brainstem dysfunction is discerned through testing of the cranial nerves. Spinal cord lesions can be differentiated from lower motor neuron disorders by the type and quality of paralysis, reflexes, muscle tone, clonus, atrophy, fasciculation, and reactions of degeneration.

Deep tendon reflexes help the examiner locate the lower motor neuron lesion and differentiate it from an upper motor neuron lesion. The deep tendon reflexes are listed in the box on page 3.

Superficial reflexes differentiate lower motor neuron lesions from upper motor neuron lesions. The superficial reflexes are listed in the box on page 3.

Pathologic reflexes determine the presence of upper motor neuron lesions. These reflexes include the following: Hoffmann's, Babinski's, Chaddock's, Oppenheim's, Bechterew-Mendel's, Rossolimo's, Gordon's, and Schaeffer's.

Cranial nerve function is determined by testing brainstem activity. The box on page 3 lists the cranial nerves and the basic function of each nerve.

Mensuration of body parts is used to determine atrophy

Deep Tendon Reflexes

Scapulohumeral C5-C6	Ulnar C8-T1
Biceps C5-C6	Patellar L2-L4
Radial C5-C6	Hamstring L4-S1
Triceps C7-C8	Achilles S1-S2
Wrist C7-C8	

Superficial Reflexes

Corneal III,V	Cremasteric	T12-L2
Upper abdominal T7-T9	Gluteal	L4-L5
Lower abdominal T10-T12	Plantar	S1-S2

Cranial Nerves and Basic Functions

I	Smell	VII	Facial muscle (taste)
II	Vision	VIII	Auditory (balance)
III	Light accommodation	IX	Taste (gag)
III,IV,VI	Eye movement	X	Voice (swallow)
V	Sensation (wink)	XI	Shoulder (shrug)
XII	Tongue (motor)		

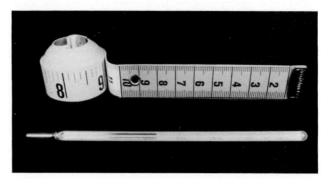

Fig. 1-5 Soft linen tape is marked in inches on one side and centimeters on the other. The fast reading clinical thermometer is made of heat-tempered, fully aged Corning glass and has permanent markings. A break-resistant bulb encloses triple-distilled mercury, and a precise constriction chamber allows for softer, easier shakedown.

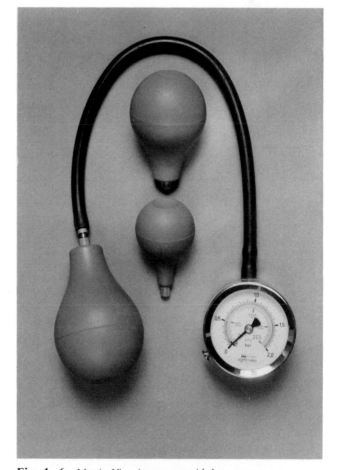

Fig. 1-6 Martin Vigorimeter aneroid dynamometer.

and functional and anatomic abnormalities. Common areas of mensuration are listed below:

1. Excursion of the chest during inspiration and expiration.
2. Upper extremity circumference (brachium and antebrachium) as measured in the noncontracted and contracted state.
3. Lower extremity circumferences (thigh and calf) as measured in the noncontracted and contracted states.
4. Leg length (standing versus supine or prone). This is to differentiate a functional short leg from an anatomic short leg.

Grip strength testing examines the function of the median nerve and can help determine malingering activity. Cervical intrinsic muscle testing relates to the cervical spine functions of flexion, extension, lateral flexion, and rotation. The box on page 4 identifies the cervical extrinsic muscles and their specific nerve root levels.

Thoracolumbar intrinsic muscle function is associated with trunk flexion and extension and lateral flexion and rotation. The box on page 4 identifies the thoracolumbar extrinsic musculature and the associated nerve root levels.

Testing of the gross sensory modalities allows for evalua-

Cervical Spine Extrinsic Musculature with Specific Nerve Roots Noted

Deltoid C5	Wrist flexors C7
Biceps C6	Finger extensors C7
Wrist extensors C6	Finger flexors C8
Triceps C7	Finger abductors T1

Thoracolumbar Extrinsic Musculature and Specific Associated Nerve Root Levels

Hip flexors L2-L3	Hip extensors L4-L5
Knee extensors L3-L4	Knee flexors L5-S1
Ankle extensors L4-L5	Ankle flexors S1-S2

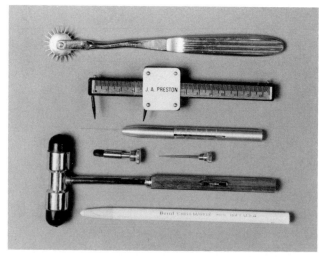

Fig. 1–7 From top to bottom the Wartenberg pinwheel, Boley two-point discrimination gauge, von Frey anesthesiometer, Buck's camel hair brush, pin, and neurological hammer and a Berol China Marker.

tion of the sensory dermatomes involved in superficial sensations, deep sensations, and proprioception.

The superficial sensations include light touch, pain, and temperature. Light touch is mediated by the dorsal columns and is easily examined with a cotton ball. Pain receptors are mediated by the lateral spinothalamic tracts and are tested by a pin prick and hot and cold temperatures. Temperature, or thermal sensation, is mediated by the dorsal columns and is tested with warm (not hot) and cool (not cold) temperatures.

The deep sensations are vibration and deep pressure perception. Vibration is tested with a C-128, or lower frequency, tuning fork and is mediated by the dorsal columns of the spinal cord. Deep pressure is tested by squeezing any muscular part of the body and is also mediated in the dorsal columns.

Proprioception, or joint sense, is mediated by the dorsal columns and can be tested by having the patient point to a particular part of the body while keeping the eyes closed.

RANGE OF MOTION

Range of motion can be tested for any movable joint in the body, including the spine. Range of motion is assessed bilaterally by comparing findings with a given set of normal values. Normal values can vary dramatically, depending on the reference source used. A physician must exercise careful professional judgment to ensure objectivity. The physician must ask: Is the motion demonstrated by the patient consistent with the nature of the injury? Is the motion also consistent with the x-rays, other tests, and objective findings? Is the motion consistent in repeated testing? The patient should be tested both actively and passively. The location, quality, and grade of pain should be noted.

Any range of motion that is less than normal may indicate or be the result of muscle spasm, sprain, strain, joint subluxation, general arthritic degeneration, postsurgical condition, or obesity.

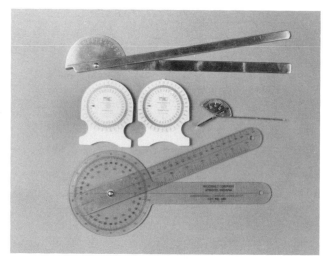

Fig. 1–8 From top to bottom, stainless steel goniometer measures movement of joints from 0 degrees to 180 degrees. Inclinometers measure the angular motion from 0 degrees to 360 degrees. Finger or small joint goniometer measures the movement of interphalangeal joints of fingers and toes. Plastic radiographic goniometer provides standard orthopedic measurements of joint motion and neutral position.

CLINICAL LABORATORY

For the physician concerned with musculoskeletal disorders, differential diagnosis becomes a challenge. Complete blood and urine tests can help determine a diagnosis. Diseases of the heart, liver, kidney, pancreas, and prostate are but a few that mimic back pain of spinal origin. The boxes on page 5 list tests that, at differing times, aid in the differential diagnosis related to spinal dysfunction.

Individual Blood and Urine Tests

HLA-B27
Acid phosphates
Alkaline phosphatase
Amylase
Cholestrol
Creatinine
Creatinine phosphokinase
Glucose
Lactic Dehygrogenase (LDH) Compression Test II
Anti-nuclear antibody (ANA)
Antistreptolysin-O titer
Urinalysis
Bilirubin
Sodium
Hemoglobin
Hematocrit
Blood urea nitrogen (BUN)

Calcium
Chloride
Leucine aminopeptidase (LAP)
Latex agglutination
Lupus erythematosus (LE) cell prep
Lipase
Lipids
Bence-Jones protein
Phosphorus
Potassium
Protein-bound iodine
RA latex
Serum glutamate oxoaloacetate tranaminase (SGOT)
Uric acid
White blood cell (WBC) count
Red blood cell (RBC) count
Heavy metal screens

Blood and Serum Panels That are Useful in the Differential Diagnosis

Bone Panel

Total protein
Calcium
Serum protein electrophoresis
Complete blood count (CBC)
Ionized calcium
Alkaline phosphatase

Arthritis Panel

RA Latex
Uric acid
ANA screen
C-reactive protein (CRP)

Liver Function Tests

Total protein—albumin and globulin
Bilirubin—total and direct
Cholesterol
SGOT
Gamma-glutamyltranspeptidase (GGT) or peptidase
Alkaline phosphatase
Serum glutamate pyruvate transaminase SGPT
LDH

Parathyroid Function and Calcium Metabolism

Serum calcium
Alkaline phosphatase
Urine calcium
Serum phosphorus
Total protein

Pancreas Function Tests

CBC
Glucose tolerance
Lipase
Amylase

Joint Pain or Swelling Tests

CBC
Sedimentation rate
Synovial fluid analysis, including culture
Heavy metal screen
RA latex
ANA screen
Uric acid

Thyroid Profile

Triiodothyronine (T_3)
Thyroxine (T_4)
Free thyroxine index (FTI)
Thyroid-stimulating hormone (TSH)

Prostate Profile

Prostatic acid phosphatase
Prostate-specific antigen

Hypertension (Coronary Risk Profile)

Cholesterol
High-density lipoprotein (HDL) cholesterol
Coronary risk indicator
Triglycerides
Low-density lipoprotein (LDL) cholesterol

Health Screen

Glucose
Creatinine
Uric acid
Triglycerides
Calculated LDL
Calcium
Phosphorus
Albumin
Albumin-globulin (A/G) ratio
Alkaline phosphatase
LDH
GGT
Potassium
Total CO_2
T_4 radioimmunoassay (RIA)
BUN
BUN-creatinine ratio
Cholesterol
HDL
Cholesterol-HDL ratio
Ionized calcium
Total protein
Globulin
Bilirubin—total
SGOT
SGPT
Sodium
Chloride
Anion GAP
CBC

ORTHOPEDIC TESTS

Orthopedic tests are based on the kinetic activity of the patient. The tests and procedures illustrated in this text are specific for the outcome noted. The tests are positive, or a sign is present, when the procedure duplicates the patient's complaint or symptom. If the testing causes different pain or symptoms it may indeed be significant, but such a result is not positive for the findings the test was designed to elicit. Specificity of findings is the key. A subjective complaint, when consistent with an objective finding, becomes another objective finding.

During an examination, the physician must employ examination techniques that account for the human tendency to exaggerate. The physician should conduct many tests so that the patient is not aware of which specific faculty or sensory modality is being examined. Using a little skepticism during the examination aids in differentiating the organic complaint from one that may have a psychologic or hysteric basis.

DIAGNOSTIC IMAGING PROCEDURES FOR THE SPECIALIST

Diagnostic imaging procedures are important to the diagnosis and to the management of the case. The decision to use any diagnostic imaging procedure should be based on a demonstrated need and should only be used after obtaining an adequate medical history and conducting a physical examination. The decision to use any imaging procedure must be based on the assumption that the results of the examination, even if negative, will significantly affect the treatment of the patient. The value of the information gained from the imaging examination must be worth the possible detrimental effects of the procedure, and the information must be worth the expense incurred. In procedures that use ionizing radiation—plain film radiography, fluoroscopy, and CT—the possible effect of radiation on the patient or future offspring must be considered.

Plain Film Radiography

Spinal radiographs are nearly always produced to rule out fracture, dislocation, anomaly, or bone pathology. The radiographs are also used in biomechanical analysis to establish an initial course of treatment for the patient.

Radiographs of the extremity skeletal structures may be produced to rule out primary extremity pathologic processes.

Soft-tissue views, or plain film radiographs of body systems other than skeletal structures, may be ordered to aid the differential diagnosis.

Studying any skeletal region requires two views, preferably at right angles to each other (such as an anteroposterior (AP) and a lateral view). Follow-up spot views also should be produced when any region on the initial study is not clear or needs further investigation.

The patient's history and clinical evaluation are guides that help determine which portion(s) of the body should be radiographed and how many different views should be

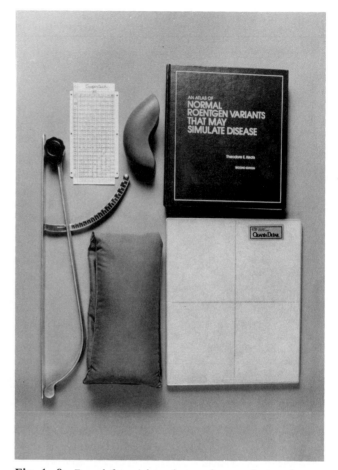

Fig. 1–9 From left to right and top to bottom, Supertech x-ray factoring computer, gonadal shielding, *An Atlas of normal roentgen variants that may simulate disease*, by Theodore E. Keats, radiographic calipers, sandbag, DuPont *Quanta Detail* Rare Earth x-ray cassette screens and compatible film.

produced. Unnecessary structures should not be included in the study of neighboring regions.

Tomography

Conventional tomography is also known as thin section radiography, planography, and linear tomography. Conventional tomography is ordered as an advanced diagnostic procedure when further analysis of a suspected pathologic process is required. Conventional tomography is largely supplanted by computed tomography. However, there are circumstances, such as evaluating subtle alterations of bone density and ruling out fracture, when conventional tomography is indicated.

Computed tomography (CT), formerly called a CAT scan, is a valuable computerized, thin-section, axial x-ray procedure. A CT scan is used for more detailed appreciation of skeletal pathologic processes, which can help evaluate suspected intervertebral disc protrusions or herniations, facet disease, or central canal and lateral recess stenosis. Such a scan is not a routine procedure. If spinal disease is suspected and is not well identified on plain films and the patient is not responding to care, a CT scan is indicated. A CT scan is especially useful for the appreciation of bone and calcifications and surpasses magnetic resonance imaging (MRI) in this regard.

Magnetic Resonance Imaging (MRI)

The MRI is a computerized, thin-section imaging procedure that uses a magnetic field and radio frequency waves rather than ionizing radiation. MRI can produce thin-section images in the sagittal, coronal, or axial planes as well as any other oblique plane desired. The MRI can image neurologic structures and other soft tissues and can reveal disc degeneration before any other imaging method. The MRI gives a null (negative) image of cortical bone, but the marrow fat in medullary bone is well visualized. Bone disease is appreciated, but often not as well as by CT.

However, indications for MRI are similar to CT. MRI is superior for the evaluation of suspected spinal cord tumors or damage, intracranial disease, and various types of central nervous system disease, such as multiple sclerosis. MRI is rapidly replacing myelography in the evaluation of disc herniation and protrusion. MRI is especially useful in the identification of small differences among similar soft tissues and surpasses CT in this regard.

Radionuclide Scanning

Several radioisotopes that have an affinity for certain tissues can be injected intravenously for distribution within target tissues. The bone scan (osteoscintigraphy) is usually the only radionuclide study of benefit in orthopedics. Bone scans are valuable for the evaluation of early bone disease. Plain film radiography is not sensitive to early bone disease because lesions in medullary bone are not radiographically visible until there is a 30% to 50% loss of bone. However, a bone scan will reveal many types of bone disease as early as 4% to 7% bone loss.

Radionuclide bone scanning is the method of choice in searching for lytic bone diseases. Bone scans are also indicated for detecting bone infection and fracture. A bone scan will be positive within 2 days of a fracture and will continue to demonstrate increased uptake for as long as 6 months following the fracture.

Video Fluoroscopy

Video fluoroscopy is used when a function study of the joint is warranted. Video fluoroscopy should be used when there is biomechanical abnormality that is not adequately demonstrated by plain film stress surveys or other examination methods.

Video fluoroscopy is used only when there is clinical

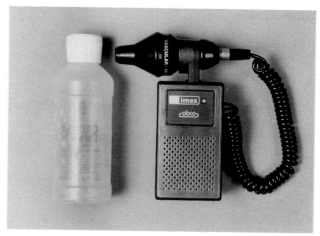

Fig. 1–10 The pocket Doppler (right) audibly monitors pulses in noisy environments when palpation is questionable or is not possible or when the pulse is especially weak or rapid. The Doppler also aids in the assessment of circulation distal to fractures, burns, and other injuries to quickly determine the extent of injury. Transmission gel (left) is used to couple the Doppler head to the skin surface and eliminate air gaps that can degrade sound transmission.

indication of significant instability (hypermobility) or in cases of fixation or marked hypomobility.

Diagnostic Ultrasound

Diagnostic ultrasound, a sound wave echo study, is particularly useful for the evaluation of soft tissues. Because of technical improvements in the use of ultrasound some facilities are now using ultrasound to study the spine. The diagnostic ultrasound does not provide the same quality of image as the CT or MRI, but the ultrasound is fast, noninvasive, and much less expensive.

Thermography

The thermographic examination is conducted with the use of contact liquid crystal detectors or sophisticated infrared scanners. Thermography is extremely sensitive to microvascular changes in the skin that accompany many pathologic conditions, and it is chiefly known for its effectiveness in demonstrating spinal radiculopathy and peripheral neuropathy. Thermography is now considered the test of choice for revealing reflex sympathetic dysfunction. The procedure also has usefulness in the evaluation of thoracic outlet syndrome and many generalized neuromuscular conditions. Thermography is also excellent for differentiating between a neurologic and vascular abnormality.

Thermography has a greater degree of sensitivity in documenting neurovascular abnormality than any of the other imaging systems because it is a test of physiology rather than a test of anatomy, but thermography has a lesser degree of specificity of image resolution than CT or MRI, and a greater degree of specificity than the radionuclide bone scan.

Bibliography

American Medical Association: *Guides to the evaluation of permanent impairment,* ed 3, 1990, Chicago.

Apley AG, Solomon L: Concise system of orthopaedics and fractures, London, 1988, Butterworth-Heinemann.

Banks SD: The use of spinographic parameters in the differential diagnosis of lumbar facet and disc syndromes, *J Manipulative Physiol Ther,* 6:111–13, 1983.

Bronfort G, Josumsen OH: The functional radiographic examination of patients with low back pain: A study of different forms of variations, *J Manipulative Physiol Ther,* 7:89–97, 1984.

Carmichael JP: Inter- and intra-examiners reliability of palpation for sacroiliac joint dysfunction, *J Manipulative Physiol Ther,* 10:164–171, 1987.

Cipriano JJ: *Photographic manual of regional orthopaedic and neurological tests,* ed 2, Baltimore, 1991, Williams & Wilkins.

Cox WA: Gonstead concepts of fullspine radiography, *Eur J Chir, 30:140–145, 1982.*

D'Ambrosia, RD: *Musculoskeletal disorders: Regional examination and differential diagnosis,* Philadelphia, 1977, JB Lippincott.

Dandy DJ: *Essential orthopaedics and trauma,* Edinburgh, 1989, Churchill Livingstone.

DeBoer KF, Harmon RO, Savoie S, Tuttle CD: Inter-and intra-examiner reliability of leg length differential measurement: A preliminary study, *J Manipulative Physiol Ther,* 6:61–66, 1983.

Doherty M, Doherty J: *Clinical examination in rheumatology,* London, 1992, Wolfe Publishing.

Henderson DJ, Domon TJ: Functional roentgenometric evaluation of the cervical spine in the sagittal plane, *J Manipulative Physiol Ther,* 8:219–227, 1985.

Hildebrandt RW: Chiropractic spinography and postural roentgenology, part 1: History of development, *J Manipulative Physiol Ther,* 3:87–92, 1980.

Jackson BL, Barker W, Bentz J, Gamble AG: Inter-and intra-examiner reliability of the upper cervical x-ray marking system: A second look, *J Manipulative Physiol Ther,* 10:157–163, 1987.

Jahn WT: Standardization of orthopedic testing of the cervical and cervicobrachial regions, *J Manipulative Physiol Ther,* 1:32–45, 1978.

Jahn WT: Standardization of orthopedic testing of the upper extremity, *J Manipulative Physiol Ther,* 4:85–92, 1981.

Katz, WA: Rheumatic diseases diagnosis and management, Philadelphia, 1977, JB Lippincott.

Kendall HO, Kendall FP, Wadsworth GE: Muscles testing and function, ed 2, Baltimore, 1971, Williams & Wilkins.

Magee DJ: Orthopedic physical assessment, Philadelphia, 1987, WB Saunders.

Mazion JM: *Illustrated manual of neurological reflexes/signs/tests, part I; orthopedic signs/tests/maneuvers for office procedure, part II* Orlando, 1980, Daniels Publishing Co.

McRae R: *Clinical orthopaedic examination,* ed 3, Edinburgh, 1990, Churchill Livingstone.

Medical Economics Books: *Patient care flow chart manual,* ed 3, Oradell, NJ, 1982, Medical Economics Books.

Schram SB, Hosek RS: Error limitations in x-ray kinemathics of the spine, *J Manipulative Physiol Ther,* 5:5–10, 1982.

Sherman R: Chiropractic x-ray rationale, *J Can Chir,* 30:33–35, 1986.

Stokes HM: The seriously injured hand-weakness of grip, *J Occup Med,* 25:683–4, 1983.

Sweere JJ: Method of physiological testing in the differential diagnosis of acute mechanical low back pain, *Ortho Brief,* CCO (ACA), Sept, 1984.

Sweere JJ: The chiropractic industrial physical examinations, *J Chir,* 16:39–62, 1982.

Thurston SE: *The little black book of neurology,* Chicago, 1987, Mosby.

Turek SL: *Orthopaedics principles and their application,* ed 3, Philadelphia, 1977, JB Lippincott.

~ 2 ~
Cardinal Symptoms and Signs

*T*he description of the steps in the following clinical examination is intended only as a guide. The actual technique of examination will vary according to individual preference. Nevertheless, it is useful to develop and stick to a particular routine. Familiarity with such a routine will ensure that no step in the examination is forgotten.

The part to be examined should be adequately exposed and in good light. Many mistakes are made simply because the examiner does not insist on the removal of enough clothing to allow proper examination. When an extremity is being examined, the uninvolved extremity should always be used for comparison.

Visual inspection should be carried out systematically, with attention to these four areas: (1) **Bones**—Observe the general alignment and position of the parts to detect any deformity, shortening, or unusual posture; (2) **Soft tissues**—Observe the soft tissue contours, comparing bilaterally and noting any visible evidence of general or local swelling or muscle wasting; (3) **Color and texture of the skin**—Look for rubor, cyanosis, pigmentation, shininess, loss of hair, or other changes; (4) **Scars or sinuses**—If a scar is present, determine from its appearance whether it was caused by operation (linear scar with suture marks), injury (irregular scar), or suppuration (broad, adherent, puckered scar).

In palpation there are also four points to consider. (1) **Skin temperature**—by careful bilateral comparison, determine whether there is an area of increased warmth or of unusual coolness. An increase of local temperature denotes increased blood flow; the usual cause is an inflammatory reaction. A rapidly growing tumor also may cause marked local hyperemia. (2) **Bones**—The general shape and outline of the bone should be investigated. Palpate in particular for thickening, abnormal prominence, or disturbed relationship of the normal landmarks. (3) **Soft tissue**—Direct attention to the muscle (spasm, atrophy), joint tissue (synovial membrane, joint distension), and to the detection of any local or general swelling of the part. (4) **Local tenderness**—The exact borders of any local tenderness should be delineated. An attempt should be made to relate this tenderness to a particular structure.

CARDINAL SYMPTOMS

Pain and Sensibility

Pain is usually the most important symptom for the patient. The examiner must be certain of the site and distribution of pain. The patient's verbal description may be misleading. The patient should point to the site of maximum intensity and map out the area over which pain is experienced.

Articular or periarticular pain may radiate widely and may be felt in a spot distant from the originating structure. Such referred pain is a perceptual error occurring at the sensory cortex, and it reflects shared innervation by structures derived from the same embryonic segment. This innervation divides into dermatome, myotome, and sclerotome. Cortical cells most commonly receive stimuli from the skin. When the same cells receive, for the first time, a painful stimulus from a deeply situated myotomal/sclerotomal structure, they interpret the signal based on experience, and the patient feels pain in the area of the skin (dermatome) that shares the connection. An important difference is that referred pain is felt deeply, rather than in the skin itself, and its boundaries are indistinct. Referred pain radiates segmentally without crossing the midline and, because the dermatome often extends more distally than the myotome, the pain is mainly referred distally. The more distal the originating structure, the more accurate the pain localization is likely to be. In addition to pain referral, tenderness also may be experienced at a distant site. Dermatomes are variable between individuals. For example, the precise area of pain referral may differ between patients with the same musculoskeletal problem. The more superficial a soft tissue structure is, the more precise its pain localization will be. Massage over the area of referred pain may improve rather than worsen the pain, and pressure over the originating structure may reproduce the pain.

The patient's description of the quality of the pain is often not helpful in diagnosis. Exceptions include sharp, shooting pain that travels a distance and is characteristic of root entrapment and extreme pain, which is typical of crystal synovitis. Although topographic localization is at the sensory cortex level, pain appreciation and severity is determined by cells in the supraorbital region of the frontal lobe. This explains why the patient's emotional state has such an influence over the severity of the pain. The memory of pain is retained in the temporal lobe. Duration, rather than severity, determines recall.

Factors that exacerbate or ameliorate the pain are important. Pain during usage suggests a mechanical problem, particularly if it worsens during use and quickly improves when resting. Pain while at rest and pain that is worse at the beginning rather than at the end of usage implies a marked inflammatory component. Night pain is a distressing symptom that reflects intraosseous hypertension and accompanies serious problems, such as avascular necrosis or bone collapse adjacent to a severely arthritic joint. Persistent bony pain is characteristic of neoplastic invasion.

It is appropriate to test sensibility to both light touch and pinprick throughout the affected area. In unilateral afflictions the opposite side should be similarly tested. The precise area of any blunting or loss of sensibility should be carefully delineated. From knowledge of the cutaneous distribution of the peripheral nerves, the particular nerves may be identified.

The sense of pain is complex because it involves not only a sensation but also feelings and emotions. The neurophysiology of pain involves structures not normally considered part of the sensory nervous system.

The sense of pain is served by free nerve endings located in the skin and certain visceral tissues. Pain can be caused by stimuli of different natures. Strong mechanical stimuli (intense pressure), very hot and very cold stimuli (thermal and certain chemical stimuli, such as acidic substances), all can cause pain. Pain receptors have a high threshold of stimulation. These receptors are usually activated when stimulus strength is very high. Because such strong stimuli are usually noxious, the evoked sensation is also called nociception (pain sense). The pain receptors activated by nociceptive stimuli are called nociceptors. One view holds that all nociceptive stimuli cause tissue damage, the extent of which may vary from the slight effects of a simple pinch to the severe consequences of burns.

Tissue damage results in the local release of certain internal nociceptive substances—such as serotonin, pressor substance (substance-P), histamine and kinin peptides (bradykinin)—in the injured area. These substances then act on the free nerve endings, activating pain signals.

Sharp pain is conveyed by thin, myelinated, fast, type A-delta fibers. Dull, aching, and hurting pain is conveyed by unmyelinated, slow, conducting type C fibers.

Stiffness

Stiffness is a subjective sensation of resistance to movement that probably reflects fluid distension of the limiting boundary of the inflamed tissue. This stiffness is most noticeable when arising from bed and after inactivity or rest. As normal usage resumes, fluid clears from the inflamed structures and stiffness wears off. The duration and severity of early morning stiffness and inactivity stiffness reflect the degree of local inflammation.

Disability and Handicap

Disability is present when a tissue, organ, or system cannot function adequately. A handicap exists when disability interferes with a patient's daily activities or social/occupational performance. A marked disability does not necessarily cause handicap. Conversely, minor disability may produce a major handicap. Both conditions require separate assessment.

Systemic Illness

Inflammatory musculoskeletal disease may trigger a marked acute phase response and cause nonspecific symptoms of systemic upset. Symptoms may include fever, reduced appetite, weight loss, fatigue, lethargy, and irritability. The patient might not volunteer specific complaints but might report feeling ill. Note that florid acute inflammation may cause confusion, especially in the elderly.

Sleep Disturbance

Several factors may interfere with normal sleep patterns and cause anxiety and depression. These factors include chronic pain, triggering of the acute phase response, reasonable anxiety concerning deformity and morbidity, central nervous system (CNS) side effects from pain-relieving drugs, and severe arthropathy. These factors may further compromise sexual function and contribute to marital/social disharmony. Features of masked or overt depression should be sought, particularly in those with severe musculoskeletal disease. A poor sleep pattern is also a feature of fibromyalgia.

REFERRED SYMPTOMS

When the source of the symptom is still in doubt after careful examination of the part, attention must be directed to possible extrinsic disorders. Determination of extrinsic disorders requires examination of other regions of the body that might be responsible. For instance, in a case of pain in the shoulder, it might be necessary to examine the neck for evidence of a lesion interfering with the brachial plexus. It might be necessary to examine the thorax and abdomen for evidence of diaphragmatic irritation. Either of these conditions may be a cause of shoulder pain. For pain in the thigh, the examination will often have to include a study of the spine, abdomen, pelvis, and genitourinary system, as well as a local examination of the hip and thigh.

The afferent pain fibers originating from the same area demonstrate extensive convergence onto the dorsal horn relay cells. In certain cases, the convergence may take place by fibers from different areas, causing the relay cell to be activated by pain originating in different body parts. Usually one part is a visceral area or organ. This mechanism may underlie the phenomenon of referred pain. Pain originating in the heart is often felt at the inner aspects of the left arm. Referred pain is either due to convergence of pain fibers from both zones onto the same spinal relay cell or due to facilitation of somatic signals during excessive pain traffic from the visceral source.

Phantom pains originate from an amputated limb. Irritation of severed endings of pain fibers at the site of the amputation signal pain to the same areas of the cortex. These signals are projected to their original source in the limb or body, creating a phantom sensation.

CARDINAL SIGNS

Posture

The way the patient positions an affected region is important. A joint with synovitis has intraarticular hypertension and is most comfortable in the position that minimizes pressure increase. Such a position is mainly determined by the configuration of the capsule. Glenohumeral synovitis is most comfortable with the arm adducted and internally rotated, as if in a sling. The opposite movements, abduction and external rotation, are the earliest movements affected and the most uncomfortable, because they maximize intraarticular hypertension. The attitude and pattern of restricted movement may suggest the underlying problem.

Tenderness

Precise localization of tenderness is the most useful sign in determining the cause of the problem. Joint line/capsular tenderness signifies arthropathy or capsular disease around the whole margin. Localized joint line tenderness suggests intracapsular pathologic processes. Periarticular point tenderness, away from the joint line, usually signifies bursitis or enthesopathy.

Changes in Dimension of the Part

Measurement of length is often necessary, especially in the lower extremities. Measurement of the circumference of an extremity provides an index of muscle atrophy, soft-tissue swelling, or bony thickening.

Fixed Deformity

Although deformity may be observed at rest, most deformities become more apparent when the limb is bearing weight or being used. The examiner should determine if the deformity is correctable or noncorrectable. Many conditions are associated with characteristic deformities, but no deformity is pathognomonic of one disease. Shorthand terms are used for combined deformities, such as "swan-neck" finger deformity for hyperextension at the proximal and fixed flexion at the distal interphalangeal joints.

Fixed deformity exists when a joint cannot be placed in the neutral (anatomic) position. The degree of fixed deformity at a joint is determined by moving the joint, as near as it will come, to the neutral position and then measuring the remaining angle. In valgus deformity, the distal part of the extremity is deviated laterally (outward) in relation to the proximal part. In hallux valgus the first metatarsal is deviated outward in relation to the foot. In genu valgum the lower leg is deviated outward in relation to the thigh. Varus deformity is the opposite. The distal part of an extremity is deviated medially (inward) in relation to the proximal part.

Diffuse Joint Swelling

Patients may notice swelling, discoloration, or abnormal contour or alignment of the joint. Although deformity describes any abnormality, the term is usually restricted to malalignment or subluxation/dislocation.

A diffuse swelling of the joint as a whole can only have three causes: (1) thickening of the bone end; (2) fluid within the joint; or (3) thickening of the synovial membrane. In some cases two or all three causes may be combined. These causes can always be differentiated by palpation.

Bony thickening is detected by deep palpation through the soft tissues. The bone outlines are compared bilaterally. A fluid effusion gives a clear sense of fluctuation in the examiner's hands. Synovial thickening gives a characteristic spongy sensation, as if a layer of soft sponge-rubber had been placed between the skin and the body. Synovial thickening is always accompanied by a well-marked increase in local tissue warmth. This increase is because the synovium is a very vascular membrane.

Swelling may be due to the presence of fluid, soft tissue, or bone. Fluid within a joint collects initially and maximally at the site of least resistance within the capsular confines, producing characteristic swelling.

For small fluid volumes in a confined cavity, a bulge sign may be produced. Larger volumes produce a balloon sign (fluctuance), where pressure over one point causes ballooning at other parts of the swelling. This is the most specific sign of fluid. Capsular swelling is the most specific sign of synovitis. The swelling is delineated by the capsular confines and becomes firmer toward the extremes of movement.

Movement

Synovitis reduces most or all joint movements, but tenosynovitis and periarticular lesions affect movement in only one plane. Synovitis and arthropathy cause a similar reduction of active and passive movement.

The pattern of pain during movement is of diagnostic significance. Pain that is absent or minimal in the midrange but increases toward the extremes of restricted movement is stress pain. Universal stress pain is the most sensitive sign of synovitis. Selective stress pain, occurring in one plane of movement only, is characteristic of a localized intraarticular or periarticular lesion. Pain uniformly present throughout a range of movement reflects mechanical rather than inflammatory problems.

Ranges of motion are age and sex dependent. Attempts to measure degrees of movement can be inaccurate and can have poor reproducibility, and are not recommended for routine examination purposes.

A useful method for demonstrating periarticular problems is resisted, active (isometric) movement. This method requires the patient to push against the examiner's restraining hand, to contract the muscle of interest, without moving the adjacent joints. If the patient's pain is reproduced and no joint has moved, the pain probably arises from muscle, tendon, or tendon insertion. Conversely, passive stress tests reproduce pain by stretching the responsible ligament or tendon.

In the examination of joint motion, information must be obtained concerning the following four points: (1) range of active movement, (2) passive versus active movement, (3) pain during movement, and (4) movement crepitation.

In measuring the range of motion, the norm varies from patient to patient. It is appropriate to use the unaffected extremity for comparison. Limitation of movement in all directions suggests some form of arthritis. Selective limitation of movement in some directions, with free movement in others, suggests a mechanical derangement.

Passive movement range is usually equal to the active range. The passive range will exceed the active only when the muscles responsible for movement are paralyzed and when the muscles or their tendons are torn, severed, or unduly slack.

Stability

Localized ligamentous or capsular instability may result from traumatic or inflammatory lesions. Arthropathy, particularly inflammatory, may produce instability via cartilage loss and capsular inflammation, as well as by ligamentous rupture. Stability is determined by demonstration of excessive movement on stressing the joint. Comparison with the unaffected side is helpful.

The stability of a joint depends partly on the integrity of its articulating surfaces and partly on intact ligaments. When a joint is unstable there is abnormal mobility. When testing for abnormal mobility, it is important to ensure that the muscles controlling the joint are relaxed. A muscle in strong contraction can often conceal ligamentous instability.

Crepitation

Crepitation is palpable crunching that is present throughout the movement of the involved structure. Fine crepitation may be audible by stethoscope and is not transmitted through the adjacent bone. Fine crepitation may accompany inflammation of the tendon sheath, bursa, or synovium. Coarse crepitation may be audible at a distance and is palpable through the bone. Coarse crepitation usually reflects cartilage or bone damage. Other noises include (1) ligamentous snaps—usually single, loud, and painless—that are common around the upper femur as a clicking hip; (2) cracking by joint distraction, which is common at the finger joints and is caused by production of an intraarticular gas bubble (such cracking cannot be repeated until the bubble has reformed); and (3) reproducible clunking noises that occur at irregular surfaces, such as when the scapula moves on the ribs.

Weakness

Muscle atrophy is a common sign but can be difficult to detect, particularly in the elderly. Synovitis quickly produces local spinal reflex inhibition of muscles acting across the joint. Atrophy can be rapid (within several days) in septic arthritis. Severe arthropathy produces widespread periarticular wasting. Localized atrophy is more characteristic of a mechanical tendon or muscle problem or nerve entrapment. Power is more important than bulk in the proximal musculature. Functional capabilities are more important in the distal muscles.

Muscle strength is determined by instructing the patient to move the joint while the examiner provides isometric resistance. With careful bilateral comparison, it is possible to detect gross impairment of muscle power.

In the occasional instance when more precise information is required, muscle strength can be measured against weights, spring balances, or deflection bars.

Skin Changes

Overlying scars or skin disease may be important clues to causation of deeper rheumatic symptoms. Erythema, commonly followed by desquamation, is an important sign, reflecting periarticular inflammation. Although this may occur in several conditions, a red joint or bursa should always raise the suspicion of sepsis or crystals.

Causes of erythema overlying a joint include sepsis, crystals (gout, pseudogout, calcific periarthritis), palindromic rheumatism, acute Reiter's or reactive arthropathy, early Heberden's or Bouchard's nodes, inflammatory (erosive) osteoarthritis of the hands, and rheumatic fever.

Warmth

Warmth is one of the cardinal signs of inflammation. The back of the examiner's hand is a sensitive thermometer for comparing skin temperature above, over, and below an inflamed structure.

Decreased Circulation

Symptoms in an extremity may be associated with impairment of the arterial circulation. Time should be spent in assessing the state of the circulation by examining the color and temperature of the skin and the texture of the skin and the nails and by measuring the arterial pulses. This examination is particularly important in the lower extremities.

Impairment of Gait

It is difficult to find a spinal or lower extremity orthopedic or neurologic disorder that does not produce abnormalities of gait at some time during its course. Gait impairments of predominant neurologic origin include, in descending order of frequency, disorders of the corticospinal pathways (spasticity), basal ganglia (Parkinsonism), cerebellum and connections (ataxia), cerebral cortex (gait apraxia), neuromuscular system (weakness), and sensation (ataxia).

Bladder Control

Incontinence and other disturbances of urinary bladder function are occasionally the first manifestation of disease of the spinal cord, as well as the rest of the nervous system.

The physiology of micturition is complex. The terms

atonic bladder or *spastic bladder* are no longer useful in describing different levels of neurologic involvement because they are related mainly to local factors in the bladder wall. Localization of impaired micturition depends on (1) loss of bladder sensation, (2) perineal sensory loss, (3) patulous anal sphincter, (4) absence of the bulbocavernosus and anocutaneous reflexes, and (5) sensory, motor, and reflex changes in the lower extremities. An associated history of impotence or rectal incontinence should clearly suggest the presence of a common neurogenic cause for urinary incontinence. The additional presence of sacral pain should suggest tumor in the sacral region.

Bibliography

Adams JC: *Standard orthopedic operations,* Edinburgh, 1985, Churchill Livingstone.

Adams RD: *Disease of muscle,* ed 3, London, 1985, Henry Kimpton.

American Academy of Orthopaedic Surgeons: *Atlas of limb prosthetics,* St. Louis, 1981, Mosby.

Apley AG, Solomon L: *Concise system of orthopaedics and fractures,* London, 1988, Butterworth-Heinemann.

Bassett, ed: *Instructional course lectures,* vol 37, Chicago, 1988, American Academy of Orthopaedic Surgeons.

Birch R: The place of microsurgery in orthopaedics. In Catterall A: *Recent advances in orthopaedics,* vol 5, Edinburgh, 1981, Churchill Livingstone.

Bobowick AR, Brody J: Epidemiology of motor-neuron diseases, *N Eng J Med,* 88: 1047–1055, 1973.

Burnett W: *Clinical science for surgeons,* London, 1981, Butterworth.

Campbell WC: *Operative orthopaedics,* ed 7, Edmonson and Crenshaw, London, 1987, Henry Kimpton.

Campion GV, Dixon A J: *Rheumatology,* Oxford, 1989, Blackwell.

Catterall A: *Recent advances in orthopaedics* vol 5, Edinburgh, 1987, Churchill Livingstone.

Cipriano JJ: *Photographic manual of regional orthopaedic and neurological tests,* ed 2, Baltimore, 1991, Williams & Wilkins.

Cruess RL, Rennie W: *Adult orthopaedics,* New York, 1984, Churchill Livingstone.

Currey JLF: *Essentials of rheumatology,* ed 2, Edinburgh, 1988, Churchill Livingstone.

Cyriax JH: *Textbook of orthopaedic medicine,* ed 8, London, 1983, Bailliere Tindall.

D'Ambrosia RD: *Musculoskeletal disorders regional examination and differential diagnosis,* Philadelphia, 1977, JB Lippincott.

Dandy DJ: *Essential orthopaedics and trauma,* Edinburgh, 1989, Churchill Livingstone.

Doherty M, Doherty J: *Clinical examination in rheumatology,* London, 1992, Wolfe Publishing.

Duthie RB, Bentley G, eds: *Mercer's orthopaedic surgery,* ed 8, London, 1983, Edward Arnold.

Eastcott HHG: *Arterial surgery,* ed 2, London, 1973, Pitman.

Galasko CSB, ed: *Neuromuscular problems in orthopaedics,* Oxford, 1987, Blackwell.

Galasko CSB, Noble J, eds: *Current trends in orthopaedic surgery,* Manchester, 1988, Manchester University Press.

Gartland JJ: Orthopaedic clinical research, *Bone Joint Surg,* 70A: 1357, 1988.

Griffin MJ: *Instructional course lectures,* vol 36, Chicago, 1988, American Academy of Orthopaedic Surgeons.

Hughes S, Benson MKD, Colton CL: *The principles and practice of musculoskeletal surgery,* Edinburgh, 1987, Churchill Livingstone.

Jepsen RH et al: Differential diagnosis of infantile hypotonia, *Am J Dis Child,* 101: 8–17, 1961.

Katz WA: *Rheumatic diseases diagnosis and management,* Philadelphia, 1977, JB Lippincott.

Kendall HO, Kendall FP, Wadsworth GE: *Muscles testing and function,* ed 2, Baltimore, 1971, Williams & Wilkins.

Kuru M: Nervous control of micturition, *Physiol Rev,* 45: 425–494, 1965.

Magee DJ: *Orthopedic physical assessment,* Philadelphia, 1987, WB Saunders.

Mazion JM: *Illustrated manual of neurological reflexes/signs/tests, part I; orthopedic signs/tests/maneuvers for office procedure, part II;* Orlando, 1980, Daniels Publishing.

McKibbin B, ed: *Recent advances in orthopaedics,* vol 4, Edinburgh, 1983, Churchill Livingstone.

McRae R: *Clinical orthopaedic examination,* ed 3, Edinburgh, 1990, Churchill Livingstone.

Medical Economics Books: *Patient care flow chart manual,* ed 3, Oradell, NJ, 1982, Medical Economics Books.

Moll JMH: *Manual of rheumatology,* Edinburgh, 1987, Churchill Livingstone.

Noble J, Galasko CSB: *Recent developments in orthopaedic surgery,* Manchester, 1987, Manchester University Press.

O'Donoghue DH: *Treatment of injuries to athletes,* ed 3, Philadelphia, 1976, WB Saunders.

Omer GE, Spinner M: *Management of peripheral nerve problems,* Philadelphia, 1980, WB Saunders.

Owen R, Goodfellow J, Bullough P, eds: *Scientific foundations of orthopaedics and traumatology,* London, 1980, Heinemann.

Plum F: Bladder dysfunction, *Mod Trends Neuro-surg,* 111: 151–172, 1962.

Rang M, ed: *The growth plate and its disorders,* Edinburgh, 1969, Livingstone.

Renshaw TS: *Paediatric orthopaedics,* Philadelphia, 1987, Saunders.

Roach HI, Shearer JR, Archer C: The choice of an experimental model: A guide for research workers, *J Bone Joint Surg,* 71B: 549, 1989.

Rothman RH, Simeone FA: *The spine,* vol 1, Philadelphia, 1975, WB Saunders.

Scott JT, ed: *Copeman's textbook of the rheumatic diseases,* ed 6, Edinburgh, 1986, Churchill Livingstone.

Stewart JDM, Hallett JP: *Traction and orthopaedic appliances,* Edinburgh, 1983, Churchill Livingstone.

Thurston SE: *The little black book of neurology,* Chicago, 1987, Mosby.

Turek SL: *Orthopaedics principles and their application,* ed 3, Philadelphia, 1977, JB Lippincott.

Williams PF, ed: *Orthopaedic management in childhood,* Oxford, 1982, Blackwell.

∼ 3 ∼

The Cervical Spine

Cervical spine syndromes are extremely common and are probably the fourth most common cause of pain. At any given time, 9% of men and 12% of women have neck pain with or without arm and hand pain and 35% of the population can remember having had neck pain at some time.

The cervical spine is the origin of a large proportion of shoulder, elbow, hand, and wrist disorders. Most people who develop pain in the neck do not seek medical attention because they regard such pain as a part of life, so they just wait for it to disappear. Neck discomfort commonly appears abruptly after some unusual motion of the neck. Such discomfort may also occur following prolonged effort at a task, such as painting a ceiling, or with unusual use of the arm, forearm, and hand. The pain usually occurs in the middle of the back of the neck. Cervical spine motion (extension and lateral flexion) increases the pain.

The neck is the most mobile segment of the spine. Many delicate and vital structures pass through this cylinder that connects the head to the thorax. The structures include carotid and vertebral arteries, the spinal cord, and the spinal nerves, all of which require great protection.

Normal function of the cervical spine requires that all movements are accomplished without injury to the spinal cord and the millions of nerve fibers that pass through it. The spinal cord has the capacity to adapt itself to marked alteration in the length of the cervical spinal canal. Flexion of the neck lengthens the spinal canal, and extension shortens it. From person to person, there is considerable variation in thickness of the cervical spinal cord and in the diameter of the spinal canal.

Diagnostic possibilities include cardiovascular disease, myocardial infarction, aortic dissection, meningitis, cervical osteoarthritis, hypertension, temporal arteritis, polymyalgia rheumatica, a spectrum of neurologic diseases and syndromes, various metabolic bone diseases, primary and metastatic cancer, infection, lymphoma, and myeloma.

Index of Tests

Bakody sign
Barre-Lieou sign
Bikele's Sign
Brachial plexus tension test
Dejerine's sign
DeKleyn's test
Distraction test
Foraminal compression test
Hallpike maneuver
Hautant's test
Jackson cervical compression test
Lhermitte's sign
Maximum cervical compression test
Naffziger's test
O'Donoghue maneuver
Rust's sign
Shoulder depression test
Soto-Hall sign
Spinal percussion test
Spurling's test
Swallowing test
Underburg's test
Valsalva maneuver
Vertebrobasilar artery functional maneuver

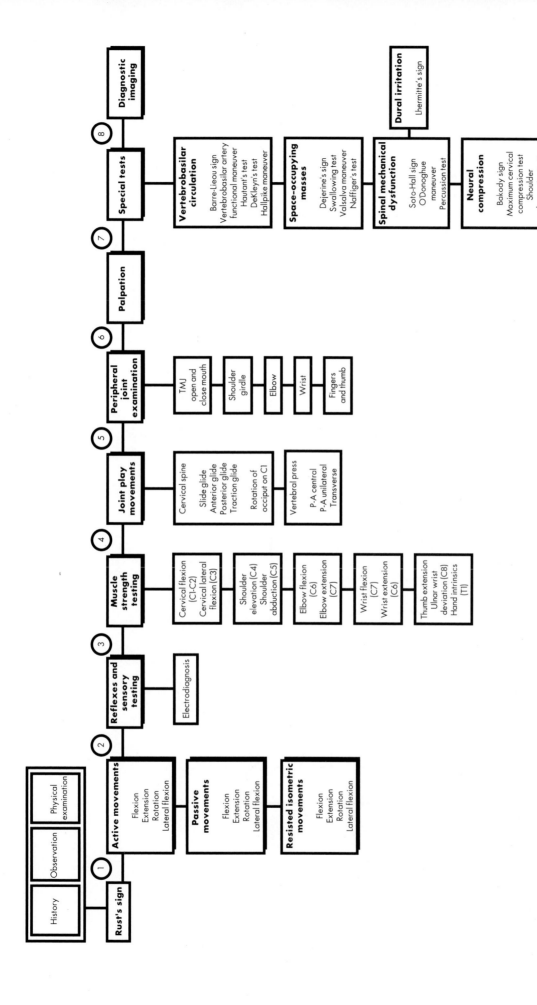

Fig. 3-1 Cervical spine assessment chart.

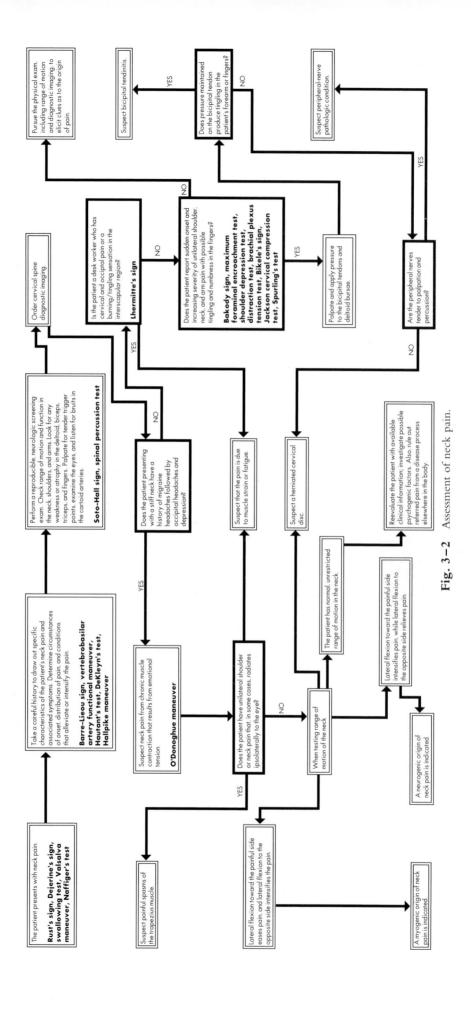

Fig. 3-2 Assessment of neck pain.

RANGE OF MOTION

In evaluating cervical spine range of motion, the examiner observes not only the total range of movement but also the smoothness and comfort with which the patient accomplishes the motions.

The first motions tested are the active movements of the cervical spine. This testing is performed while the patient is in the sitting position. The examiner looks for differences in range of motion and differences in the patient's willingness to perform the movement. The most painful movements should be performed last. The examiner should also differentiate between movement in the upper and lower cervical spine. Isolated movement can occur between C1 and C2 alone but not between the other pairs of cervical vertebrae.

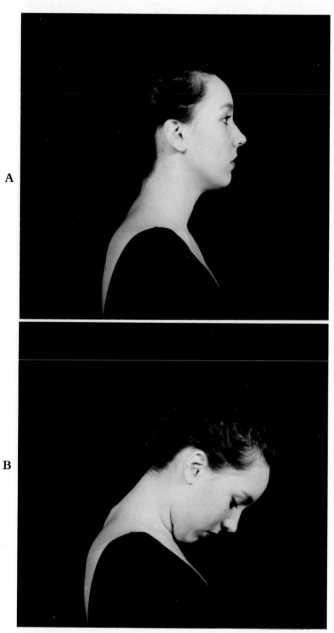

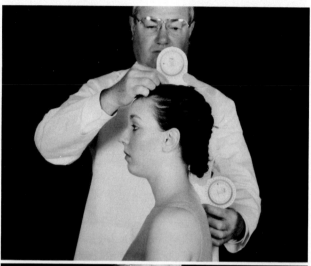

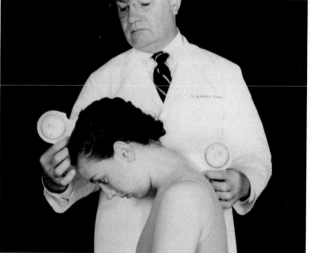

Fig. 3–3 Flexion. **(A)** To assess cervical range of motion, the examiner has the patient sit with the head upright, **(B)** then instructs the patient to tuck the chin in toward the chest. For flexion the maximum range of motion is 80 to 90 degrees. The extreme of the range is when the chin can reach the chest while the mouth is closed. Up to two finger widths distance between the chin and the chest is normal. Forty degrees or less of retained cervical flexion is an impairment of neck function in the activities of daily living.

Fig. 3–4 Flexion assessed with an inclinometer. **(A)** With the patient seated and the cervical spine in the neutral position, the examiner places one inclinometer over the T1 spinous process, in the sagittal plane. The second inclinometer is placed at the superior aspect of the occiput, or on top of the head, also in the sagittal plane. Both inclinometers are zeroed in these positions. **(B)** The patient flexes the head and neck forward. The examiner records both angles. The T1 inclination is subtracted from the cranial inclination to determine the cervical flexion angle. The expected range of motion is 60 degrees or greater from the neutral position.

(Continued).

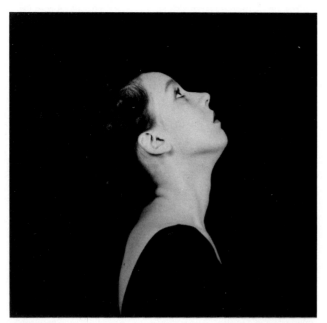

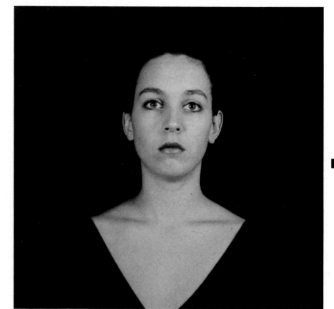

Fig. 3–5 Extension. Extension is normally 70 degrees. Because there is no anatomic block to stop movement going past this point, excessive and forceful excursions may often lead to problems similar to whiplash or cervical strain. Normally, the plane of the nose and forehead should be nearly horizontal during maximum extension. Fifty degrees or less of retained cervical extension is an impairment of neck function in the activities of daily living.

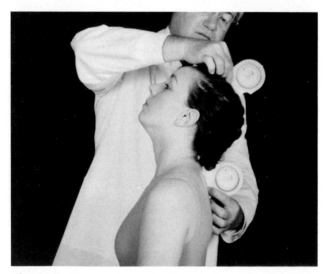

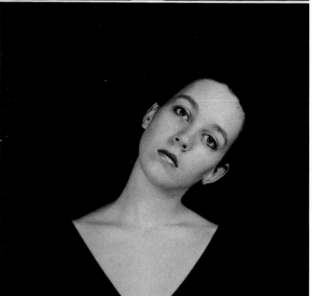

Fig. 3–6 Extension assessed with an inclinometer. The patient is seated with the cervical spine in the neutral position. The examiner places one inclinometer slightly lateral to the T1 spinous process, in the sagittal plane. The second inclinometer is placed at the superior aspect of the occiput, or on top of the head, in the sagittal plane. Both inclinometers are zeroed in these positions. The patient extends the head and neck, and the examiner records the angle of both inclinometers. The T1 inclination is subtracted from the occipital inclination to determine the cervical extension angle. The expected range of motion is 75 degrees or greater from the neutral position.

Fig. 3–7 Lateral flexion. **(A)** The patient begins with the cervical spine in the neutral position. **(B)** Lateral flexion of the cervical spine is normally about 20 to 45 degrees to the right and left. Most of the side flexion occurs between the occiput and C1 and between C1 and C2. In this movement the ear moves to the shoulder—not the shoulder to the ear. Thirty degrees or less of retained lateral flexion is an impairment of neck function in the activities of daily living.

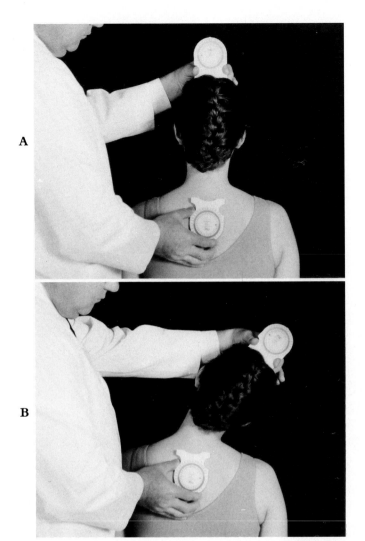

A

B

Fig. 3–8 Lateral flexion assessed with an inclinometer. **(A)** With the patient seated and the cervical spine in a neutral position, the examiner places one inclinometer on the T1 spinous process, in the coronal plane. The examiner places the second inclinometer at the superior aspect of the occiput, or on top of the head, also in the coronal plane. Both instruments are then zeroed. **(B)** The patient laterally flexes the head and neck to one side. The examiner records the angles of both instruments. The T1 inclination is subtracted from the occipital inclination to determine the cervical lateral flexion angle. The expected range of motion is 45 degrees or greater from the neutral position. The procedure should be repeated for the opposite side.

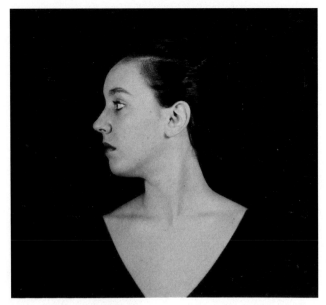

Fig. 3–9 Rotation. Normally rotation of the cervical spine is 70 to 90 degrees to the right and left. With cervical rotation the chin does not quite reach the plane of the shoulder. This combined movement may or may not be visible, depending on the movement tested. Sixty degrees or less of retained cervical rotation is an impairment of the cervical spine in the activities of daily living.

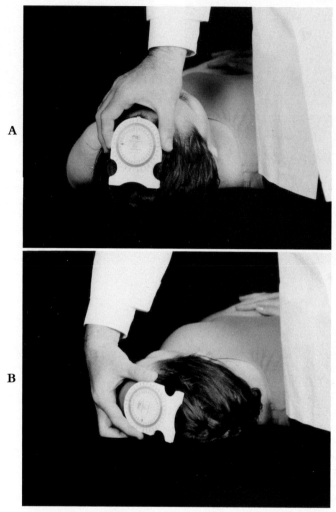

Fig. 3–10 Rotation assessed with an inclinometer. **(A)** With the patient in a supine position the examiner places the inclinometer at the crown of the head, in the coronal plane. The instrument is zeroed. **(B)** The patient rotates the head to one side, and the examiner records the angle indicated on the instrument. This angle is the cervical spine rotation angle. Repeat the procedure for the opposite side. The expected range of motion is 80 degrees or greater from the neutral position.

MUSCLE TESTING

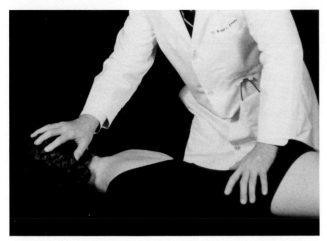

Fig. 3–11 Posterolateral head and neck extensors. The muscles included in this test are chiefly the splenius capitis and cervicis, semispinalis capitis and cervicis, and cervical erector spinae. The patient is prone on the examining table. Slight fixation is necessary. The patient tries a posterolateral extension with the face turned toward the side tested. The upper trapezius, also a posterolateral neck extensor, is tested in a similar manner with the face turned away from the side examined. The examiner applies pressure in an anterior direction against the posterolateral aspect of the head.

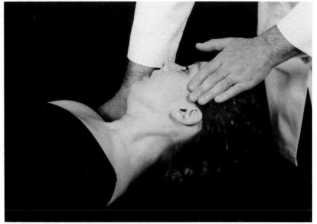

Fig. 3–12 Anterolateral head and neck flexors. The muscles acting in this test are chiefly the sternocleidomastoid and scaleni. The patient is supine on the examination table. If the patient's anterior abdominal muscles are weak, the examiner can give fixation by firm downward pressure on the thorax. The patient attempts anterolateral neck flexion. The examiner applies pressure to the temporal region of the head in an obliquely posterior direction. If the neck muscles are strong enough to hold the head but not strong enough to flex completely, the patient may try to lift the head from the table by raising the shoulders. This occurs especially in the tests for right and left neck flexors because the patient attempts to aid the maneuver by taking some weight on the elbow or hand, allowing the shoulder to rise from the table. To avoid this, the examiner holds the patient's shoulder flat on the table.

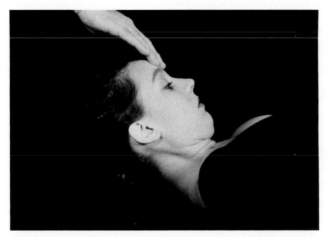

Fig. 3–13 Anterior head and neck flexors. The patient is resting on the examination table in the supine position with elbows bent and hands over the head. The anterior abdominal muscles must be strong enough to give anterior fixation of the thorax to the pelvis. This strength allows the head to be raised by the neck flexors. If the abdominal muscles are weak, the examiner can provide fixation by applying firm, downward pressure on the thorax. Children 5 years or younger should always have fixation of the thorax provided by the examiner. The patient tries to flex the cervical spine by lifting the head from the table toward the sternum while keeping the mouth closed and the chin depressed. The examiner applies pressure to the forehead in a posterior direction.

❧ Bakody Sign ❧
SHOULDER ABDUCTION TEST
CERVICAL FORAMINAL COMPRESSION TEST

Comment

Although cervical nerve root compression is a part of the syndrome of cervical osteoarthritis, particularly with zygapophyseal and Luschka joint involvement, faulty posture of the cervical spine may contribute to the cervical nerve root compression or it may be the primary etiology of compression.

Hyperextension of the cervical spine, performed with the chin in a forward position, compresses the zygapophyseal joints and Luschka joints on the posterior surfaces of the cervical vertebrae, and is the etiology and pathogenesis of the compression.

There are neither specific genetic and environmental factors nor are there specific epidemiologic factors for cervical compression.

In cervical hyperextension syndromes, radiographic characteristics may include those typical of cervical osteoarthritis in addition to other postural factors.

A cervical nerve root compression syndrome may result from direct trauma to the nerve roots from the pincerlike action of the foraminal architecture during an acute hyperextension trauma, from chronic irritation from hypertrophic spurring, or from disc disease. This latter source may be a traumatic aggravation of chronic disc disease or an acute herniation or prolapse of disc material. Symptoms of nerve root compression are distinctly different from those of neurovascular compression syndromes or reflex sympathetic dystrophy. These symptoms include proximal (root) pain and neck pain, distal paresthesia in dermatome patterns, muscle weakness in one or several muscles supplied by a single root, loss of deep tendon reflexes, muscle fasciculation, and radiating pains that are further aggravated by movements of the neck.

Irritation of the cervical nerve roots may cause pain, sensory changes, muscle atrophy, or spasm and alteration of the tendon reflexes anywhere along the segmental distribution.

Any condition causing a narrowing of the intervertebral canals may cause a compression of the nerve roots and the spinal branches of the vertebral arteries, venous congestion and irritation, and compression of the recurrent meningeal nerves.

Encroachment, or narrowing, of the intervertebral canals may be the result of some involvement of the proximate soft tissue structures or the bony structures. Any condition that causes inflammation and swelling of the dural sleeves of the nerve roots may also cause neural compression.

Procedure

While in the seated position, the patient actively places the palm of the affected extremity on top of the head, raising the elbow to a height approximately level with the head. By elevating the suprascapular nerve, traction of the lower trunk of the brachial plexus is relieved. Overall, this maneuver decreases stretching of the compressed nerve root. The sign is present when the radiating pain is lessened or disappears with this maneuver. The test is as reliable as Spurling's test, and is less painful for the patient to endure.

Confirmation Procedures

Dejerine's sign, Valsalva maneuver, Naffziger's test, reflexes, maximum foraminal compression test, distraction test, brachial plexus tension test, Bikele's sign, Jackson cervical compression test, Spurling's test, electrodiagnosis, diagnostic imaging

---

Reporting Statement

A cervical nerve root compression is indicated by Bakody sign on the right.

A cervical nerve root compression syndrome is suspected in the presence of Bakody sign on the right.

❧ Clinical Pearl ❧

Patients with moderate to severe radicular symptoms usually do not have to be directed into the Bakody sign position because it also is an antalgic pain-relieving posture. The more difficult it is for the patient to lower the arm, the more difficult the condition will be to treat conservatively. If the patient cannot lower the arm without severe exacerbation of pain, surgery is probably indicated.

Patients suffering from moderate to severe cervical nerve root compression find the most comfortable sleeping positions to be those that involve abduction and elevation of the arm. Again, this position relieves the traction of the neural elements and is an antalgic position for someone experiencing cervical nerve root compression. It is not uncommon for a patient to voluntarily assume the Bakody sign position while in the examination room.

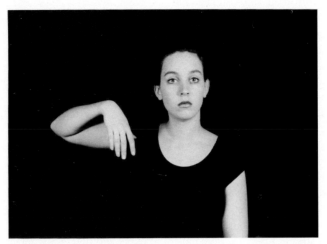

Fig. 3−14 The patient abducts and externally rotates the ipsilateral shoulder by moving the hand toward the head.

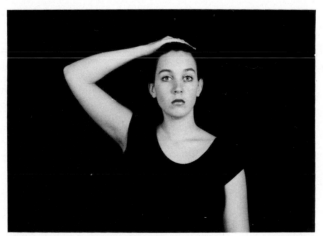

Fig. 3−15 The hand is placed on top of the head. If this position relieves radicular pain, then this is a positive sign that indicates a nerve root syndrome.

Comment

Rotation of the neck to one side usually decreases the circulation in the atlantoaxial portion of the contralateral vertebral artery. Such movement when there is kinking of the artery, atheromata, or osteoarthritis reduces the circulation even more. Other mechanisms that could alter the blood supply to the brainstem are carotid sinus compression, use of a surgical collar, manipulation of the neck that causes the release of emboli from atheromatous plaques in the great vessels, or thrombosis with infarction of the cerebellum or brainstem.

Vertebral artery insufficiency, whether permanent or transitory, has been identified as the explanation for some of the symptomatology seen with hyperextension/hyperflexion injuries. The course of the vertebral artery in the cervical spine is tortuous and the artery passes through, over, and around structures that may become malaligned after trauma. Abnormal pressures or tractional stresses may impede circulation through these arteries. The vertebral arteries also may be compressed as a result of chronic degenerative disease of the cervical spine. This compression may occur at any point along its usual course from C6 to C2 and may become symptomatic following cervical spine trauma. Three mechanisms of compression have been described: (1) osteophytes from the lateral disc margin, (2) anteriorly extending osteophytes from the facet joint, and (3) compression from the inferior facet due to posterior subluxation and a scissoring effect by the adjacent superior facet. Increased tissue pressures from myospasm, edema, or hemorrhage may also compromise the flow of blood through the vertebral artery. This is especially true when patency is already compromised because of atherosclerosis or congenital anomaly. Arterial spasm may also occur.

Three areas in which the vertebral artery is most susceptible to trauma are (1) the posterior atlanto-occipital membrane, which is dense and inelastic and may become calcified (firmly attached to the artery); (2) the space between the occiput and posterior arch of the atlas, especially during extension; and (3) between the lateral mass of the atlas and the transverse process of the axis, especially during extension and rotation. Older patients with preexisting atherosclerotic disease are at a greater risk of injury that results in vertebral artery syndrome, or of vertebrobasilar artery insufficiency.

Procedure

While the patient is in a seated position, the examiner instructs the patient to slowly rotate the head from side to side. Rotating the head causes compression of the vertebral arteries. Vertigo, dizziness, visual disturbances, nausea, syncope, and nystagmus are all signs of a positive test. A positive finding indicates a buckling of the ipsilateral vertebral artery.

Confirmation Procedures

Vertebrobasilar artery functional maneuver, Hautant's test, DeKleyn's test, Hallpike maneuver, Underburg's test, vascular investigation, diagnostic imaging

---

Reporting Statement

Barre-Lieou sign is present on the right. This finding suggests vertebrobasilar insufficiency on the right side.

Barre-Lieou sign is present on the right. This result indicates the presence of vertebrobasilar insufficiency.

~ Clinical Pearl ~

The patient with a positive Barre-Lieou sign is a poor risk for aggressive cervical spine manipulation. Such manipulation should not be undertaken until all vascular etiologies have been investigated. Aggravation of the sympathetic ganglia of the cervical spine can produce many, if not all, of these symptoms (vertigo, dizziness, visual disturbances, nausea, syncope, and nystagmus), in which case cervical spinal manipulation is warranted.

In 1926 Barre studied and established a syndrome that was further described in 1928 by his student Lieou. So diverse and widespread is the combination of symptoms and signs that some people no longer regard the syndrome as a disorder associated with the cervical spine. Rather, they view the syndrome as one caused by vertebral artery insufficiency and its multivariant characteristics. The symptoms of this syndrome include pain in the head, neck, eye, ears, face, sinuses, and throat; sensory disturbances in the pharynx and larynx; paroxysmal hoarseness and aphonia; tinnitus that is synchronous with the pulse; various auditory hallucinations, such as whistling and humming; deafness; visual disturbances, (such as blurring, scintillating scotomata, photophobia, blepharospasm, squinting sensations, and a peculiar pulling at the back of the eyes; flushing, sweating, salivation, lacrimation, nausea, vomiting, and rhinorrhea.

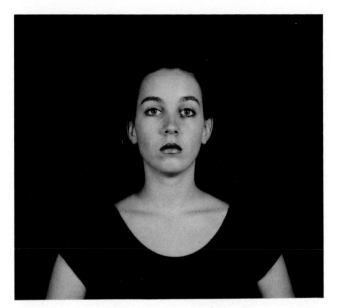

Fig. 3–16 The patient is seated as comfortably and as erect as possible. The blood pressure and pulse are examined and recorded before starting the test.

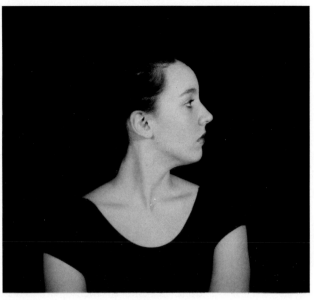

Fig. 3–17 The patient rotates the head maximally from side to side. This move is performed slowly at first and then accelerated until the patient's tolerance is reached.

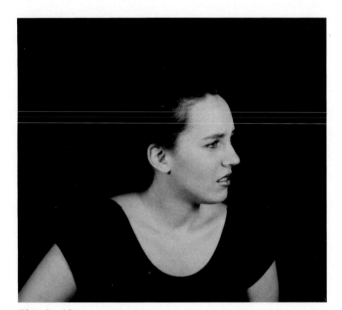

Fig. 3–18 A vertebral artery syndrome is indicated by vertigo, blurred vision, nausea, syncope, or nystagmus. These symptoms may occur singly or in combination.

Comment

Brachial plexus lesions result in motor and sensory syndromes of muscles of the upper extremities. The brachial plexus is made up of the anterior primary rami of the four lower cervical nerves, C5 through C8, and the greater part of T1. The C5 and C6 rami form the upper trunk; the C7 ramus forms the middle trunk; and the C8 and T1 rami form the lower trunk. Trunks are placed in the supraclavicular fossa distal to the anterior scalene muscle. Each trunk splits into an anterior and a posterior division, with derivation of three cords from them. The lateral cord is formed by the anterior division of the upper and middle trunks, the medial cord by the anterior division of the lower trunk (C8 and T1), and the posterior cord by the posterior divisions of all three trunks and nerves. The upper trunk branches to the supraclavicular nerve, innervating the supraspinatus and infraspinatus muscles as well as the subclavius muscles. The lateral cord branches to the lateral anterior thoracic nerve, innervating the greater pectoral muscle. The medial cord becomes the medial anterior thoracic cord, which goes to the pectoral muscles and the medial antebrachial and brachiocutaneous nerves. The posterior cord branches to the subscapular nerve, which innervates the subscapular and teres major muscle, and the thoracodorsal nerve, which innervates the latissimus dorsi muscles. Terminal branches of the posterior cord are the axillary and radial nerves, and the terminal branches of the lateral cord are the musculocutaneous (bicep) component and the lateral component of the median nerve. The terminal branches of the medial cord are the ulnar nerve and the medial component of the median nerve.

Procedure

With the arm held upward and backward and the elbow fully flexed, the patient extends the elbow. If such movement meets with resistance and increases radicular pain from the cervicodorsal region, then the test is positive. This finding indicates brachial plexus neuritis or meningitis because this maneuver stretches the brachial plexus nerve roots or coverings.

Confirmation Procedures

Reflexes, sensory testing, Bakody maneuver, Dejerine's sign, Valsalva maneuver, maximum foraminal encroachment testing, shoulder depression test, distraction test, brachial plexus tension test, Jackson cervical compression test, Spurling's test, electrodiagnosis, diagnostic imaging

When reflex sympathetic symptoms are present, additional tests may be indicated. These tests include matchstick testing, pilomotor response testing, and thermography

---

Reporting Statement

Bikele's sign is present on the right. This result suggests brachial plexus neuritis.

Bikele's sign is positive on the right. Because the patient is afebrile, this sign indicates brachial plexus neuritis.

≈ **Clinical Pearl** ≈

Injury to the C8 and T1 roots, the lower trunk, or the medial cord of the brachial plexus may be caused by tumors, by disease of the pulmonary apex, or by a fractured clavicle or cervical rib. Aneurysm of the arch of the aorta, fracture or dislocation of the humeral head, or unusually abrupt and severe upward traction of the arm may also injure the nerves.

Although Bikele's sign does not usually produce a profound finding in minor cervical nerve root compression syndromes, the maneuver often produces startling results in lower brachial plexopathy in the thoracic outlet. Reflex sympathetic changes may be present with the plexopathy and should be correlated with other physiologic findings.

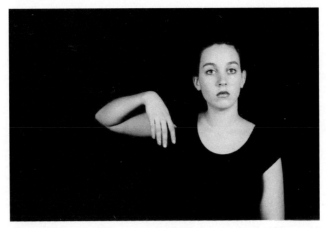

Fig. 3—19 The patient is seated and abducts the shoulder to 90 degrees. The shoulder is externally rotated.

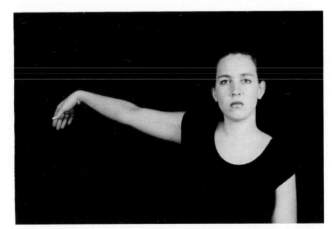

Fig. 3—20 The arm is fully extended at the elbow, and the patient attempts to reach behind. In the presence of radiculopathy or plexopathy, this maneuver produces the radicular pain.

～ Brachial Plexus Tension Test ～

Comment

A direct traumatic insult to the nerve roots causes inflammation in the dural sleeves and perineural tissues. This inflammation may result in fibrosis. Adhesions may occur between the dural sleeves and the adjacent capsular tissues. Normally, the nerve roots are free in the intervertebral canals and can move ¼ to ½ of an inch. Nerve roots that are injured or compressed by capsular thickening or bony encroachments cannot move within the intervertebral canals. Nerve roots subjected to compressive forces by osteophytic encroachments have varying amounts of distortion and perineural fibrosis.

In many instances at least one fiber of a nerve root fails to continue in that particular nerve root. This fiber descends to join the adjacent distal nerve root. For instance, one of the fourth cervical nerve root fibers that leaves the cord at that level may actually leave the spinal canal with fibers of the fifth cervical nerve root. If the fourth cervical nerve root is irritated within the foramen of the fifth cervical nerve root, the examiner may find that the fourth cervical nerve is also involved.

The fifth cervical nerve root is the one irritated most frequently, and the sixth, fourth, third, second, and seventh roots become irritated in that order of frequency. Irritation or compression of a nerve root may cause pain-sensory changes anywhere along its distribution. Localized areas of tenderness and muscle spasm will be found at the site of the pain. Frequently, the examiner finds some areas of segmental tenderness of which the patient is not aware. These myalgic areas are found only by deep palpation because hyperalgesia, or superficial tenderness, is not present.

In cases affecting the fifth cervical root, the pain extends from the scapular area to the front of the arm and forearm and can extend as far as the radial side of the hand. However, the pain does not reach the thumb, and the pins-and-needles sensation is absent. The weak muscles are the two spinati, the deltoid, and the biceps. The biceps reflex may be sluggish or absent, and the brachioradialis reflex is sluggish, absent, or inverted.

Procedure

The patient fully elevates the shoulders through abduction. The patient extends the elbows to a point just short of the onset of pain and maintains this position. The patient then externally rotates the shoulders to the point just short of the onset of pain and maintains this position. The examiner supports the shoulder and forearm in this position, while the patient flexes the elbow. Reproduction of symptoms implies problems originating in the cervical region, probably at the C5 nerve root. In addition, if the cervical spine is then flexed, symptoms will increase.

Confirmation Procedures

Dejerine's sign, Valsalva maneuver, reflex testing, Bakody sign, maximum foraminal encroachment test, shoulder depression test, distraction test, Bikele's sign, Jackson cervical compression test, Spurling's test, diagnostic imaging

---

Reporting Statement

The brachial plexus tension test is positive on the right. This result suggests a C5 nerve root syndrome.

～ Clinical Pearl ～

Although the brachial plexus tension test involves a shoulder joint movement, it also provides maximum stretch on the brachial plexus, which affects the lower branches of the cervical spine (C5) the most. If this test is positive, the early stages of a C5 nerve root disorder may also be present along with the subtle signs of a positive doorbell sign (pain that occurs at the superior scapulovertebral border and radiates with the use of deep palpation of the C5 segment), and pain in the deltoid area. The deltoid pain is often misconstrued as an articular problem of the shoulder.

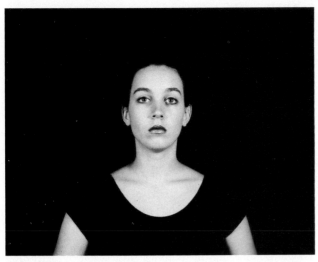

Fig. 3–21   The patient is sitting erect. An alternative is to have the patient assume the supine position on the examination table.

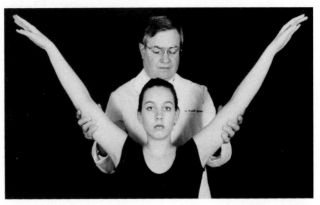

Fig. 3–22   The patient fully elevates the shoulders through abduction to the end-point of joint play. The elbows are fully extended. The examiner supports the patient's arms in this position.

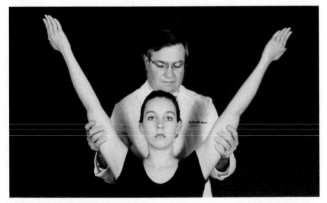

Fig. 3–23   The patient externally rotates the shoulders to the end-point of joint play or to the onset of discomfort. The examiner supports the patient's arms in this position.

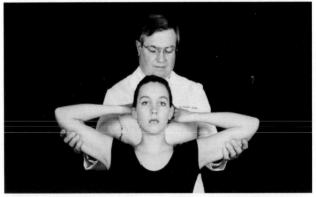

Fig. 3–24   As the shoulders are supported in this position, the patient flexes the elbows. Reproduction of the radicular symptoms suggests a nerve root syndrome that probably involves C5. If symptoms do not appear, a final maneuver is the flexion of the cervical spine.

≈ Dejerine's Sign ≈

DEJERINE'S TRIAD
TRIAD OF DEJERINE

Comments

Infections and tumors, benign or malignant, are rare occurrences in the cervical spine. The cervical spine is unique, anatomically and physiologically, with its concentration of crowded, critical structures. Rapid clinical catastrophe is a constant threat unless early diagnosis and optimum management of tumor and infection are instituted. Neurologic structures have little tolerance to mechanical compression. The possibilities of quadriplegia, spinal cord stroke, and death are always in the background. The close anatomic and physiologic relationships among the spinal cord, nerve roots, and peripheral nervous system and the structurally confining implications of the skeletal and soft tissues make early diagnosis mandatory in these rare cervical spinal disorders.

Space-taking lesions in or around the spinal canal cause a broad spectrum of clinical syndromes ranging from neck pain, radiculitis, and paresthesia to quadriparesis and death. Cervical cord compression can be caused by the gross space occupation of an expanding abscess; a rapidly growing vertebral, medullary, or extramedullary tumor; or the fracture, collapse, and dislocation of the supporting structures. These structures include the bones, discs, joints, ligaments, and tendons. Therapeutic choices require identification of either or both destructive pathologic processes. Critical structures that are at risk when tumors and infections of the cervical spine are present include the lower brainstem, cervical spinal cord, nerve roots and rootlets, ganglia and common spinal nerves, vertebral arteries, carotid artery, trachea, and esophagus.

Cervical spine, shoulder, and arm pain that radiates and is accompanied by tenderness, muscle spasms, and decreased cervical spine movements may be the only clinical manifestations of a benign, space-occupying mass. Torticollis is more common in masses involving the upper cervical spine. Mass enlargement or bony displacement may cause clinical symptoms and signs of radiculitis or spinal cord compression. Spinal stroke occurs when the radicular arteries, the end arteries in the cord itself, or the anterior and posterior spinal arteries are constricted.

Clinical manifestations of cervical disc disease are highly variable. Patients may have a variety of complaints and physical findings. Generally, signs and symptoms can be categorized as neurogenic or discogenic. Neurogenic symptoms result from pressure on the cervical nerve roots or the spinal cord by disc material or by posterior or posterolateral osteophytes. The patients may have radicular symptoms alone, or they may have signs and symptoms of nerve root and spinal cord compression simultaneously.

Patients with discogenic symptoms have no objective neurologic findings. The patients complain of intermittent, chronic pain in the posterior cervical region and the shoulder, chest wall, and scapular region. Occipital headaches are frequent. It is postulated that the pain experienced by the patients with discogenic symptoms results from the stimulation of the sensory receptors of the sinuvertebral nerve. The sinuvertebral nerve is located in the fibrous ring of the intervertebral disc and in the posterior and anterior longitudinal ligament.

Root pain is frequently produced or aggravated by coughing, sneezing, or straining, such as during defecation, or any other measures that suddenly increase intrathoracic and intraabdominal pressure. Such pressure increases block the venous flow from the epidural space through the intervertebral veins or permit a retrograde flow of blood because these veins do not contain valves. This pressure increase causes a distention of the veins in the epidural space, which in turn forces the dura, which envelops the nerve roots, toward the spinal cord. Because the nerve roots are fixed to the spinal cord proximally and peripherally at the intervertebral foramen, the displacement of the dura results in a stretching of the involved nerve root, which may result in pain. In addition, distention of the intervertebral vein may result in direct compression of the nerve root.

Procedure

Coughing, sneezing, and straining during defecation may cause aggravation of radiculitis symptoms. This aggravation is due to the mechanical obstruction of spinal fluid flow. Dejerine's sign is present when one of the following exists: herniated or protruding intervertebral disc, spinal cord tumor, or spinal compression fracture. The course of the radiculitis helps identify the location of the lesion.

Confirmation Procedures

Swallowing test, Valsalva maneuver, Naffziger's test, vascular assessment, diagnostic imaging, such as magnetic resonance imaging (MRI)

Reporting Statement

Dejerine's sign is present and suggests a space-occupying mass at the C5 level.

Dejerine's sign is present with reproduced radicular symptoms on the right in the C5 dermatome. This result suggests a space-occupying mass at that vertebral level.

~ **Clinical Pearl** ~

Patients suffering from radicular symptoms and pronounced Dejerine's sign, especially if it is in the lumbar spine, will appreciate being told to bend the knees and lean into a wall during a cough or sneeze. This maneuver reduces intradiscal pressure and minimizes the effect of the cough or sneeze on the nerve root.

A more worrisome situation is the sudden, unexpected absence of Dejerine's sign when all other clinical findings indicate an active, nerve root compression. The loss of the sign indicates fragmentation of the disc with momentary decompression of the nerve.

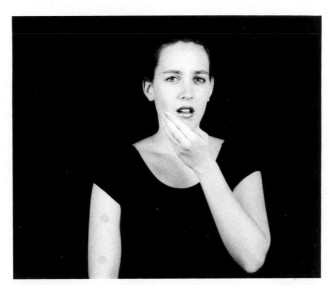

Fig. 3–25   Coughing, sneezing, or straining during defecation causes a reproduction of radicular symptoms, which suggests a space-occupying mass that is creating neurologic compression.

Comment

Vertebral artery syndrome (also known as vertebral artery compression syndrome or vertebral-basilar artery insufficiency) is characterized by recurring transient episodes of cerebral symptoms. The notable cerebral symptoms include vertigo, nystagmus, and sudden postural collapse without unconsciousness. These symptoms are precipitated by rotation and hyperextension of the neck and are due to temporary occlusion of the vertebral artery. This mechanical action produces ischemia at the base of the brain. A combination of cerebrovascular arteriosclerosis and cervical spondylosis is fundamental in this syndrome.

The main tributaries to the basilar artery at the base of the brain are the internal carotid and vertebral arteries. Occlusive arterial disease gradually reduces blood flow to a certain critical point. Any further reduction in the caliber of the vessel, unless an adequate collateral supply has developed, will result in ischemia and cerebral symptoms.

Normally, hyperextension and rotation of the neck compresses and may occlude the vertebral artery on the contralateral side at the level of the atlas and axis. However, symptoms do not develop because collateral circulation is adequate. When vessels are occluded by atheromatous plaque and compressed by osteophytes, collateral blood flow may be insufficient and symptoms may develop as the vertebral artery becomes blocked momentarily during the rotation and hyperextension movement of the cervical spine.

Various causes of dizziness must first be ruled out, particularly those due to labyrinthine or cerebellar disease. The drop attack must be differentiated from epilepsy, syncope, and the Stokes-Adams syndrome. Carotid sinus sensitivity, with its cardioinhibitory and vasodepressor reflexes, can be identified by an electrocardiogram (ECG) that is conducted while the carotid sinus is massaged.

The subclavian steal syndrome must be ruled out because its symptoms are due to basilar artery insufficiency. However, syncopal episodes are precipitated by exertion of the upper extremity. With the subclavian steal syndrome, occlusion occurs at the portion of the subclavian artery that is proximal to the origin of the vertebral artery. Because of this occlusion, blood flow is diverted from the opposite vertebral artery into the artery on the obstructed side, which results in perfusion of the distal subclavian bed with blood that was intended for cerebral circulation.

Procedure

With the patient in the supine position and the patient's head off the table, the examiner instructs the patient to hyperextend and rotate the head and hold this position for 15 to 45 seconds. The patient repeats this maneuver with the head rotated and extended to the opposite side. Vertigo, blurred vision, nausea, syncope, and nystagmus are signs of a positive test. The test indicates vertebral, basilar, or carotid artery stenosis or compression at one of the following sites: (1) between C1 and C2 transverse processes, where the vertebral arteries are fixed in the C1 and C2 transverse foramina; (2) at the level of the superior articular facet of C3, on the ipsilateral side of head rotation; (3) at the C1 transverse process and the internal carotid artery; (4) at the atlanto-occipital aperture near the posterior arch of the atlas and the rim of the foramen magnum or anteriorly by folding of the atlanto-occipital joint capsule and posteriorly by the atlanto-occipital membrane; (5) at the C4-C5 or C5-C6 levels, due to arthrosis of the joints of Luschka, with compression on the ipsilateral side of head rotation; (6) at the transverse foramen of the atlas or axis between the obliquus capitis inferior and transversarii during rotary movements; and (7) before entering the C6 transverse process by the longus colli muscle or by tissue communicating between the longus colli and scalenus anterior muscles.

Confirmation Procedures

Hautant's test, George's screening procedure, Underburg's test, Hallpike maneuver, vertebrobasilar artery functional maneuver, Barre-Lieou sign, vascular assessment, vascular imaging, MRI

Reporting Statement

DeKleyn's test is positive following cervical rotation to the right with hyperextension. This result suggests vertebral artery syndrome on the ipsilateral side.

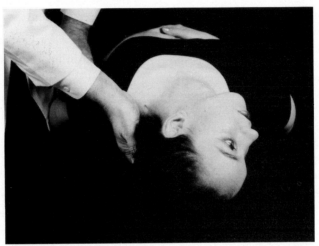

Fig. 3–26   The patient is supine with the head extending off the end of the examination table. The patient rotates and hyperextends the neck to one side and holds this position for 15 to 45 seconds. The examiner may provide minimal support for the weight of the skull. The maneuver is repeated for the opposite side. The production of vertigo, visual disturbance, nausea, syncope, or nystagmus indicates vertebrobasilar circulation compromise.

∽ Distraction Test ∽

Comment

The intervertebral foramina are short tunnels bounded ventromedially by the disc, with its covering of the posterior longitudinal ligament, and the uncovertebral joint (joint of Luschka), and dorsolaterally by the zygapophyseal joint and the superior articular process of the subjacent vertebra. The shape of the foramen resembles a figure eight or the sole of a shoe with the heel positioned inferiorly. The foramina are largest at the C2-C3 level, becoming progressively smaller down to the C6-C7 level. The average vertical diameter is 10 mm, and the transverse is 5 mm. The intervertebral foramina enclose and transmit the lateral termination of the anterior and posterior nerve roots, spinal radicular arteries, intervertebral veins, and plexuses, and an extension of the epidural space with areolar and fatty tissue. Small arteries, veins, and lymphatics provide a protective cushion for the nerves. The roots occupy one quarter to one third of the foraminal space. The anterior root lies anterior and inferior to the posterior root near the uncovertebral joint. The posterior root is close to the zygapophyseal joint and especially to the superior articular process of the subjacent vertebra. The roots lie nearer the upper vertebral pedicle at the medial end of the foramen and nearer the lower vertebral pedicle at the lateral end.

Procedure

With the patient seated, the examiner exerts upward pressure on the patient's head. This removes the weight of the patient's head from the neck. Generalized, increased pain indicates muscle spasm. Relief of pain indicates intervertebral foraminal encroachment or facet capsulitis. The examiner continues the distraction for 30 to 60 seconds.

This test provides some prediction of the effect of cervical spine traction in relieving pain or paresthesia. Nerve root compression may be relieved, with disappearance of the symptoms and signs, if the intervertebral foramina are opened or the disc spaces extended. Pressure on the joint capsules of the apophyseal joints is also decreased by distraction.

Confirmation Procedures

Bakody sign, maximum foraminal encroachment test, shoulder depression test, brachial plexus tension test, Bikele's sign, Jackson cervical compression test, Spurling's test, reflexes, diagnostic imaging

---

Reporting Statement

Distraction test is positive in relieving the C5 radicular pain on the right. This result suggests nerve root compression syndrome at that level, on the right.

∽ Clinical Pearl ∽

The procedure not only indicates the nature of the patient's complaint but also identifies the merit of cervical traction in the treatment regimen. It should also be noted that the higher the poundages of *static* cervical traction required for relief, the more unstable the nerve compression syndrome is. Indeed, the higher poundage requirement is often an indicator of the need for surgical resolution.

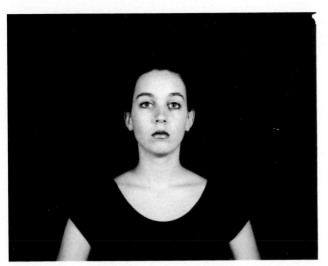

Fig. 3–27 The patient is seated comfortably, with the spine erect and the head and neck in a neutral position.

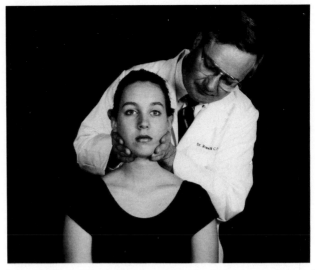

Fig. 3–28 With the hands cupping the patient's mandible and occiput, the examiner lifts the patient's head. A positive finding is the relief of the patient's localized or radicular pain. The sign is confirmed if the symptoms return when the weight of the head is returned to the neck.

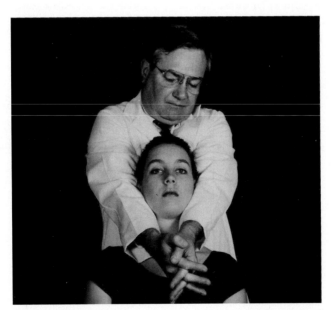

Fig. 3–29 Alternatively, the examiner can lift the patient's head by clasping the forearms under the patient's mandible. In this procedure the back of the patient's head is fixed against the examiner's chest. In both methods the lift or distraction is maintained for as many seconds as possible but not beyond patient tolerance.

Comment

A disc whose internal structure is damaged may be a source of pain that is referred to an area that is embryologically related to that disc.

The outer fibers of the annulus fibrosis of the cervical intervertebral discs are richly supplied with sensory receptors from which impulses are transmitted by way of the sinuvertebral nerve. When the anterior fibers of each of the cervical discs from C3 to C7 are stimulated on one side of the midline, pain is referred to the vertebral border of the scapula on the ipsilateral side (doorbell sign). Pain from the upper cervical discs develops a more cephalad level along the inner border of the scapula. Pain from the lower disc develops at a more caudad level. When the anterior peripheral fibers are stimulated in the midline, pain develops in the interscapular area.

If the disc is ruptured in a posterior or posterolateral direction, the resulting pain is of three types.

In discogenic pain, the disc rupture extends to but not through the peripheral fibers. Pain develops first at the medial scapular border, then spreads to the shoulder and down the posterior surface of the arm as far as the elbow. This produces a deep, dull, aching sensation, which may be severe and which subsides in 5 to 10 minutes.

In neurogenic pain, the peripheral fibers of the disc are lacerated with or without herniation of disc fragments into the spinal canal. Fluid pressure is transmitted through the defect resting against the nerve root and spinal cord. Neurogenic pain that is the result of nerve root irritation has a sharper, more intense quality that is described as an electric shock or a hot burning sensation. This type of pain shoots into the arm, forearm, and hand along a dermatome distribution.

Myelogenic pain results from a central posterior defect, which permits a midline protrusion and spinal cord compression, allowing the pressure of the disc to be transmitted to the spinal cord. This pain produces a momentary shocklike sensation (Lhermitte's sign) that shoots downward along the spine and may spread into one or several extremities.

Procedure

With the patient in the seated position, the examiner rotates the patient's neck while exerting strong downward pressure on the head. The test is then repeated bilaterally with the head in a neutral position. When the neck is rotated and downward pressure is applied, closure of the intervertebral foramen occurs. Localized pain indicates foraminal encroachment. Radicular pain indicates pressure on the nerve root. If nerve root involvement is suspected, the neurologic level must be evaluated.

Confirmation Procedures

Bakody sign, maximum foraminal encroachment test, shoulder depression test, distraction test, brachial plexus tension test, Bikele's sign, Jackson cervical compression test, Spurling's test, reflex and sensory testing, electrodiagnosis, diagnostic imaging

---

Reporting Statement

Foraminal compression testing is positive on the right, in the C5 dermatome. This result suggests nerve root encroachment.

∼ Clinical Pearl ∼

This test, as well as other compression maneuvers, often produces a cervical collapse sign in addition to radicular complaints. In the presence of capsular sprain with radicular components, compression overcomes the modicum of muscular strength that remains in the neck and is required for postural control. This condition means that the neck will collapse or buckle during the test. This collapse is found in grade II or greater sprain syndromes.

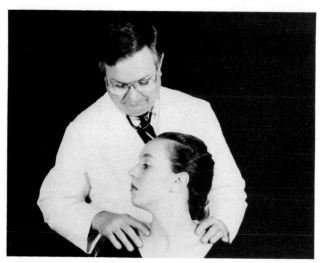

Fig. 3–30 The seated patient actively rotates the head from side to side. Localization of any discomfort is noted.

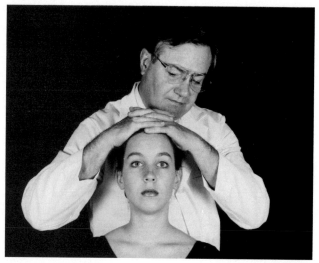

Fig. 3–31 With the patient seated and the head and neck returned to a neutral position, the examiner exerts progressively increasing downward pressure (compression) on the head and neck. Symptoms may lateralize and localize at this point.

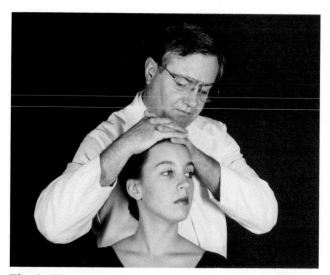

Fig. 3–32 The head is rotated toward the side of complaint and similar compression is applied. Reproduction of the complaint is a positive finding and indicates foraminal encroachment.

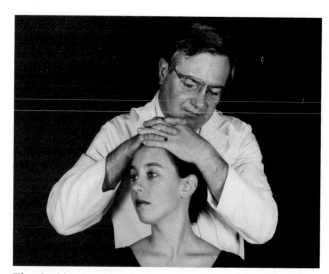

Fig. 3–33 The maneuver is repeated for the opposite side.

Comment

In cerebral transient ischemic attacks the symptoms vary according to which area of the brain is ischemic. There are two main groups of symptoms: those associated with partial or total ischemia of a cerebral hemisphere and those associated with ischemia of the brainstem. The symptoms most often include transient contralateral weakness of the lower face, fingers, hand, arm, or leg. Such patients may also experience fleeting sensory symptoms, such as tingling, paresthesia, or numbness, in parts of the body contralateral to the ischemia. Ischemia in the dominant hemisphere may cause dysphasia with impairment of speech and, at times, a transient lack of understanding.

Patients with ischemia in the portion of the brain that is supplied by the posterior cerebral artery may suffer blurred vision or may notice transient hemianopic or altitudinal visual field defects or impairment of visual acuity.

Ischemia or insufficiency due to internal carotid artery stenosis often produces transient retinal ischemia which results in monocular blindness or reduced acuity on the side of the stenosis combined with contralateral weakness of the face, arm, or leg.

Ischemic attacks that involve the section of the brain that is supplied by the vertebral and basilar arteries have an extremely wide range of symptoms. Common symptoms include vertigo, tinnitus, diplopia, dysarthria, dysphagia, and dysphonia. Patients may complain of unilateral or bilateral face, arm, and leg weakness and unilateral or bilateral sensations of numbness and tingling in the face, arms, or legs. There may be tinnitus, hearing loss, and ataxia. In addition, patients with brainstem ischemia experience drop attacks in which they suddenly lose postural tone and fall to the ground without losing consciousness, then immediately regain postural control and rise quickly. Dizziness is the most common complaint with transient ischemic attacks that are caused by vertebrobasilar insufficiency. However, dizziness is commonly associated with other physiologic disturbances and is rarely the only symptom of brainstem ischemia.

Although the symptoms of vertebral basilar artery ischemia vary they tend to occur in combinations that aid diagnosis. Vertigo, ataxia, dysarthria, paresthesia, diplopia, tinnitus, and dysphagia and focal weakness of the face, jaw, or pharynx tend to coexist, although not always in the same sequence or combination. Another grouping of symptoms is that of unilateral or bilateral weakness of the extremities with drop attacks and diplopia. The reason for these differences in symptom combinations can be found by referring to any diagram of the blood supply of the brainstem. Ischemia of the dorsal and lateral portions of the brainstem, which are supplied by the circumferential arteries, produces the first group of symptoms. Ischemia of the more ventral portions, supplied by the medial perforating arteries, causes the second group of symptoms.

Procedure

The Hallpike maneuver is an enhanced DeKleyn's test and must be performed with extreme caution.

The patient is lying supine with the head extending off the end of the examination table. The examiner provides support for the weight of the skull. The examiner brings the patient's head into positions of reclination (extension), rotation and lateral flexion. The patient's eyes are open so that the examiner may look for nystagmus and other neurovascular signs. The test is repeated for the opposite side. These positions are held for 15 to 45 seconds.

In a final maneuver the patient's head is allowed to hang freely in extreme extension (hyperextension) off the end of the examination table. Vertigo, blurred vision, nausea, syncope, and nystagmus are signs of a positive test. The test indicates vertebral, basilar, or carotid artery stenosis or compression at one of the following sites: (1) between C1 and C2 transverse processes, where the vertebral arteries are fixed in the C1 and C2 transverse foramina; (2) at the level of the superior articular facet of C3, on the ipsilateral side of the head rotation; (3) at the C1 transverse process and the internal carotid artery; (4) at the atlantoocipital aperture near the posterior arch of the atlas and the rim of the foramen magnum or anterior by folding of the atlantooccipital joint capsule and posterior by the atlantoocipital membrane; (5) at the C4-C5 or C5-C6 levels because of arthrosis of the joints of Luschka with compression on the ipsilateral side of head rotation; (6) at the transverse foramen of the atlas or axis between the obliquus capitis inferior and transversarii during rotary movements; (7) and before entering the C6 transverse process, by the longus colli muscle or by tissue communicating between the longus colli and scalenus anterior muscles.

Confirmation Procedures

Barre-Lieou sign, vertebrobasilar artery functional maneuver, Hautant's test, DeKleyn's test, Underburg's test, vascular assessment, vascular imaging (MRI)

Reporting Statement

Hallpike maneuver is positive. This result suggests vertebrobasilar arterial insufficiency.

∼ **Clinical Pearl** ∼

Cervical spine manipulation and adjunctive therapeutic techniques are safe to use. Nevertheless, the patient's welfare is always of prime concern, and screening tests will help identify those who may be predisposed to cerebrovascular problems. During these procedures, symptoms of vertigo, nystagmus, dizziness, fainting, nausea, vomiting, visual blurring, headache (onset), or other sensory disturbances may identify a possible vertebrobasilar insufficiency. Problems in the cervical spine apart from the vertebral arteries may cause the same signs and symptoms. In suspected vertebral artery constriction, resisted neck extension may be painful and prolonged cervical extension may produce a feeling of faintness. The transverse processes of the atlas are often tender on the side of involvement.

These symptoms may be significantly improved by using manipulative procedures. Therefore manipulation should not necessarily be abandoned. Rather, the manipulative technique should be modified so that simultaneous extension and rotation are not used.

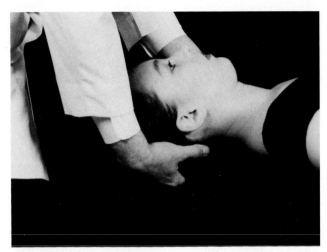

Fig. 3–34 The patient is lying supine with the head extending off the end of the examination table. The examiner provides support for the weight of the skull.

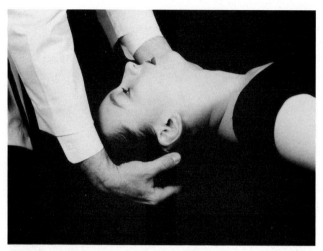

Fig. 3–35 The examiner brings the patient's head into the reclination (extension) position.

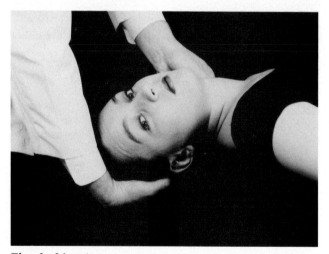

Fig. 3–36 The examiner then moves the patient's head into rotation and lateral flexion. The patient's eyes are open so that the examiner may look for nystagmus and other neurovascular signs.

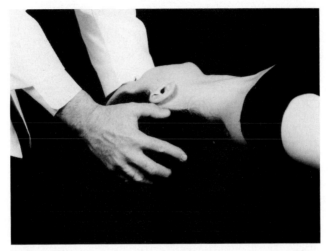

Fig. 3–37 The test is repeated for the opposite side. These positions are held for 15 to 45 seconds.

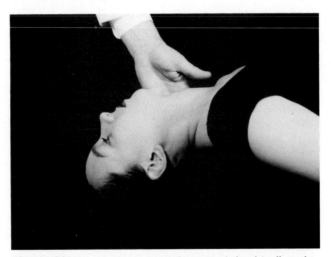

Fig. 3–38 In a final maneuver the patient's head is allowed to hang freely in extreme extension (hyperextension) off the end of the examination table. Vertigo, blurred vision, nausea, syncope, and nystagmus are signs of a positive test. The test indicates vertebral, basilar, or carotid artery stenosis or compression.

Hautant's Test

Comment

The atlantoaxial joints (C1–C2) constitute the most mobile articulations of the spine. Flexion and extension involve a move of approximately 10 degrees, and lateral flexion involves a move of approximately 5 degrees. Rotation, which involves a move of approximately 50 degrees, is the primary movement of these joints. During rotation the height of the cervical spine decreases as the vertebrae approximate. This decrease is due to the shape of the facet joints. The odontoid process of C2 acts as a pivot point for the rotation. This middle, or median, joint is classified as a pivot (trochoidal) type of joint. The lateral atlantoaxial, or facet, joints are classed as plane joints. If a patient can talk and chew, there is probably some motion occurring at C1–C2.

Rotation of the cervical spine past 50 degrees to one side may lead to kinking of the contralateral vertebral artery. The ipsilateral vertebral artery may kink at 45 degrees of rotation. This kinking of the ipsilateral vertebral artery may lead to vertigo, nausea, tinnitus, drop attacks, visual disturbances, stroke, or death.

If an osteophyte developing on the neurocentral joint extends laterally, the vertebral artery foramen may be encroached and the vertebral artery may become compressed to a significant degree. Minor degrees of vertebral artery compromise may be responsible for the so-called vertebral artery syndrome. Occasionally, a neurocentral osteophyte may produce severe kinking of the artery, which eventually results in vertebral artery thrombosis. Thrombosis may extend superiorly and involve the posteroinferior cerebellar artery. Occlusion of this artery leads to the development of Wallenberg's syndrome. Wallenberg's syndrome is associated with the following symptom complex:

1. Dysphagia, ipsilateral palatal weakness, and vocal cord paralysis from involvement of the nucleus ambiguous of the vagus
2. Impairment of sensation to pain and temperature on the same side of the face from involvement of the descending root and nucleus of the fifth cranial nerve
3. Horner's syndrome in the homolateral eye from the involvement of the descending sympathetic fibers
4. Nystagmus due to the involvement of the vestibular nuclei
5. Cerebellar dysfunction in the ipsilateral arm and leg from interference of the function of the midbrain and cerebellum
6. Impairment of sensation to pain and temperature on the side of the body opposite from the involvement of the spinothalamic tract

Procedure

With the patient seated and the eyes closed, the patient extends the arms out in front with the palms up. The patient extends and rotates the head to one side. The patient repeats the maneuver with the head extended and rotated to the opposite side. Drifting of the arms, vertigo, blurred vision, nausea, syncope, and nystagmus are signs of a positive test. The test indicates vertebral, basilar, or carotid artery stenosis or compression.

Confirmation Procedures

Barre-Lieou sign, vertebrobasilar artery functional maneuver, DeKleyn's test, Hallpike maneuver, Underburg's test, vascular testing or imaging, diagnostic imaging

Reporting Statement

Hautant's test is positive on the right. This result suggests vertebral artery syndrome on the ipsilateral side.

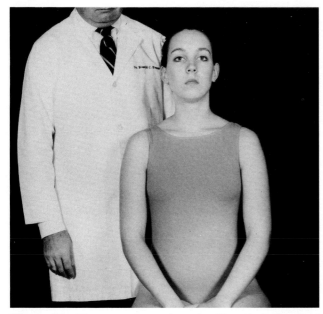

Fig. 3–39 The patient is seated comfortably with the head and neck in the neutral position.

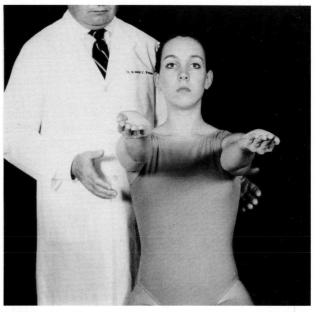

Fig. 3–40 The patient extends the arms forward and elevates them to shoulder level. The hands are supinated. The patient maintains this position for a few seconds.

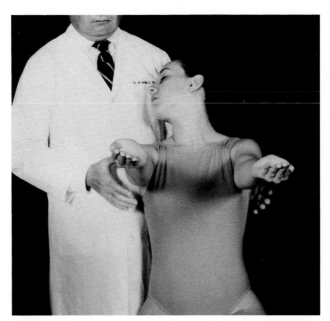

Fig. 3–41 The patient closes the eyes, rotates the head to one side, and hyperextends the neck. The examiner observes for any significant drifting of the arms from their original position. Drifting of the arms is a positive sign for vertebrobasilar vascular compromise.

Comment

Patients who are symptomatic from cervical disc degeneration usually suffer from compression of a nearby nerve root or the spinal cord. Acute herniation of degenerated disc material produces such compression and resembles an acute lumbar disc herniation. The various syndromes related to chronic disc degeneration, with herniation and insidious compression or degenerative subluxation, make the condition deceptive during clinical presentation. Typical of the confusion surrounding the problem of chronic disc degeneration are its many partial synonyms: osteoarthritis, chronic herniated disc, chondroma, spur formation, and others. Recently the term *cervical spondylosis* has gained favor and may be used interchangeably for chronic cervical disc degeneration.

From C3 through C7 the average anteroposterior measurement of the cervical canal is 17 mm. Spinal cord compression will occur only if this figure is reduced to 11 mm or less. In cervical spondylosis some reduction will usually take place in the anteroposterior diameter of the spinal canal and, when associated with a canal that is initially small, myelopathy can occur.

The dorsal and ventral nerve roots pass through the subarachnoid space and converge to form the spinal nerve at approximately the level of its respective intervertebral foramen.

Root pain may awaken the patient after several hours of sleep and may be relieved approximately 15 to 30 minutes after the patient sits up. The patient may learn to prevent the pain by sleeping in a chair. However, in contrast to peripheral neuritis, the antalgic position is the important determining factor. If the patient lies down for awhile during the day, the pain would occur as it does during the night. This feature of root pain occurs because the spinal column lengthens when the patient lies down and shortens when the patient sits up. Because the length of the spinal *cord* remains the same regardless of the patient's position, the lengthening of the spinal column results in a tensing of, or traction on, the nerve roots.

Procedure

Cervical compression is commonly performed by having the patient sit up and bend the head obliquely backward while the examiner applies downward pressure on the vertex. However, with the Jackson cervical compression test, the head is only slightly rotated to the involved side. In either case, the sign is positive if localized pain radiates down the arm. A positive sign indicates nerve involvement from a space-occupying lesion, subluxation, inflammatory swelling, exostosis of degenerative joint disease, tumor, or disc-herniation.

Confirmation Procedures

Bakody sign, maximum foraminal encroachment test, shoulder depression test, distraction test, brachial plexus tension test, Bikele's sign, Spurling's test, foraminal compression test, reflexes, sensory testing, diagnostic imaging

---

Reporting Statement

Jackson cervical compression is positive on the right and elicits pain in the C5 dermatome.

∽ **Clinical Pearl** ∽

Closure of the intervertebral foramina occurs on the side of flexion in this maneuver. This test should be performed without excessive discomfort. The collapse sign may be present.

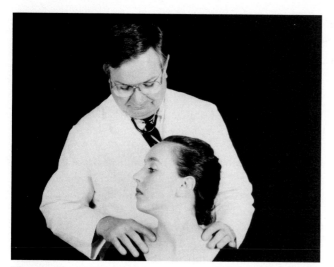

Fig. 3–42 While seated, the patient rotates the head from side to side. Localization of any complaint is noted.

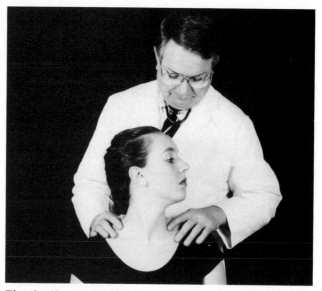

Fig. 3–43 Pain on the side opposite of rotation suggests muscular strain, while pain on the side of rotation suggests facet or nerve root involvement.

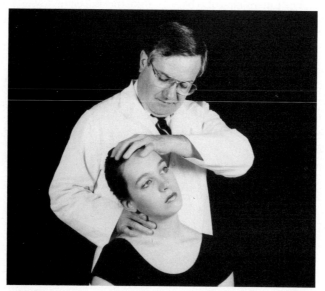

Fig. 3–44 The head is laterally flexed in an attempt to approximate the ear to the shoulder. This position is held, and the examiner exerts downward pressure on the patient's head. An exacerbation of the local or radicular pain indicates a positive test.

Comment

Peripheral neuropathy is a disorder that affects the peripheral motor, sensory, or autonomic nerves to a variable degree. If only one nerve is affected, it is considered a mononeuropathy. If several nerves are involved in a distal symmetric or asymmetric fashion, it is characterized as a polyneuropathy. If there are multiple, single-peripheral nerves or their branches involved, then this pattern is called mononeuritis multiplex.

Patients who suffer any form of peripheral neuropathy will often describe their symptoms similarly, using words such as prickling, burning, or jabbing. These symptoms often indicate whether disease exists in the peripheral nerves.

In most patients with polyneuropathy, distal weakness is more prominent than proximal weakness and usually there is an accompanying sensory abnormality. With mononeuropathy, muscles innervated by a single peripheral nerve are weak and atrophic. This pattern must be differentiated from that in a patient with a radiculopathy, in which only the muscles supplied by a single root are affected. The pattern must also be differentiated from that of a patient with a plexopathy, in which the pattern of motor and sensory dysfunction is in a multiple root or peripheral nerve distribution.

Neuropathies that develop abruptly and are associated with pain are usually of an ischemic origin, such as in rheumatoid arthritis and polyarteritis nodosa. Neuropathies that evolve over a few days may be due to industrial intoxications, such as those associated with the use of thallium or triorthocresyl phosphate. A neuropathy evolving over many weeks or months should suggest several possibilities: exposure to toxic agents or drugs, nutritional deficiencies, a chronically abnormal metabolic state, a remote effect of a malignant disease, or even a genetic polyneuropathy, which may have an insidious onset at any age.

Primary diseases of muscle are not usually confused with peripheral neuropathies, but in some cases electrophysiologic studies are required for differentiation. Distal symmetric or asymmetric paresthesia in the extremities without a significant component of muscle weakness should be differentiated from multiple sclerosis, cervical spondylitic myelopathy, or occasionally from extradural tumors of the cervical cord. Constant and severe pain in the neck or pain while flexing the neck (Lhermitte's sign) usually indicates cervical cord disease. Sometimes symptoms or signs of spasticity may occur later in these myelopathies, and this creates a problem in diagnosis. Electrophysiologic testing usually resolves the issue.

Procedure

The patient is in the seated position on the examining table. The examiner passively flexes the patient's head. A positive test is indicated by a sharp pain down the spine and into the upper or lower limbs. This result indicates dural irritation in the spine. The test is similar to a combination of Brudzinski's sign and double straight leg raising tests.

Confirmation Procedures

Soto-Hall sign, reflexes and sensory testing, electrodiagnosis, MRI

Reporting Statement

Lhermitte's sign is present. This result suggests myelopathy of the cervical spine.

∾ Clinical Pearl ∾

Although Lhermitte's sign is often construed as a pathognomonic test for multiple sclerosis (MS), it is not. However, Lhermitte's sign does reveal or suggest myelopathy due to MS, stenosis, tumor, or disc herniation.

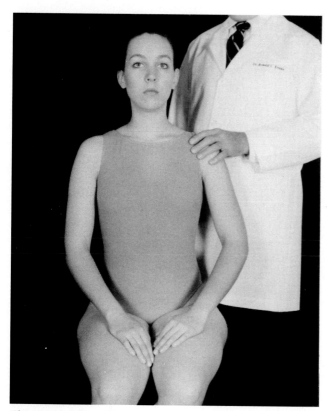

Fig. 3–45 The patient sits comfortably but erect with the head and neck in the neutral position.

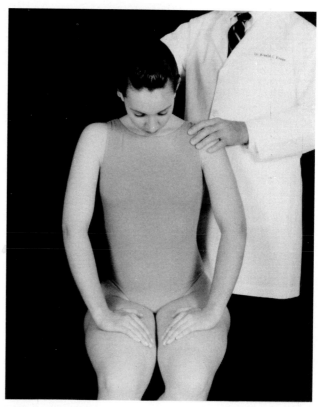

Fig. 3–46 The head and neck are passively flexed toward the patient's chest.

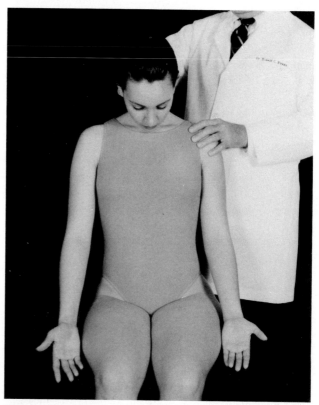

Fig. 3–47 The patient may experience a sharp, radiating pain or paresthesia along the spine and into one or more extremities. The presence of these symptoms suggests myelopathy and constitutes a positive test.

Comment

Acute injury (sprain) of a joint produces synovial effusion, histamine release, capsular or ligamentous stretch or tear, bleeding, and associated clinical disabilities. Some of these conditions are visible and palpable in joints of the extremities but not the spine. With repetition of the traumatic process or with chronic stress on the joint from shearing and other forces, a chronic synovial reaction is established. This reaction extends to the underlying articular cartilage. The cartilage softens then becomes rough and eroded. Stresses in the capsule and periosteum result in marginal osteophytosis, which may encroach on the underlying nerve root. A loose body may develop in the joint cavity, or an osteophytic process may fracture and lie free or loosely attached in or near the foramen. The facetal bone may thicken or become hypertrophic, and the laminae may do so as well. Degenerative enlargement of facets with irritative compression of one or more cervical roots may also occur.

Trauma to the cervical spine may injure the nervous tissue and related structures in several ways. During the hyperextension phase of an injury, nerve roots may suffer a compression injury at the point of exit from the neural foramina. The nerve root may become contused enough to produce actual disruption of axons and resulting axonotmesis. However, because the internal structure is fairly well preserved, recovery is spontaneous. Neurapraxic injury is more common and is clinically manifested as the transient paresthesia that is seen most often approximately a week following the trauma. The spinal cord, dura, and arachnoid may also be contused. During the hyperflexion phase, traction injury may occur.

The nerve supply to the capsular and ligamentous structures of the cervical spine is of significance in the interpretation of painful conditions. The capsules of the atlantoaxial joints and those of the posterior or apophyseal joints are supplied by the capsular branches of the medial divisions of the posterior primary rami of the cervical spine nerves. The posterior longitudinal ligament and the capsular structures of the lateral interbody joints receive their nerve supply from the recurrent spinal meningeal nerves (the sinuvertebral nerves), which contain afferent somatic sensory fibers and efferent sympathetic fibers.

Chronic cervical strain is the most common cause of neck pain that mimics cervical spondylosis. This mimicry has led to unnecessary myelography because the associated patterns of referred pain and neuralgia are so similar between the two conditions.

Procedure

While in the seated position, the patient is instructed to approximate the chin to the shoulder and extend the neck. The test is performed bilaterally. Pain on the concave side indicates nerve root or facet involvement. Pain on the convex side indicates muscular strain.

Confirmation Procedures

Dejerine's sign, swallowing test, Valsalva maneuver, Naffziger's test, Bakody sign, shoulder depression test, distraction test, brachial plexus tension test, Bikele's sign, Jackson cervical compression test, Spurling's test, foraminal compression test, reflexes, sensory testing, diagnostic imaging

---

Reporting Statement

Maximum cervical compression on the right is positive on the right. This result suggests neural compression at C5.

Maximum cervical compression on the right is positive on the left. This result is consistent with muscular strain of the cervical paraspinals.

∽ Clinical Pearl ∽

The patient with lower cervical nerve root compression syndrome has already discovered that looking up or down with the head rotated is uncomfortable and produces neck and arm pain. If these positions are already pain producing, then attempts to use manipulative procedures incorporating these positions will be difficult for the patient to tolerate.

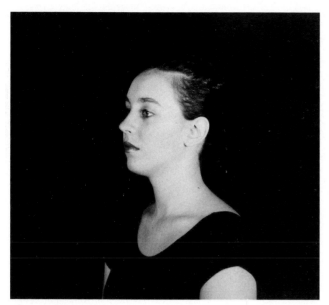

Fig. 3–48 The patient is seated comfortably with the head and neck in the neutral position.

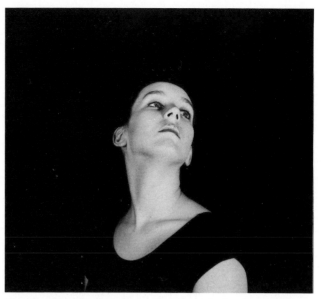

Fig. 3–49 The patient actively rotates the head and hyperextends the neck toward the side of radicular complaint. Reproduction of symptoms suggests foraminal encroachment. The maneuver is repeated for the opposite side.

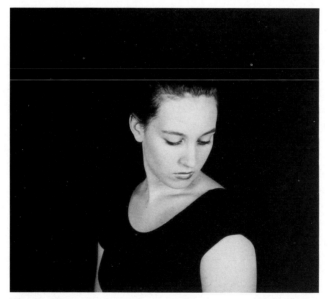

Fig. 3–50 A slight variation of this test requires rotation and maximum flexion of the neck toward the side of radicular complaint, as if looking into a shirt pocket. Reproduction of the radicular complaint suggests foraminal encroachment of a nerve root.

Comment

Although spinal cord tumors are rare, they are always a part of the differential diagnosis of neck pain. These tumors arise within the spinal cord from cells that may be metastatic. Such tumors can be primary or secondary, extradural or intradural. Intradural tumors require further sorting into extramedullary or intramedullary.

Of the intradural tumors, 71% are extramedullary, and 32% of these are meningiomas and 38% are schwannomas. The remaining tumors found in this location are sarcomas, angiomas, chordomas, lymphomas, lipomas, epidermoids, melanomas, and neuroblastomas. Other kinds of lesions occur very rarely. Virtually any kind of tumor may metastasize to the intradural space, but such spread is distinctly unusual.

Of meningiomas, 15% are either completely extradural or both intradural and extradural, and 85% are intradural and extramedullary. Meningiomas are found in the cervical region in about 13% of the cases. The tumors are usually nodular, well circumscribed, and less well encapsulated than neurofibromas. The histology of cervical meningiomas is not different from that of meningiomas elsewhere, and malignant tumors are very rare. The tumors begin growing at the dorsal root entry zone and are clinically indistinguishable from neurofibromatosis. It is uncommon for the pain to be localized. An unusual meningioma involves the upper cervical area as well as the intracranial cavity and is called a foramen magnum tumor. Tumors in this area are very difficult to diagnose and are most commonly meningiomas.

Symptoms of meningiomas are bizarre and often variable. Patients with these tumors often have their complaints dismissed as psychiatric. A nondescript headache is an early complaint. Weakness and paresthesia in the lower extremities may occur, but the complaints and locations often vary from examination to examination. Muscular atrophy and fibrillation in the hands and forearms are common and probably result from compression of the anterior spinal arteries. A mistaken diagnosis of lower motor neuron disease in the cervical region is common. The course of the illness is relentlessly progressive and the nature of the disease frequently becomes apparent only when quadriparesis is evident.

Changing position, coughing, or sneezing or a rise in cerebrospinal fluid pressure results in increased pain.

Procedure

Naffziger's compression test is performed by having the patient sit erect while the examiner holds digital pressure over the jugular veins for 30 to 40 seconds. The patient is then instructed to cough deeply. Pain along the distribution of a nerve may indicate nerve root compression. Although this test is more commonly used for lower back involvements, cervical or thoracic root compression may also be aggravated. Local pain in the spine does not positively indicate nerve compression but may indicate the site of a strain or sprain injury or other lesion. The sign is always positive in the presence of cord tumors, particularly spinal meningiomas. The resulting increased spinal fluid pressure above the tumor causes the growth to compress or pull on certain sensory nerve structures, which produces radicular pain. The test is *contraindicated* for a geriatric patient, and extreme care should be taken when performing this test on anyone suspected of having atherosclerosis. In all cases, the patient should be alerted that jugular pressure may result in light-headedness or dizziness.

Confirmation Procedures

Dejerine's sign, swallowing test, Valsalva maneuver, Barre-Lieou sign, vertebrobasilar artery functional maneuver, Hautant's test, DeKleyn's test, Hallpike maneuver, Underburg's test, vascular assessment

---

Reporting Statement

Naffziger's test is positive. This result suggests a space-occupying mass in the cervical spine.

∾ Clinical Pearl ∾

This is not a good test for a geriatric or atheromatous patient to endure. The resulting increase in cerebrospinal fluid (CSF) pressure is uncomfortable, and the momentary circulatory obstruction may result in significant syncope.

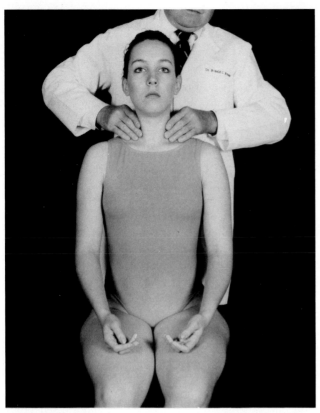

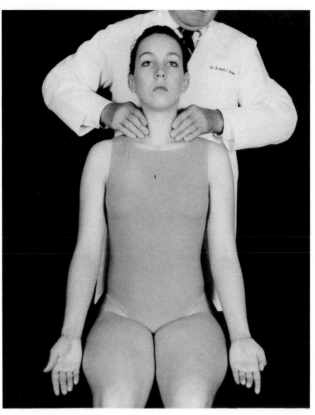

Fig. 3–51 With the patient seated comfortably, the examiner occludes the jugular veins bilaterally for 30 to 40 seconds.

Fig. 3–52 The patient may experience radicular pain or localized pain in the spine. The finding is nonspecific but does suggest a space-occupying mass in the spinal column.

Comment

A strain is damage to a muscle or tendon as a direct result of a sudden forcible contraction or violent stretching. Muscle strain includes those cases of overuse and overstretching that are just short of actual muscular rupture. The mechanism of injury is usually one of the following: (1) athletic participation, which is by far the most frequent means of sustaining a strain injury, (2) overuse; (3) overstretching; (4) contraction of the muscle against resistance; and (5) direct blow.

Strains are divided into three categories according to the degree of damage. A mild strain is a low-grade inflammatory reaction accompanied by no appreciable hemorrhage, minimal amounts of swelling and edema, and some disruption of adjacent fibers. A moderate strain involves laceration of fibers and appreciable hemorrhaging into the surrounding tissue (hematoma), followed by an inflammatory reaction with swelling and edema. A severe strain is the consequence of a single, violent incident that results in complete disruption of the muscle unit. These strains occur when a tendon is torn from the bone or pulled apart, when the musculotendinous junction ruptures, or when the muscle ruptures through its belly. In all varieties of strain, contraction of the muscle against resistance will increase pain. This response is a characteristic finding of strains and differentiates the injury from sprains.

A sprain is an injury to a ligamentous tissue that results in some degree of damage to the fibers of the ligament or its attachments.

Fundamentally, motion that exceeds the tolerance of a ligament is sufficient to produce a sprain. The extent of damage depends on the amount and duration of the applied force. As the abnormal force is applied, the ligament becomes tense and gives way at one or more of its attachments or at a point within its substance. A sprain also may involve injury to the periosteum, muscles, tendons, blood vessels, supporting soft tissue, and nerves in the adjacent area.

Sprain is divided into four categories according to the severity of the injury. A mild sprain describes an injury in which only a few of the ligamentous fibers are severed. A moderate sprain may be defined as a more severe tearing but less than a complete separation of the ligament. A severe sprain describes a complete tearing of a ligament from its attachments or a complete separation within its substance. A sprain-fracture has occurred when the ligamentous attachment pulls loose with a fragment of bone (avulsion).

Initially the examination of a sprain will reveal discomfort when an attempt is made to stretch the ligament or the mechanism of injury is repeated. This one maneuver, when positive, will differentiate a sprain injury from a strain injury.

Procedure

While the patient is sitting, the cervical spine is actively moved through resisted range of motion then through passive range of motion. Pain during resisted range of motion, or isometric contraction, signifies muscle strain. Pain during passive range of motion signifies ligamentous sprain.

Confirmation Procedures

Soto-Hall sign, spinal percussion test, diagnostic imaging

Reporting Statement

O'Donoghue maneuver is positive for sprain of the cervical spine.

O'Donoghue maneuver is positive for muscular strain of the cervical spine.

∼ Clinical Pearl ∼

This maneuver can be applied to any joint or series of joints to determine ligamentous or muscular movement. By remembering that resisted range of motion stresses mainly muscles and passive range of motion stresses mainly ligaments, the examiner should be able to differentiate between strain and sprain, and should be able to determine if a combination of both is present.

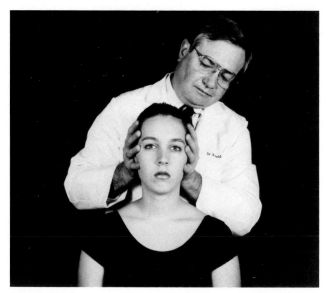

Fig. 3–53 The patient is seated comfortably, with the head and neck in the neutral position. The examiner grasps the patient's head with both hands.

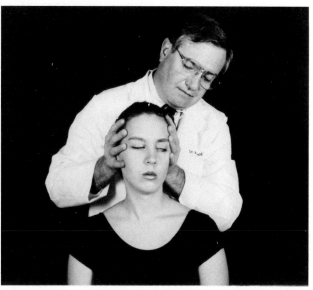

Fig. 3–54 The patient actively attempts rotation of the head to one side against isometric resistance. Pain production at this stage suggests muscular strain of the activated musculature. The test is repeated for the opposite side.

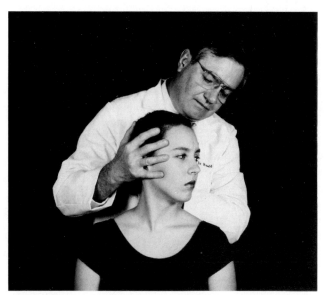

Fig. 3–55 If isometric testing is negative, the examiner passively rotates the patient's head and neck to one side to the limit of joint play. Pain produced in this maneuver suggests ligamentous injury. The maneuver is performed bilaterally.

Comment

Of the three areas in the upper cervical spine in which fracture can be identified, the most common is the odontoid fracture, then the so-called hangman's fracture, followed by Jefferson's fracture. Anatomic areas, such as transverse processes, spinous processes, and lamina and lateral masses, may also be injured. Compression fractures of the upper three vertebral bodies do occur, but these fractures are uncommon. Upper cervical fractures are usually associated with injury to the head or face and not to the neck itself. Most patients with upper cervical vertebral fractures sustain minimal neurologic damage because a severe spinal cord injury results in death from respiratory arrest before the patient can be treated. Pathologic fractures of the upper cervical spine occur in osteomyelitis, tuberculosis, osteogenic sarcoma, and metastatic carcinoma, as well as in association with nasopharyngeal infections (Grisel's disease). Untreated fractures of the upper cervical spine may produce serious neurologic sequelae.

Most patients with upper cervical spine fractures have sustained the trauma from automobile accidents, diving injuries, or falls. A large percentage of patients exhibit neck rigidity and complain of painful torticollis that is sometimes out of proportion to the injury. Such complaints, either immediately following an injury or as long as several weeks later, should alert the physician to the possibility of an upper cervical spine fracture. Examination reveals neck rigidity, and there is often tenderness over the upper cervical spine and occasionally paraparesis or quadriparesis. The symptoms and signs may be puzzling and atypical. For instance, sleep attacks have been described.

Atlantoaxial subluxation is the most common and significant manifestation of rheumatoid involvement of the cervical spine. Long duration of disease, advanced patient age, and peripheral joint erosive instability are associated with more frequent and severe C1-C2 instabilities.

The instability pattern of rheumatoid involvement of the atlantoaxial joint complex is usually one of two types: anterior atlantoaxial subluxation or upward translocation of the odontoid (which is also called superior migration, verti

cal subluxation, and downward luxation of the atlas on the axis). Posterior subluxation of the atlantoaxial joint does not occur in rheumatoid arthritis unless there is an associated fracture of the odontoid or nearly complete arthritic erosion and destruction of the odontoid. The anterior and posterior contact points of the odontoid are true synovial joints. Synovitic destruction of the front or back of the odontoid on the anterior arch of C1 produces some instability.

The clinical presentation of rheumatoid atlantoaxial instability results from a combination of (1) local arthritic and mechanical instability and pain, (2) neurologic dysfunction of brainstem, cord, and peripheral nerve (root), and (3) vertebral artery insufficiency. Pain in the cervical area is common and usually of moderate severity. Subjective sensory symptoms of paresthesia in the hands, "electric shock" sensations (Lhermitte's sign), and transient feelings of weakness are commonly noted. When palpating the upper cervical spine, joint crepitus and instability may be felt in the form of a "clunk" as C1 moves forward subluxing on C2 and producing an increasing prominence of C2 posteriorly. This clunk test, or Sharp and Purser test, is to be avoided or at least cautiously undertaken.

Procedure

If the patient spontaneously grasps the head with both hands when lying down or when arising from a recumbent position, then this is a positive sign that indicates severe sprain, rheumatoid arthritis, fracture, or severe cervical subluxation.

Confirmation Procedure

Diagnostic imaging

Reporting Statement

Rust's sign is present. This result suggests severe upper cervical (atlantoaxial) instability.

~ **Clinical Pearl** ~

No other physical finding is as important or as revealing as Rust's sign. The presence of this sign mandates that (1) no further passive or active testing be undertaken, (2) imaging is performed immediately, and (3) the neck is adequately supported by using a cervical collar. Rust's sign has never been observed in conditions of minor consequence.

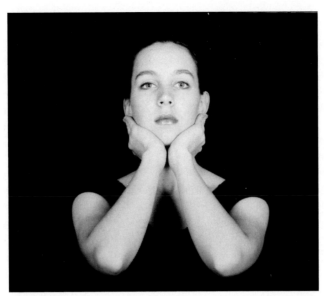

Fig. 3–56   The patient presents with a markedly splinted cervical spine and holds the weight of the head with both hands.
Removal of this support cannot be tolerated. This implies gross
instability of the upper cervical spine due to fracture or severe
sprain.

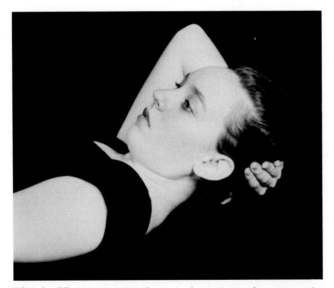

Fig. 3–57   No less significant is the patient who cannot rise
from the supine position without lifting the head manually. This
suggests gross upper cervical spine instability due to fracture or
severe sprain.

Comment

Following trauma, scar formation will occur with regularity around the dura and nerve roots. The reasons this will cause symptoms in one patient and not in others are not well understood. One explanation is that the scar tissue can act as a tethering force as well as a constricting force around the nerve roots. A direct traumatic insult to the nerve roots causes inflammation in the dural sleeves and perineural tissues. This inflammation may result in fibrosis, and adhesions may occur between the dural sleeves and the adjacent capsular structures. Normally the nerve roots are free in the intervertebral canals and can be moved approximately ¼ to ½ of an inch. Nerve roots that have been injured or have been compressed by capsular thickening or bony encroachments cannot move within the intervertebral canals.

Nerve roots subjected to compressive forces by osteophytic encroachments have varying degrees of distortion and perineural fibrosis.

Procedure

With the patient seated, the examiner depresses the patient's shoulder on the affected side and laterally flexes the cervical spine away from that shoulder. This sign is positive if radicular pain is produced or aggravated. A positive sign indicates adhesions of the dural sleeves, spinal nerve roots, or adjacent structures of the joint capsule of the shoulder.

Confirmation Procedures

Bakody sign, maximum foraminal encroachment test, distraction test, brachial plexus tension test, Bikele's sign, Jackson cervical compression test, Spurling's test, foraminal compression test, reflexes, sensory testing, diagnostic imaging

Reporting Statement

Shoulder depression testing is positive on the right. This result suggests dural sleeve adhesion at C5.

∼ Clinical Pearl ∼

As with cervical distraction testing, this maneuver helps predict the viability of cervical traction in therapy. A sharply positive finding usually means that the patient will not tolerate cervical traction. The traction may aggravate the dural sleeve adhesion instead of relieving it.

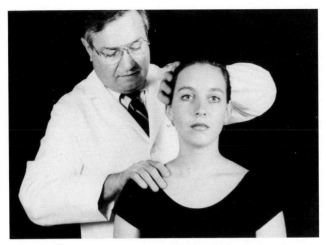

Fig. 3–58 The patient is seated and the head and neck are in the neutral position. On the side of complaint, the examiner uses the contact points of the lateral skull and superior shoulder.

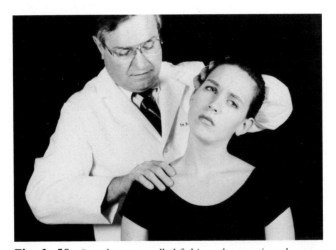

Fig. 3–59 In a slow, controlled fashion, the examiner depresses the shoulder while flexing the head toward the opposite shoulder. Reproduction of symptoms suggests a brachial plexitis or dural sleeve adhesion.

Comment

Local neck pain is usually described as a nonradiating, aching, deep, dull soreness of the neck muscles and is associated with a variable degree of spasm that is influenced by posture. Local pressure or percussion may elicit tenderness.

Most local cervical spinal pain is secondary to involvement of the vertebral bodies, intervertebral discs, and ligamentous structures and the associated spasms of the paravertebral muscles. Too often the symptoms of neck pain are translated into evidence for diagnosis of arthritis or disc disease without adequate examination of the patient or full consideration of the various possible causes of this symptom.

During infancy and childhood, neck pain is uncommon, but when it occurs, the possibilities are intriguing. Diskitis is an important consideration when it occurs as a local bacterial infection of the disc space in the cervicothoracic region and is accompanied by x-ray changes that are characteristic but late to develop. Meningismus, or meningitis, particularly in infants and very young children, whose sensorium may be difficult to evaluate, can present as neck pain due to meningeal inflammation and associated muscle spasm. Lymphomatous infiltration or an abscess in the epidural space may become painful well before neurologic symptoms are evident. A herniated disc may also be symptomatic.

Although infections in the cervical spine are rare, the consequences of failing to diagnose such infections are so ominous that infection is a necessary consideration even in instances of slightly aberrant cervical spine syndromes. About 15% of bone infections involve the spine, but the spine is the most common site of tuberculosis of bone. Of the entire spine—cervical, thoracic, lumbar, and sacral—the cervical spine is the most uncommon site for infection. Although all age groups may have infections in the spine, people in their teens or 40s and older have the highest rates of incidence.

Procedure

The patient is placed supine. The examiner places one hand on the sternum of the patient and exerts slight pressure so no flexion can take place at either the lumbar or thoracic regions of the spine. The examiner places the other hand under the patient's occiput and flexes the head toward the chest. The test is primarily employed when fracture of a vertebra is suspected. The flexion of the head and neck on the sternum progressively produces a pull on the posterior spinous ligaments. When the spinous process of the injured vertebra is reached, the patient experiences a noticeable local pain. A positive result indicates subluxation, exostoses, disc lesion, sprain or strain, vertebral fracture, or meningeal irritation (there must be an elevated temperature for corroboration).

Confirmation Procedures

O'Donoghue maneuver, spinal percussion, Lhermitte's sign, Dejerine's sign, swallowing test, Valsalva maneuver, Naffziger's test, reflexes, sensory testing, diagnostic imaging

---

Reporting Statement

Soto-Hall (afebrile) sign is positive with pain elicited at the C5 level.

Soto-Hall (febrile) sign is positive with nuchal rigidity noted and Kernig's, or Brudzinski's, sign, which suggests meningeal irritation or inflammation.

∾ Clinical Pearl ∾

Soto-Hall Sign is often misapplied in the assessment of fractures and sprains for the entire spine. The sign is a non-specific test with limited capacity to localize conditions of the cervical and upper thoracic spine. The use of this sign to draw conclusions below T8 is largely guesswork.

With the Kernig/Brudzinski phenomena in this test, the patient's temperature must be assessed. A febrile patient with Kernig's, or Brudzinski's, sign—a variation of Soto-Hall sign—is a high-risk candidate for meningitis.

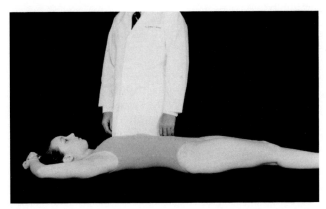

Fig. 3–60   The patient rests on the examining table in a supine position with the legs fully extended and the arms extended over the head.

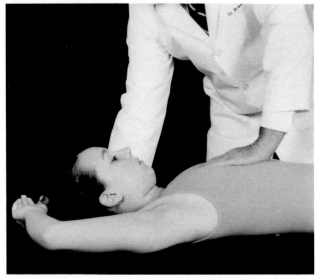

Fig. 3–61   The examiner supports the patient's head with one hand while stabilizing the patient's chest with the other hand.

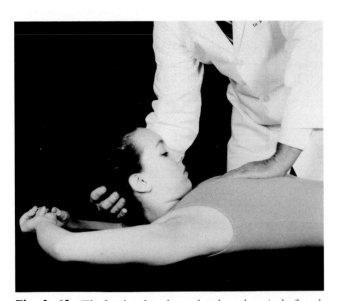

Fig. 3–62   The head and neck are sharply and passively flexed, approximating the patient's chin to the chest. Any tendency for the shoulders to rise from the table is countered with downward sternal pressure. Pain that is localized to the cervicothoracic spine suggests subluxation, exostoses, disc lesion, sprain, strain, or fracture of vertebrae.

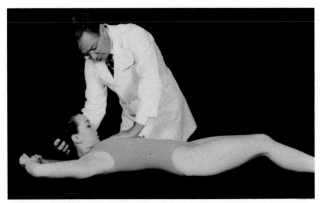

Fig. 3–63   While the head is flexed toward the chest, a reflex flexion of the knees and thighs may be produced. This reflex is equivalent to a Kernig's or Brudzinski's sign and suggests meningitis.

Comment

Vehicular accidents are a common source of trauma to the lower cervical spine and may cause a wide variety of fractures and dislocations. Compression fractures at the anterior edge of the vertebral bodies may be caused by a hyperflexion motion alone or in combination with a vertical compression. The stability of these fractures depends on the degree of vertebral compression and the presence of posterior ligamentous damage.

Traumatic injuries of the cervical spine are among the most common causes of severe disability and death following trauma. Often these injuries are not diagnosed in the emergency room situation. Approximately one third of the injuries to the cervical spine are due to motor vehicle accidents, one third to falling, and the remaining one third to some type of athletic injury or wound inflicted by a missile or falling object.

The incidence of cervical spine injuries peaks during adolescence, young adulthood, and again during the sixth and seventh decades. Because of the nature of accidents resulting in cervical spine injuries, the majority involve young, healthy persons who are very active. This includes those who engage in physically dangerous activities and occasionally those who exhibit sociopathic personality traits. People in their fifth and sixth decades make up the second largest group of cervical spinal injury patients. Cervical spondylosis and a preexisting narrow spinal canal are closely associated with injury in this age group. Lesser forces may result in severe spine and spinal cord injury in this group.

Procedure

With the patient seated and the head slightly flexed, the examiner percusses the spinous processes and associated musculature of each of the cervical vertebra with a neurologic reflex hammer. Evidence of localized pain indicates a possible fractured vertebra. Evidence of radicular pain indicates a possible disc lesion. Due to the nonspecific nature of this test, other conditions will also elicit a positive pain response. A ligamentous sprain will cause pain when the spinous processes are percussed. Percussing the paraspinal musculature will elicit a positive sign for muscular strain.

Confirmation Procedures

Soto-Hall sign, O'Donoghue test, Dejerine's sign, swallowing test, Valsalva maneuver, Naffziger's test, Lhermitte's sign, diagnostic imaging

---

Reporting Statement

Spinal percussion elicits pain on the spinous process of C5. This result suggests osseous injury at that level.

Spinal percussion elicits pain at the paraspinal muscle on the right at C5. This result suggests soft tissue injury at that level.

∽ Clinical Pearl ∽

When soft-tissue percussion reproduces the pain, the examiner may expect the same phenomenon from applications of ultrasound to the tissue. This pain represents spasmophilia, and the uses of such therapies may need to be delayed until the soft tissue is no longer reactive to percussion

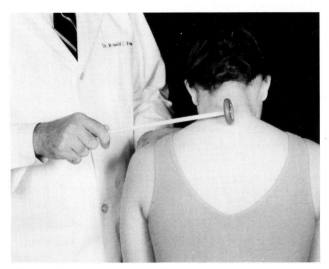

Fig. 3−64 In the seated position, the patient flexes the cervical spine forward, exposing the spinous processes as much as possible. The examiner percusses the spinous processes of each vertebra. Localized pain is evidence of a fracture or severe sprain. Radiating pain suggests an intervertebral disc syndrome.

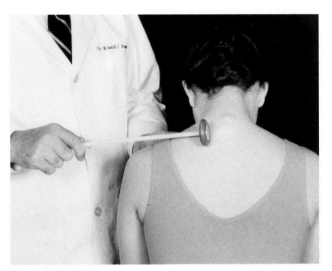

Fig. 3−65 The paravertebral tissues are percussed. Pain elicited in the soft tissues suggests muscular strain and highly sensitive myofascial trigger points.

Comment

Narrowing of the intervertebral foramina, pressure and shearing forces on the zygapophyseal joint surfaces, intervertebral disc compression, and pressure on stiff ligamentous and muscular structures may all cause pain. A pain pattern may be perfectly reproduced, which allows for identification of the neurologic level. If radicular pain or paresthesia with referral to the upper extremity occurs, nerve root irritation is present. If the pain is confined to the neck, then soft, connective tissues or joints are more likely to be the pain-sensitive structures.

Root pain may be aggravated by those spinal motions that narrow the intervertebral foramen through which the diseased nerve root passes. In cervical nerve root disease, simultaneous extension and lateral flexion of the neck toward the affected side, or a blow to the vertex of the head (Spurling's test) may result in sudden aggravation of neck and dermatomal arm pain, paresthesia, or both.

Sometimes this test is of value in the diagnosis of a laterally herniated intervertebral disc in the cervical region.

Procedure

The test is performed with the patient seated. The examiner places one hand on top of the patient's head and gradually increases downward pressure. The patient notes any pain or paresthesia and the distribution thereof. Pressure may also be applied while the head is laterally flexed to either side and extended. Pressure should be maintained for 30 to 60 seconds. This maneuver closes the intervertebral foramina on the side of the flexion and reproduces the familiar pain or paresthesia.

Confirmation Procedures

Bakody sign, maximum foraminal encroachment test, shoulder depression test, distraction test, brachial plexus tension test, Bikele's sign, Jackson cervical compression test, foraminal compression test, reflex and sensory testing, electrodiagnosis, diagnostic imaging

Reporting Statement

Spurling's test is positive on the right with pain and paresthesia elicited in the C5 dermatome.

❧ Clinical Pearl ❧

Spurling's test is an aggressive cervical compression test and the patient should be informed of each step as it is introduced. However, the examiner should not cue the patient for pain responses. Spurling's test elicits collapse sign quite easily.

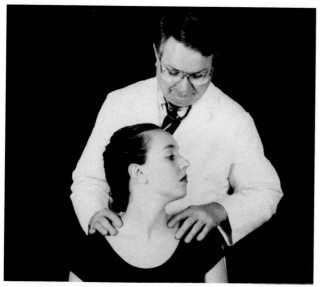

Fig. 3–66 While seated comfortably and with an erect posture, the patient actively rotates the head from side to side. Localization of pain is noted.

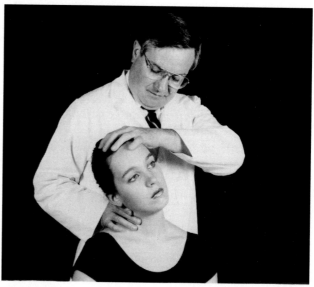

Fig. 3–67 The patient's head is laterally flexed toward the side of complaint. The examiner applies gradually progressive downward pressure to the head and neck. Reproduction of symptoms or collapse sign at this point constitutes a positive test. The balance of the test should not be completed.

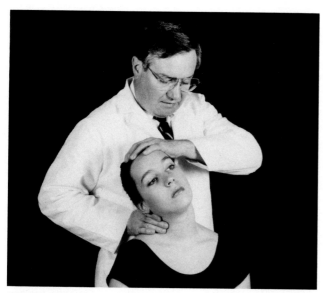

Fig. 3–68 From the laterally flexed position, the neck is extended as far as the patient can tolerate. The examiner applies progressive downward pressure. Reproduction of radicular symptoms suggests nerve root compression. Localized spinal pain suggests facet involvement.

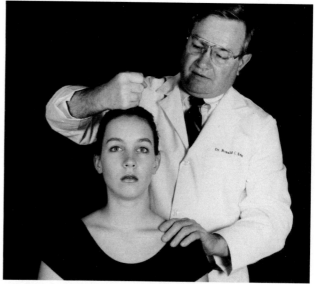

Fig. 3–69 A vertical blow is delivered to the uppermost portion of the cranium. The examiner may wish to interpose a hand between the concussing hand and the patient's skull. The head and neck are first in a neutral position for this procedure and then positioned into lateral flexion and extension for a repeated procedure. The test will stimulate any nerve root irritation or other pain-sensitive structures related to disc disease and cervical spondylosis. Use of this modification should not be a surprise to the patient.

Comment

Dysphagia may be of prognostic significance and is often indicative of esophageal injury, pharyngeal hemorrhage or edema, or retropharyngeal hemorrhage. Dysphagia may also result from severe muscle spasm.

When dysphagia is present, the clinician should look for ligamentous disruption, dislocation, subluxation, or fracture and should make careful use of cineradiography, tomography, and CT or bone scanning to uncover the true nature and extent of injuries.

Anterior osteophytes from the cervical vertebrae, particularly C5, C6, and C7, may compress the posterior wall of the esophagus and may irritate the tissues and smooth muscle. The symptom may be either dysphagia or simply an annoying awareness of swallowing.

Procedure

While seated, the patient is instructed to swallow. Presence of pain or difficulty swallowing indicates a space-occupying lesion ligamentous sprain, muscular strain, or fracture, such as disc protrusion, tumor, or osteophyte at the anterior portion of the cervical spine.

Confirmation Procedures

Dejerine's sign, Valsalva maneuver, Naffziger's test, Lhermitte's sign, reflexes and sensory testing, diagnostic imaging

---

Reporting Statement

A positive swallowing test indicates that dysphagia is present. This result suggests esophageal irritation.

∼ **Clinical Pearl** ∼

Dysphagia is often observed following hyperextension trauma of the cervical spine. Coupled with other sympathetic nervous system phenomena, the patient attributes the sore throat or hoarseness to a cold. The dysphagia is fleeting but serves as a more conclusive sign as to the extent of soft-tissue involvement in the injury.

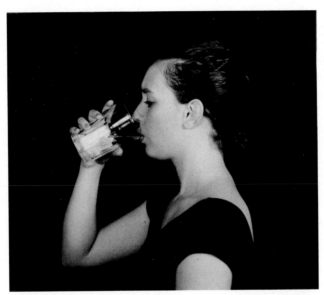

Fig. 3–70 The patient is seated and instructed to swallow. A beverage or small food item may be needed to induce this activity. The presence of pain indicates esophageal irritation due to direct trauma or a retroesophageal space-occuyping mass.

Comment

The blood supply of the vital neck structures—including bony spine, spinal cord, nerve roots, coverings, and posterior cranial fossa and cerebral visual cortex—is derived from the vertebral arteries. The tortuous course these arteries take and the susceptibility of their intimate coverings to structural change places the arteries in a vulnerable position. In most instances the protective mechanism is amazingly adequate. However, when changes, such as atheromatous cracks, develop within the vessels, circulation may be compromised or temporarily obstructed.

The artery is intimately related to the Luschka joints medially and the apophyseal joint posterolaterally so that osteophyte formation at either site may encroach on the artery's usual course. The efficiency of the vertebral artery system is related to the anastomosis at the circle of Willis with the internal carotid system. A weak point in one area may influence the other.

Contrast studies have been used to show that head and neck movement, primarily involving rotation, may alter flow in the vertebral artery. Pathologic changes in the vertebral artery may favor ischemia. The flow between C6 and C2 may be diminished on the side to which the head and neck is turned, and the flow may be increased in the opposite vessel at the point where the artery twists over the arch of the atlas. Changes in such a mechanism would explain transient attacks of vertigo that are attributed to vertebrobasilar ischemia.

Procedure

The patient is standing and is instructed to outstretch the arms, supinate the hands, and close the eyes. The patient marches in place and extends and rotates the head while continuing to march. The test is repeated with the head rotated and extended to the opposite side. The examiner watches for a loss of balance, dropping of the arms, and pronation of the hands. If this occurs, then the examiner should suspect vertebral, basilar, or carotid artery stenosis or compression.

Confirmation Procedures

Barre-Lieou sign, vertebrobasilar artery function test, Hautant's test, DeKleyn's test, Hallpike maneuver, vascular diagnosis, diagnostic imaging

---

Reporting Statement

Underburg's test is positive. This result suggests vertebrobasilar artery syndrome.

∼ Clinical Pearl ∼

If the patient loses equilibrium at any time while the eyes are closed, cerebellar circulation must be evaluated. In this procedure the patient may lose equilibrium as soon as the head is rotated to one side. The examiner must be prepared to keep the patient from falling.

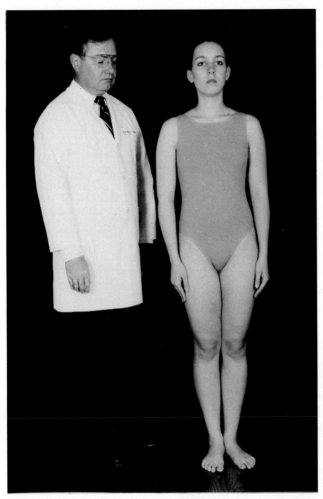

Fig. 3–71 The patient stands with the eyes open and the arms resting at the sides. The postural base is narrowed. The examiner observes for any equilibrium difficulty. It is important for the examiner to remain close to the patient throughout this procedure.

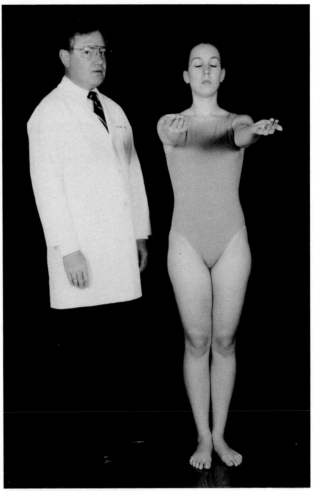

Fig. 3–72 The patient closes the eyes and elevates the extended arms forward to shoulder level. The patient's hands are fully supinated. While the patient maintains this position with the narrowed postural base, the examiner observes for loss of equilibrium or drift of the arms and pronation of the hands.

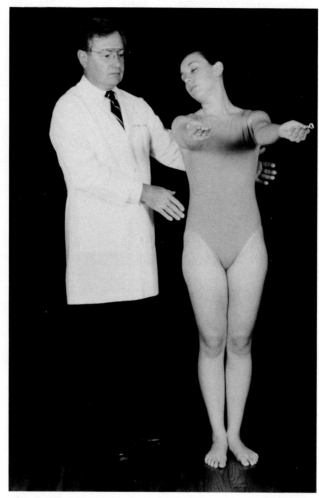

Fig. 3–73   The patient extends the neck and rotates the head to one side while maintaining a narrowed postural base, elevating the arms, and supinating the hands. The eyes remain closed. The examiner observes for difficulty in the performance of each segment of the test.

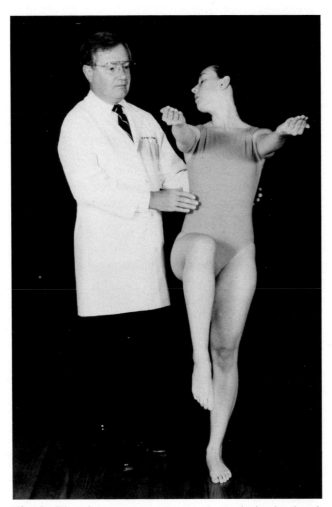

Fig. 3–74   The patient attempts to maintain the head and neck rotation or extension, arm elevation, and hand supination while marching in place. Loss of balance, dropping or drifting of the arms, or pronation of the hands is indicative of vertebrobasilar or carotid artery stenosis or compression. The test is repeated with the head and neck rotated to the opposite side.

Comment

Disc compression of the nerve root is influenced by changes in volume and consistency of the disc as well as changes in position of the motion segment. These factors form the basis for a number of diagnostic measures. During infantile and adult stages, the intervertebral disc is not stiff and inflexible. Rather, the disc is a connective tissue structure, which can physiologically change its form and volume by loading and unloading. The remaining parts of the motion segment, including the nerve fibers, adjust themselves to these changes. There is sufficient space between the dural sac and its nerve roots in relation to the posterior part of the intervertebral disc. Changes in the form of the disc as well as changes in the position of the nerve roots during spinal movement will not influence the spinal nerves. The epidural space, which is filled with fatty tissue and venous plexus, varies in width. As a rule, the intervertebral foramen is large enough to allow ample space for the passage of nerves. When the spinal space becomes diminished by disc protrusions, osteophytes, engorged vessels, or stenosis (a narrowing of the spinal canal), the nerve roots come under pressure. When the nerve roots come in contact with a disc surface that has its consistency by physiologic changes, the nerve roots can no longer alter their position, which, in turn, makes them more sensitive to the mechanical influence.

Symptoms of extramedullary lesions may include local tissue destruction, radicular involvement by space-occupying mass or bony compression, or by spinal cord compression secondary to bony collapse or tumor. Radicular pain is common, and the spinal cord level is usually discrete. Sensory loss is uniform, and motor loss is frequently uniform, also. Simple guidelines for quick localization are as follows: if the deltoid muscle is spared, the lesion is likely to be at C4-C5; if the biceps are spared, the lesion is likely to be at C5-C6; if the triceps are spared, the lesion is likely to be at C6-C7; and if the hands are spared, the level is likely to be C7-T1 or below. Radicular complaints follow the roots involved and are similar to those associated with disc herniation.

Procedure

The examiner asks the patient to take a deep breath and hold it while bearing down, as if moving the bowels. A positive test is indicated by increased pain, which may be due to increased intrathecal pressure. This increased pressure within the spinal cord is usually due to a space-occupying lesion, such as a herniated disc, a tumor, or osteophytes. However, test results may be subjective. The test should be done with care and caution because the patient may become dizzy and pass out while or shortly after performing this test because the procedure can block the blood supply to the brain.

Confirmation Procedures

Dejerine's sign, swallowing test, Naffziger's test, Bakody sign, maximum foraminal encroachment test, shoulder depression test, distraction test, brachial plexus tension test, Bikele's sign, Jackson cervical compression test, Spurling's test, foraminal compression test, reflexes and sensory testing, diagnostic imaging

---

Reporting Statement

Valsalva maneuver is positive. This result elicits radicular pain on the right in the C5 dermatome.

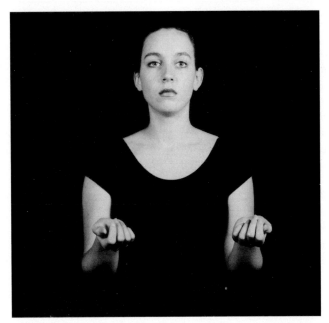

Fig. 3–75 The patient is seated comfortably. The arms may be slightly flexed at the elbows. The patient is instructed to take a deep breath and hold it.

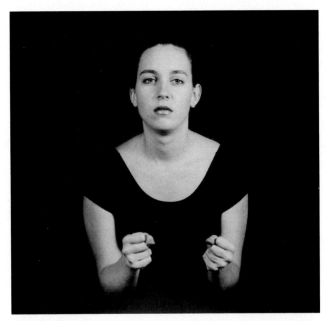

Fig. 3–76 While holding the deep breath, the patient bears down to create greater intraabdominal pressure. Reproduction of radicular pain is indicative of nerve root compression by a space-occupying mass in the spine.

Comment

The vertebral arteries are vulnerable to injury in the foramina of the lower cervical vertebra, at the junction between C1 and C2, and as they pass over the arch of C1 through the atlanto-occipital membrane. Intimal disruption may lead to acute, complete thrombotic occlusion, subintimal hematoma, dissection of the artery, or pseudoaneurysm formation. Obviously, atlanto-occipital dislocation usually causes total disruption of the vertebral basilar system and results in death.

The mechanism of injury seems to be cervical hyperextension accompanied by excessive rotation. Severely diminished flow in one of the vertebral arteries may well lead to occlusion of the posterior inferior cerebellar artery on that side, resulting in a lateral medullary infarction, (Wallenberg's syndrome). This syndrome is characterized by the ipsilateral loss of cranial nerves V, IX, X, and XI and by cerebellar ataxia, Horner's syndrome, and contralateral loss of pain and temperature sensation.

With increasing severity of injury, vascular involvement can ascend to the basilar, superior cerebellar, and posterior cerebral arteries. Sudden death, quadriplegia, or the "locked-in" syndrome (quadriplegia accompanied by the loss of lower cranial nerves, which allows eye blinking only) can ensue. These symptoms should alert the examiner to the possibility of vascular injury, which means that immediate cerebral arteriography is recommended to obtain an accurate diagnosis.

Symptoms of vertebrobasilar insufficiency include paroxysmal symptoms induced by certain head movements, mainly rotation, extension, and lateral flexion. Dizziness, diplopia, drop attack, syncope, and spinal stroke increase in frequency and intensity with increasing magnitudes of cervical osteoarthritis, atheromatosis in vessels, and advanced age. Manipulation of the neck in patients with those characteristics is hazardous.

There is marked pathophysiologic involvement of the Luschka and zygapophyseal joints when encroachment of the vertebral artery occurs, especially at the occipito-atlantoaxial level, but this involvement may occur at any level. Atheromatous plaques with calcification may be noted in the carotid artery (specifically at the siphon) and in the walls of the vertebral artery. There is occasionally a rare aneurysm of the vertebral or carotid artery in the cervical spine. Angiography discloses varying magnitudes of obstruction or complete obstruction such as that caused by thrombosis.

Procedure

With the patient in a seated position, the examiner palpates the carotid and subclavian arteries and auscultates for pulsations and bruits. If neither of these exist, the patient is instructed to rotate and hyperextend the head to one side and then the other. This second maneuver should be performed only if initial palpation and auscultation did not reveal bruits or pulsations. The test is considered positive if either maneuver reveals pulsations or bruits. The rotation and hyperextension portion of this test places motion-induced compression on the vertebral arteries. Vertigo, dizziness, visual blurring, nausea, faintness, and nystagmus are all signs of a positive test, which indicates vertebral, basilar, or carotid artery stenosis or compression.

Confirmation Procedures

Barre-Lieou sign, Hautant's test, DeKleyn's test, Hallpike maneuver, Underburg's test, reflex and sensory testing, vascular assessment, vascular imaging, MRI

Reporting Statement

The vertebrobasilar artery functional maneuver is positive. This result suggests arterial stenosis or compression at the upper cervical level.

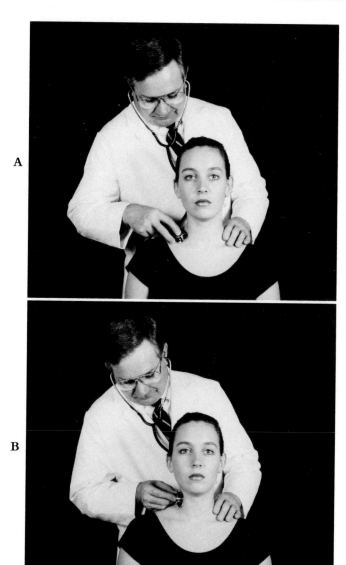

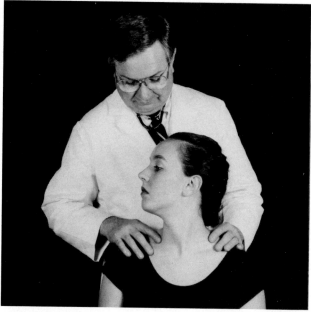

Fig. 3–78 If bruits are not found, the patient rotates and hyperextends the head and neck, both to the right and left. The production of vertigo, visual disturbances, nausea, syncope, or nystagmus is indicative of vertebral, basilar, or carotid artery stenosis or compression.

Fig. 3–77 While the patient is in a seated position, the subclavian (**A**) and then the carotid (**B**) arteries are auscultated for bruits. This is followed by palpatation of the arteries for pulse assessment. If bruits are present, the balance of the test is not completed, and the test is considered positive.

Bibliography

Alexander E Jr, Davis CH: Reduction and fusion of fracture of the odontoid process, *J Neurosurg*, 31:580-582, 1969.

Allen BL, Ferguson RL, Lehmann TR, O'Brien RP: A mechanistic classification of closed indirect fractures and dislocations of the lower cervical spine, *Spine*, 7(1): 1-27, 1982.

American Medical Association: Guides to the evaluation of permanent impairment, ed. 3, Chicago, 1990, The Association.

Ames MD, Schut L: Results of treatment of 171 consecutive myelomeningoceles, *Pediatrics*, 50:466-470, 1972.

Amyes EW, Anderson FM: Fracture of the odontoid process of the axis, *J Bone Joint Surg*, 56A:1663-1674, 1974.

Apley AG, Solomon L: *Concise system of Orthopaedics and fractures*, London, 1988, Butterworth-Heinemann.

Askenasy HM, Braham MJ, Kosary IZ: Delayed spinal myelopathy after atlanto-axial fracture dislocation, *J Neurosurg*, 17:1100-1104, 1960.

Bailey RW, Badgley CE: Stabilization of the cervical spine by anterior fusion, *J Bone Joint Surg*, 42A:565, 1960.

Barre JA: Le syndrome sympathique cervical posterieur et sa cause frequente, l'artherite cervicale, *Rev Neurol* (Paris), 33:1246, 1926.

Bateman JE: *The shoulder and neck,* Philadelphia, 1972, WB Saunders.

Bettmane EH, Neudorfer RJ: Cervical disc pathology resulting in dysphagia in an adolescent boy, *NY State J Med*, 60:2465, 1960.

Bland JH: Disorders of the cervical spine diagnosis and medical management, Philadelphia, 1987, WB Saunders.

Bland JH: Rheumatoid arthritis of the cervical spine, *J Rheumatol*, 1:319, 1974.

Bocchi L, Orso CA: Whiplash injuries of the cervical spine *Ital J Orthop Traumatol*, 171-181, November 9, 1983.

Bohlman HH: The neck. In D'Ambrosia R (ed): *Regional examination and differential diagnosis of musculoskeletal disorders*, Philadelphia, 1977, JB Lippincott.

Bohlman HH: Late anterior decompression and fusion for the spinal cord injuries: Review of 100 cases with long term results, *Orthopaedic Transactions*, 4 (1):42, 1980.

Bohlman HH: Indications for late anterior decompression and fusion for cervical spinal cord injuries. In Tator CH (ed): Early management of acute cervical spinal cord injury, *Seminars in Neurological Surgery*, New York, 1982, Raven Press.

Bohlman HH, Bahniuk E, Field G, Raskulinecz G: Spinal cord monitoring of experimental incomplete cervical spinal cord injury, *Spine*, 6:428, 1981.

Bohlman HH, Ducker TB, Lucas JT: Spine and spinal cord injuries. In Rothman RH, Simeone FA (eds), *The Spine*, ed 2, Philadelphia, 1982, WB Saunders.

Bohlman HH, Eismont FJ: Surgical techniques of anterior decompression and fusion for spinal cord injuries, *Clin Orthop*, 138:154-57, 1981.

Bohlman HH, Riley L Jr, Robinson RA: Anterolateral approaches to the cervical spine. In Ruge D, Wiltse LL (eds), *Spinal disorders*, Philadelphia, 1977, Lea & Febiger.

Brain WR: Some unsolved problems in cervical spondylosis, *Br Med Bull* 1:711, 1963.

Brieg A: Biomechanics of the central nervous system, Chicago, 1960, Mosby.

Brieg A, Turnbull IM, Hassler O: Effects of mechanical stresses in the spinal cord in cervical spondylosis, *J Neurosurg* 25:45, 1966.

Cervical Spine Research Society: *The cervical spine*, Philadelphia, 1983, JB Lippincott.

Cipriano JJ: *Photographic manual of regional orthopeadic and neurological tests*, ed. 2, Baltimore, 1991, Williams & Wilkins.

Cloward, RB: The clinical significance of the sinu-vertebral nerve or the cervical spine in relation to the cervical disc syndrome, *J Neurol Neurosurg Psychiatry*, 23:321-326, November, 1960.

Conlon, PW, Isdale IC, Rose BS: Rheumatoid arthritis of the cervical spine: An analysis of 333 cases, *Ann Rheum Dis*, 25:120, 1966.

Crellin RQ, MacCabe JJ, Hamilton EB: Surgical management of the cervical spine in rheumatoid arthritis, *J Bone Joint Surg*, 52B(2):244, 1970.

D'Ambrosia, RD: *Musculoskeletal disorders: regional examination and differential diagnosis*, Philadelphia, 1977, JB Lippincott.

Dandy DJ: *Essential orthopaedics and trauma*, Edinburgh, 1989, Churchill Livingstone.

Daniels L, Worthington C: *Muscle Testing: Techniques of manual examination*, Philadelphia, 1980, WB Saunders.

Davidson RI, Dunn EJ, Metzmaker W: The shoulder abduction test in the diagnosis of radicular pain in cervical extradural compressive monoradiculopathies, *Spine*, 6:441, 1981.

DeJong RH: *The neurologic examination*, ed. 3, New York, 1967, Harper & Row.

de Kleyn A, Versteegh C: Uber verschledene formen von nemieres syndrome, *Dtsch Z Nervenheilkd*, 132:157, 1933.

Doherty M, Doherty J: *Clincial examination in rheumatology*, London, 1922, Wolfe Publishing.

Ehni G: Degenerative motion segment encroachments, In *Cervical arthrosis: Diseases of the cervical motions segments*, p 54, Chicago, 1984, Mosby.

Ford JS: *Posttraumatic headache*, Med Recertification Associates. 1985, Chicago.

Foreman SM, Croft AC: *Whiplash injuries: The cervical acceleration/deceleration syndrome*, Baltimore, 1988, Williams & Wilkins.

Ganguly DN, Roy, KKS: A study on the craniovertebral joint in man, *Anat Anz*, 114:433, 1964.

Gowers, WR: *Diseases of the nervous system*, ed 2, London, 1969, Churchill.

Hall CW, Danoff D: Sleep attacks-apparent relationship to atlanto-axial dislocation, *Arch Neurol*, 32:57-58, 1975.

Hann CL: Detropharyngeal-tendinitis, *AJR Am J Roentgenol*, 130:1137-1140, 1978.

Hastings D, McNab I, Lawson V: Neoplasms of the atlas and axis, *Can J Surg*, 11:290, 1968.

Howe JR, Taren JA: Foramen magnum tumors: pitfalls in diagnosis, *JAMA*, 225:1060, 1973.

Isdale IC, Corrigan B: Backward luxation of the atlas, *Ann Rheum Dis*, 29:6, 1970.

Jackson R: *The Cervical Syndrome*, ed 3, Springfield, IL, 1966, Charles C Thomas.

Katz, WA: *Rheumatic diseases diagnosis and management*, Philadelphia, 1977, JB Lippincott.

Keiser RP, Grimes HA: Intervertebral disc space infections in children, *Clin Orthop*, 30:163-166, 1963.

Kendall HO, Kendall FP, Wadsworth GE: *Muscles testing and function*, ed 2, Baltimore, 1971, Williams & Wilkins.

Keuter EJW: Non-traumatic atlanto-axial dislocation associated with nasopharyngeal infections (Grisel's disease), *Acta Neurochirurg*, 21:11-22, 1969.

Kramer J: *Intervertebral disc diseases,* Chicago, 1981, Mosby.

Lambert EH, Rooke ED: Myasthenic state and lung cancer, In Brain RL, Norris FH (eds): *The remote effects of cancer on the nervous system,* p 67, New York, 1965, Grune & Stratton.

Levick JR: An investigation into the validity of subatmospheric pressure recordings from synovial fluid and their dependence on Joint Angle, *J Physiol,* 289:55, 1979.

Lhermitte J: Etude de la commotion de la moelle, *Rev Neurol (Paris),* 1:210, 1932.

Lhermitte J, Bollak P, Nicholas M: Les douleurs a type de decharge electrique dans la sclerose en plaques. Un cas e forme sensitive de la sclerose multiple, *Rev Neurol* (Paris), 2:56, 1924.

Lieou YC: *Syndrome sympathique cervical posterieur et arthrite cervicale chronique: Etude clinique et radiologique,* Strasbourg, 1928, Schuler and Minh.

Lipson SJ: Fractures of the atlas associated with fractures of the odontoid process and transverse ligament ruptures, *J Bone Joint Surg,* 59A:940, 1977.

Lorber J: Spina bifida cystica, *Arch Dis Child,* 47:854-873, 1972.

Macnab I: Acceleration extension injuries of the cervical spine, In Rothmann RH, Simeone FA (eds): *The spine,* vol 2, ed 2, Philadelphia, 1982, WB Saunders.

Magee DJ: Orthopedic physical assessment, Philadelphia, 1987, WB Saunders.

Maitland GD: *Vertebral manipulation,* London, 1973, Butterworths.

Markhashov AM: Variations in the arterial blood supply of the spine, *Vestn Khir,* 94:64-74, 1965.

Martel W: The Occipito-atlanto-axial Joints in Rheumatoid Arthritis and Ankylosing Spondylitis, *AJR Am J Roentgenol,* 86:233, 1961.

Mayo Clinic & Mayo Foundation: *Clinical examination in neurology,* Philadelphia, 1981, WB Saunders.

Mazion JM: *Illustrated manual of Neurological reflexes/signs/tests, part I orthopedic signs/tests/maneuvers for office procedure, part II,* Orlando, 1980, Daniels Publishing.

McRae R: *Clinical orthopaedic examination,* ed 3, Edinburgh, 1990 Churchill Livingstone.

Medical Economics Books: *Patient care flow chart manual,* ed 3, Ordell, 1982, Medical Economics Books.

Norris SH, Watt I: The prognosis of neck injuries resulting from rear-end vehicle collisions, *J Bone Joint Surg,* 65B(5):608-611, 1983.

O'Donoghue DH: *Treatment of injuries to athletes,* ed 3, Philadelphia, 1976, WB Saunders.

Office Orthopedic Practice: *The orthopedic clinics of north america,* vol 13, Number 3, Philadelphia, July 1982, WB Saunders.

Omer GE, Spinner M: *Management of peripheral nerve problems,* Philadelphia, 1981, WB Saunders.

Payne EE et al: The cervical spine, *Brain,* 80:571-596, 1957.

Prineas J: Polyneuropathies of undetermined cause, *Acta Neurol Scand,* 46(suppl 44):1, 1970.

Rana NA, Hancock DO, Taylor AR et al: Upward translocation of the dens in rheumatoid arthritis, *J Bone Joint Surg,* 55B(3):471, 1973.

Ranawat CS, O'Leary P, Pellicci P et al: Cervical spine fusion in rheumatoid arthritis, *J Bone Joint Surg,* 61A(7):1003, 1979.

Robbins SL: Blood vessels, In Robbins SL (ed): *Pathologic basis of disease,* 604, Philadelphia, 1974, WB Saunders.

Rothman RH, Simeone FA: *The spine,* vol 1, Philadelphia, 1975, WB Saunders.

Schneider RC, Livingston KE, Cave AJE: "Hangman's fracture" of the cervical spine, *J Meirpsirg,* 22:141-145, 1965.

Sharp J, Purser DW: Spontaneous atlanto-axial dislocation in ankylosing spondylitis and rheumatoid arthritis, *Ann Rheum Dis,* 20:47, 1961.

Smith PH, Benn RT, Sharp J: Natural history of rheumatoid cervical luxations, *Ann Rheum Dis,* 31 (6):431, 1972.

Smith PH, Sharp J, Kellgren JH: Natural history of rheumatoid cervical subluxations, *Ann Rheum Dis,* 31(3), 1972.

Sprou G: Basilar artery insufficiency secondary to obstruction of left subclavian artery, *Circulation,* 28:259, 1963.

Spurling RG, Scoville WB: Lateral rupture of the cervical intervertebral discs, *Syn Gyn Obst,* 78:350, 1944.

Stein S, Schut L, Borns P: Lacunar skull deformity (Lukenschadel, LDS) and intelligence in myelomeningocele, *J Neurosurg,* 1974.

Thurston SE: *The little black book of neurology,* Chicago, 1987, Mosby.

Turek SL: *Orthopaedics principles and their applications,* ed 3, Philadelphia, 1977, JP Lippincott.

Van Beusekom GT: The neurological syndrome associated with cervical luxations in rheumatoid arthritis, *Acta Orthop Belg,* 58(1):38, 1972.

White A: Biomechanical stability of the cervical spine, *Clin Orthop,* 109:85, 1975.

Wickstrom J, LaRocca H: Trauma: Head and neck injuries from acceleration-deceleration forces, In Ruge D, Wiltse LL (eds): *Spinal disorders: diagnosis and treatment,* Philadelphia, 1977, Lea & Febiger.

Wilkinson M: The anatomy and pathology of cervical spondylosis, *Proc Roy Soc Lond [Belg],* 57:159-162, 1964.

Yashon D: *Spinal injury,* New York, 1978, Appleton-Century-Crofts.

CHAPTER

~ 4 ~

The Shoulder

*T*he shoulder is a system of joints, and many movements of this system involve the neck. Completely independent action of the shoulder is possible, but independent, simultaneous action of the shoulder and neck is not. Primary functions can be identified in both areas, and a natural synchrony may be defined supplementing these. The shoulder exists so the hands can be used to advantage. The neck is built so that the properties of the special senses can be used to advantage.

Three primary functions of the shoulder can be identified: suspension of the upper limb, fixation for motion, and provision of a fulcrum for the upper extremity.

The arm lever is useless unless it has a fixed base. The fixed base comes largely from the layers of flat muscles piled one on top of another and attached to all surfaces of the scapula.

Paralytic disorders implicating these muscles come into clinical focus when weakness in the fixation mechanism is demonstrated. The serratus anterior, when paralyzed, allows the scapula to swing backward and loosen its attachment to the chest. The trapezius allows the scapula to spin like a pinwheel, which contributes to the loss of fixation.

The mobility of this part of the body results from the configuration of the bony parts and the mechanically advantageous attachment of the multiple muscles. The shallow socket and ball head favor frictionless spinning, and the main joint has four accessory articulating zones that compliment and enhance the action of the shoulder. Shoulder motion, therefore, can be fully appreciated only by understanding both the main and the accessory zone phases.

Shoulder motion is interpreted through excursion of the arm from the body and is recorded according to the anatomic planes. However, for practical purposes the action of lifting the arm, regardless of the plane, is the vital function because rotation of the body or rotation of the trunk converts what began as a simple lift into flexion or abduction, depending on the position the body assumes. The summation of shoulder motion (flexion, extension, abduction, adduction, or internal and external rotation) is reached by circumduction, which is an example of integrated joint action and muscle control. Most shoulder movement occurs at the glenohumeral joint, but this is appreciably enhanced by contributions from the sternoclavicular, acromioclavicular, and scapulothoracic mechanisms.

Everyday activities are made up of acts such as lifting, holding, pushing, turning, and shoving. It is through such common and accepted motions that clinical disorders are manifested. These are combined pattern motions with contributions from many parts of the shoulder complex. Individual joint and muscle contribution may be analyzed in these acts to aid localization and understanding of injury and disease. Consideration must also be given to the part that the elbow and hand play in shoulder function. Shoulders are used unconsciously during actions of the hand, wrist, and elbow. Injury or disease may hamper normal action of any of these areas, so increased replacement effort is sought from the shoulder. For example, loss of rotatory range, as in arthrodesis of the wrist or elbow, unconsciously results in increased rotation at the shoulder. Weakness or disorder of one muscle group evokes replacement effort in another group. For example, the hunching motion by the trapezius that follows attempted abduction is a replacement effort associated with paralysis of the deltoid. Scrutiny of these purposeful patterns is of great help for understanding disability in this region.

Index of Tests

Abbott-Saunders test

Adson's test

Allen maneuver

Apley's test

Apprehension test

Bryant's sign

Calloway's test

Codman's sign

Costoclavicular maneuver

Dawbarn's sign

Dugas' test

George's screening procedure

Halstead maneuver

Hamilton's test

Impingement sign

Ludington's test

Mazion's shoulder maneuver

Reverse Bakody maneuver

Roos' test

Shoulder compression test

Speed's test

Subacromial push button sign

Supraspinatus press test

Transverse humeral ligament test

Wright's test

Yergason's test

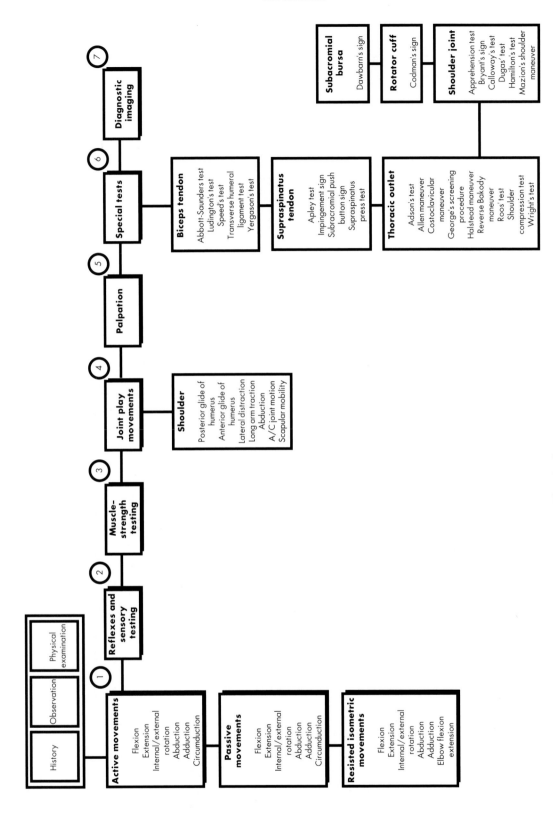

Fig. 4–1 Shoulder joint assessment.

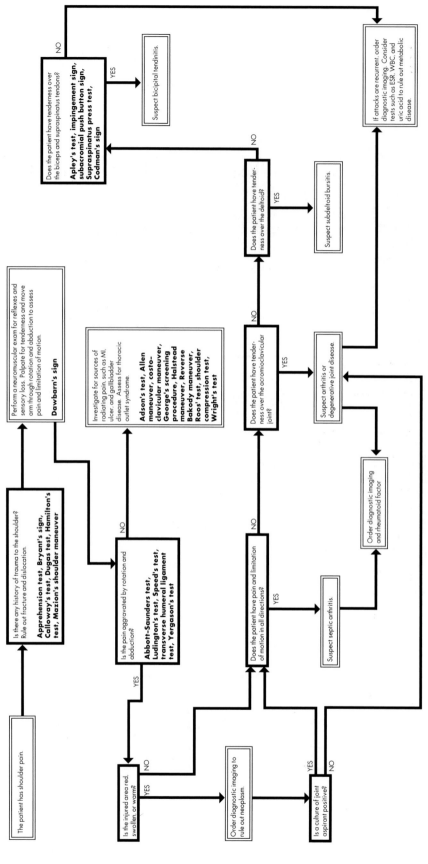

Fig. 4-2 Assessment of shoulder pain.

RANGE OF MOTION

A   B

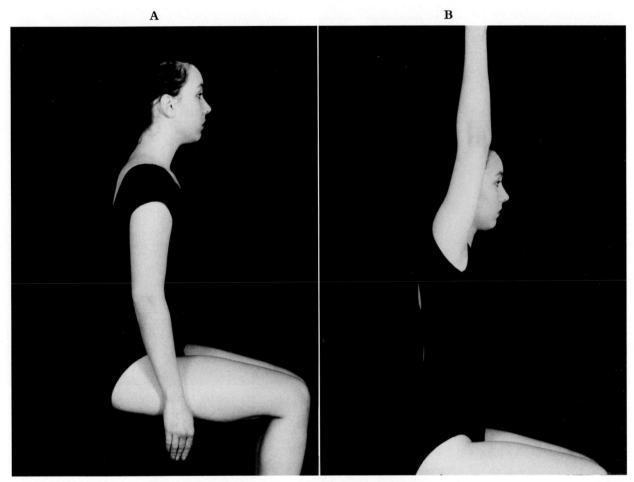

Fig. 4–3 **(A)** The patient sits with the shoulder in a neutral position and the arm hanging straight at the side. **(B)** The arm may be flexed 110 degrees at the shoulder and carried on up to 180 degrees in circumduction flexion. In this movement the head of the humerus does not encounter the same obstructions from the coracoacromial arch that occurs during abduction. The scapula is fixed to the chest initially and then moves forward around the chest wall during the 90 degrees of elevation, ending up farther in front than during the motion of abduction. Flexion is accomplished by the anterior deltoid, pectoralis major, coracobrachialis, and biceps. A retained flexion range of motion that is 160 degrees or less is an impairment of the shoulder in the activities of daily living.

Continued.

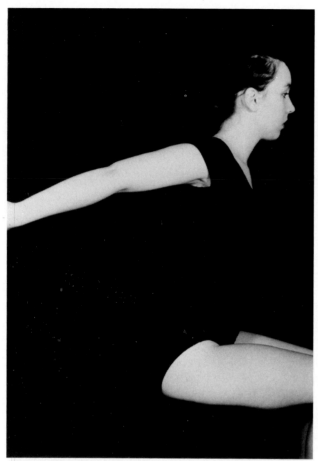

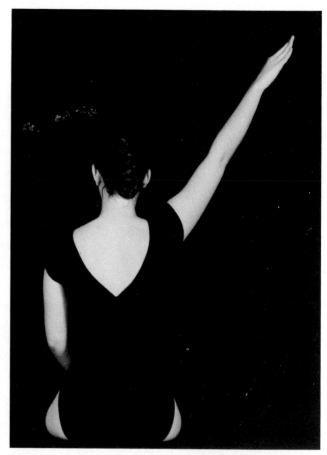

Fig. 4–4   The arm may be extended at the shoulder behind the line of the body for 50 degrees. In this action the clavicle rotates downward a little on its long axis and moves backward, with the sternoclavicular joint as the fulcrum. The scapula shifts backward and tilts upward a little on the chest wall. Extension is accomplished by the posterior deltoid, latissimus, teres major and minor, infraspinatus, and triceps muscles. Adhesive joint disorders and arthritis in the glenohumeral joint interfere with extension. Forty degrees or less of retained extension range of motion is an impairment of the shoulder in the activities of daily living.

Fig. 4–5   Abducting the arm from the side of the body to over the head is a complex procedure. The normal range of motion is 180 degrees and is accomplished largely at the glenohumeral joint, but all the axillary joints contribute. The muscles chiefly concerned are the trapezius, the serratus anterior, and the deltoid and rotator cuff group. Less than 160 degrees of retained abduction range of motion is an impairment of the shoulder in the activities of daily living.

A   B

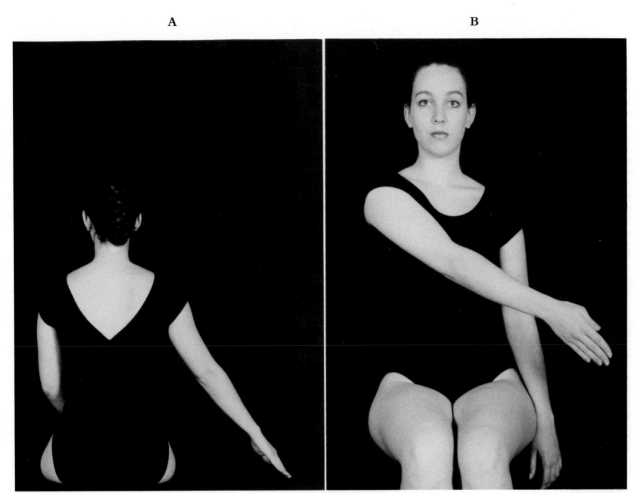

Fig. 4–6 From 180 degrees circumduction the arm may be pulled down to the side **(A)**, and at the end of the excursion the arm can be adducted in front of the chest 50 degrees farther **(B)**. This action takes place with the assistance of gravity, and when resistance is added, the latissimus dorsi, teres major, and pectoralis major are the movers. As the arm descends from 180 degrees circumduction, the clavicle rotates downward on its long axis. The scapula moves on the chest wall during the middle 90 degrees, starting at 45 degrees from the top and stopping at 45 degrees from the bottom. The motion is largely at the glenohumeral joint, as the head of the humerus rotates internally and follows a linear arc from the bottom to the top of the glenoid. This motion reverses the route taken during abduction. A retained adduction range of motion of 30 degrees or less is an impairment of the shoulder in the activities of daily living.

Continued.

A   B

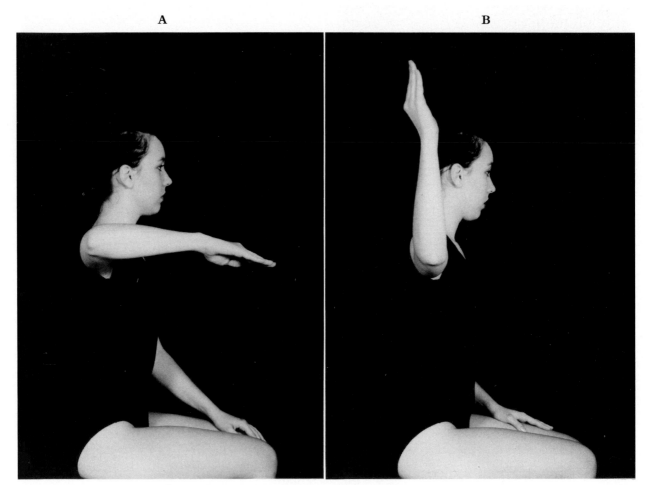

Fig. 4–7 From the midposition, which involves horizontal abduction of the arm at the side **(A)**, the shoulder may be externally rotated almost 90 degrees **(B)**. Nearly all of this movement occurs at the glenohumeral joint. When the arm is at the side, this action is accomplished by the infraspinatus, teres minor, and posterior deltoid. When the arm is horizontal, the supraspinatus also contributes. External rotation is the most important action, and when this rotation is lost, shoulder action is seriously compromised. Sixty degrees or less of retained external rotation is an impairment of the shoulder in the activities of daily living.

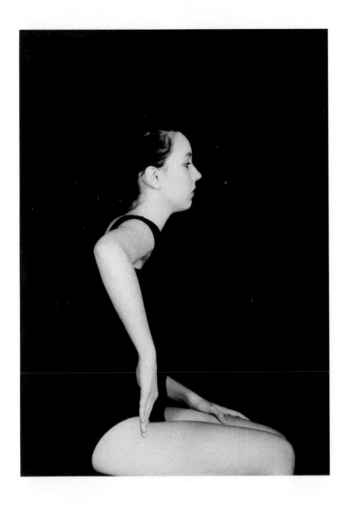

Fig. 4–8, left. The arm may be turned inward a little more than 90 degrees in both horizontal and vertical planes. This movement occurs chiefly at the glenohumeral joint and is powered by the subscapularis, pectoralis major, latissimus dorsi, and teres major muscles. The motion is an action that synchronizes with adduction as a striking blow and is hindered mainly by paralytic deformities. Sixty degrees or less of retained internal rotation is an impairment of the shoulder in the activities of daily living.

MUSCLE TESTING

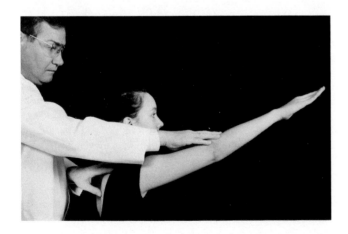

Fig. 4–9, left. The prime movers of flexion of the shoulder are the anterior portion of the deltoid muscle (axillary nerve, C5, and C6) and the coracobrachialis muscle (musculocutaneous nerve, C5, and C6). The accessory muscles to flexion are the middle fibers of the deltoid, the clavicular fibers of the pectoralis major, and the biceps brachii. To test flexion of the shoulder the examiner immobilizes the patient's scapula on the side being tested. The examiner achieves immobilization by grasping and holding the lower border with one hand. The patient flexes the arm anteriorly to 90 degrees while the forearm is pronated and the elbow slightly flexed. The examiner's free hand provides graded resistance just above the elbow. Rotation, adduction, or abduction of the arm should be prevented while flexion is being tested.

Continued.

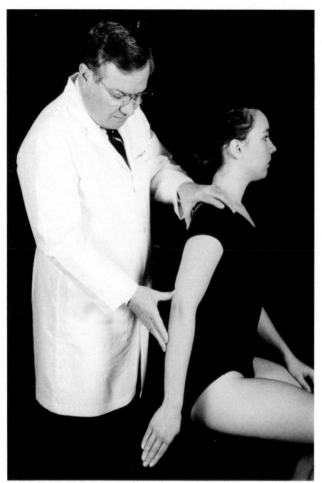

Fig. 4–10 The prime movers involved in shoulder extension are the latissimus dorsi (thoracodorsal nerve and C6 through C8), teres major (lowest subscapular nerve, C5, and C6), and deltoid (axillary nerve, C5, and C6) muscles. The teres minor and the long head of the triceps muscles are accessory to this motion. Extension of the shoulder is tested with the patient's elbow straightened and the forearm fully pronated (palm posterior) to prevent lateral rotation and adduction. The examiner fixes the scapula as described for testing flexion, and the patient extends the arm posteriorly through the range of motion. The examiner's other hand, which is placed just above the elbow, provides graded resistance.

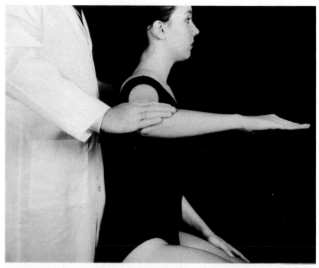

Fig. 4–11 The prime movers involved in abduction are the middle fibers of the deltoid (axillary nerve, C5, and C6) and the supraspinatus (suprascapular nerve and C5) muscles. The accessory muscles involved in abduction are the anterior and posterior fibers of the deltoid and serratus anterior muscles. The latter muscle functions by direct action of the scapula. Abduction of the shoulder is tested while the patient's arm is at the side, while the forearm is between pronation and supination (palm medial), and while the elbow is flexed a few degrees. The examiner stabilizes the scapula as described for flexion. The patient abducts the arm to 90 degrees. This abduction occurs against graded resistance applied by the examiner's other hand, which is placed proximal to the patient's elbow.

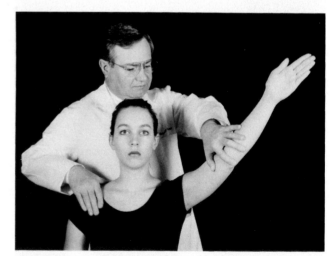

Fig. 4–12 The prime mover involved in adduction of the shoulder is the pectoralis major muscle (medial and lateral pectoral nerves, C5 through C8, and T1). The anterior fibers of the deltoid muscle are accessory to this motion. Adduction also occurs mainly at the glenohumeral joint and is assessed with the patient's arm abducted to 90 degrees. The patient adducts the arm anteriorly through the horizontal plane of motion and against graded resistance. This resistance is applied by the examiner's other hand, which is placed over the front of the arm and proximal to the patient's elbow.

Continued.

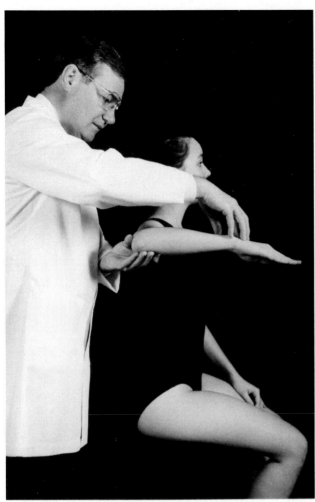 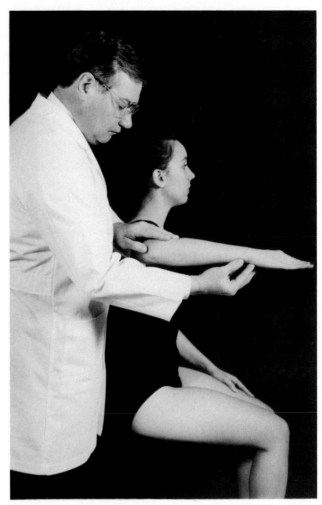

Fig. 4–13 The prime movers involved in external rotation are the infraspinatus (suprascapular nerve, C5, and C6) and teres minor (axillary nerve and C5). The posterior fibers of the deltoid muscle are accessory to this motion. The external rotation of the shoulder is assessed with the patient's arm abducted to 90 degrees (or at the patient's side, if abduction is not possible), with the elbow flexed to 90 degrees, and with the hand and fingers pointing forward. The examiner supports the patient's elbow by holding it with one hand while the patient rotates the arm upward (or outward, if shoulder abduction is not possible) against graded resistance that is applied by the examiner's other hand, which is placed on the patient's forearm proximal to the wrist.

Fig. 4–14 The prime movers of internal rotation of the shoulder are the subscapularis (upper and lower subscapular nerves, C5, and C6), pectoralis major (medial and lateral pectoral nerves, C5 through C8, and T1), and teres major (lowest subscapular nerve, C5, and C6) muscles. The anterior fibers of the deltoid muscle are accessory to this motion. Internal rotation of the shoulder is tested with the arm abducted to 90 degrees (or at the side, if abduction is not possible), the elbow flexed to 90 degrees, and the hand pointed forward. The examiner supports the patient's elbow with one hand, as described previously, while the patient rotates the arm downward (or inward, if the shoulder abduction is not possible) against graded resistance that is applied by the examiner's other hand, which is placed on the patient's forearm proximal to the wrist.

〜 Abbott-Saunders Test 〜

Comment

Rupture or stretching of the fascial covering of the bicipital groove permits the tendon to subluxate from the groove. This may occur as an acute injury. The predisposing factor for this condition is a congenitally shallow bicipital groove. The intertubercular groove not only may be shallow but may be broader than normal. This permits the tendon to flatten out and slide back and forth within the groove itself. The patient complains of a snap that occurs anteriorly in the shoulder and is accompanied by pain. The pain is followed by residual soreness along the bicipital groove. The soreness is elicited by the same motions that cause pain with tenosynovitis. Rupture or stretching of the fascial covering of the bicipital groove is indistinguishable from tenosynovitis. In a muscular patient, it may be difficult to palpate the subluxing tendon. If the condition becomes chronic, as a result of a defect in the roof of the groove with redundant tissue, chronic synovitis usually occurs. Movement of the shoulder results in painful snapping as the tendon slips back and forth out of the groove, particularly during rotation of the arm.

Procedure

With the patient in the seated position, the examiner fully abducts and externally rotates the patient's arm. The examiner then lowers the arm to the patient's side. A palpable or audible click indicates a subluxation or dislocation of the biceps tendon.

Confirmation Procedures

Ludington's test, Speed's test, transverse humeral ligament test, Yergason's test

Reporting Statement

Abbott-Saunders test is positive for the right shoulder. This result indicates subluxation or dislocation of the biceps tendon.

〜 Clinical Pearl 〜

The biceps tendon will not rupture or dislocate under ordinary stresses unless it is already weak. The predisposing factor to rupture or dislocation is age-degeneration, which is probably accelerated by oft-repeated friction and angulation at the point where the tendon enters the bicipital groove of the humerus.

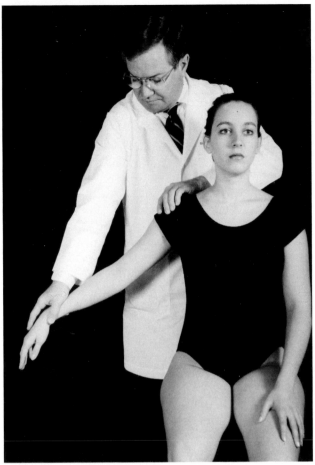

Fig. 4–15 With the patient in the seated position, the examiner fully abducts the patient's arm.

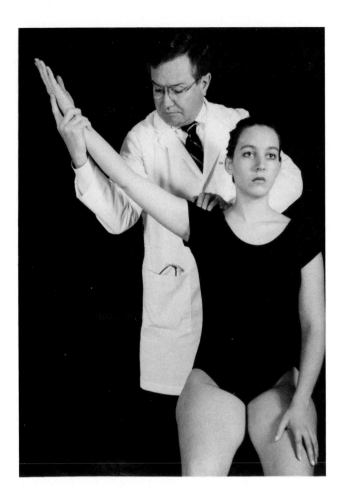

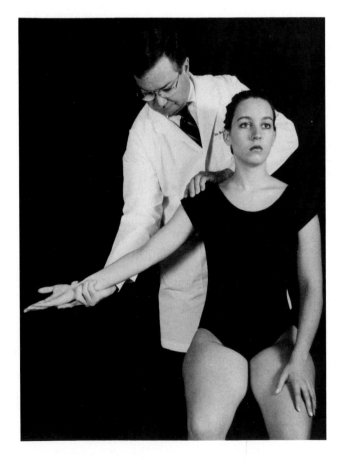

Fig. 4–16, above right. The examiner externally rotates the patient's arm when the arm is at the top of the abduction maneuver.

Fig. 4–17, below right. While maintaining the arm in external rotation, the examiner then lowers the arm to the patient's side. A palpable or audible click is a positive finding, which indicates a subluxation or dislocation of the biceps tendon.

~ Adson's Test ~

Comment

The brachial plexus and the subclavian artery can be compressed as they pass between the anterior and medial scalene muscles and the first rib, yielding a characteristic neurovascular syndrome—the anterior scalene syndrome.

All three scalene muscles originate from the transverse processes of the cervical vertebrae and insert on the first and second ribs. The anterior and medial scalene muscles insert on the respective tubercles on the first rib and sandwich the subclavian artery into a sulcus. The posterior scalenus muscle is fixed to the second rib. A variable scalenus minimus muscle may exist and insert between the anterior and medial scalenus muscles. The scalene muscles raise the first and second rib during inspiration. Unilateral contraction inclines the head to the side of action and turns the face to the opposite side. Bilateral contraction flexes the cervical spine. The anterior and medial scalene muscles form one side of the scalene foramen, with the sternocleidomastoid muscle and the first rib forming the other sides. Bounded by the anterior scalene muscle, the first rib, and the medial scalene muscle, the posterior scalene foramen admits the brachial plexus and the subclavian artery to the costoclavicular space. The posterior foramen can range from 0.4 to 3.5 cm in width.

The subclavian artery bends over and passes through a sulcus in the first rib. Composed of nerve roots from C5 to C8 and T1, the brachial plexus represents the innervation of the entire upper extremity and lies tautly stretched and without bony protection in this region.

Neurovascular compression can occur when disease or anatomic variations narrow a tight foramen. In the development of the anterior scalene syndrome, some anatomic variations are very important.

The anterior scalene syndrome has many similarities with the costoclavicular syndrome, also known as the syndrome of the cervical rib.

Under normal circumstances, there is enough room in the posterior scalene foramen of the brachial plexus and the subclavian artery. However, many anatomic variations and consequent changes in the functional anatomy of the shoulder and upper extremity can cause the development of the clinical symptoms. Many embryologic, anatomic, and physiologic factors create a disposition for development of compression in the posterior scalene foramen.

The neurovascular symptomatology depends on the frequency, duration, and degree of compression of the subclavian artery and the brachial plexus. The lower roots of the brachial plexus (C8-T1) are at higher risk than the more superior roots, due to their location in the plexus. The symptoms include pain in the fingers, hand, forearm, arm, and shoulder and paresthesia and hyperesthesia, especially in the eighth cervical and first thoracic nerve root dermatomes. Numbness occurs most often in the fingers, hand, and forearm. Depending on the degree of arterial compression, ischemic symptoms of numbness, cold, weakness, and skin color changes appear.

Procedure

The following procedure is probably the most common means of testing for thoracic outlet syndrome. The patient's head is rotated to face the tested shoulder. The patient then extends the head while the examiner externally rotates and extends the shoulder. The examiner locates the radial pulse and the patient is instructed to take a deep breath and hold it. A disappearance of the pulse indicates a positive test. If the maneuver is negative, it is repeated by having the patient turn the head to the opposite side. The test is significant for identifying neurovascular compression of the subclavian artery and brachial plexus of the ipsilateral side, which are commonly caused by scalenus anticus or cervical rib thoracic outlet syndromes.

Confirmation Procedures

Allen maneuver, costoclavicular maneuver, George's screening procedure, Halstead maneuver, reverse Bakody maneuver, Roos' test, shoulder compression test, Wright's test

---

Reporting Statement

Adson's test is positive on the right. This result indicates thoracic outlet syndrome due to scalenus anticus syndrome or cervical rib syndrome.

~ Clinical Pearl ~

Radiographic demonstration of a cervical rib does not prove that it is the cause of the symptoms. The condition has to be distinguished (1) from other causes of pain and paresthesia in the forearm and hand, (2) from other causes of muscle atrophy in the hand, and (3) from other causes of peripheral vascular changes in the upper extremity.

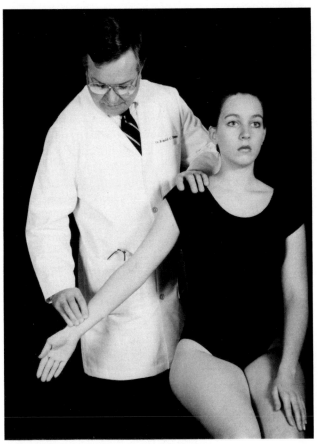

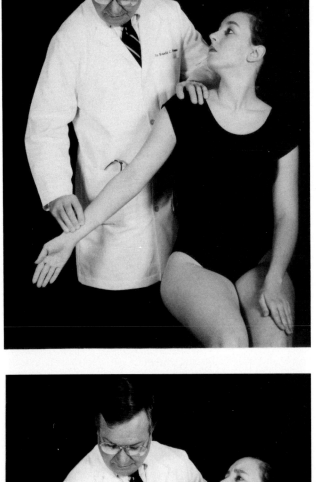

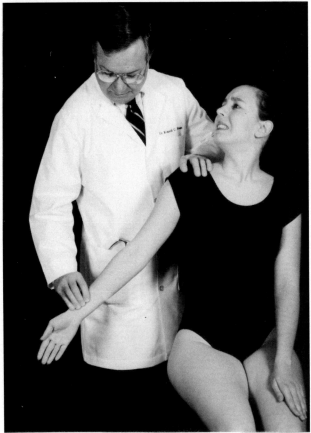

Fig. 4–18 The patient is seated comfortably with the arms at the sides. The examiner slightly abducts the affected arm and palpates the radial pulse.

Fig. 4–19, above right. The patient rotates the head toward the affected shoulder. The patient then extends the head, and the examiner externally rotates and extends the shoulder slightly.

Fig. 4–20, below right. The patient is instructed to take a deep breath and hold it. A disappearance of the pulse indicates a positive test. If the test is negative, the procedure is repeated with the patient turning the head to the opposite side (modified Adson's test). The test is significant for neurovascular compression of the subclavian artery and brachial plexus of the ipsilateral side, commonly caused by the scalenus anticus or cervical rib thoracic outlet syndrome.

Comment

Multiple etiologic possibilities, complex anatomic considerations, and a variety of neurogenic and vascular symptoms engage the interest of many disciplines that encounter the thoracic outlet neurovascular compression syndromes. Static and dynamic anatomic relationships within the thoracic outlet dictate morbid aberrations in blood perfusion and neural function.

Usually a contributory anatomic element that underlies each of the compression syndromes can be identified. Therefore the usual clinical maneuvers used to bracket the level of compression can be equivocal. Often patients do not have one single complaint or set of complaints that unfailingly point to a compression syndrome. In fact, symptoms of several compression syndromes may be similar.

The anatomic areas of potential neurovascular compression are the interscalene space, near the thoracic rib; the costoclavicular space; and the axilla between the coracoid process and pectoralis minor tendon.

There are additional considerations that may affect these levels of compression. Movement of the head and neck; deep inspiration; and clavicular, scapular, and humeral movement—when performed in concert—can simultaneously alter structural relationships at one level or several levels and can cause impingement of nerves and vessels. Muscle hypertrophy, due to occupational stress and obesity, may compromise otherwise patent spaces. Loss of muscle tone and strength from a variety of causes; pain from unrelated but adjacent structures; chest deformity as a result of emphysema; postural portrayal of depressed mental status; bad working posture; and middle-age disuse atrophy, either singly or in combination, may alter potential spaces through sagging or displacement of the anatomic members.

Clavicular fractures with excessive callus or residual displacement of fragments and subacromial humeral luxation, blunt trauma to the upper thorax, postirradiation fibrosis, and the use of vibrating tools may either stretch part of the brachial plexus or damage vessel walls and result in thrombotic vessel wall complications. A cervical rib with or without a prefixed brachial plexus, a bifid clavicle, abnormal bony protuberances from the first thoracic rib, a fibrous remnant of the scalenus minimus muscle, abnormal scalene insertions on the first rib, and abnormal splitting of the scalenus medius by all or part of the brachial plexus may contribute to compression symptoms. Either postural, dynamic, traumatic, or arteriosclerotic factors must be added to precipitate patient symptoms.

Procedure

The examiner flexes the patient's elbow to 90 degrees while the shoulder is abducted and externally rotated. The patient then rotates the head away from the test side. The examiner palpates the radial pulse, which disappears when the head is rotated. The disappearance of the pulse indicates a positive test result for thoracic outlet syndrome. When doing any thoracic outlet test, the examiner must find the pulse before positioning the patient. In a normal individual, the pulse may be diminished.

Confirmation Procedures

Adson's test, costoclavicular maneuver, George's screening procedure, Halstead maneuver, reverse Bakody maneuver, Roos' test, shoulder compression test, Wright's test

---

Reporting Statement

Allen maneuver is positive on the right. This result indicates thoracic outlet syndrome.

∼ Clinical Pearl ∼

Altered relative position of the shoulder girdle to the neurovascular bundle, or vice versa, is a common element of thoracic outlet syndrome. However, a group of symptoms may be separated, in which there may be a static or gradual process underway that appears as a more general development without specific, separate, irritating incidents. Such a condition is labeled "postural," because of the alteration of the normal girdle relationship to the rest of the body.

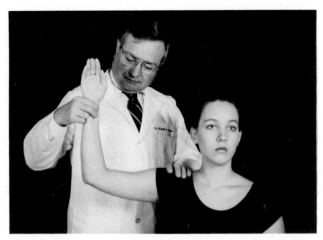

Fig. 4–21 The patient is seated. The examiner abducts the affected shoulder to 90 degrees. The patient's elbow is flexed to 90 degrees, and the shoulder is externally rotated. The radial pulse is located and recorded.

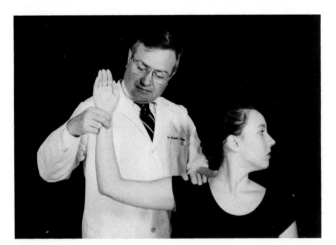

Fig. 4–22 The patient rotates the head to the opposite side. If the pulse disappears during this maneuver, the test is positive. The test is significant for thoracic outlet syndrome. When doing any thoracic outlet test, the examiner must find the pulse before positioning the patient or completing the maneuver. Even in a normal individual, the pulse may be diminished.

Comment

Supraspinatus tendinitis is the most common type of tendinitis in the upper limb. This condition occurs most frequently in swimmers and tennis players or athletes in any other sport requiring repeated overhead movement of the arm.

The supraspinatus tendon passes beneath the acromion and inserts on the greater tubercle of the humerus, passing beneath the coracoacromial ligament that forms a fibrous arch over the tendon. Between the tendon and the overlying structures is the subacromial bursa.

Repeated abduction of the shoulder, unless it is maintained in external rotation, causes impingement of the tendon within the very narrow space between the humerus and the overlying acromion and ligament. This disorder is often called impingement syndrome. It has also been called swimmer's shoulder.

The microvasculature of the supraspinatus tendon is reduced where the tendon is wrung out by pressure during abduction. This site corresponds to that of tears in the supraspinatus tendon of geriatric patients. These tears may be the result of poor healing because of impaired circulation. Although tears are not as common in younger patients, the area affected is the same. Sometimes calcification occurs at this site.

The etiology of this tendinitis is well defined and can be confirmed by horizontally adducting the patient's arm across the body. This move causes further impingement and reproduces the painful symptoms.

Procedure

The patient is seated and is instructed to place the affected hand behind the head and touch the opposite superior angle of the scapula. The patient is then instructed to place the hand behind the back and attempt to touch the opposite inferior angle of the scapula. Exacerbation of the patient's pain indicates degenerative tendinitis of one of the tendons of the rotator cuff, usually the supraspinatus tendon.

Confirmation Procedures

Impingement sign, subacromial push button sign, supraspinatus test

Reporting Statement

Apley's scratch test (superior or inferior) is positive on the right. This result indicates tendinitis of the supraspinatus tendon.

Clinical Pearl

Apley's inferior is a useful test of internal rotation and extension. With severe restriction the patient will not be able to get the hand behind the back at all. This movement is commonly affected in adhesive capsulitis.

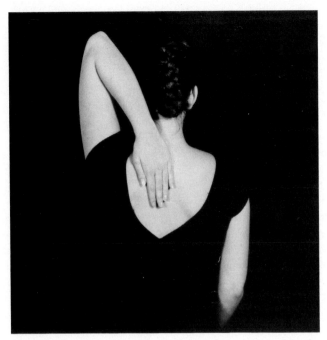

Fig. 4–23 The patient is seated and is instructed to place the hand of the affected arm behind the head and touch near the opposite scapula (Apley's scratch superior).

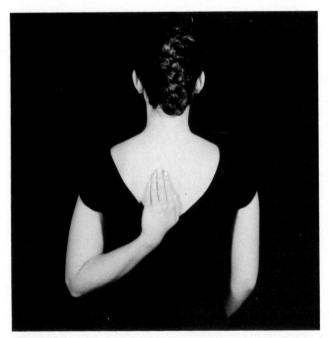

Fig. 4–24 The patient is then instructed to place the hand of the affected shoulder behind the back and attempt to touch near the opposite scapula (Apley's scratch inferior). If either position exacerbates the patient's pain, this indicates degenerative tendinitis of one of the tendons, usually the supraspinatus, of the rotator cuff.

Comment

Dislocation of the shoulder follows the loss of function of the restraining structures around the shoulder. This dislocation is a result of the same mechanism that causes subluxations. By far, the most common type of dislocation of the shoulder in young patients is anterior–inferior. This is pure dislocation, unaccompanied by fracture. As age advances, the ligaments become firmer and the bone less strong, so the dislocation may be accompanied by avulsion fracture, rather than a tear of the ligament. In the young patient it is always the ligament or muscle that gives way. As the arm is forced into abduction and external rotation, the humeral head is thrust against the anterior portion of the glenohumeral joint. The coracoacromial ligament forces the humeral head downward, and it then emerges anteriorly and inferiorly into the redundant area of the capsule, which is protected by the glenohumeral ligaments. These ligaments give way when they are torn from the glenoid labrum because of avulsion of the labrum or actual disruption of the ligaments. The head of the humerus slips over the glenoid rim and immediately slides forward to lodge between the rim of the glenoid and coracoid process, and the arm drops toward the side but not against it. This is the classic dislocation of the shoulder in young patients. The damage to the ligament may be a transverse tear across the capsule, and in addition, the capsular reinforcements known as the glenohumeral ligaments may split, with one passing above the humeral head and the other below it. In some instances the ligaments actually grasp the humeral head to impede its reduction.

Posterior dislocation of the shoulder is uncommon. The cause is a direct driving force against the lower end of the humerus with the arm flexed forward. This force is transmitted up the arm and drives the head out posteriorly. No gross deformity of the shoulder is evident. The patient resists any motion of the shoulder, and on careful palpation the examiner can feel less fullness of the humeral head in front and some increased fullness behind. There is also increased prominence of the coracoid. Such a dislocation is readily determined only if it is palpated very early, because within a short time the swelling that is around the shoulder and that occurs from this extremely disabling injury will mask any physical findings.

Procedure

The examiner abducts and externally rotates the patient's shoulder. A positive test is indicated when the patient shows apprehension or alarm and resists further motion. The patient also may state that such rotation elicits a feeling that resembles the pain felt when the shoulder was previously dislocated. This test must be performed slowly. If the test is done too quickly, there is a chance that the humerus will dislocate. A positive test indicates anterior shoulder dislocation trauma.

In determining the trauma resulting from posterior shoulder dislocation, the examiner flexes and internally rotates the patient's shoulder. The examiner then applies a posterior force on the patient's elbow. A positive result is indicated if the patient exhibits a look of alarm or feeling of apprehension and resists further motion. A positive test indicates a posterior dislocation of the humerus.

Confirmation Procedures

Bryant's sign, Calloway's test, Dugas' test, Hamilton's test, Mazion's shoulder maneuver, diagnostic imaging

---

Reporting Statement

Apprehension test is positive for the right shoulder in the anterior portion. This result indicates shoulder dislocation trauma.

Apprehension test is positive for the right shoulder in the posterior portion. This result indicates shoulder dislocation trauma.

∼ Clinical Pearl ∼

These maneuvers are also known as the drawer tests of Gerber and Ganz. Any movements, clicks, or patient apprehension support the diagnosis of recurrent shoulder dislocation. Axial diagnostic images are made to confirm the diagnosis.

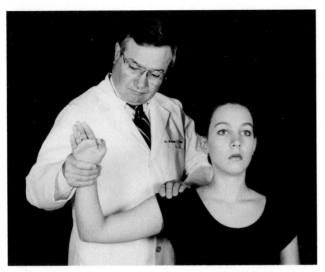

Fig. 4–25 The patient is seated comfortably with the arms at the sides. The examiner slowly abducts and externally rotates the patient's affected shoulder.

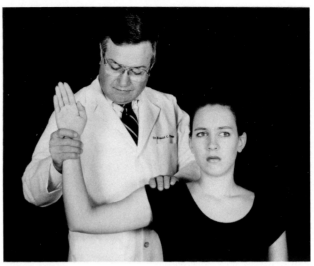

Fig. 4–26 A positive test is indicated by a look or feeling of apprehension or alarm on the patient's face. The patient will usually resist further motion. The patient also may state that this maneuver duplicates the feeling of the previous dislocation. This test must be done slowly. If the test is done too quickly, there is a chance that the humerus will dislocate. A positive test indicates anterior shoulder dislocation trauma.

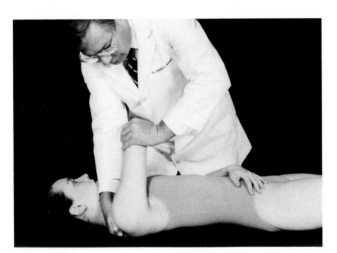

Fig. 4–27 For determining the trauma resulting from posterior shoulder dislocation, the patient should be supine. The examiner flexes and internally rotates the patient's affected shoulder. The examiner then applies a posterior force on the patient's elbow (forcing the humeral head posterior on the glenoid). A positive test is indicated by a look of apprehension or alarm on the patient's face. The patient will resist further motion. A positive test indicates posterior dislocation of the humerus.

Comment

Two common dislocations of the shoulder occur at the acromioclavicular and glenohumeral joints. Of all glenohumeral dislocations, 95% are anterior dislocations and occur most often in young adult males. These dislocations are the result of forced abduction and external rotation of the shoulder. This type of dislocation occurs when the head of the humerus leaves the glenohumeral joint through a tear in the anterior inferior capsule, a defect that usually does not heal. The patient is then subject to recurrent dislocations that occur whenever the extremity is abducted and externally rotated. With an acute lesion there is a history of trauma with pain and of considerable discomfort in the glenohumeral joint when the patient attempts to move the upper extremity. Careful and early inspection reveals flattening and loss of the normal curvature of the shoulder, but swelling obliterates these findings later. Diagnostic imaging is needed to confirm the diagnosis. When shoulder dislocation is suspected, an axillary view is paramount to distinguish the exact position of the head of the humerus in relation to the glenoid process. Anterior dislocations of the shoulder can often be recognized in an anteroposterior diagnostic image, but posterior dislocations of the shoulder may frequently be in line with the glenoid process and indistinguishable in this view.

Dislocations of the shoulder are occasionally accompanied by injury to the axillary nerve with resulting loss of function of the deltoid muscle. With shoulder dislocations the function of the deltoid and any sensory disturbance in the skin overlying the deltoid must be ascertained. The area over the deltoid is innervated by the axillary nerve and assessment of the skin sensation will aid in predicting the recovery of the nerve. Dislocations of the shoulder rarely result in injury to other nerves and vessels of the upper extremity, but injuries of the posterior cord of the brachial plexus have been reported.

Procedure

View the characteristic lowering of the axillary fold (anterior and posterior pillars of the armpit) that is seen after trauma when dislocation of the glenohumeral articulation ensues.

Confirmation Procedures

Apprehension test, Calloway's test, Dugas' test, Hamilton's test, Mazion's shoulder maneuver, diagnostic imaging

---

Reporting Statement

Bryant's sign is present in the right shoulder. This result indicates shoulder dislocation trauma.

∾ Clinical Pearl ∾

With dislocations of the shoulder the axillary nerve may be injured. The patient is unable to contract the deltoid muscle, and there may be a small patch of anesthesia over the muscle. This anesthesia is usually a neurapraxia, which recovers spontaneously after a few weeks or months. Occasionally the posterior cord of the brachial plexus is injured. This occurrence is somewhat alarming, but it usually recovers with time.

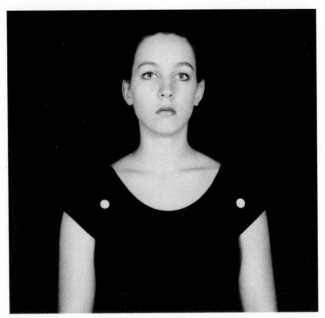

Fig. 4–28 The patient is seated with the arms comfortably at the sides.

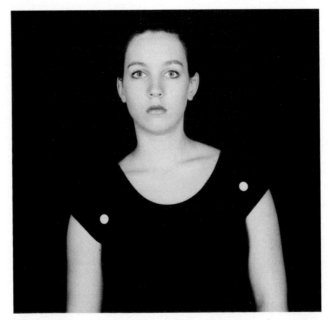

Fig. 4–29 If the sign is present, there is a characteristic lowering of the axillary fold (anterior and posterior pillars of the armpit) on the affected side. The sign is present when dislocation of the glenohumeral articulation has occurred.

Comment

Shoulder dislocation at the glenohumeral joint occurs anteriorly in 95% of the cases. The remaining 5% dislocate posteriorly. The incidence of anterior dislocation is attributed to the anatomic weakness of the anterior aspect of the joint.

The joint capsule is thin and loose. The capsule is reinforced by folds called glenohumeral ligaments. These ligaments attach from the humerus and fan out to attach to the superior anterior aspect of the glenoid fossa, partly to the glenoid labrum, and partly to a portion of the bone of the scapula. An opening in the capsule frequently exists between the superior and middle glenohumeral ligaments. This opening is called Weitbrecht's foramen. The opening may be a frank perforation or may be covered by a thin layer of the capsule. The articular cavity connects with the subscapular fossa through Weitbrecht's foramen. The humeral head dislocates through this opening, and dislocations may recur due to fraying or actual destruction of the middle glenohumeral ligament.

With dislocations the glenoid labrum may be partially or completely detached and a tear may occur in the anteroinferior aspect. The glenoid labrum contains no fibrocartilage and is a redundant fibrous fold of the anterior capsule that disappears when the humerus is externally rotated. This pouch invites dislocation. The humeral head can protrude into this pouch, especially if an anatomic variant of the middle humeral ligament exists.

There are five types of dislocation, and the most common is the subcoracoid dislocation. The subclavicular and subglenoid types are less frequent and may be a progression of the subcoracoid type. All anterior types of dislocations can change into any of the other anterior types. The fifth type of dislocation—the posterior, or subspinous—is rare. The type of dislocation is determined by the location of the humeral head in relation to the glenoid seat when the diagnosis is made.

Primary anterior dislocations occur with equal frequency regardless of age, but recurrence of a dislocation is highest in the young and decreases after age 45. There is less recurrence in cases in which the primary dislocation was severe and resulted in greater hemorrhage and therefore greater scar formation in healing.

Procedure

The test consists of measuring the girth of the shoulder joints bilaterally. This test is helpful in the examination of obese patients. The examiner loops a flexible tape measure through the axilla. The girth is measured at the acromial tip. In a positive test the girth of the affected joint is increased. The test is significant for dislocation of the humerus.

Confirmation Procedures

Apprehension test, Bryant's sign, Dugas' sign, Hamilton's test, Mazion's shoulder maneuver, diagnostic imaging

---

Reporting Statement

Calloway's test demonstrates an increased shoulder axillary circumference on the right. This increase is consistent with shoulder dislocation trauma.

~ **Clinical Pearl** ~

With shoulder dislocation the pain is severe. The patient supports the arm with the opposite hand and is hesitant to permit any kind of examination. The lateral outline of the shoulder may be flattened and, if the patient is not too muscular, a small bulge may be seen and felt just below the clavicle. The arm must always be examined for nerve and vessel injury.

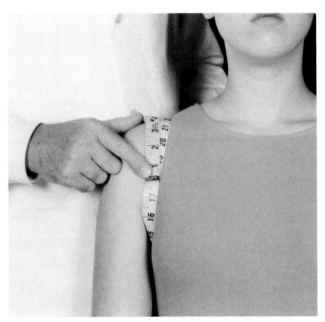

Fig. 4–30 The patient is seated comfortably with the arms at the sides. The examiner loops a flexible tape measure through the axilla and measures the girth of the affected shoulder at the acromial tip. The girth of the affected shoulder is compared with the girth of the unaffected shoulder. In a positive test, the girth of the affected joint is increased. The test is significant for dislocation of the humerus.

~ Codman's Sign ~
DROP ARM TEST

Comment

Complete tears of the tendinous cuff must be distinguished from incomplete tears. The clinical effects of the tears are different. An incomplete tear is one cause of the painful arc syndrome, and a complete tear seriously impairs the patient's ability to abduct the shoulder.

The tendon gives way under a sudden strain, usually caused by a fall or by overexertion. Age attrition of the tendon is a predisposing factor.

A tear of the tendinous cuff is mainly of the supraspinatus tendon, but it may extend into the adjacent subscapularis or infraspinatus tendons. Such a tear is close to the insertion of the tendons and usually involves the capsule of the joint, into which the tendons are blended. The edges of the rent retract, leaving a gaping hole that establishes a communication between the shoulder joint and the subacromial bursa.

With complete tears of the Supraspinatus tendon the patient is usually a male older than 60. After a strain or fall, the patient's complaints include pain at the tip of the shoulder and down the upper arm and an inability to raise the arm.

Examination reveals local tenderness below the margin of the acromion. When the patient attempts to abduct the arm, no movement occurs at the glenohumeral joint, but a range of 45 to 60 degrees of abduction can be achieved entirely by scapular movement. However, there is a full range of passive movement. If the arm is abducted with assistance beyond 90 degrees, the patient can sustain the abduction by deltoid action. The essential and characteristic feature in cases of torn supraspinatus tendon is inability to initiate glenohumeral abduction. The usual explanation is that the early stages of abduction demand combining the action of the supraspinatus with the action of the deltoid muscle. This combined action supplies the main abduction force and the supraspinatus action that stabilizes the humeral head in the glenoid fossa.

A complete tear of the tendinous cuff must be distinguished from other causes of impaired glenohumeral abduction, especially the painful arc syndrome and paralysis of the abductor muscles (poliomyelitis or nerve injury). Inability to initiate glenohumeral abduction accompanied by enough power to sustain abduction once the limb has been raised passively is characteristic of a widely torn supraspinatus. With the painful arc syndrome, the power of abduction is retained but the movement is painful. In a case of complete tear, arthrography will demonstrate communication between the joint and the subacromial bursa. The tear also may be visualized by ultrasound scanning.

Procedure

The patient's arm is passively abducted. The examiner suddenly removes support at some point above 90 degrees, which makes the deltoid contract suddenly. If shoulder pain occurs and there is a hunching of the shoulder due to the absence of rotator cuff function, the sign is present for rotator cuff tear or, more specifically, rupture of the supraspinatus tendon.

In a slight modification of the test the examiner abducts the patient's shoulder to 90 degrees and then instructs the patient to slowly lower the arm to the side in the same arc of movement. The test is positive if the patient is unable to return the arm to the side slowly or has severe pain. A positive test indicates a tear in the rotator cuff complex.

Confirmation Procedures

Apley scratch test, impingement sign, subacromial push button sign, supraspinatus test

---

Reporting Statement

Codman's drop arm sign is present on the right. This result indicates a tear in the rotator cuff complex.

~ Clinical Pearl ~

The cardinal sign of cuff rupture is persistent weakness. The patient may be conscious of this weakness, but often the examiner must point it out. Sometimes the weakness is easily overlooked. The patient may be able to lift the arm into full abduction or beyond the point of a full-thickness cuff tear. However, if this action is resisted a little, sometimes by as little as the pressure of one finger, even a very strong patient may be unable to abduct or flex the shoulder well.

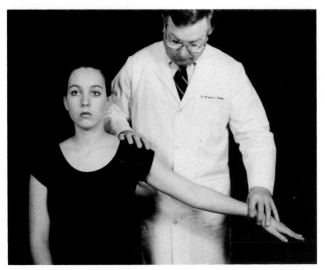

Fig. 4–31 The patient is seated. The examiner passively abducts the patient's affected arm.

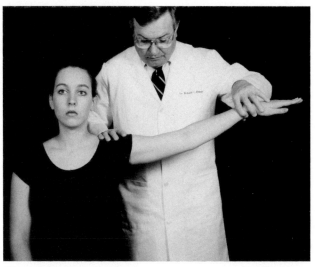

Fig. 4–32 The passive abduction is carried to a range slightly above 90 degrees.

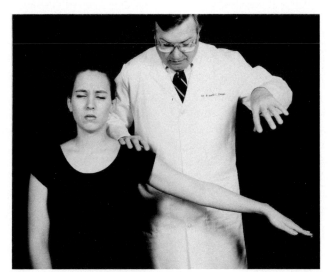

Fig. 4–33 The examiner suddenly removes support, making the deltoid contract suddenly. If the sign is present, shoulder pain and a hunching of the shoulder occur due to the absence of rotator cuff function. The sign is significant for rotator cuff tear (rupture of the supraspinatus tendon).

Comment

As the neurovascular bundle enters the axillary canal, it runs through a narrow cleft beneath the clavicle and on top of the first rib. This cleft is a slit-like aperture over which the subclavius muscle arches sometimes with a sharp, fusiform lower margin. Alterations and abnormalities in this cleft can compress the neurovascular bundle. Because the vein is the most medial structure running into the arm and lies in the narrowest part of the cleft, it suffers the most from any narrowing that develops. Abnormalities, fractures, and dislocations of the medial third of the clavicle or fractures of the first rib followed by excessive callus formation can constrict this space. The resulting symptoms are a sense of fullness in the hand and fingers, and an aching, crampy pain in the forearm and hand. Vague shoulder or shoulder-arm discomfort may be mentioned, but the radiating pain is emphasized. The hand may be intermittently swollen, and sometimes superficial veins around the shoulder are engorged. There is no limitation of shoulder movement, which contrasts with shoulder-arm-hand syndrome, in which gross shoulder immobilization is prominent and hand symptoms are present. The radiating discomfort has the typically diffuse vascular pattern, which means the discomfort is not localized to nerve root or peripheral nerve distribution.

In addition to those patients with obvious abnormality of the rib and clavicle, some patients develop this disturbance from a sagging shoulder girdle and atonic musculature. Normally it is difficult to encroach upon the neurovascular bundle beneath the clavicle, but it is conceivable that some sagging occurs, and when tension in the bundle and enveloping sheath is added, the vessels may be compressed.

This costoclavicular disturbance can be separated from scalene and cervical rib disturbances by several findings. There is no relation to cervical spine movements and no scalene or supraclavicular tenderness. The diagnostic images are different, because no cervical rib is present. Arterial symptoms are occasionally prominent, but most of the disturbance is the result of venous obstruction. Costoclavicular compression can be differentiated from postural compression by the absence of any significant relation to body position either at work or while sleeping. Costoclavicular compression is also clearly differentiated from hyperabduction compression by the lack of significant correlation to shoulder movement.

Procedure

The examiner palpates the radial pulse while drawing the patient's shoulder down and into extension. The patient flexes the cervical spine (chin to chest). The test is positive if the pulse is absent. A positive result is more pronounced in patients who complain of symptoms while wearing a backpack or a heavy coat. A positive test suggests thoracic outlet syndrome.

Confirmation Procedures

Adson's test, Allen maneuver, George's screening procedure, Halstead maneuver, reverse Bakody maneuver, Roos' test, shoulder compression test, Wright's test

---

Reporting Statement

The costoclavicular maneuver is positive on the right. This result indicates costoclavicular thoracic outlet compression syndrome.

∿ Clinical Pearl ∿

Radiating discomfort due to neurovascular compression can be associated with sleep or recumbency. This discomfort is a common disturbance that has many descriptive terms applied to it. These terms include Wartenberg's nocturnal dysesthesia, sleep tetany, waking numbness, nocturnal palsy, and morning numbness.

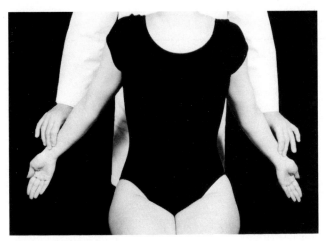

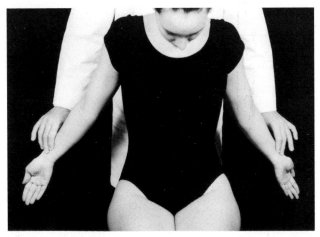

Fig. 4–34 The patient is seated comfortably with the arms at the sides. The examiner bilaterally palpates the radial pulse.

Fig. 4–35 The examiner extends the patient's shoulders as the patient flexes the cervical spine (chin to chest). The test is positive if the radial pulse of the affected arm disappears. A positive test indicates thoracic outlet syndrome.

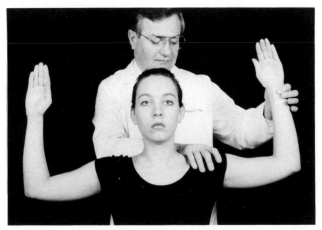

Fig. 4–36 An alternative is to have the patient actively abduct the shoulders and flex the elbows to 90 degrees. The examiner palpates the radial pulse of the affected arm and externally rotates the arm. The test is positive if the pulse disappears. A positive test indicates thoracic outlet syndrome. Before the arm is externally rotated in this position, a subtle sign of thoracic outlet syndrome may occur. This sign involves blanching of the hand of the affected arm. The examiner should use the unaffected side as a control.

Comment

A painful shoulder is a complaint that is common to all age groups in both sexes. To treat these patients effectively, the exact cause must be determined in each case. The use of bursitis as an all-inclusive term denoting the diagnosis and basis for therapy in the painful shoulder syndrome is irrational.

Excluding traumatic causes, shoulder pain may radiate from a lesion of the cervical spine or may be the result of irritation from some other organ, such as the gallbladder or heart. However, most frequently shoulder pain originates as some derangement of the subacromial mechanism in the shoulder joint proper.

The subacromial mechanism of the shoulder joint is bounded above by the acromion and the coracoacromial ligament and below by the humeral head. The component structures of the shoulder include the subacromial, or sub-deltoid, bursa; the musculotendinous, or rotator, cuff; the articular capsule of the shoulder joint; and the tendon sheath gliding mechanism of the long head of the biceps brachii muscle.

The majority of patients with shoulder pain will be found to have some lesion involving a component of this mechanism. The use of the blanket term *bursitis* to explain all the derangements of the subacromial mechanism is the most important factor against successful management of the painful or stiff shoulder. All lesions of the subacromial mechanism may secondarily involve the subdeltoid bursa. It is rare that true, primary subdeltoid bursitis is encountered. The most frequent derangements of the subacromial mechanism that cause shoulder pain are calcific deposits in the musculotendinous cuff, bicipital tendinitis, lesions of the acromioclavicular joint, and adhesive capsulitis of the shoulder joint.

Procedure

With the patient's arm comfortably at the side, deep palpation of the shoulder by the examiner elicits a well-localized, tender area. With the examiner's finger still on the painful spot, the patient's arm is passively abducted by the examiner's other hand. The sign is present if, as the arm is abducted, the painful spot under the examiner's nonmoving finger disappears. The sign is significant for subacromial bursitis.

Confirmation Procedure

Diagnostic imaging

Reporting Statement

Dawbarn's sign is present in the right shoulder. This result indicates subacromial bursitis.

～ Clinical Pearl ～

Subacromial bursitis is not common as a primary condition. The condition may be caused by a direct blow over the shoulder. This blow causes an inflammatory reaction that is aggravated by further motion. Bursitis is usually a secondary reaction. The examiner should search for a primary lesion before commencing treatment.

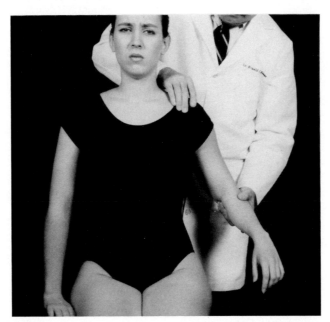

Fig. 4–37 The patient is seated with the arms comfortably at the side. The examiner palpates the affected shoulder deeply. A well-localized, tender area at the subacromial bursa is found.

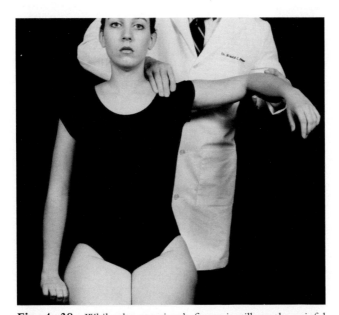

Fig. 4–38 While the examiner's finger is still on the painful spot, the patient's arm is passively abducted by the examiner's other hand. The sign is present when, as the arm is abducted, the painful spot disappears under the examiner's nonmoving finger. The sign is significant for subacromial bursitis.

Comment

Anterior dislocation is by far the most common pattern of shoulder dislocation. This type of dislocation occurs when the head of the humerus slips off and in front of the glenoid when the arm is abducted and extended.

Once off the glenoid, the head slips medially when the arm is lowered. This slipping produces the characteristic profile of a dislocated shoulder. Because the head of the humerus is not lying in its normal position, the shoulder has a flatter appearance than usual and the elbow points outward. If the tip of the acromion and the lateral epicondyle can be joined by a straight line (Hamilton's test), the shoulder is dislocated.

This appearance and the observation that the patient supports the injured arm with the other hand makes it possible for the examiner to diagnose a dislocated shoulder from the other end of the examination room. A similarly flattened contour is also seen in patients with atrophied deltoid muscles and in displaced fractures of the surgical neck. However, in these patients the humeral head is still in its normal position and the ruler test is negative.

Damage to the axillary nerve that occurs as it runs around the neck of the humerus causes partial or complete paralysis of the deltoid. The axillary nerve should be examined with an electromyogram (EMG) three and six weeks after the injury. If the examiner finds no change in pathologic findings between the two examinations, the nerve has been damaged and specific treatment may be necessary.

Brachial plexus injuries also occur if there has been a violent abduction strain.

If dislocation occurs and causes neurologic damage, the results are often poor.

The axillary artery can be damaged by traction at the time of injury or by pressure from the humeral head. The radial pulse should be checked, and its presence should be recorded.

The humeral head occasionally buttonholes through the subscapularis. This action makes reduction impossible.

Procedure

The patient places the hand of the affected shoulder on the opposite shoulder and attempts to touch the chest with the elbow. The test is positive if the patient cannot touch the chest wall with the elbow. The test is positive in shoulder dislocation.

Confirmation Procedures

Apprehension test, Bryant's sign, Calloway's test, Hamilton's test, Mazion's shoulder maneuver, diagnostic imaging

Reporting Statement

Dugas' test is positive on the right shoulder. This result indicates shoulder dislocation.

～ Clinical Pearl ～

In exceptional circumstances the humeral head can become jammed below the glenoid with the arm pointing directly upward (luxatio erecta), presenting a spectacular appearance sometimes mistaken for hysteria. This condition is a true, inferior dislocation. In contrast to anterior dislocation, the humeral head in this situation lies against the vessels and can cause ischemia. The rotator cuff is always damaged.

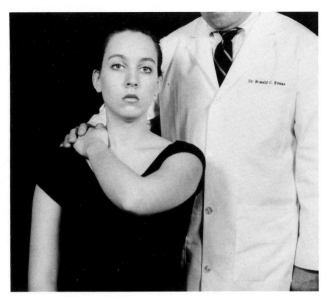

Fig. 4—39 The patient is seated comfortably with the arms at the sides. The patient places the hand of the affected shoulder on the opposite shoulder and attempts to touch the chest with the elbow.

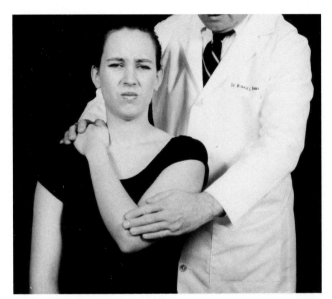

Fig. 4—40 If the patient cannot touch the chest wall with the elbow, the examiner confirms this by gently applying pressure to the elbow, attempting to approximate the elbow to the chest. Inability to move the elbow or increased pain is a positive sign. A presence of the sign indicates shoulder subluxation or dislocation.

Comment

Thoracic outlet syndrome describes the signs and symptoms resulting from proximal compression of the neurovascular structures supplying the upper limb.

The normal anatomy of the thoracic outlet, which extends from the intervertebral foramina and superior mediastinum to the axilla, must be considered not only in one plane but also in three dimensions to appreciate the potential mechanisms of compression.

The scalene muscles, which are the flexors and rotators of the neck, were formerly considered major causes of compression. This belief led not only to the term *scalenus anticus syndrome* but also to therapy directed solely at the release of these structures (scalenotomy). This method of therapy is a simple procedure with a high failure rate.

With many potential causes for compression, the three structures at risk—the subclavian artery, the vein, and the lower trunk of the brachial plexus—may be affected to significantly different degrees. The typical patient is likely to be a woman between the ages of 20 and 40. The ratio of women with thoracic outlet syndrome to men with the syndrome is 5:1. Complaints are often vague and hard to define.

Procedure

With the patient seated, the examiner assesses the patient's blood pressure bilaterally and records it. The examiner also assesses the character of the patient's radial pulse bilaterally. A difference of 10 mm Hg between the two systolic blood pressures and a feeble or absent radial pulse suggests possible subclavian artery stenosis or occlusion on the side of the feeble or absent pulse. If the test is negative, the examiner places a stethoscope over the supraclavicular fossa and auscultates the subclavian artery for bruits. If bruits are present, subclavian artery stenosis or occlusion is suspected.

Confirmation Procedures

Adson's test, Allen maneuver, costoclavicular maneuver, Halstead maneuver, reverse Bakody maneuver, Roos' test, shoulder compression test, Wright's test

Reporting Statement

The results of George's screening procedure suggest subclavian artery stenosis or occlusion on the right.

∾ Clinical Pearl ∾

The shoulder joint can be linked with the hand in a symptom complex presenting the features of a reflex sympathetic disturbance. The shoulder symptoms may be due, in part, to the neurovascular upset that develops as a result of sympathetic stimulation. Usually the shoulder complaint is secondary to some other factor, but the reflex dystrophy phenomenon has become so predominant that it is mislabeled as the cause when it is actually a result.

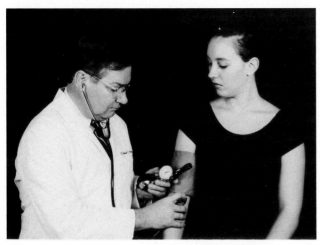

Fig. 4–41 The patient is seated. The examiner bilaterally assesses the patient's blood pressure and records the findings.

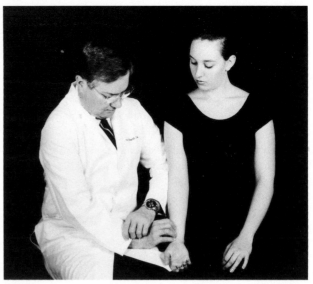

Fig. 4–42 The examiner bilaterally determines the character of the patient's radial pulse. A difference of 10 mm Hg between the two systolic blood pressures and a feeble or absent radial pulse suggests subclavian artery stenosis or occlusion on the side of the feeble or absent pulse.

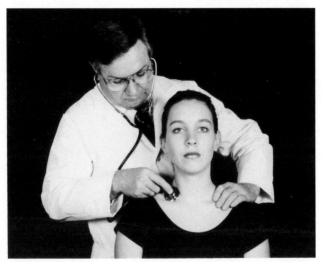

Fig. 4–43 If the first two procedures are negative, the examiner places a stethoscope over the supraclavicular fossa and auscultates the subclavian artery for bruits. If bruits are present, the screening procedure suggests a possible subclavian artery stenosis or occlusion.

Comment

Further out from the spinal cord, the nerve roots are grouped into trunks and cords that become intimately associated with the vascular bundle of the arm. The union takes place above the clavicle at a point where an additional cervical rib or tight scalenus anterior muscle may partially block the combined neurovascular bundle.

Compression of this bundle results in radiating discomfort and shoulder pain. However, the character of the pain changes from a well-defined neural pattern to a broad, more-vague discomfort because of the vascular association. The general properties of both these pain conditions should be appreciated. Both conditions produce an aching neck and shoulder pain, a feeling of numbness, and tingling down the arm to the fingers. The inner aspect of the forearm and hand is the site usually involved, as opposed to the outer aspect of the thumb and index finger in the common cervical root lesions. The tingling that occurs frequently involves all the fingers and produces a sense of fullness in the hand. If motor and sensory signs develop, they involve the ulnar supply most often because of pressure on the medial cord of the plexus. The small muscles of the hand may be involved, but either median or ulnar groups are singled out. This distribution of atrophy, following a definite peripheral nerve pattern, is in contrast to progressive muscular atrophy, in which there is generalized involvement that does not follow a specific pattern.

Shoulder and arm movements are not particularly involved in either cervical rib or scalenus anticus disorders.

Points of tenderness and soreness may be identified in the supraclavicular region away from the shoulder area proper and lying above the clavicle. When neck pain is present, it tends to be at the front, which is in contrast to the posterior discomfort of fibrositis and postural disorders.

Procedure

The examiner finds the radial pulse of the affected arm and applies downward traction on the extremity. The patient then hyperextends the neck. The absence, disappearance, or noted decrease in pulse pressure indicates a positive test. If the test is negative, it is repeated with the patient rotating the head to the opposite side. A positive test indicates thoracic outlet syndrome.

Confirmation Procedures

Adson's test, Allen maneuver, costoclavicular maneuver, George's screening procedure, reverse Bakody maneuver, Roos' test, shoulder compression test, Wright's test

---

Reporting Statement

Halstead maneuver is positive on the right shoulder. This result suggests the existence of thoracic outlet syndrome.

∼ Clinical Pearl ∼

Raynaud's disease, acroparesthesia, and thromboangiitis obliterans may be confused with thoracic outlet compression syndromes, but actually the former three conditions differ profoundly from outlet compression syndromes because Raynaud's disease, acroparesthesia, and thromboangiitis obliterans are not accompanied by shoulder discomfort, have no correlation to arm or shoulder movement, and are not affected by body posture.

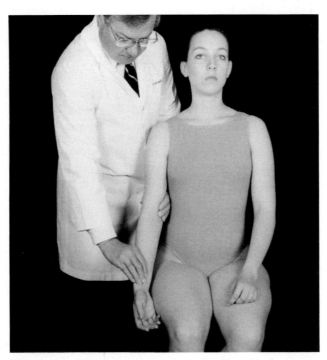

Fig. 4–44   The patient is seated comfortably with the arms at the sides. The examiner palpates the radial pulse of the affected arm.

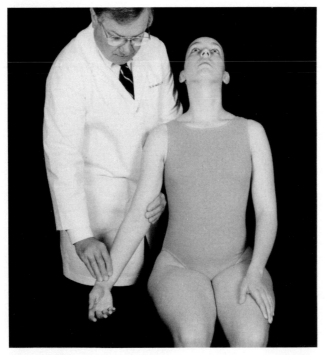

Fig. 4–45   The examiner applies downward traction on the affected extremity while the patient hyperextends the neck. Disappearance of the pulse is a positive test. A positive test indicates thoracic outlet syndrome. If the pulse does not disappear, the test is repeated with the patient's head rotated to the opposite side.

Comment

One of the tributes exacted for the superb mobility of the shoulder is frequent dislocation. A dislocated shoulder is an injury of the young, in whom it occurs more often than fracture of the neck of the humerus. Solid, healthy bone withstands abduction and twisting strain, but the weak capsule of the young gives way. Later in life the bone becomes soft and the capsule contracts, so abduction and twisting result in shaft breaks while the joint remains intact. Young adults suffer this injury often. The most common accident that causes a dislocated shoulder is a fall with the arm outstretched for protection. The contribution of the elbow and body weight have been somewhat overlooked in explaining the mechanism of this injury. The essential episode is that the head of the humerus is forced against the weak, anterior or anteroinferior capsule. In a fall the outstretched hand absorbs the impact while the elbow is extended. As long as this extension is retained, a solid strut transmits the force to the superior or posterosuperior joint structures. The weight of the body alters this situation. As full weight is applied, momentary giving way or buckling of the elbow is inevitable. This breaks the solid strut, and the elbow must flex, which tilts the upper end of the humerus downward and forward. As the fall continues, the head slips off the glenoid rim easily. At this point the extremity is in abduction and external rotation, exposing the posterosuperior part of the humeral head to the glenoid rim. The rim usually gets cut or creased. It is understandable that with repeated similar trauma, less and less force is needed to dislocate the humeral head. The humeral head commonly comes to lie at the front of the glenoid, resting on the rib. Occasionally the humeral head lies higher, just below the clavicle.

Procedure

If a straight edge (ruler or yardstick) can rest simultaneously on the acromial tip and the lateral epicondyle of the elbow, the test is positive. The positive test is significant for dislocation of the shoulder.

Confirmation Procedures

Apprehension test, Bryant's sign, Calloway's test, Dugas' test, Mazion's shoulder maneuver

---

Reporting Statement

Hamilton's test is positive for the right shoulder. This result indicates dislocation trauma of the shoulder.

~ **Clinical Pearl** ~

Fractures of the humeral head that result in several fragments are usually accompanied by dislocation. Fracture dislocations of the humeral head present several problems: (1) the fragment may obstruct reduction and make open reduction necessary, (2) the reduction will be very unstable, (3) soft-tissue damage and hemorrhage into and around the shoulder lead to joint stiffness, and (4) avascular necrosis of the humeral head can follow fractures through the anatomic neck.

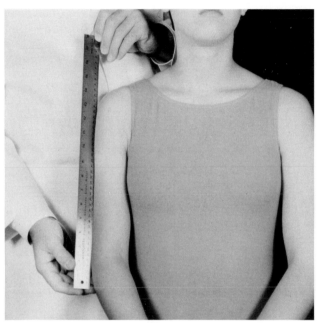

Fig. 4—46   The patient is seated comfortably with the arms at the sides. The examiner places a straight edge (ruler) at the lateral border of the affected shoulder from the acromion to the elbow. The test is positive if the straight edge can rest simultaneously on the acromial tip of the shoulder and the lateral epicondyle of the elbow. The test is significant for dislocation of the shoulder.

Comment

Tenosynovitis of the long head of the biceps is a common cause of shoulder pain in adults older than 40. This condition also may occur in young athletes, from repeated strains, such as those caused by the throwing motion. The basic lesion is an inflammation of the tendon and its sheath in the bicipital groove. The disorder may be primary or secondary to disease of the overlying rotator cuff.

The biceps tendon may rupture as a result of advanced degeneration from chronic tendinitis. The rupture is usually complete and may follow a forceful contraction of the biceps muscle.

The biceps tendon may occasionally dislocate from the bicipital groove. The usual cause is a tear in the overlying subscapularis tendon as the result of degenerative changes. The condition also may result from a congenitally shallow groove. The disorder also may occur in the young patient after forceful external rotation and abduction of the shoulder. Recurrences are frequent and may be reproducible by the patient. Tenosynovitis frequently develops and leads to pain and stiffness.

Procedure

The patient's arm is slightly abducted and moved fully through flexion by the examiner, causing a jamming of the greater tuberosity against the anteroinferior acromial surface. Pain in the shoulder is a positive test result. The test indicates an overuse injury to the supraspinatus and sometimes to the biceps tendon.

Confirmation Procedures

Apley's test, subacromial push button sign, supraspinatus press test, Codman's sign

---

Reporting Statement

Impingement sign is present in the right shoulder. This result indicates an overuse injury of the supraspinatus or biceps tendon.

~ **Clinical Pearl** ~

The old-fashioned concept of the hunching girdle rhythm as the telltale mark of supraspinatus rupture needs to be discarded. Without resistance a decrease in the range of motion may not be apparent. Always assess the motion against resistance. The presence of consistent weakness helps differentiate a tear from simple chronic tendinitis.

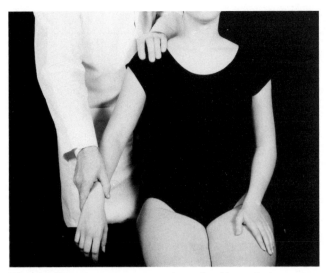

Fig. 4–47 The patient is seated comfortably with the arms at the sides. The examiner slightly abducts the patient's affected arm moving it through forward flexion.

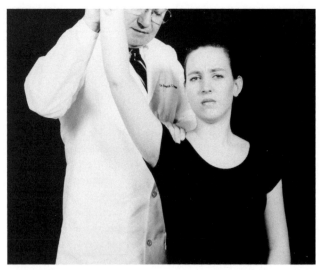

Fig. 4–48 Forward flexion causes jamming of the greater tuberosity against the anteroinferior acromial surface. Pain in the shoulder is a positive result. A positive test indicates an overuse injury to the supraspinatus and sometimes the biceps tendon.

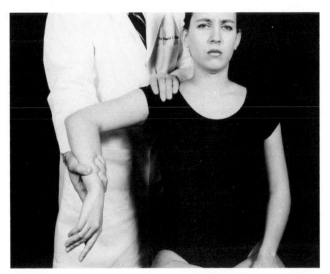

Fig. 4–49 The examiner can, as an alternative, internally rotate the affected shoulder. This rotation occurs while the shoulder is abducted to 90 degrees and flexed at the elbow. The arm also can be moved into flexion, which will produce the same jamming effect.

Comment

The tendon of the long head of the biceps arises from the tubercle on the superior rim of the glenoid fossa. The tendon passes in close approximation to the articular surface of the humeral head, toward the bicipital groove. Where it enters the groove, the tendon is covered by the transverse humeral ligament that extends between the tuberosities. The tendon becomes enveloped by a prolongation of the synovium, which enters the bicipital groove with the tendon. At the distal end of the bicipital groove the synovium is reflected backward to cover the extraarticular portion of the tendon. The groove is covered over by fascia extensions of the subscapularis tendon at the upper end and of the pectoralis major at the lower end. Before the tendon enters the groove, the intraarticular portion of it is superficially close to the capsule and the coracohumeral ligament. The coracohumeral ligament lies medially and laterally between the subscapularis and the supraspinatus. When movement occurs at the glenohumeral joint, the tendon glides within the groove. During abduction and forward flexion, the tendon glides distally. During adduction, extension, and external rotation, the tendon glides proximally into the joint.

Acute rupture of the biceps tendon occurs as a result of forceful contraction of the biceps muscle or forceful movement of the arm while the biceps muscle is contracted. The injury may be an avulsion of the tendon from the muscle belly or the tendon may rupture anywhere along its course or be pulled free from its attachment to the glenoid. The history is one of immediate, sharp pain, followed by tenderness along the course of the long head of the biceps. Diagnosis can be made by having the patient contract the biceps with the arm abducted and externally rotated with the elbow at 90 degrees. If the tear is complete, the muscle belly moves away from the rupture.

Procedure

The patient clasps both hands on top of or behind the head, allowing the interlocking fingers to support the weight of the upper limbs. This action allows maximum relaxation of the biceps tendon in its resting position. The patient then alternately contracts and relaxes the biceps muscles. While the patient completes the contractions and relaxations, the examiner palpates the biceps tendons. The tendon will be felt on the uninvolved side but not on the affected side. The absence of the tendon is a positive test result. A positive test indicates a rupture of the long head of the biceps tendon.

Confirmation Procedures

Abbott-Saunders test, Speed's test, transverse humeral ligament test, Yergason's test

---

Reporting Statement

Ludington's test is positive on the right. This result indicates disruption of the biceps tendon.

～ **Clinical Pearl** ～

Sometimes a double defect occurs, with the cuff giving way from the tuberosity on both sides of the tendon. Cuff laxity at this point seriously interferes with biceps function, and the tendon may slip medially, over the lesser tuberosity and off the head.

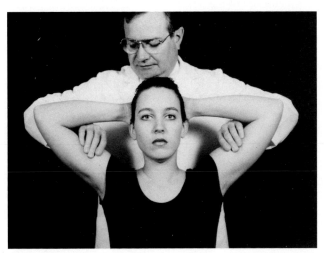

Fig. 4–50   While seated, the patient clasps both hands on top of or behind the head, allowing the interlocking fingers to support the weight of the upper limbs. The patient alternately contracts and relaxes the biceps muscles. While the patient completes the contractions and relaxations, the examiner palpates the biceps tendons. If the examiner can feel the tendon on the uninvolved side but not on the affected side, the test is positive. A positive test indicates a rupture of the long head of the biceps tendon.

Mazion's Shoulder Maneuver
SHOULDER ROCK TEST

Comment

Pain felt in the cervicobrachial area may extend from the occiput to the arm or, at times, to the upper anterior chest and back.

Muscle strain and nerve root compression often follow this distribution. Tendinitis, arthritis, and trigger points usually cause a more localized discomfort that enables the patient to pinpoint the source of the pathologic process. One notable exception is the pain of acute subdeltoid bursitis. In this condition the patient thinks that the discomfort can be located precisely in the musculature of the upper arm, but tenderness is always over the inflamed area, several centimeters higher, and beneath the acromion. Having the patient characterize the onset of the pain, including whether or not it was precipitated by acute or repeated trauma to the shoulder and neck, narrows the differential diagnosis. For example, continuous use of the arm above the head predisposes it to bursitis or tendinitis. Acute injury, of course, can result in obvious fractures or dislocations. Lacerations of the rotator cuff may be more elusive. Sudden lifting of a heavy object is all that is needed to tear the subacromial tendons.

Shoulder pain brought on by exertion, especially if the upper extremities are not being used, is more apt to be caused by coronary insufficiency than by localized pathologic process.

The clinical history may be the key to diagnosis. For example, adhesive capsulitis follows immobilization of the joint; shoulder-arm-hand syndrome is a complication of myocardial infarction; and fibromyositis is associated with emotional tension. Shoulder pain of arthritis and polymyalgia rheumatica is insidious at the onset. The pain from both of the conditions is worse in the morning, when the patient arises from sleep. Other disorders may be worse during the day. The temporal relationships of the pain are important to the diagnosis. Pain severity, constancy, and migratory nature are also important.

Procedure

While standing or sitting, the patient places the palm of the affected upper limb over the top of the opposite clavicle. From this position the patient moves the elbow from the chest to the forehead, giving it an inferior to superior rocking motion. The maneuver is positive if this action produces or aggravates shoulder or arm pain on the ipsilateral side. The pain of any significant pathologic process of the shoulder will be intensified and localized by this maneuver.

Confirmation Procedures

Apprehension test, Bryant's sign, Calloway's test, Dugas' test, Hamilton's test, diagnostic imaging

---

Reporting Statement

Mazion's shoulder maneuver is positive on the right. This result indicates significant pathologic process of the shoulder.

∼ Clinical Pearl ∼

Adhesive capsulitis is a common but ill-understood affliction of the glenohumeral joint. Capsulitis is characterized by pain and uniform limitation of all movements but without radiographic change and with a tendency to a slow spontaneous recovery. There is no evidence of inflammatory or destructive change.

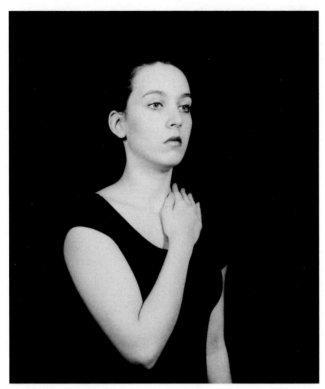

Fig. 4–51 While seated, the patient places the palm of the hand of the affected shoulder over the top of the opposite clavicle.

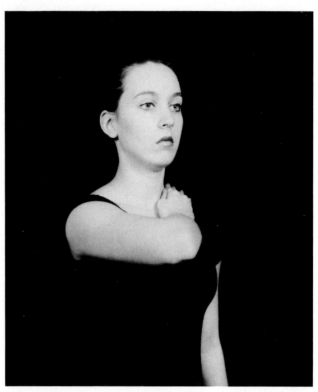

Fig. 4–52 The patient moves the elbow of the affected side from the chest toward the forehead.

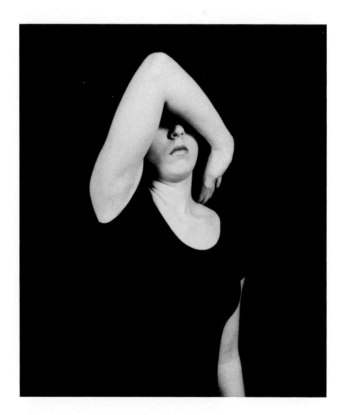

Fig. 4–53, right. This movement provides an inferior to superior rocking motion. The maneuver is positive if this action produces or aggravates shoulder or arm pain on the ipsilateral side. This maneuver will intensify and localize the pain of any significant shoulder pathology.

Comment

A cervical rib is a congenital overdevelopment, bony or fibrous, of the costal process of the seventh cervical vertebra. A cervical rib often exists, especially in the young, without causing symptoms. However, in adult life the tendency for gradual drooping of the shoulder girdle may lead to neurologic or vascular disturbance in the upper limb.

The overdeveloped costal process may be unilateral or bilateral, and it can range in size from a small bony protrusion, often with a fibrous extension, to a complete supernumerary rib. The subclavian artery and the lowest trunk of the brachial plexus arch over the rib. In some cases the nerve trunk suffers damage at the site of pressure against the rib. This accounts for the neurologic manifestations. The vascular changes are accounted for by local damage to the subclavian artery, from which thrombotic emboli may be repeatedly discharged into the peripheral vessels of the upper limb.

A cervical rib is often symptomless. When symptoms occur, they usually begin during adult life. They may be neurologic, vascular, or combined.

The sensory symptoms are pain and paresthesia in the forearm and hand. These symptoms are most marked toward the medial (ulnar) side and are often relieved temporarily by changing the position of the arm. The motor symptoms include increasing weakness of the hand with difficulty carrying out the finer movements.

There is usually an area of sensory impairment and sometimes complete anesthesia in the forearm and hand. The affected area does not correspond in distribution to any of the peripheral nerves but may be related to the lowest trunk of the brachial plexus. There may be atrophy of the muscles of the thenar eminence or of the interosseous and hypothenar muscles.

The vascular changes that have been observed range from dusky cyanosis of the forearm and hand to gangrene of the fingers. The radial pulse may be weak or absent.

The important alternative causes are (1) central lesions, such as tumors involving the spinal cord or its roots, (2) plexus lesions, such as tumors at the thoracic inlet (Pancoast tumor), (3) distal nerve lesions, such as friction neuritis of the ulnar nerve at the elbow, and (4) pressure on the median nerve in the carpal tunnel.

Occasionally the neurologic manifestations characteristic of a cervical rib occur without a demonstrable skeletal deformity. The manifestations may have been ascribed to trapping of the nerves between the first rib and the clavicle (costoclavicular compression) or between the first rib and the scalenus anterior muscle, or to stretching of the lowest trunk of the brachial plexus over the normal first rib. More often, they are caused by a tough fibrous band in the scalenus medius muscle that may lead to kinking of the lowest trunk of the brachial plexus. The symptoms are easily confused with those from a prolapsed intervertebral disc between C7 and T1.

Procedure

While in the seated position, the patient actively places the palm of the affected extremity on top of the head, raising the elbow to a height approximately level with the head. By elevating the arm, interscalene compression increases. The sign is present when the radiating pain appears or is worsened with this maneuver. The sign helps differentiate between cervical foraminal compression and interscalene compression.

Confirmation Procedures

Adson's test, Allen maneuver, costoclavicular maneuver, George's screening procedure, Halstead maneuver, Roos' test, shoulder compression test, Wright's test

---

Reporting Statement

The presence of brachial plexus compression is indicated by the presence of a reverse Bakody sign on the right.

~ Clinical Pearl ~

Radiographs will show the abnormal rib. If it is small, it is clearly observed in the oblique projections. In cases of suspected vascular obstruction, arteriography is required.

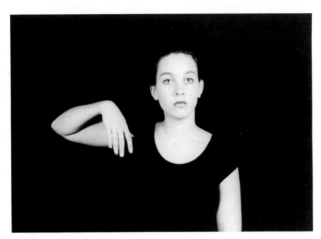

Fig. 4–54 While seated, the patient abducts and externally rotates the affected shoulder, moving the hand toward the top of the head.

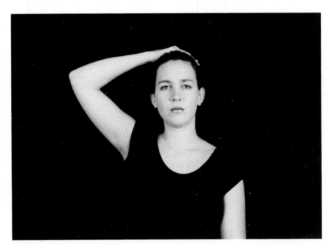

Fig. 4–55 The hand is placed on top of the head. The increase of pain in this position is a positive sign and indicates interscalene compression of the lower branches of the brachial plexus.

Comment

Costoclavicular syndrome occurs with compression of the subclavian artery, subclavian vein, and brachial plexus as they pass between the clavicle and the first rib. This syndrome is separate from the anterior scalene syndrome due to the vascular involvement.

The triangular costoclavicular space connects the cervical spine with the upper extremity and is called the canalis cervicoaxillaris. The boundaries of this space are the following: anteriorly, the medial third of the clavicle and the subclavius muscle; posteriorly, the upper margin of the scapula; and posteromedially, the anterior third of the first rib and the insertions of the anterior and medial scalene muscles. The neurovascular bundle runs in the medial angle of this triangle. The subclavian vein lies medially in front of the anterior scalenus insertion on the first rib and deep to the costoclavicular ligament and thickening of the clavipectoral fascia, which extends from the coracoid process to the first rib (costocoracoid ligament). The subclavian artery briefly enters this space via the posterior scalene foramen to lie lateral to the subclavian vein. Passing between the anterior and medial scalene muscles, the brachial plexus joins the vascular bundle in the costoclavicular space.

When the costoclavicular space becomes narrowed by disease or dynamic compression, the neuromuscular structures are compromised. Although congenital anomalies are associated with thoracic outlet syndrome, functional or dynamic anatomy predominates as an etiology for clinical disease. The following actions narrow the space: (1) raising the arm rotates the clavicle posteriorly into the space, (2) displacing the shoulder posteriorly and interiorly rotates the clavicle posteriorly, and (3) inhaling deeply raises the first rib into the space, because the clavicle does not rise with inspiration.

Patients with costoclavicular syndrome present similar subjective complaints as those with the anterior scalene syndrome (scalenus anticus syndrome). Although the neurologic complaints of pain, paresthesia, and hyperesthesia dominate in the anterior scalene syndrome, vascular symptoms dominate in the costoclavicular syndrome. Vein compression leads to temporary or permanent edema.

Clinical examination relies on the radial pulse evaluation, which occurs when the patient thrusts the chest forward and posteriorly and interiorly pulls the shoulders. Typically the pulse weakens or disappears.

Procedure

While in the seated position, the patient positions both arms at 90 degrees and abducts and externally rotates them. The patient repeatedly opens and closes the fists for 3 minutes. If this maneuver reproduces the usual symptoms of discomfort, the patient probably has thoracic outlet syndrome.

Confirmation Procedures

Adson's test, Allen maneuver, costoclavicular maneuver, George's screening procedure, Halstead maneuver, reverse Bakody maneuver, shoulder compression test, Wright's test

---

Reporting Statement

Roos' test is positive on the right. This result suggests thoracic outlet syndrome.

～ Clinical Pearl ～

Because all the neurologic, arterial, and venous symptoms are consistently aggravated by both exercise and arm elevation, the most reliable test for the diagnosis of thoracic outlet syndrome is the 3-minute, elevated-arm stress test.

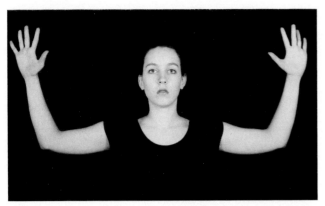

Fig. 4–56 While in the seated position, the patient places both arms in the 90 degree abducted and externally rotated position.

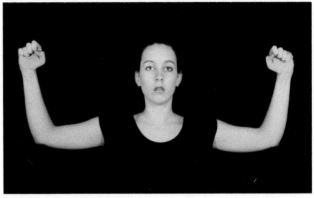

Fig. 4–57 The patient repeatedly opens and closes the fists slowly for three minutes.

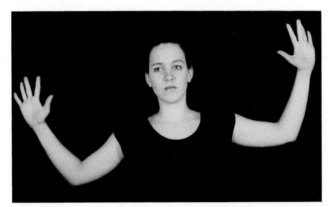

Fig. 4–58 If the test is positive, the usual symptoms are reproduced and the affected arm weakens. A positive test indicates thoracic outlet syndrome.

Comment

Clavipectoral compression syndrome is a disorder that produces shoulder and other radiating symptoms but does not belong to the cervical root or scalenus or cervical rib classes. The syndrome resembles the latter because the findings suggest a vascular or neurovascular etiology. Many forms of clavipectoral compression have been erroneously called scalene or cervical rib lesions. However, there are further distinguishing features that separate these conditions. The complete etiology and pathology have not been firmly established, so clinical attributes are largely relied upon for classification.

The symptom common to the group as a whole is paresthesia, or numbness and tingling, in the hand and fingers. Paresthesia develops after vague shoulder discomfort. The peripheral portion of the extremity—forearm, hand, and fingers—quickly becomes the seat of the prominent discomfort, and the shoulder symptoms fade. The paresthesia follows no well-defined distribution and the pattern is indistinct, particularly compared with the pain or numbness of peripheral nerve lesions. Frequently both sides are involved. The vascular contribution is manifested by coldness, cyanotic hue, and crampy pain on effort. Writer's cramp is an example. Many of the symptoms and disorders have a striking relation to the position of the arm or the head. In many instances the abducted position of the arm at work or rest is a potent irritant.

The fundamental pathologic process common to the group is stretching and compression of the neurovascular bundle at some point in the periclavicular, not clavicular, course. This possibility above the clavicle has been acknowledged in cervical rib and scalene lesions, but generally it has not been recognized that a similar disturbance may arise behind and below the clavicle as well. Pressure on the neurovascular bundle along the cervicoaxillary canal may develop directly behind the clavicle, below the clavicle, or behind the pectoralis minor. The bundle lies on a firm bed along its entire course, but the structures on top of it move in three separate zones. Superiorly, the clavicle rolls up and down and may pinch vessels on the first rib. Lower down, the costocoracoid membrane, as a remnant of the precoracoid primitive forms, may tighten on the bundle through its connections with the enveloping fascia. Still more distally,

the sharp edge of the pectoralis minor may become the compressing force or fulcrum. A soft bundle on a hard bed is easily crushed by these structures. Several special types of compression may be recognized: costoclavicular, postural, and hyperabduction. These conditions are to be differentiated from the carpal tunnel syndrome, in which there is no shoulder involvement, and the numbness and tingling are clearly confined to the median nerve distribution.

Patients with the hyperabduction syndrome are usually young males of short, stocky stature, who work long hours with the arms held above the shoulder level. Shoulder pain and finger paresthesia develop. In some instances the discomfort appears without extreme abduction. Some patients are more prone than others to develop these symptoms. Patients prone to this condition are easily separated from the rest by their medical history, their youth, and the characteristically easy obliteration of the pulse during abduction.

Procedure

While the patient is seated upright, the examiner palpates the distal apex of the coracoid process and marks it with a flesh pencil. With a hypothenar contact the examiner applies downward pressure over the marked area. Production of symptoms that are similar to neurovascular compression of the subclavian artery and brachial plexus constitutes a positive test. The test is significant for coracoid pressure syndrome, which is identical to the hyperabduction type of thoracic outlet syndromes.

Confirmation Procedures

Adson's test, Allen maneuver, costoclavicular test, George's screening procedure, Halstead maneuver, reverse Bakody maneuver, Roos' test, Wright's test

---

Reporting Statement

Shoulder compression test on the right is positive. This result indicates thoracic outlet compression due to coracoid pressure.

℘ Clinical Pearl ℘

The neurovascular bundle may be compressed in the zone distal to the clavicle as the bundle passes beneath the costocoracoid membrane and pectoralis minor. The pectoralis minor has a particular contribution in this process and is a significant factor in creating the shoulder and radiating symptoms.

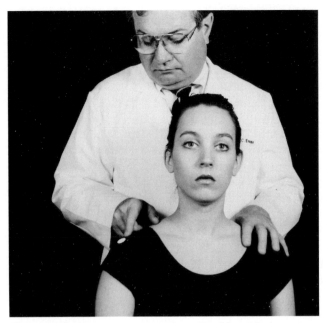

Fig. 4–59   The patient is seated comfortably with the arms at the sides. The examiner palpates the distal apex of the coracoid process and marks it.

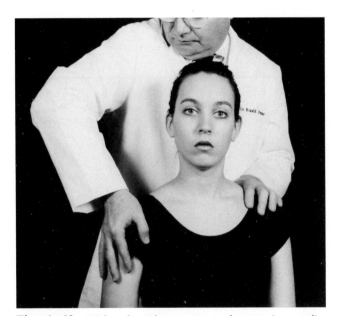

Fig. 4–60   With a hypothenar contact the examiner applies downward pressure over the marked area. If the symptoms produced are similar to neurovascular compression of the subclavian artery and brachial plexus, then this constitutes a positive test. The test is significant for coracoid pressure syndrome, which is identical to the hyperabduction-type of thoracic outlet syndromes.

Comment

The long head of the biceps arises by a long, narrow tendon from the supraglenoid tubercle of the scapula. The long head passes through the shoulder joint and emerges from it to lie in the intertubercular sulcus (bicipital groove), where it is restrained by the transverse humeral ligament. The long head of the biceps is subject to the same type of impingement as the supraspinatus tendon, and it is difficult, at first, to differentiate between the two. One distinguishing feature relates to internal and external rotation of the shoulder. In cases of bicipital tendinitis, rotation during abduction is usually painful, especially if the examiner applies slight pressure to the tendon in its groove while the patient's arm is passively maneuvered. In patients with supraspinatus tendinitis, the internally rotated position may be painful, but this pain will disappear when the humerus is rotated outward, because the greater tubercle of the humerus no longer impinges on the acromion process.

The slight difference in the mechanics of these two types of tendinitis means that bicipital tendinitis occurs more often in patients who participate in activities involving throwing or paddling. Of course bicipital tendinitis may occur in swimmers or other patients as well. Bicipital tendinitis is sometimes secondary to supraspinatus tendinitis because the latter may be accompanied by inflammation that involves the nearby biceps.

Procedure

The examiner resists flexion of the shoulder by the patient. The patient's forearm is supinated and the elbow is completely extended. A positive test reveals increased tenderness in the bicipital groove, which indicates bicipital tendinitis.

Confirmation Procedures

Abbott-Saunders test, Ludington's test, transverse humeral ligament test, Yergason's test

---

Reporting Statement

Speed's test is positive on the right. This result indicates bicipital tendinitis.

~ Clinical Pearl ~

Tenosynovitis in the bicipital groove may develop into complete adherence of the tendon. This interdicts any extensive range of motion of the shoulder. The shoulder motion may remain restricted or the biceps may rupture proximal to the groove.

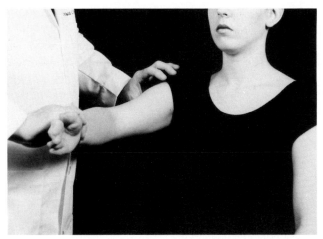

Fig. 4−61 While seated, the patient flexes the affected shoulder, and the examiner provides resistance.

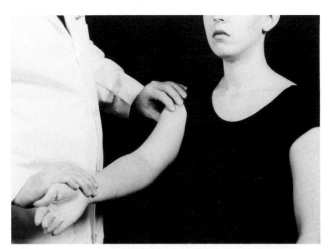

Fig. 4−62 While flexing the shoulder, the patient supinates the forearm, and completely extends the elbow. A positive test elicits increased tenderness in the bicipital groove and indicates bicipital tendinitis.

Subacromial Push Button Sign

MAZION'S CUFF MANEUVER

Comment

The rotator cuff is an almost complete tissue annulus that is attached to the humerus in the region of the anatomic neck and is formed by the fusion of the joint capsule with the musculotendinous insertions of the subscapularis in front, the supraspinatus above, and the teres minor and infraspinatus behind. The most important of these structures is the supraspinatus, which runs through a tunnel formed by the acromion and the coracoacromial ligament. The supraspinatus is separated from the acromion by part of the subdeltoid bursa.

The rotator cuff may suffer a large tear as a result of sudden traction to the arm. Such a tear occurs most readily in middle-age patients because of degenerative changes in the rotator cuff. Most commonly the supraspinatus region is involved, and the patient has difficulty initiating abduction of the arm. In other cases a torn or inflamed rotator cuff impinges the acromion during abduction, causing a painful arc of movement. Although the range of passive movement is not initially disturbed, limitation of rotation supersedes, so many of these cases become indistinguishable from those suffering adhesive capsulitis.

Procedure

The patient is seated with the upper extremities hanging limply at the sides. The examiner exerts strong finger or thumb pressure toward the midline at the clavicle, at a point even with the scapular spine. The production or increase of shoulder pain indicates a positive test. The test is significant for rotator cuff tear of the supraspinatus tendon.

Confirmation Procedures

Apley's test, impingement sign, supraspinatus press test, Codman's sign

---

Reporting Statement

Subacromial push button sign is positive on the right. This result indicates a rotator cuff tear of the supraspinatus tendon.

∽ Clinical Pearl ∽

Degenerative changes in the supraspinatus tendon may be accompanied by the local deposition of calcium salts. This process may continue without symptoms, although radiographic changes are obvious. However, sometimes the calcified material causes inflammatory changes in the subdeltoid area and results in sudden, severe, and incapacitating pain. When this occurs, the shoulder is acutely tender and is often swollen and warm to the touch.

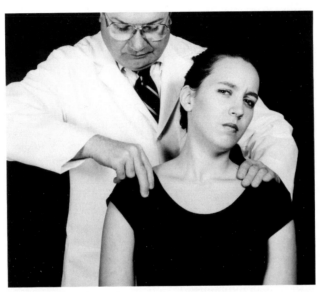

Fig. 4-63 The patient is seated with the upper extremities hanging limply at the sides. The examiner exerts strong finger or thumb pressure toward the midline of the clavicle, at a point even with the scapular spine. The production or increase of shoulder pain is a positive test. The test is significant for a rotator cuff tear, specifically a tear of the supraspinatus tendon.

Comment

Supraspinatus syndrome (painful arc syndrome) is characterized by pain in the shoulder and upper arm during midrange abduction of the glenohumeral with freedom from pain at the extremes of the range. The syndrome is common to five distinct shoulder lesions (supraspinatus tendon tear, supraspinatus tendon inflammation, calcific deposits in the supraspinatus tendon, subacromial bursitis, and undisplaced fracture of the greater tuberosity).

The pain is produced mechanically by nipping of a tender structure between the tuberosity of the humerus and the acromion process and coracoacromial ligament.

Even in the normal shoulder, the clearance between the upper end of the humerus and the acromion process is small during abduction between the range of 45 and 160 degrees. If a swollen and tender structure is present beneath the acromion, pain occurs during the arc of movement because the clearance is so small. In the neutral position and in full abduction, the clearance is greater and pain is less marked or absent.

Although five primary lesions cause the syndrome, these lesions only represent variations of the degeneration that is the underlying defect.

1. In minor tearing of the supraspinatus tendon, tearing or strain of a few degenerate tendon fibers causes an inflammatory reaction with local swelling. Power is not as significantly impaired as it is after a complete tear of the rotator cuff.

2. With supraspinatus tendinitis there is an inflammatory reaction provoked by the degeneration of the tendon fibers.

3. Calcific deposits in the supraspinatus tendon occur when a white, chalky deposit forms within the degenerate tendon, and the lesion is surrounded by an inflammatory reaction. Pain occurs when the calcified material bursts into the surrounding tissue.

4. With subacromial bursitis, the bursal walls are inflamed and thickened by mechanical irritation.

5. With injury to the greater tuberosity, a contusion or undisplaced fracture of the greater tuberosity is a frequent cause.

Whatever the primary cause, the clinical syndrome has the same general features, although they vary in degree. With the arm dependent, pain is absent or minimal. During abduction of the arm, pain begins at about 45 degrees and persists up to 160 degrees of movement. Above 160 degrees, the pain lessens or disappears. Pain is experienced again during descent from full elevation, in the middle arc of the range. Often the patient will twist or circumduct the arm grotesquely to lower it as painlessly as possible. The severity of the pain varies from case to case. When the calcified deposit is in the supraspinatus tendon, the pain may be so intense that the patient is scarcely able to move the shoulder and is driven to seek emergency treatment.

Procedure

The patient's shoulder is abducted to 90 degrees, and the examiner provides resistance to this abduction. The shoulder is then medially rotated and angled 30 degrees forward, so the patient's thumbs point to the floor. The examiner again provides resistance to abduction while observing for weakness or pain. If the patient exhibits weakness or experiences pain, the test is positive, which indicates a tear of the supraspinatus tendon or muscle.

Confirmation Procedures

Apley's test, Codman's sign, impingement sign, subacromial push button sign

---

Reporting Statement

Supraspinatus test is positive on the right. This result indicates a tear of the supraspinatus tendon.

∿ **Clinical Pearl** ∿

Painful arc syndrome is sometimes confused with arthritis of the acromioclavicular joint, which also causes pain during a certain phase of the abduction arc. However, with acromioclavicular arthritis, the pain begins later in abduction (not below 90 degrees) and increases, rather than diminishes, as full elevation is achieved.

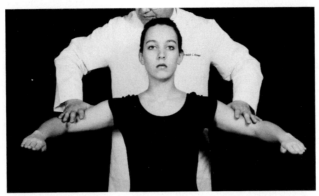

Fig. 4–64 While the patient is seated, the shoulders are abducted to 90 degrees with the arm in neutral rotation. The examiner provides resistance to abduction.

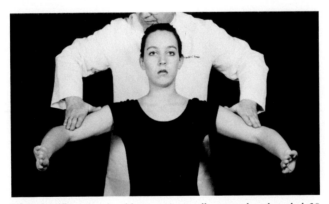

Fig. 4–65 The shoulders are internally rotated and angled 30 degrees forward, so the patient's thumbs point to the floor. The examiner again provides resistance to abduction. A positive test is indicated by pain or weakness in the affected shoulder, compared to the unaffected side. A positive test indicates a tear of the supraspinatus tendon or muscle.

Comment

Below and medial to the coracoacromial ligament, the long head of the biceps may be palpated beneath the capsule. The long head of the biceps is held in the groove by the transverse humeral ligament, a thickened prolongation of the capsule extending between the lesser and greater tuberosities. The critical zones in the structure are (1) the point at which the tendon arches over the humeral head and (2) the point where the floor on which the tendon glides changes from bony cortex to articular cartilage.

Dimensions of the groove vary widely. Deep narrow apertures favor constriction of the tendon, and shallow flat grooves allow slipping and subluxation of the tendon. If the cuff zone at the top of the groove is torn, the tendon may slip out of the groove, particularly if the arm is abducted and externally rotated. Similarly, if strong force is applied while the arm is abducted and externally rotated, the tendon may be wrenched out of the groove.

Procedure

The patient's shoulder is abducted and internally rotated by the examiner. The examiner's fingers are then placed along the bicipital groove and the patient's shoulder is externally rotated. If the examiner feels the tendon snap in and out of the groove as the external rotation occurs, this is an indication of a positive test. A positive test indicates a torn transverse humeral ligament.

Confirmation Procedures

Abbott-Saunders test, Ludington's test, Speed's test, Yergason's test

---

Reporting Statement

Transverse humeral ligament test is positive on the right. This result indicates a torn transverse humeral ligament.

∼ Clinical Pearl ∼

Conditions involving the bicipital tendon and the bicipital groove are particularly pertinent to athletes because many sports involve the throwing motion of the arm. These athletes include the baseball pitcher, the football quarterback, the batter, and the tennis player. The throwing motion is especially inhibited by bicipital tendon problems. It is especially pertinent to recognize if the defect is an adhesive tenosynovitis, fraying of the tendon, or subluxation or dislocation of the tendon.

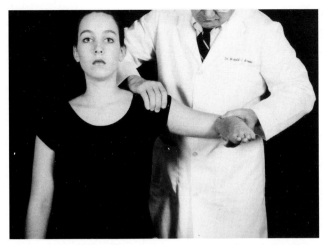

Fig. 4–66 The patient is seated, and the affected shoulder is abducted with the elbow flexed to 90 degrees.

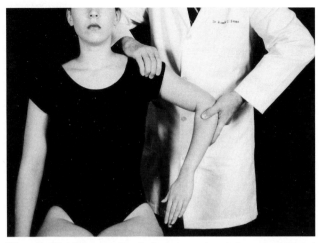

Fig. 4–67 The examiner's fingers are placed along the bicipital groove, and the patient's shoulder is internally rotated.

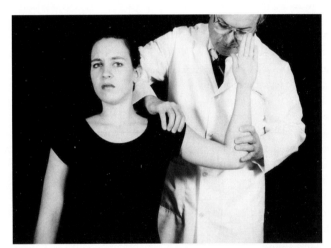

Fig. 4–68 While maintaining palpation of the bicipital groove, the examiner externally rotates the shoulder. If the examiner feels the tendon snap in and out of the groove as the external rotation occurs, this is a positive test. A positive test indicates a torn transverse humeral ligament.

Comment

With repetitive or prolonged hyperabduction of the arm, the neurovascular bundle in the axilla can be stretched under the pectoralis minor tendon and the coracoid process, resulting in symptoms of neurovascular compression.

When leaving the costoclavicular space, the three cords of the brachial plexus, the subclavian artery, and the subclavian vein pass under the insertion of the pectoralis minor muscle on the coracoid process. As this neurovascular bundle enters the axillary fossa, the artery and vein become known as the axillary artery and the axillary vein. As the upper extremity is abducted to 180 degrees, the neurovascular bundle is stretched around a fulcrum, which consists of the tendon of the pectoralis minor, the coracoid process, and the humeral head. The bundle almost reaches an angle of 90 degrees around the fulcrum. Unfortunately, the neurovascular bundle's course remains fixed, allowing no motion of the bundle. Compression at the fulcrum and tension along its components is the only way the bundle can compensate. Abduction of the arm produces a 30 degree elevation and a 35 degree posterior displacement of the clavicle, thereby narrowing the costoclavicular tunnel. The tunnel's anterior wall—consisting also of the pectoralis minor muscle, the subclavius muscle, and the costoclavicular ligament (the thickening of the clavipectoral fascia)—is stretched and brought posteriorly further, pushing the neurovascular bundle against the fulcrum.

There are two critical anatomic points where compression of the neurovascular bundle may occur when the arm is hyperabducted. The first is where the bundle passes through the costoclavicular tunnel, or slit. The second is where the bundle passes under the pectoralis minor tendon at its insertion on the coracoid process. During abduction of the arm the fixed neurovascular bundle can be compressed by the tendon of the pectoralis minor muscle as well as by the humeral head. The characteristic position that produces this compression is 180 degrees abducted and elbow flexion. This position commonly occurs during sleep or in certain occupations, such as that of electricians, painters, bricklayers, dry-wall hangers, or masons.

Pain, paresthesia, and numbness develop first in the fingers and later in the hand. In some patients transitory ischemia and edema develop. These symptoms may resemble Raynaud's disease, and are present in 38% of the patients with hyperabduction syndrome. Neurologic symptoms are usually absent in hyperabduction syndrome because as paresthesia and pain develop, the patient corrects the arm position, so the nerve compression only lasts for a short time. If the arm is abducted to 180 degrees in patients with hyperabduction syndrome, symptoms can increase. The radial artery pulse may weaken or disappear. However, just as tests for the anterior scalene syndrome or the costoclavicular syndrome can be positive in a normal position, the same results can be found when testing for the hyperabduction syndrome.

Procedure

Before this test is started, the Allen test at the wrist is performed to establish patency of the radial arteries.

The patient is seated, with both arms hanging at the sides. The examiner palpates the patient's radial pulse. Both arms, in turn, are passively abducted to 180 degrees. The examiner notes the angle of abduction at which the radial pulse diminishes or disappears on the affected side. The examiner compares the results with those on the unaffected side. The test is significant for neurovascular compromise of the axillary artery, as seen in the hyperabduction thoracic outlet syndromes. Many patients have cessation of the radial pulse upon abduction without the hyperabduction syndrome being present. If the nonaffected limb demonstrates radial pulse dampening or cessation, at the same approximate degree of abduction as the affected side, the test is not positive for hyperabduction syndrome.

Confirmation Procedures

Adson's test, Allen maneuver, costoclavicular maneuver, George's screening procedure, Halstead maneuver, reverse Bakody maneuver, Roos' test, shoulder compression test

Reporting Statement

Wright's test is positive on the right. This result indicates hyperabduction thoracic outlet compression syndrome.

∾ Clinical Pearl ∾

In most instances of compression hyperabduction of the shoulder obliterates the radial pulse, but obliteration of the radial pulse also may occur in the normal extremity. However, there is a difference. On the affected side the marginal position is reached sooner than on the normal side. The marginal position is the level of abduction just below that which produces obliteration of the pulse. Frequently the patient is aware of the exact level of abduction at which the symptoms occur.

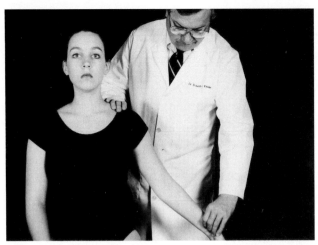

Fig. 4–69   The patient is seated with both arms hanging at the sides. The examiner palpates the radial pulse of the affected arm.

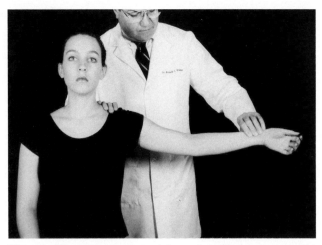

Fig. 4–70   The examiner abducts the affected arm to 180 degrees.

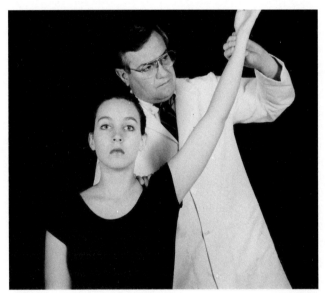

Fig. 4–71   The examiner notes the angle of abduction at which the radial pulse on the affected side diminishes or disappears. This angle is compared with the angle obtained on the unaffected side. The test is significant for neurovascular compromise of the axillary artery, as seen in the hyperabduction thoracic outlet syndromes. If the nonaffected arm demonstrates radial pulse dampening or cessation at the same approximate angle of abduction, the test is not positive for hyperabduction syndrome.

Comment

The long head of the biceps follows a tortuous and hemmed-in course from its origin in the muscle belly to the supraglenoid tubercle. The type of trauma that usually produces tenosynovitis (for example, in the wrist) is one heavy blow or repeated blows, resulting in constrictive adhesions. This is not the mechanism commonly encountered at the long head of the biceps. The bicipital area is not nearly so vulnerable to direct trauma as the more distal regions of the extremity, so tendinitis and tenosynovitis may develop gradually without definite acute episodes of injury.

Following an activity such as the first game of the season for badminton or tennis or a jerking strain after lifting with outstretched arms, discomfort is noted in the shoulder. At first the ache is indefinite and is not plainly related to motions that use the biceps tendon. Later more acute pain develops and the patient avoids lifting and keeps the arm at the side with the elbow flexed because this is the position of maximum comfort.

Examination reveals tenderness at the top and front of the shoulder. This tenderness is related to the tendon course across the upper end of the humerus. The tenderness follows into the bicipital groove and along the tendon into the arm. Deep palpation at the medial border of the deltoid delineates tenderness when pressure is applied along the tendon as the arm is rotated externally and internally. Flexion of the elbow and supination of the hand against resistance may produce pain that is referred to the front and inner aspects of the shoulder. In all shoulder lesions in which involvement of the biceps mechanism is suspected, diagnostic images that show the groove in profile should be acquired. With tendinitis or tenosynovitis, bony abnormalities are not unusual, but any abnormal contour of the groove may predispose the patient to development of the condition. If the groove is too flat or shallow, the tendon may slip out. If the groove is too deep, the tendon is roughened and squeezed. If there is spur formation, the tendon may become frayed.

Procedure

The patient flexes the elbow while seated. The examiner resists the patient's attempt to supinate the hand. Then the patient resists the examiner's efforts to extend the affected upper extremity. The test is positive if pain over the intertubercular groove develops or is aggravated. A positive sign indicates tenosynovitis or involvement of the transverse humeral ligament. This test is not conclusive because motion does not occur between the tendon and the bicipital groove during the test. Biceps tendon pain tends to occur during motion rather than during tension.

Confirmation Procedures

Abbott-Saunders test, Ludington's test, Speed's test, transverse humeral ligament test

---

Reporting Statement

Yergason's test is positive on the right. This result indicates bicipital tenosynovitis or a torn transverse humeral ligament.

~ Clinical Pearl ~

The concept that the biceps tendon moves up and down the groove during motion at the glenohumeral joint is questionable. With the bicipital tendon and groove exposed under anesthesia, the biceps tendon remains fixed in the groove during motion. However, the head of the humerus glides up and down the tendon. Contraction of the biceps muscle, by supinating the forearm or flexing the elbow, makes the tendon taut but produces no motion of the tendon in the groove. All movements of the shoulder joint, regardless of the plane in which the arm is elevated, are accompanied by gliding motions of the humerus on the tendon.

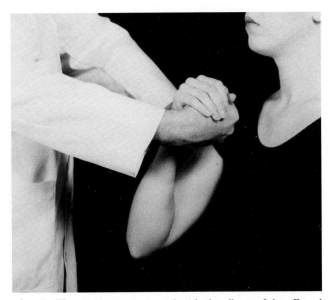

Fig. 4–72   The patient is seated with the elbow of the affected arm flexed. The patient resists the examiner's efforts to extend the upper extremity.

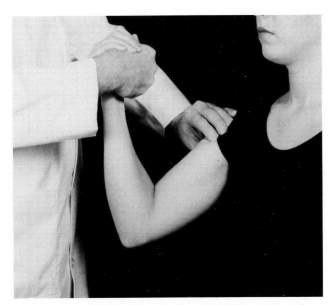

Fig. 4–73   The examiner resists the patient's attempt to supinate the forearm. The test is positive if pain develops or is aggravated over the intertubercular groove. A positive test indicates biceps tenosynovitis or involvement of the transverse humeral ligament.

Bibliography

American Medical Association: *Guides to the evaluation of permanent impairment,* ed 3, 1990, Chicago.

Apley AG, Solomon L: *Concise system of orthopaedics and fractures,* London, 1988, Butterworth-Heinemann.

Bateman JE: The diagnosis and treatment of ruptures of the rotator cuff, *Surg Clin North Am,* 43:1523, 1963.

Bateman JE: *The shoulder and neck,* ed 2, Philadelphia, 1978, WB Saunders.

Bateman JE: *Trauma to nerves in limbs,* Philadelphia, 1962, WB Saunders.

Bland JH, Merrit JA, Boushey DR: The painful shoulder, *Semin Arthritis Rheum,* 7:21–47, 1977.

Bozyk Z: Shoulder-hand syndrome in patients with antecedent myocardial infarctions, *Revmatologiia (mosk),* 6:103–106, 1968.

Bush LH: The torn shoulder capsule, *J Bone Joint Surg,* 57A:256, 1975.

Cailliet R: *Shoulder pain,* Philadelphia, 1966, FA Davis.

Cinquegranao D: Chronic cervical radiculitis and its relationship to "chronic bursitis", *Am J Phys Med Rehabil,* 47:23–30, 1968.

Cipriano JJ: *Photographic manual of regional orthopaedic and neurological tests,* ed 2, Baltimore, 1991, Williams & Wilkins.

Codman EA: *The shoulder,* Boston, 1934, published by author.

Curwin S, Stanish WD: *Tendinitis: Its etiology and treatment,* Lexington, 1984, The Collamore Press.

D'Ambrosia RD: *Musculoskeletal disorders regional examination and differential diagnosis,* Philadelphia, 1977, JB Lippincott.

Dandy DJ: *Essential orthopaedics and trauma,* Edinburgh, 1989, Churchill Livingstone.

Debeyre J, Patte D, Elmelik E: Repair of ruptures of the rotator cuff of the shoulder, *J Bone Joint Surg,* 47B:36, 1965.

DePalma AF: *Surgery of the shoulder,* ed 2, Philadelphia, 1973, JB Lippincott.

Doherty M, Doherty J: *Clinical examination in rheumatology,* London, 1992, Wolfe Publishing.

Engelman RM: Shoulder pain as a presenting complaint in upper lobe bronchogenic carcinoma: Report of 21 cases, *Conn Med* 30:273–276, 1966.

Finke J: Neurologic differential diagnosis: The lower cervical region, *Dtsch Med Wochenschr,* 90:1912–1917, 1965.

Gascon J: A current problem: Diagnosis of the shoulder pain syndrome, *Union Med Can,* 94:463–469, 1965.

Goldie I: Calcified deposits in the shoulder joint produced by calciphylaxis and their inhibition by triamcinolone: an experimental model, *Bull Soc Int Chir* 23:91, 1965.

Hale MS: *A practical approach to arm pain,* Springfield, IL, 1971, Charles C Thomas.

Hawkins RJ, Kennedy JC: Impingement syndrome in athletics, *Am J Sports Med,* 8:141, 1980.

Katz WA: *Rheumatic diseases diagnosis and management,* Philadelphia, 1977, JB Lippincott.

Kendall HO, Kendall FP, Wadsworth GE: *Muscles testing and function,* ed 2, Baltimore, 1971, Williams & Wilkins.

Kessel L, Watson M: The painful arc syndrome: Clinical classification as a guide to management, *J Bone Joint Surg,* 59B:166, 1977.

Lain TM: The military brace syndrome: A report of 16 cases of Erb's palsy occurring in military cadets, *J Bone Joint Surg,* 51A:557–560, 1969.

Leffert RD et al: Infra-clavicular brachial plexus injuries, *J Bone Joint Surg,* 47B:9–22, 1965.

Lucas DB: Biomechanics of the shoulder joint, *Arch Surg,* 107:425–432, 1973.

Magee DJ: *Orthopedic physical assessment,* Philadelphia, 1987, WB Saunders.

Mazion JM: *Illustrated manual of neurological reflexes/signs/tests, Part I; Orthopedic Signs/Tests/Maneuvers For Office Procedure, Part II,* Orlando, 1980, Daniels Publishing.

McLaughlin HL: The "frozen" shoulder, *Clin Orthop,* 20:126, 1961.

McRae R: *Clinical orthopaedic examination,* ed 3, Edinburgh, 1990, Churchill Livingstone.

Medical Economics Books: *Patient care flow chart manual,* ed 3, Oradell, NJ, 1982, Medical Economics Books.

Mercier LR, Pettid FJ: *Practical orthopedics,* Chicago, 1982, Mosby.

Merle D'Aubigne R: Nerve injuries in fractures and dislocations of the shoulder, *Surg Clin North Am,* 43:1685–1689, 1963.

Moseley HF: *Shoulder lesions,* ed 3, Baltimore, 1969, Williams & Wilkins.

Neer CS: Anterior acromioplasty for the chronic impingement syndrome in the shoulder, *J Bone Joint Surg,* 54A:41, 1972.

Neviaser JS: Musculoskeletal disorders of the shoulder region causing cervicobrachial pain: Differential diagnosis and treatment, *Surg Clin North Am,* 43:1703–1714, 1963.

O'Donoghue DH: *Treatment of injuries to athletes,* ed 3, Philadelphia, 1976, WB Saunders.

Omer GE, Spinner M: *Management of peripheral nerve problems,* Philadelphia, 1980, WB Saunders.

Parsons TA: The snapping scapula and subscapular exostosis, *J Bone Joint Surg,* 55B:345, 1963.

Pecina MM, Krompotic-Nemanic J, Markiewitz AD: *Tunnel syndromes,* Boston, 1991, CRC Press.

Polley HF, Hunder GG: *Rheumatologic interviewing and physical examination of the joints,* ed 2, Philadelphia, 1978, WB Saunders.

Quigley TB: The nonoperative treatment of symptomatic calcareous deposits in the shoulder, *Surg Clin North Am,* 43: 1495, 1963.

Roos DB et al: Thoracic outlet syndrome, *Arch Surg,* 93:71–74, 1966.

Selye H: The experimental production of calcified deposits in the rotator cuff, *Surg Clin North Am,* 43:1483–1488, 1963.

Steinbrocher O: The painful shoulder, in Hollander JL, McCarty DJ, eds: *Arthritis and allied conditions,* ed 8, Philadelphia, 1972, Lea & Febiger.

Thurston SE: *The little black book of neurology,* Chicago, 1987, Mosby.

Turek SL: *Orthopaedics principles and their application,* ed 3, Philadelphia, 1977, JB Lippincott.

Wright IS: Neurovascular syndrome produced by hyperabduction of the arms, *Am Heart J,* 29:I, 1945.

Wright IS et al: The subclavian steal and other shoulder girdle syndromes, *Trans Am Clin Climatol Assoc,* 76:13–25, 1964.

Wright IS: *Vascular diseases in clinical practice,* Chicago, 1948, Mosby.

Wright V: The shoulder-hand syndrome, *Rep Rheum Dis,* 24:1–2, 1966.

Yergason RM: Supination sign, *J Bone Joint Surg,* 12:160, 1931.

~ 5 ~

The Elbow

*A*lthough the number of diseases that affect the elbow with any degree of frequency is small, examining the joint often provides clues to diagnosis of specific rheumatic diseases. Pain is the symptom that focuses attention on this joint and prompts the patient to seek medical attention. Although the pain usually reflects a localized process at the elbow, the pain may be referred from the hand and wrist or from the shoulder and neck. Most actions of the elbow can be compensated for by the shoulder; therefore even moderate compromises of motion, provided they are painless, do not result in disability. Subtle flexion contractures may develop over a period of years without the patient even being aware of them. In contrast, significant pain at the elbow can incapacitate the entire arm. Sleeves adequately cover the elbows, so swellings and deformities are cosmetically important only when they are exaggerated.

The elbow's primary role in the upper limb complex is to help position the hand in the appropriate location to perform its functions. Once the shoulder has positioned the hand in a gross fashion, the elbow allows for adjustments in height and length of the limb. In addition, the forearm rotates to place the hand in the most effective position to perform its function.

The elbow consists of a complex set of joints that require careful assessment for proper treatment. Six tissues that work in concert make the upper extremity an organ of movement. The most obvious and accessible tissue is skin, evaluated first by inspection and then by palpation. The most vital tissues are vascular and neural and should be evaluated next. If these tissues are not responsible for presenting symptoms, then the examiner shifts to joints and their supporting tissues, tendon, muscle, and bone.

Pain of lateral elbow origin is usually diagnosed as radiohumeral bursitis, epicondylitis, or tennis elbow. This pain involves either the wrist extensors in the form of tendinitis or, occasionally, the radial nerve in the form of impingement by musculotendinous structures crossing the elbow joint.

A similar problem may occur on the medial elbow epicondyle because all the wrist flexors and pronators originate from this epicondyle. Affected individuals use flexor-pronator muscle groups repetitively, isometrically, or isokinetically. Such movement is unusual because forceful, wrist-flexor power is seldom used. The most powerful hand grasping is accomplished in the dorsiflexed wrist position.

Intraarticular abnormalities, such as osteochondritis dissecans of the capitellum, may result in lateral elbow pain. However, the loss of wrist-extensor power in the absence of point epicondylar tenderness rules out this condition. An extremely minor fracture of the radial head might cause pain that could be confused with tennis elbow.

Pain in the elbow—particularly if it extends along the entire arm—without objective findings at the joint suggests psychogenic rheumatism. Other diseases that refer pain to the elbow include myocardial infarction, cervical root lesions, thoracic outlet syndromes, or even subdeltoid bursitis. Psychogenic rheumatism is also suggested by a history of neurosis or strange behavior or a history that is bizarre and inconsistent. Diagnostic imaging and laboratory tests are as unimpressive as the physical findings. Carpal tunnel syndrome may cause retrograde radiation of pain to the elbow.

Index of Tests

Cozen's test
Elbow flexion test
Golfer's elbow test
Kaplan's sign
Ligamentous instability test
Mills's test
Tinel's sign at the elbow

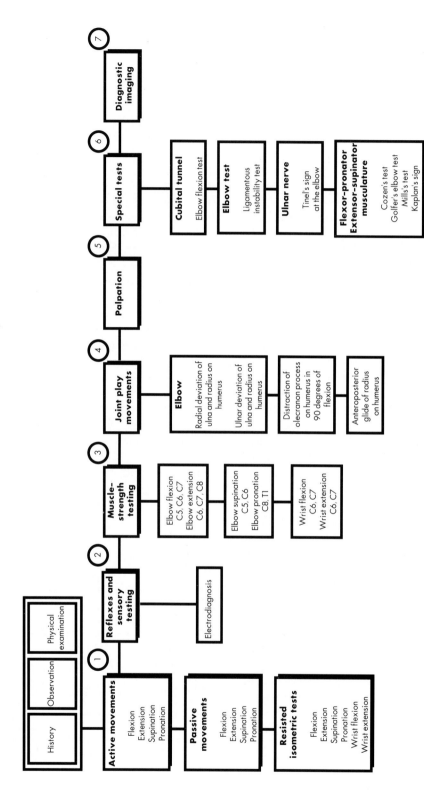

Fig. 5–1 Elbow joint assessment.

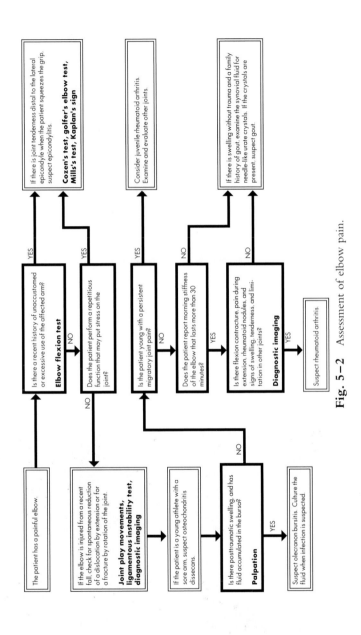

Fig. 5-2 Assessment of elbow pain.

RANGE OF MOTION

Range of motion evaluation of the elbow is performed while the patient is in the seated position. Active movements are performed first, and the most painful movements are performed last. The active movements of the elbow include flexion, extension, supination, and pronation.

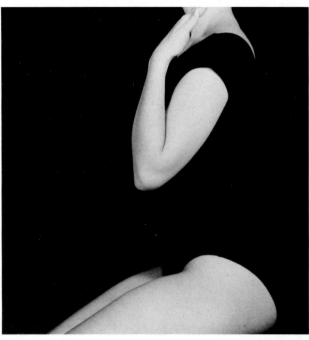

Fig. 5–3 Elbow flexion is limited to 140 to 150 degrees because of tissue approximation. In thin individuals, the end feel may be bone to bone as a result of the coronoid process hitting against the coronoid fossa. Retained flexion motion of 130 degrees or less is an impairment in the activities of daily living.

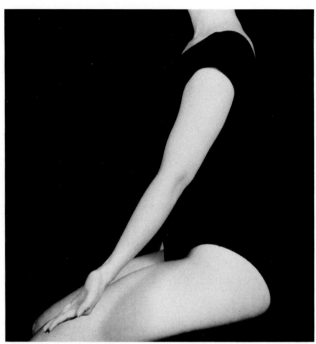

Fig. 5–4 Elbow extension is 0 degrees, although up to 10 degrees of hyperextension may be exhibited, especially in women. The hyperextension is considered normal if it is equal bilaterally and if there is no history of trauma. The inability to return the elbow to within 10 degrees of the neutral position is an impairment in the activities of daily living.

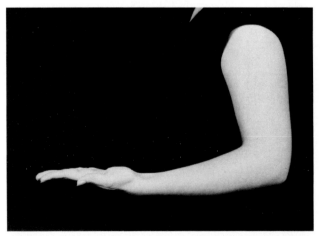

Fig. 5–5 Supination of the elbow is limited, by tissue stretch, to 90 degrees. Retained supination motion of 60 degrees or less is an impairment in the activities of daily living.

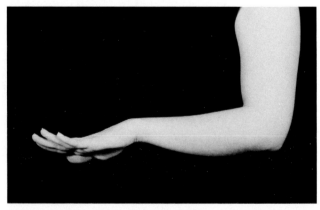

Fig. 5–6 Elbow pronation range of motion, 80 to 90 degrees, is approximately the same as supination. The end feel is tissue stretch. For both supination and pronation, only about 75 degrees occurs in the forearm articulations. The remaining 15 degrees is the result of wrist action. Retained pronation motion of 70 degrees or less is an impairment in the activities of daily living.

MUSCLE TESTING

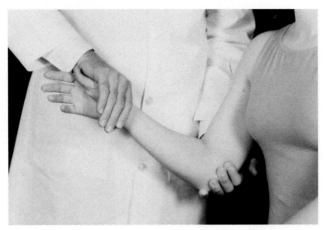

Fig. 5–7 The prime movers in flexion of the elbow are the biceps brachii (musculocutaneous nerve, C5, and C6), brachialis (musculocutaneous nerve, C5, and C6), and brachioradialis (radial nerve, C5, and C6) muscles. The flexor muscles of the forearm that arise from the medial epicondyle of the humerus are the accessory muscles. For testing flexion of the elbow, the patient sits with the arm at the side, the elbow slightly flexed, and the forearm supinated. The examiner stabilizes the patient's arm by grasping it with one hand. The patient is instructed to flex the elbow through its range of motion against graded resistance applied by the examiner. The examiner's other hand is just proximal to the patient's wrist. If the biceps and brachialis are weak, as in a musculocutaneous lesion, the patient will pronate the forearm before flexing the elbow. With this type of lesion, the patient is using the brachioradialis, extensor carpi radialis longus, pronator teres, and wrist flexors.

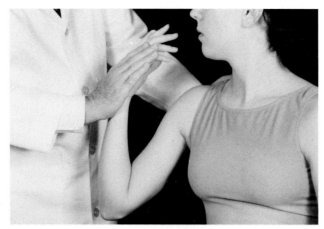

Fig. 5–8 The prime mover in extension of the elbow is the triceps brachii muscle (radial nerve, C7, and C8), and the anconeus muscle is an accessory. The patient is seated. To test extension of the elbow, the examiner fixes the patient's arm as described for flexion, and the patient is instructed to move the elbow through the range of extension motion against graded resistance provided by the examiner's other hand just proximal to the patient's wrist. When the arm is horizontally abducted, the long head of the triceps is shortened over the shoulder joint. When the shoulder is flexed, the long head of the triceps is shortened over the elbow joint and elongated over the shoulder joint.

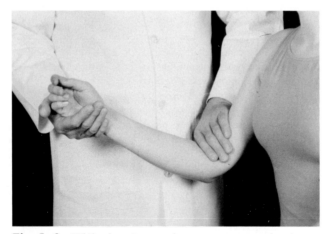

Fig. 5–9 While the triceps and anconeus act together in extending the elbow joint, the two muscles can be differentiated. The belly of the anconeus muscle is below the elbow joint and is easily distinguished from the triceps by palpation. The branch of the radial nerve that innervates the anconeus arises near the midhumeral level and is long. It is possible for a lesion to involve only this branch, leaving the triceps unaffected. Paralysis of the anconeus materially reduces the strength of elbow extension. The muscle grade of *good* in elbow extension strength is actually the result of a normal triceps and a zero anconeus function.

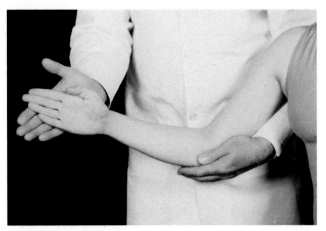

Fig. 5–10   The primary supinators are the biceps brachii and the supinator. The accessory muscle in this movement is the brachioradialis. In addition to its role in supination, the biceps also functions as an elbow flexor. Its total biceps function is well illustrated in the act of twisting a corkscrew into the cork of a bottle and then pulling the cork out of the bottle. In testing supination the examiner stabilizes and supports the elbow at the side of the patient. This support will prevent the substitution of shoulder adduction and external rotation for forearm supination. The thenar eminence of the examiner's resisting hand is placed upon the dorsal surface of the patient's hand and wrist. The patient begins supination from a position of pronation and as the arm is moved into supination, the resistance is gradually increased.

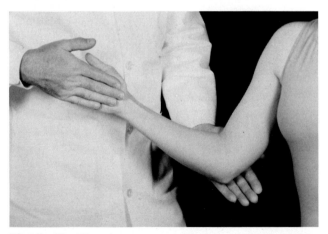

Fig. 5–11   The primary pronators are the pronator teres and the pronator quadratus. The accessory muscle in this movement is the flexor carpi radialis. The examiner stabilizes the patient's elbow just proximal to the joint. This stabilization prevents the substitution of shoulder abduction and internal rotation for pure forearm pronation. The resisting hand is adjusted so the thenar eminence presses against the volar surface of the hand. This adjustment requires only that the examiner turn the resisting hand from the dorsal to the volar surface of the patient's hand. The patient begins forearm pronation from a position of supination. As the patient moves into pronation, the resistance is increased.

Continued.

Comment

The syndrome of chronic and disabling pain in the elbow, particularly near the radiohumeral articulation, is commonly and mistakenly designated tennis elbow rather than epicondylitis or radiohumeral bursitis. There is often a lack of specificity regarding the origin of this type of pain.

The actual cause of epicondylitis or radiohumeral bursitis is unknown. The majority of opinions indicate that the condition is caused by a partial tearing of the tendon fibers from their attachments to the epicondyle and to the epicondylar ridge. Constant muscle contractions prevent healing, creating a traumatic periostitis. Treatment is directed toward complete severance of the tendon from its attachment and firm fixation of the tendon to its origin.

The annular ligament undergoes hyaline degeneration and may be the source of pain. Other pathologic conditions include arthritis of the radiohumeral joint, radiohumeral bursitis, traumatic synovitis of the radiohumeral joint through forced extension and supination, and periostitis or osteitis of the epicondyle.

Although patients do not usually recall a specific traumatic episode, they do admit that symptoms of low-grade pain and morning stiffness were brought on or aggravated by certain repetitive activities, such as tennis, golf, and pipe fitting. A grasping motion that stretches the epicondylar muscle attachments will accentuate the pain.

Procedure

The patient is directed to clench the fist tightly, dorsiflex it, and maintain a pronated position. The examiner, while grasping the patient's lower forearm, applies a flexing force to the dorsiflexion posture of the patient's wrist. The test is positive if it reproduces acute lancinating pain in the region of the lateral epicondyle. The test is significant for epicondylitis or radiohumeral bursitis.

Confirmation Procedures

Golfer's elbow test, Mills's test, Kaplan's sign

Reporting Statement

Cozen's test is positive for the right elbow. This result suggests lateral epicondylitis or radiohumeral bursitis.

∿ Clinical Pearl ∿

Cozen's is the easiest test to perform for lateral epicondylitis. Often the patient has already discovered the pain that accompanies resisted dorsiflexion of the wrist, such as when lifting a gallon of milk. Although the pain of epicondylitis is sometimes exquisite and sharply localized, the condition does not truly differentiate itself from tendinitis or bursitis.

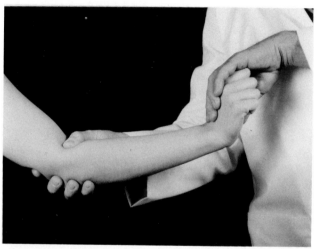

Fig. 5–12 With the patient seated and the affected elbow slightly flexed and pronated, the patient makes a fist. The patient actively dorsiflexes the hand and wrist. The examiner applies steady pressure against the dorsum of the patient's hand in an attempt to flex it. The patient resists this movement. Pain elicited at or near the lateral epicondyle suggests epicondylitis.

Comment

The ulnar nerve may be compressed at a point just distal to the medial epicondyle through the two heads of the flexor carpi ulnaris. The ulnar nerve is given off from the brachial plexus in the axilla. While medial to the brachial artery, the nerve passes down the extremity until it reaches the distal third of the arm. At this point, the nerve and the brachial artery diverge, and the nerve enters the groove between the medial epicondyle of the humerus and the olecranon. The ulnar nerve passes between the humeral and ulnar heads of the flexor carpi ulnaris muscle and descends to the wrist and hand. This path is along the ulnar aspect of the forearm.

Within the bony groove at the elbow, the nerve is susceptible to compression. The compression can result from direct trauma or changes that occur within the groove and cause gradual impingement. Sometimes a slow and progressive ulnar palsy is the delayed result of a fracture or soft-tissue injury at the elbow that has produced scarring. Changes in configuration of the groove that are due to osteoarthritis are occasionally seen with ulnar damage. In addition to severe, direct trauma that affects the elbow joint and may produce immediate or delayed ulnar palsy, repeated, mild trauma may be an overlooked factor. Habitual leaning on the elbow on a desk or constant use of the elbow as a support at work may cause tardy ulnar palsy.

The restrictive opening that the nerve passes through at the elbow is formed by an aponeurotic arch between the olecranon and the medial epicondyle. The floor of this arch is the medial ligament of the elbow joint. This unyielding passageway is somewhat snug, so tissue edema in this region may produce nerve compression.

If the ulnar nerve lesion is above the midforearm, clawing of the two fingers that are innervated by the ulnar nerve does not occur. Clawing does not occur because the extrinsic muscles producing interphalangeal joint flexion are also denervated.

Procedure

The patient is asked to completely flex the elbow and to hold it in the flexed position for 5 minutes. The test is positive if tingling or paresthesia occurs in the ulnar distribution of the forearm and hand. The test helps to determine if cubital tunnel syndrome is present.

Confirmation Procedures

Tinel's sign at the elbow, electrodiagnosis

Reporting Statement

The elbow flexion test is positive on the right. This result indicates cubital tunnel syndrome.

The elbow flexion test is positive on the right. This result suggests compression of the ulnar nerve in the cubital tunnel.

∾ Clinical Pearl ∾

Not only is this a test for cubital tunnel syndrome, but also it may reveal the mechanism that resulted in injury to the ulnar nerve. The fully flexed elbow is a common posture for the arm during sleep, natural or chemically induced. Patients may wake up with ulnar palsy symptoms that stem from prolonged neural compression and anoxia.

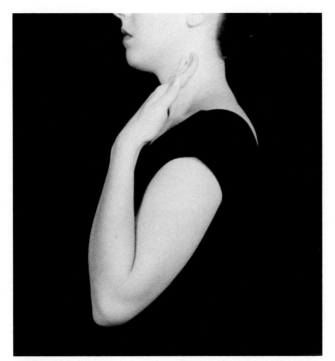

Fig. 5–13 The seated patient maintains a fully flexed elbow for as long as possible. The norm is 5 minutes or longer with no symptoms produced. Ulnar paresthesia developing in less than 5 minutes suggests cubital tunnel syndrome.

Comment

Epicondylitis is a type of involvement that is peculiar to the elbow and develops along the medial and lateral epicondyles. The extensor-supinator muscles arise along the lateral epicondyle and the flexor-pronator muscles arise along the medial epicondyle, where they have an aponeurotic attachment. Epicondylitis may occur either by contusion of the area or, more commonly, by strain. Characteristic irritation develops at the attachment of the aponeurosis to the bone. Pain, which is aggravated by gripping, occurs along the epicondyle. The pain medially or laterally extends down the corresponding group of muscles, sometimes as far as the wrist. When clenching the fist, one of the first phases of action is strong contraction of carpal extensors to fix the wrist. If this contraction did not occur, the wrist would go into flexion, and an ineffective fist would result. This is exemplified by the hand in which there is radial paralysis. A patient with this condition is unable to make a fist not because the fingers cannot be flexed but because the wrist cannot be stabilized. When the hand grasps an object, tension is placed on both the flexors and extensors of the wrist. Gripping will cause pain whether the involvement is medial or lateral. During examination there is tenderness localized to the affected epicondyle or upward along the supracondylar ridge for a short distance. The tenderness also may extend down over the radial head. In true epicondylitis the acute tenderness is directly on the epicondyle.

Although epicondylitis may follow an acute strain, it more often results from chronic degenerative changes. These changes are due to attrition of the aponeurotic fibers at the elbow. Degeneration occurs in certain types of athletes, such as baseball pitchers. If there is degenerative change, there may be calcification or even spur formation over the epicondyle. The patient complains of aching on the outer or inner side of the elbow. Active use of the forearm and hand makes the pain more severe.

Procedure

While the patient is seated, the examiner flexes the patient's elbow slightly and supinates the hand. The patient flexes the elbow against resistance. Pain over the medial epicondyle indicates medial epicondylitis.

Confirmation Procedures

Cozen's test, Kaplan's sign, Mills's test

Reporting Statement

The golfer's elbow test is positive on the right. This result suggests epicondylitis at the medial epicondyle.

The golfer's elbow test is positive on the right. This result suggests flexor-pronator aponeurosis tendinitis at the medial epicondyle.

∽ Clinical Pearl ∽

This test is a reverse procedure of Cozen's test. Cozen's test relies on resisted wrist dorsiflexion, but the golfer's elbow test relies on resisted elbow-wrist flexion. The pain associated with medial epicondylitis spreads down the forearm and is often confused with carpal tunnel syndrome symptoms.

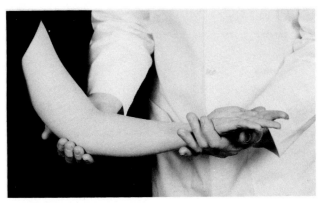

Fig. 5–14 The seated patient slightly flexes the elbow. The hand and wrist are in supination.

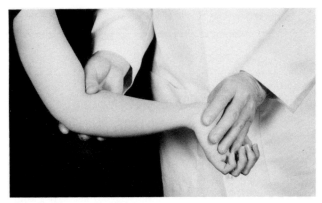

Fig. 5–15 The examiner applies steady pressure to the supinated hand in an attempt to extend the elbow. The patient resists this movement with active flexion. Pain elicited at the medial epicondyle indicates epicondylitis.

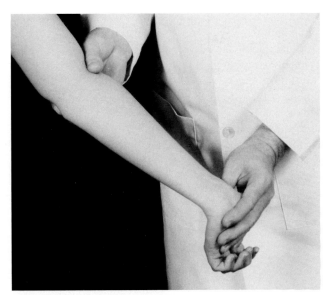

Fig. 5–16 With severe medial epicondylitis the examiner can overcome the flexor muscle groups and extend the elbow fully. With aponeurosis contractures present, the full extension localizes the lesion more sharply.

Comment

The so-called tennis elbow is a type of condition that is common in athletes, particularly part-time athletes. There are at least three distinctly different conditions that are commonly called tennis elbow. Physical examination will usually reveal which condition is present. The history is very likely to be the same for each of the conditions. Each condition may involve some unusual exertion of the grip of the hand with lateral play of the wrist. The phrase *tennis elbow* is derived from the instance of someone who plays tennis before becoming well conditioned. Pain occurs in the lateral and sometimes medial side of the elbow. The condition is aggravated by gripping and rotating. In the days before the vacuum sweeper, tennis elbow was also called *rug beater's elbow.* There are other phrases to describe the condition in relation to the activities that ordinarily involve lateral movement of the wrist, such as in tennis playing, beating a rug, or using a hammer. Overuse, such as shaking hands at a reception, can also bring on the symptoms.

The various conditions on the lateral side of the elbow that cause inflammation of the extensor-supinator aponeurotic attachment to the lateral epicondyle are (1) radioulnar synovitis, marked by development of a pannus of synovium between the radius and ulna, (2) strain that is often directly over the radial head in the aponeurosis itself, and (3) radiohumeral bursitis. Because of the proximity of the epicondyle, the radiohumeral joint, and the supinator aponeurosis, it is understandable how conditions involving these areas are often confused. Overuse of the elbow joint mechanism is often the main cause of these elbow conditions. On the medial side of the elbow, ulnar neuritis will sometimes be misclassified as tennis elbow. The phrase *tennis elbow* should be discarded in favor of a more definitive diagnosis.

Procedure

While the patient is seated, the affected upper limb is held straight out with the wrist in slight dorsiflexion. Grip strength is tested with a dynamometer. This maneuver is then repeated as the examiner firmly encircles the patient's forearm with both hands or with a strap placed approximately 1 to 2 inches below the elbow joint line. The sign is present if initial grip strength improves and lateral elbow pain diminishes. A marked lessening of pain caused by constriction of the musculature of the upper forearm also occurs.

Confirmation Procedures

Cozen's test, golfer's elbow test, Mills's test

Reporting Statement

Kaplan's sign is present on the right. This result suggests lateral epicondylitis.

∿ Clinical Pearl ∿

Kaplan's sign is a good test for discerning the efficacy of tennis-elbow support in the management of a patient's condition. Obviously if the grip does not improve while the brace is in place, the musculature and epicondylar tissues are not being supported adequately. The condition may be so severe that the use of a brace is not helpful.

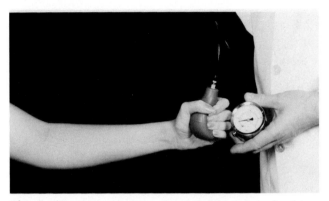

Fig. 5–17 With the elbow flexed slightly and the hand in a position of function, the seated patient grips a dynamometer. The examiner records the findings.

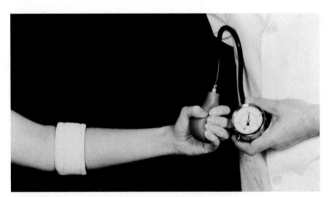

Fig. 5–18 The grip strength is tested again with the elbow supported by either a tennis elbow strap or the examiner's hands. The examiner records the findings. Increased grip strength and decreased elbow pain indicate lateral epicondylitis.

Comment

Because the elbow is a stable joint, ligament injury is uncommon. It is impossible to sprain the elbow by excessive flexion. In excessive extension the olecranon impinges against the back of the humerus, and the continuing force pulls the coronoid away from the trochlea of the humerus. This condition results in an injury to the anterior portion of the collateral ligament, particularly on the medial side. This injury may vary from a partial tear to complete rupture of the ligaments and capsule. As the force stops short of complete rupture, the elbow flexes, the tension releases, and no feeling of instability occurs at the elbow joint. This lack of instability is because of the inherent, bony stability of the elbow and because the elbow does not require the same degree of stability for bearing weight that is necessary in the knee.

The patient with an injury of excessive elbow extension will have a history of elbow hyperextension and of severe pain on the medial and sometimes the lateral side of the elbow. This pain is relieved by flexion. The symptoms at the time of examination vary according to the severity of the injury. Pain is ordinarily not a prominent factor, but there will be localized tenderness at the site of the tear, either along the ulna on the medial side or along the epicondyle. There may also be pain along the lateral collateral ligament at the site of the tear. Any attempt to extend the arm causes pain, and motion is stopped, short of complete extension, by a muscle spasm.

The collateral ligaments also may be sprained by lateral motion. Forced abduction of the extended arm will damage the medial ligaments. Forced adduction will damage the lateral ligaments. Instability is extremely infrequent. It is difficult to determine whether or not the rupture of the ligaments is complete unless there has been complete dislocation of the elbow. A sprain-fracture due to an avulsion of the ligament with a bony fragment may be revealed by diagnostic imaging. Symptoms of lateral stresses will be localized to the one side and will be accompanied by the same findings as for hyperextension. These findings include tenderness along the site of the tear, local swelling, and pain during attempts to reproduce the causative force.

Procedure

The patient's arm is stabilized with one of the examiner's hands at the elbow, the examiner's other hand is placed at the patient's wrist. With the patient's elbow slightly flexed (20 to 30 degrees) and stabilized with the examiner's hand, an adduction (varus) force is applied to the distal forearm by the examiner to test the lateral collateral ligament. The examiner applies the force several times with increasing pressure, while noting any alteration in pain or range of motion. An abduction (valgus) force at the distal forearm is then applied to test the medial collateral ligament. The examiner should note any laxity, decreased mobility, or altered pain that may be present. The examiner should compare any such findings with the uninvolved elbow.

Confirmation Procedure

Diagnostic imaging

Reporting Statement

Adduction stress is positive on the right for sprain of the lateral collateral ligaments of the elbow.

Abduction stress is positive on the right for sprain of the medial collateral ligaments of the elbow.

∽ Clinical Pearl ∽

It is not uncommon in elbow ligamentous testing for osseous reductions to be felt or heard. During this procedure the radial head may be reduced because of a minor subluxation, or simple adhesion releases may occur. The testing may become the treatment.

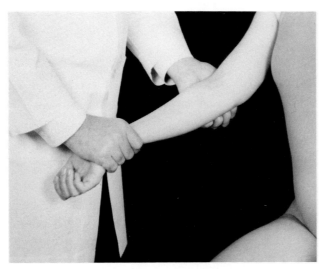

Fig. 5–19 The patient is seated comfortably with the elbow slightly flexed (20 to 30 degrees) and the hand and arm in supination. The examiner stabilizes the elbow while applying an abduction (valgus) force to the distal forearm. This tests the medial collateral ligaments. Pain indicates sprain.

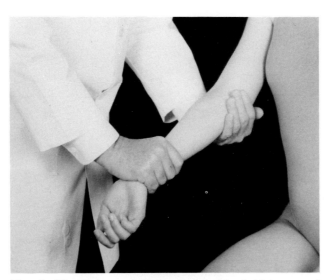

Fig. 5–20 The procedure described in Fig. 5-19 is repeated with an adduction force applied to the distal forearm while the examiner stabilizes the elbow. This procedure assesses the lateral collateral ligaments. Pain indicates sprain.

Mills's Test

Comment

Lateral epicondylitis is a symptom complex that results in pain at the elbow, especially during extension of the wrist or fingers against resistance. Lateral epicondylitis is usually due to a tear in the conjoined tendons of the extensor muscles, and it is often associated with a bone chip or spur on the lateral condyle of the humerus. Direct compression of the dorsal interosseous nerve at or distal to the level of the supinator also can give the same symptoms.

During palpation there is pain in the area of the lateral epicondyle. This pain continues down the dorsal aspect of the forearm and over the wrist extensors and the extensor digitorum communis.

Etiologic factors include direct trauma to the elbow joint in the area of the lateral epicondyle or, more commonly, a muscle strain secondary to athletic activities. If direct trauma is determined as the underlying etiology, tangential diagnostic images of the lateral epicondyle should be obtained. These images may demonstrate the presence of small osteophytes within the substance of the conjoined tendon. There also may be cortical irregularity of the epicondyle.

Occasionally medial epicondylitis is encountered. This condition usually has the same etiology as tennis elbow and involves either the medial epicondyle or the origin of the common flexor tendon.

Procedure

The patient's forearm, fingers, and wrist are passively flexed. The forearm is pronated and extended. The test is positive if elbow pain increases. A positive test indicates lateral epicondylitis (tennis elbow).

Confirmation Procedures

Cozen's test, golfer's elbow test, Kaplan's sign, diagnostic imaging

---

Reporting Statement

Mills's test is positive on the right. This result indicates lateral epicondylitis of the elbow.

Clinical Pearl

Mills's test is also a treatment maneuver. One of the principles of management for lateral epicondylitis is the sectioning of the aponeurosis from the epicondyle. In the final maneuvers of Mills's test, this separation is accomplished.

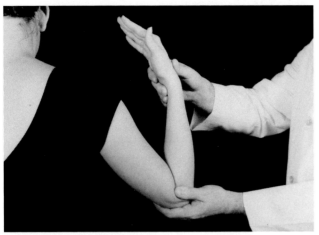

Fig. 5–21 The patient is seated. The examiner passively and fully flexes the elbow.

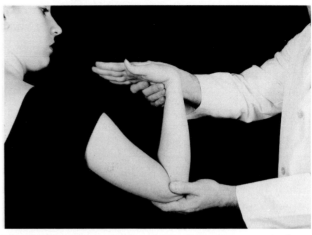

Fig. 5–22 After passively and fully flexing the patient's elbow, the examiner flexes the patient's wrist.

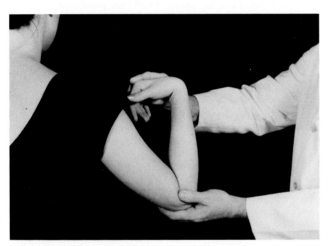

Fig. 5–23 After attaining the position described in Fig. 5-22, the patient's fingers are fully flexed. The forearm, wrist, and hand are all fully flexed in supination.

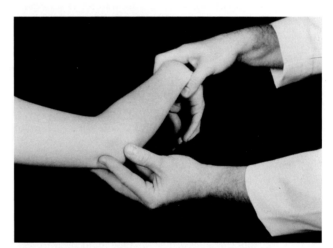

Fig. 5–24 The examiner maintains wrist and finger flexion while extending the patient's elbow.

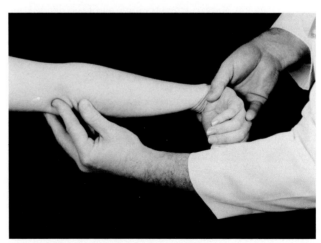

Fig. 5–25 At maximum elbow extension, with the wrist and fingers still flexed, the forearm is pronated. Pain at the lateral epicondyle indicates epicondylitis. All the movements associated with this procedure should be accomplished in a smooth continuous manner.

Tinel's Sign at the Elbow

FORMICATION SIGN
DISTAL TINGLING ON PERCUSSION (DTP) SIGN
HOFFMAN–TINEL SIGN

Comment

Nerve roots and peripheral nerves may be injured by a blunt object that causes a contusion or by a sharp object that produces a partial or complete laceration. The nerve also can be injured by a severe stretch, resulting from a traction injury. In addition, nerves are particularly vulnerable to prolonged ischemia, which can lead to necrosis.

In neuropraxia there is only slight damage to the nerve with transient loss of conductivity, particularly in its motor fibers. In neuropraxia, wallerian degeneration, which is the breakdown of the myelin sheaths into lipid material and fragmentation of the neurofibrils, does not occur. Complete recovery from neuropraxia may be expected within a few days or weeks.

In axonotmesis the injury damages axons, which are prolongations of the cells in the spinal cord, but does not damage the structural framework of the nerve. The axons distal to the injury undergo wallerian degeneration. Peripheral regeneration of the axons occurs along the intact neural tubes to the appropriate end organs. This regeneration occurs very slowly, approximately 1mm each day, or 3cm each month. If axonotmesis in a nerve occurred 9cm proximal to its site of entrance into a muscle, it would take approximately 3 months for the regenerating axons to reinnervate that muscle.

In the injury of neurotmesis, the internal neural structural framework and the enclosed axons are divided, torn, and destroyed. Wallerian degeneration occurs in the distal segment. Because the axons in the proximal segment have lost their neural tubes, natural regeneration is improbable. The neurofibrils and fibrous elements grow out of the divided end of the nerve to produce a bulbous neuroma. The only hope of recovery lies in excision of the damaged section of the nerve and accurate approximation of the freshened ends. Even under ideal circumstances recovery is less than complete.

Immediately after nerve injury, there is a loss of conductivity in motor, sensory, and autonomic fibers. The muscles supplied by the nerve root or peripheral nerve exhibit a flaccid paralysis and later undergo atrophy. A loss of cutaneous sensations, deep sensation, and position sense can be detected. The autonomic deficit is characterized by a lack of sweating (anhidrosis) in the cutaneous distribution of the nerve. There is a temporary vasodilation and resultant warm skin followed by vasoconstriction and cold skin.

The precise diagnosis concerning both the type of injury and its location can be helped by the appropriate electrical tests, which include nerve conduction, strength curve, and electromyography.

The prognosis depends on the type of injury (neuropraxia, axonotmesis, or neurotmesis). If recovery does take place, it is evidenced first by return of muscle power in the most proximally supplied muscle. Return of sensation follows a definite pattern. Deep sensation returns first, followed by pain and position sense. As regeneration of axons proceeds along the nerve, the regenerated portion becomes hypersensitive. Tapping over the injured area causes a tingling sensation. Assessing the distal limit of this phenomenon at intervals makes it possible to determine the progress of regeneration.

Procedure

While the patient is seated, the examiner taps the groove between the olecranon process and the lateral epicondyle with a neurologic reflex hammer. The same is repeated for the groove between the olecranon process and the medial epicondyle. Hypersensitivity indicates neuritis or neuroma of the respective nerve.

Confirmation Procedure

Electrodiagnosis

Reporting Statement

Tinel's sign is present in the medial epicondylar groove of the right elbow. This sign suggests ulnar neuropathy.

Tinel's sign is present in the lateral epicondylar groove of the right elbow. This sign suggests involvement of the superficial radial nerve.

∼ Clinical Pearl ∼

It must be remembered that the tingling elicited by the Tinel's sign represents regeneration. Pain and tingling represent injury and degeneration. The more distally the tingling is felt from the site of percussion, the more distally the axons have regenerated.

The Elbow

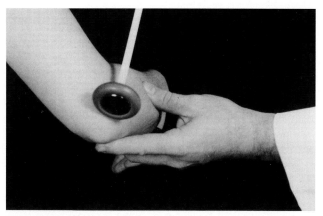

Fig. 5−26 The patient is seated comfortably with the elbow flexed to 90 degrees. The examiner percusses the nerve at the lateral epicondylar groove. Tingling that radiates down the lateral forearm indicates regeneration associated with superficial radial nerve palsy. Pain radiating down the lateral forearm is associated with injury and superficial radial nerve degeneration. The same procedure is repeated for the medial epicondylar groove and the ulnar nerve.

Bibliography

American Medical Association: *Guides to the evaluation of permanent impairment,* ed 3, 1990, Chicago.

American Orthopaedic Association: *Manual of orthopaedic surgery,* Chicago, 1972, The Association.

Apfelberg DB, Larson SJ: Dynamic anatomy of the ulnar nerve at the elbow, *Plast Reconstr Surg,* 51:76, 1973.

Apley AG, Solomon L: *Concise system of orthopaedics and fractures,* London, 1988, Butterworth-Heinemann.

Bateman JE: *Trauma to nerves in limbs,* Philadelphia, 1962, WB Saunders.

Beals RK: The normal carrying angle of the elbow, *Clin Orthop,* 119:194, 1976.

Beetheam WP, Polley HF, Slocumb CH, Weaver WF: *Physical examination of the joints,* Philadelphia, 1965, WB Saunders.

Boyd HB, McLeod AC: Tennis elbow, *J Bone Joint Surg,* 55A: 1183, 1973.

Bradley WG: *Disorders of peripheral nerves,* Oxford, 1974, Blackwell Scientific Publications.

Cipriano JJ: *Photographic manual of regional orthopaedic and neurological tests,* ed, 2 Baltimore, 1991, Williams & Wilkins.

D'Ambrosia, RD: *Musculoskeletal disorders regional examination and differential diagnosis,* Philadelphia, 1977, JB Lippincott.

Dandy DJ: *Essential orthopaedics and trauma,* Edinburgh, 1989, Churchill Livingstone.

Delagi E, Perrotto L, Iazzetti J, Morrison D: *An anatomic guide for the electromyographer,* Springfield, IL, 1975, Charles C. Thomas.

Doherty M, Doherty J: *Clinical examination in rheumatology,* London, 1992, Wolfe Publishing.

Garden RS: Tennis elbow, *J Bone Joint Surg,* 43B:100, 1961.

Gardner E: *Fundamentals of neurology,* ed 4, Philadelphia, 1963, WB Saunders.

Grant JCB: *A method of anatomy: Descriptive and deductive,* ed 5, Baltimore, 1952, Williams & Wilkins.

Grant JCB, Basmajian JV: *Grant's method of anatomy,* ed 7, Baltimore, 1965, Williams & Wilkins.

Hale MS: *A practical approach to arm pain,* Springfield, IL, 1971, Charles C. Thomas.

Hollinshead WH: *Anatomy for surgeons,* vol 3, *The back and limbs,* ed 2, New York, 1969, Hoeber Medical Division, Harper & Row.

Hoppenfeld S: *Physical examination of the spine and extremities,* New York, 1976, Appleton-Century-Crofts.

Kaplan EB: Treatment of tennis elbow (epicondylitis) by denervation, *J Bone Joint Surg,* 41A:147, 1959.

Katz, WA: *Rheumatic diseases diagnosis and management,* Philadelphia, 1977, JB Lippincott.

Kendall HO, Kendall FP, Wadsworth GE: *Muscles testing and function,* ed 2, Baltimore, 1971, Williams & Wilkins.

Magee DJ: *Orthopedic physical assessment,* Philadelphia, 1987, WB Saunders.

Mazion JM: *Illustrated manual of Neurological reflexes/signs/tests, part 1, Orthopedic signs/tests/maneuvers for office procedure, part II,* Orlando, 1980, Daniels Publishing.

McRae R: *Clinical orthopaedic examination,* ed 3, Edinburgh, 1990, Churchill Livingstone.

Medical Economics Books: *Patient care flow chart manual,* ed 3, Oradell, NJ, 1982, Medical Economics Books.

Mercier LR, Pettid FJ: *Practical orthopedics,* Chicago, 1980, Mosby.

Mills GP: The treatment of tennis elbow, *Dr Med J,* 1:12, 1928.

Mitchell SW: *Injuries of nerves and their consequences,* Philadelphia, 1972, JB Lippincott.

O'Donoghue DH: *Treatment of injuries to athletes,* ed 3, Philadelphia, 1976, WB Saunders.

Omer GE, Spinner M: *Management of peripheral nerve problems,* Philadelphia, 1980, WB Saunders.

Osborne G: Compression neuritis of the ulnar nerve at the elbow, *Hand Clin,* 2:10, 1970.

Polley HF, Hunder GG: *Rheumatologic interviewing and physical examination of the joints,* ed 2, Philadelphia, 1978, WB Saunders.

Salter RB: *Disorders and injuries of the musculoskeletal system,* Baltimore, 1970, Williams & Wilkins.

Salter RB: *Textbook of disorders and injuries of the musculoskeletal system,* Baltimore, 1970, Williams & Wilkins.

Sandifer PH: *Neurology in orthopaedics,* London, 1967, Butterworths.

Seddon H: *Surgical disorders of the peripheral nerves,* Baltimore, 1968, Williams & Wilkins.

Seddon H: *Surgical disorders of the peripheral nerves,* Edinburgh, 1972, Churchill.

Smith FM: *Surgery of the elbow,* ed 2, Philadelphia, 1972, WB Saunders.

Spinner M, Spencer PS: Nerve compression lesions of the upper extremity: A clinical and experimental review, *Clin Orthop,* 104:46, 1974.

Sunderland S: *Nerves and nerve injuries,* Baltimore, 1968, Williams & Wilkins.

Thurston SE: *The little black book of neurology,* Chicago, 1987, Mosby.

Tullos HS, King JW: Lesions of the pitching arm in adolescents, *JAMA,* 220:264, 1972.

Turek SL: *Orthopaedics principles and their application,* ed 3, Philadelphia, 1977, JB Lippincott.

Vanderpool DW, Chalmers J, Lamb DW, Whiston TR: Peripheral compression lesions of the ulnar nerve, *J Bone Joint Surg,* 50B:792, 1968.

Wadsworth TG: *The elbow,* New York, 1982, Churchill Livingstone.

Warwick R, Williams PL: *Gray's anatomy,* ed 35 Brit Philadelphia, 1973, WB Saunders.

Wiens E, Lane S: The anterior interosseous nerve syndrome, *Can J Surg,* 21:354, 1978.

Wilson, FC: *The musculoskeletal system,* Philadelphia, 1975, JB, Lippincott.

~ *6* ~

The Forearm, Wrist, and Hand

*C*hronic wrist pain has often been called the lower back pain of hand conditions. Both areas offer the clinician significant diagnostic and therapeutic challenges. As in the examination of the lower back, a precise evaluation based on thorough knowledge of regional anatomy is essential to successful management.

The wrist joint is probably the most complicated joint in the body because of its unique arrangement and articulation of the radiocarpal and intercarpal joints. Ligamentous injuries to the carpus can lead to significant and possibly permanent disability. Diagnosis may be difficult with persistent degrees of carpal instability. Definitive treatment modalities have not been perfected. As with most joint injuries, a more thorough understanding of the anatomy and pathogenesis of these injuries is useful.

Carpal injuries represent a spectrum of bony and ligamentous damage. The names given to the various injuries only describe the resultant damage apparent on radiographs. For example, lunate dislocation, perilunate dislocation, scaphoid fracture, transscaphoid perilunate fracture dislocation, or transscaphoid transtriquetral perilunate fracture dislocation. Each injury is not an entity but part of a continuum. The final injury is determined by (1) the type of three-dimensional loading, (2) the magnitude and direction of the forces involved, (3) the position of the hand at the time of impact, and (4) the biomechanical properties of the bones and ligaments.

A stable and pain-free wrist is a prerequisite for normal hand function. In contrast, a painful, unstable, or deformed wrist impairs function. The wrist, a common target of rheumatoid arthritis, is adversely affected by the reaction of synovial tissue on capsuloligamentous structures, articular cartilage, and subchondral bone. The mechanical forces of the different muscle groups acting across the wrist also contribute to deformities occurring at this level.

The initial evaluation of a patient with an injured wrist must be thorough and methodical. In recent years, increased understanding of carpal mechanics and instability patterns, with and without fractures, has increased the importance of accurate examination of the wrist. The diagnosis of "sprained wrist" is not adequate in establishing a proper treatment regimen. By taking a careful history, performing an exact examination, and utilizing appropriate diagnostic aids—such as motion views, tomography, bone scans, and arthrography—an accurate diagnosis of wrist injury can be established. It is only after an accurate diagnosis is established that a rational, therapeutic regimen can be prepared.

Index of Tests

Allen's test
Bracelet test
Bunnell-Littler test
Carpal lift sign
Cascade sign
Dellon's moving two-point discrimination test
Finkelstein's test
Finsterer's sign
Froment's paper sign
Interphalangeal neuroma test
Maisonneuve's sign
Phalen's sign
Pinch grip test
Shrivel test
Test for tight retinacular ligaments
Tinel's sign at the wrist
Tourniquet test
Wartenberg's sign
Weber's two-point discrimination test
Wringing test

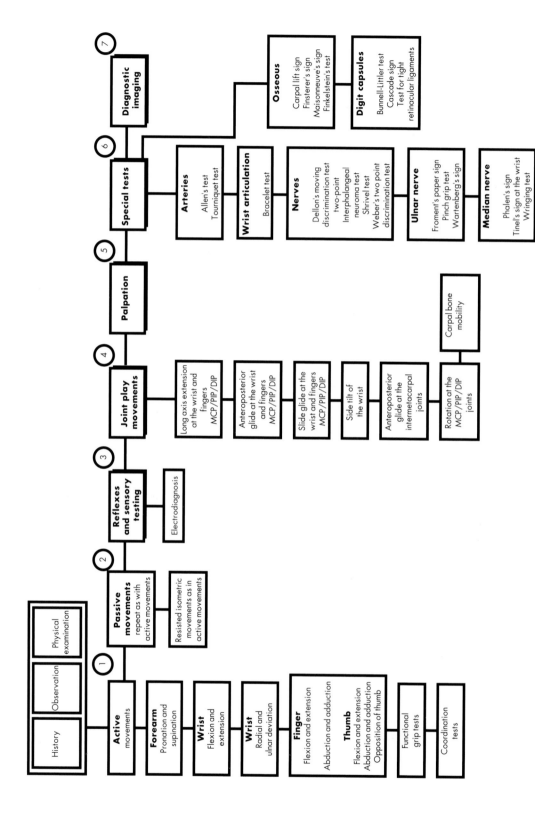

Fig. 6–1   Forearm, wrist, and hand assessment.

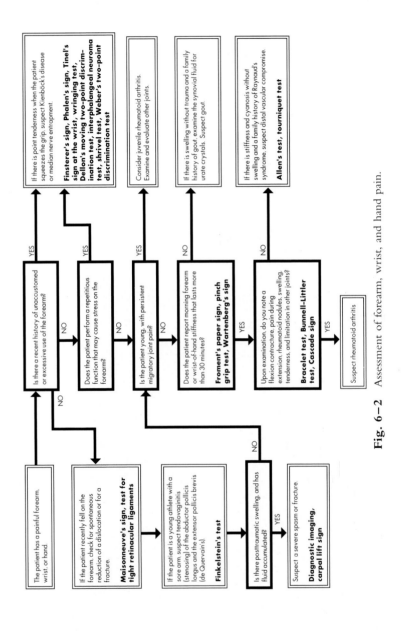

Fig. 6–2 Assessment of forearm, wrist, and hand pain.

A

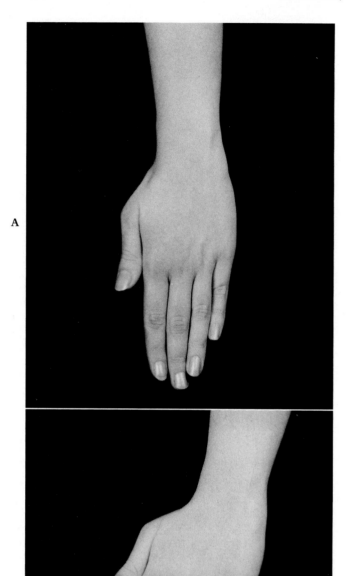

RANGE OF MOTION

Examination of the range of motion for the wrist and hand is accomplished while the patient is in the seated position. As always, the most painful movements are done last. In determination of the movements of the hand, the middle finger is considered midline. Wrist flexion will decrease as the fingers are flexed, and movement of flexion and extension are limited, usually by the antagonistic muscles and ligaments.

Finger abduction (20 to 30 degrees) occurs at the metacarpophalangeal joints. The end feel is tissue stretch. Finger adduction (0 degrees) occurs at the same joint. The loss of finger abduction or adduction active range of motion has minimal effect on the activities of daily living. The digits are medially deviated slightly in relation to the metacarpal bones. As well, the metacarpals are at an angle to each other. These positions increase the dexterity of the hand and oblique flexion of the medial four digits, and contribute to deformities seen in conditions such as rheumatoid arthritis. Thumb flexion occurs at the carpometacarpal joint, within a range of 45 to 50 degrees; the metacarpophalangeal joint, within a range of 50 to 55 degrees; and the interphalangeal joint, within a range of 80 to 90 degrees. Such flexion is associated with medial rotation of the thumb as a result of the shape of

B

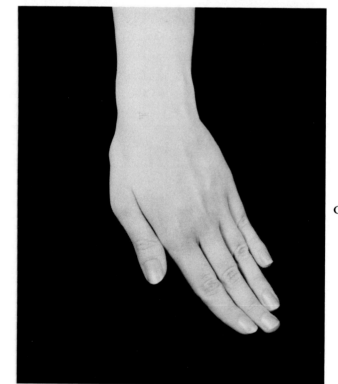

C

Fig. 6–3 **(A)** The wrist in neutral position. Radial deviation **(B)** is 15 degrees, and ulnar deviation **(C)** is 30 to 45 degrees. The normal end feel of these movements is bone to bone. Radial deviation of 15 degrees or less and ulnar deviation of 25 degrees or less are impairments of the forearm in the activities of daily living.

the carpometacarpal joint. Extension of the thumb occurs at the interphalangeal joint within a range of 0 to 5 degrees. Extension is associated with lateral rotation. Flexion and extension take place in a plane parallel to the palm of the hand. Thumb abduction is 60 to 70 degrees, and thumb adduction is 30 degrees. These movements occur in a plane at right angles to the flexion-extension plane. Seventy degrees or less of retained flexion of the thumb at the interphalangeal joint and 50 degrees or less retained flexion at the metacarpophalangeal joint are considered impairments of the thumb in the activities of daily living. Zero degrees of extension at the interphalangeal joint is considered the sole impairment of extension for the thumb. Forty degrees or less of radial abduction and 25 degrees or less of adduction are considered impairments of the thumb in the activities of daily living.

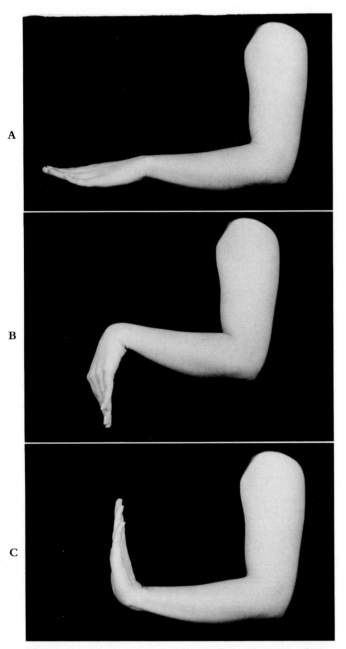

Fig. 6–4 (**A**) The wrist in the neutral position. Wrist flexion (**B**) is 80 to 90 degrees, and wrist extension dorsiflexion (**C**) is 70 to 90 degrees. The end feel of both movements is tissue stretch. Wrist flexion of 50 degrees or less and wrist extension dorsiflexion of 34 degrees or less are impairments of the forearm in the activities of daily living.

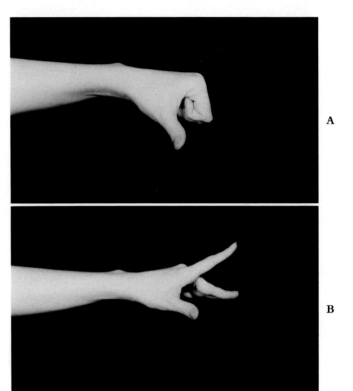

Fig. 6–5 Flexion of the fingers (**A**) occurs at the metacarpophalangeal joints (85 to 90 degrees), the proximal interphalangeal joints (100 to 115 degrees), and the distal interphalangeal joints (80 to 90 degrees). Extension (**B**) occurs at the metacarpophalangeal joints (30 to 45 degrees), the proximal interphalangeal joints (0 degrees), and the distal interphalangeal joints (20 degrees). The end feel of finger flexion and extension is tissue stretch. Retained active finger flexion of 80 degrees or less at the metacarpophalangeal joint, 90 degrees or less at the proximal interphalangeal joint, and 60 degrees or less at the distal interphalangeal joint serve as an impairment of the fingers in the activities of daily living. Retained active extension of 10 degrees or less at the metacarpophalangeal joint serves as the sole impairment of the fingers in the activities of daily living.

MUSCLE TESTING

The muscles controlling the movements of the hand are conventionally divided into two groups: (1) extrinsic muscles that originate within the arm and forearm, and (2) intrinsic muscles whose origins and insertions are entirely within the hand. This grouping of the hand muscles is convenient for descriptive purposes but has no relation to the functions of the muscles because any movement is the result of complicated integration of the actions of both groups.

Because there is no intrinsic musculature on the dorsum of the hand, the long extensor tendons lie in a loose connective tissue between the skin and the bones. The most important action of the long extensor tendons is to provide dorsal stability for the metacarpophalangeal (MCP) joint against the flexor power of both intrinsic and extrinsic muscles. The central portion of the tendon continues distally over the proximal phalanx and inserts into the base of the middle phalanx. The central portion contributes to a certain degree to the extension of the middle finger joint. The majority of this motion is accomplished by the intrinsic muscles.

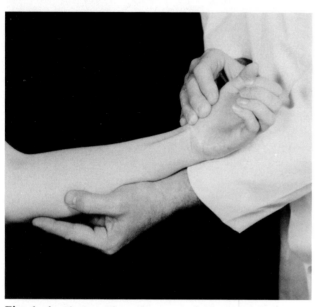

Fig. 6–6 Flexion. The prime movers for flexion of the wrist are the flexor carpi radialis (median nerve, C6, and C7) and the flexor carpi ulnaris (ulnar nerve, C8, and T1) muscles. The palmaris longus muscle is accessory to this motion. Flexion is tested while the patient sits with the forearm supinated. The arm can be resting comfortably on a table. The muscles of the thumb and other fingers should be relaxed. The examiner holds the patient's forearm in the middle with one hand for further stabilization. The patient flexes the wrist against graded resistance provided by the fingertips of the examiner's other hand placed in the patient's palm. The flexor carpi radialis muscle is tested when the examiner provides resistance on the palmar side of the base of the second metacarpal bone in the directions of extension and ulnar deviation. The flexor carpi ulnaris is tested when the examiner applies resistance on the palmar side of the base of the fifth metacarpal bone in the directions of extension and radial deviation.

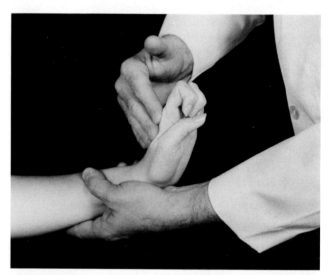

Fig. 6–7 Extension. The prime movers for extension of the wrist are the extensor carpi radialis longus (radial nerve, C6, and C7), extensor carpi radialis brevis (radial nerve, C6, and C7), and extensor carpi ulnaris (radial nerve, C7, and C8) muscles. Extension is tested while the patient sits with the arm pronated. The forearm can be resting on a table. The examiner holds the patient's forearm in the middle with one hand to stabilize it. The patient extends the wrist against graded resistance applied by the examiner's other hand to the dorsal surface of the patient's metacarpals. For testing the extensor carpi radialis longus and brevis muscles, resistance is applied by the examiner to the dorsal surface of the patient's second and third metacarpal bones in the directions of flexion and ulnar deviation. For testing the extensor carpi ulnaris muscle, resistance is applied to the dorsal surface of the fifth metacarpal bone in the directions of flexion and radial deviation. When the forearm is pronated, the extensor carpi ulnaris muscle lies lateral to the ulnar head and acts as a strong ulnar deviator.

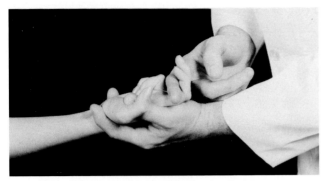

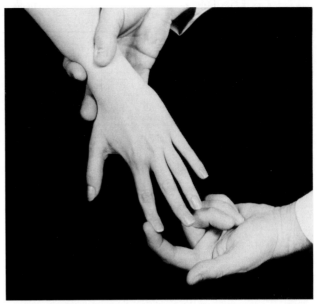

Fig. 6–8 Flexion of the interphalangeal joints of the fingers is accomplished by the long flexor tendons, entering the hand within the *ulnar bursa,* which begins just proximal to the wrist. Of the two long flexor tendons, the flexor digitorum sublimis has its main action on the middle finger joint. The flexor digitorum profundus acts on the distal finger joint. To test for sublimis action, the profundus tendon to the finger in question must be put completely out of action by passively flexing the metacarpophalangeal joint and by hyperextending the adjacent fingers. Hyperextension of these fingers will pull the profundus tendons distally as far as is possible. This apparent lengthening of the profundus tendons will effectively prevent any power from being transferred to the profundus tendon in the finger that is being examined. In tests for profundus action, the finger must be held passively extended at both the proximal and middle finger joints. Voluntary flexion of the distal finger joint will show the presence of profundus power.

Fig. 6–9 The intrinsic muscles of the hand consist of a central group containing the interossei and lumbricales and the two lateral groups of hypothenar and thenar eminences. The thenar group is composed of the opponens, flexor pollicis brevis, and abductor pollicis brevis. An additional muscle is the adductor, which arises by transverse and oblique heads. The muscles of the hypothenar eminence are concerned with the activity of the little finger. The abductor and flexor aid in abduction and flexion of the finger. The detailed anatomy of the interossei is infinitely more complicated than standard texts may lead one to believe. The seven palmar interossei have been split into four dorsal and three palmar interossei. The four lumbrical muscles are unique in that they have their origin on a flexor tendon and their insertion on an extensor tendon. Many actions have been attributed to the lumbricales, but they have no powerful individual action of their own and can only operate with the stronger interossei.

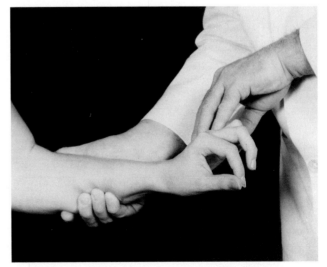

Fig. 6–10 The interosseous and lumbrical muscles are of fundamental importance in the extension of the fingers.

∽ Allen's Test ∽

Comment

The blood supply of the hand is largely anterior or palmar in position. All of the arterial supply enters on the front of the wrist, and at least half of the venous drainage leaves by the same route. Both arterial and venous systems are subject to many variations. Age has some influence on the state of the system. Arteriovenous anastomoses are poorly developed in children, and in elderly persons both the arteries and the veins become elongated, large, and tortuous.

The superficial and deep palmar arterial arches are so named because of their relationship to the flexor tendons. These arches are connected to the dorsal carpal arterial arch (which lies deep to the extensor tendons) by a proximal and distal row of perforating arteries that pass between the metacarpal shafts.

The extensive anastomoses between the various vessels allows occlusion of an arch within its length without serious risk to the distal blood supply. Even when both the radial and ulnar arteries are occluded at the wrist, the blood supply can usually be maintained through collateral circulation that, in such cases, will pass mainly through the perforating arteries. The digital arteries of a finger are of sufficient caliber to allow survival of the finger tip of one of the radial or ulnar arteries.

The veins that drain blood from the hand are either superficial or deep systems. The superficial veins start on the dorsum of the fingers and collect their blood from the plexuses on the palmar and lateral sides of the fingers. The superficial veins run in several trunks parallel to the long axis of the fingers and drain into the cephalic and basilic veins via the dorsal venous network. There is no consistent pattern for this dorsal network, but in general, the cross communications are scanty. The deep veins of the hand and forearm are small and do not drain as much blood as the superficial system.

Procedure

While seated, the patient is instructed to make a tight fist to express blood from the palm. The examiner uses finger pressure to occlude the radial and ulnar arteries. The patient opens and closes the fist to express any remaining blood. The examiner releases the arteries one at a time. The sign is negative if the pale skin of the palm flushes immediately after an artery is released. The sign is positive if the skin of the palm remains blanched for more than 5 seconds. This test, which should be performed before Wright's test, Eden's test, and the shoulder hyperabduction maneuver, is significant for revealing vascular occlusion of the artery tested.

Confirmation Procedures

Tourniquet test, vascular assessment

Reporting Statement

Allen's test is positive for the right wrist. This result suggests ulnar arterial occlusion.

Allen's test is positive after performing right wrist radial artery occlusion.

∽ Clinical Pearl ∽

This test will often elicit paresthesia when an underlying distal peripheral nerve entrapment syndrome exists (carpal tunnel syndrome). The test is used as an early indicator of other general pathologic conditions only when paresthesia is elicited.

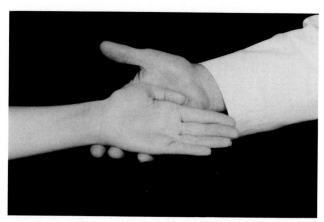

Fig. 6–11 The patient is seated with the elbow of the affected arm flexed and the forearm supinated.

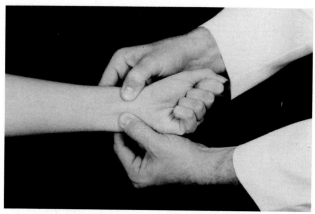

Fig. 6–12 With the patient's arm in the position of 6–11, the radial and ulnar arteries are occluded by the examiner. The examiner will use both hands to occlude the arteries.

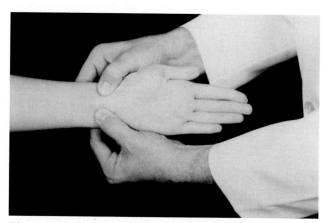

Fig. 6–13 While the radial and ulnar arteries are occluded, the patient opens and closes the hand repeatedly to express the blood from the tissue. Arterial occlusion is maintained.

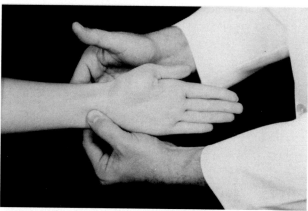

Fig. 6–14 The patient opens the hand, which should be blanched by ischemia. The examiner opens one artery, radial or ulnar. The filling time of the hand is recorded. If circulation fails to return within 5 seconds or less, this represents vascular compromise. The test is repeated for the remaining artery.

Comment

The hands and wrists are extremely important in the differential diagnosis of rheumatic diseases. Many of these disorders, which number more than 100, affect only the hands, and most of them strike at one time or another. In the two hands and wrists there are more than 60 articulations activated by dozens of muscles, tendons, ligaments, and bones an examiner may witness. In a single glance an examiner not only may witness the manifestations of one joint complex but also an entire clinical syndrome. For example, a solitary swollen ankle may hold a variety of possible diagnoses for the observer, but a conglomerate of such swellings in the hands often enables the physician to single out one disease.

It is not surprising then that the hands and the wrists may provide the necessary clues to the diagnosis of many systemic diseases. The hands are in constant motion during the waking hours and even during sleeping hours. The hands are used in a majority of activities of daily living, such as working, eating, and playing; therefore, even the slightest compromise of function will be quickly bothersome to the patient. Such a disease has an effect psychosocially too, because the hands are often noticed by others, and they cannot be concealed for long. Handshaking, dining, touching, and fondling have cardinal roles in our interpersonal relationships. No rheumatologic examination is complete without a thorough assessment of symptoms, physical findings, and functions of the hands.

Rheumatoid arthritis usually begins in the proximal interphalangeal joints (PIP) with development of typical fusiform swelling. At a later stage the metacarpophalangeal and carpal joints may be affected. There is a gradual loss of articular cartilage as evidenced by narrowing of the joint spaces, and decalcification of bone occurs, particularly at a point adjacent to the affected joint. Along with these joint changes there may be a weakness of grip due to atrophy of the intrinsic muscles. As the disease progresses, there is increasing deformity with flexion contractures of the metacarpophalangeal joints, ulnar deviation of the fingers, and adduction of the thumb.

The characteristic changes of adult rheumatoid arthritis are found most commonly in the hands. Although arthritis may present as a monarticular process, multiple joints are usually symmetrically affected. The onset of arthritis is usually gradual, and some of the early signs may be morning stiffness, weakness, paresthesia, and relative disability. Un-capping jars and holding a coffee cup may be difficult, and fastening buttons may be frustrating.

Examination of someone with arthritis reveals that the palms are moist and red while the fingers are tremulous. Fist formation, grip strength, and pinching are impaired, especially after prolonged disuse of the hands. The following findings suggest, but are not pathognomonic, of rheumatoid arthritis: symmetrical swelling of the PIP joints, boutonniere or swan-neck deformities of several PIP joints, swelling or tenderness of the MCP joints, ulnar deviation or subluxation of these MCP and PIP joints, synovitis of the wrist (especially at the distal ulna), tenderness of the distal ulna, and swelling of the extensor carpi ulnaris tendon. More than one of these makes rheumatoid arthritis a likely diagnosis. The symptom complex of MCP joint swelling with ulnar deviation of the fingers, dorsal interosseous muscle atrophy, and extensor swelling at the wrist is virtually pathognomonic of rheumatoid arthritis. Caput ulnae syndrome also has a high degree of specificity. Subcutaneous nodules in the elbow and forearm may point to early diagnosis of this syndrome. The skin is moist, warm, lightly mottled, and thin and may be transparent.

The erythrocyte sedimentation rate is elevated, but a normal value does not rule out the disease. Early in the disease the latex fixation test is most often negative, and only soft tissue swelling is found when using diagnostic imaging. The test for rheumatoid factor eventually becomes positive in 70 percent of patients. Subchondral osteoporosis, erosive changes, and joint space narrowing later appear on the diagnostic images.

Procedure

The examiner gives mild to moderate lateral compression of the lower ends of the radius and ulna. This compression causes acute forearm, wrist, and hand pain. The test is significant for rheumatoid arthritis.

Confirmation Procedures

Clinical laboratory, diagnostic imaging

> ### Reporting Statement
>
> Bracelet test is positive on the right. This result indicates rheumatoid involvement of the wrist.

∽ Clinical Pearl ∽

The bracelet test can be similar to a manual tourniquet test. The examiner must carefully compress osseous structures and not occlude arterial structures.

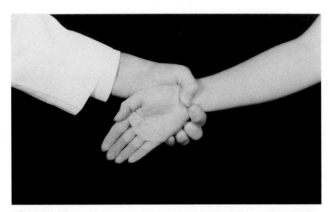

Fig. 6–15 The patient is seated with the elbow flexed. The examiner grasps the affected wrist, applying lateral compression to the distal radius and ulna. This may cause acute pain that indicates rheumatoid arthritis of the wrist.

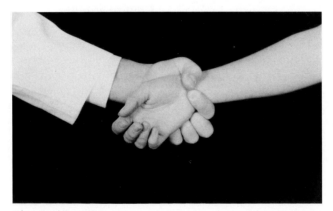

Fig. 6–16 While the examiner applies the lateral compression, the patient attempts to make a fist. This action, which will intensify the pain, will detect and localize the structures more involved in the arthritic degeneration.

Comment

Osteoarthritis is a common abnormality that affects the hands. This type of arthritis attacks the DIP joints, where bony enlargement occurs. Sometimes acute Heberden's nodes, characterized by erythematous periarticular inflammation, occur. Osseous hypertrophy of the PIP joints is characteristic of Bouchard's nodes. Heberden's and Bouchard's nodes may affect one or all the fingers, but the effects are usually symmetrical. Except for the thumb, the MCP joints are not involved. Rheumatoid arthritis usually involves the ulnar aspect of the hand and osteoarthritis involves the radial aspect. The first carpometacarpal joint (CMC) is one of the joints most commonly involved. The wrists are usually spared, except for some volar swelling that occurs when there is an associated carpal tunnel syndrome. Contrary to what is widely believed, the erythrocyte sedimentation rate is sometimes slightly elevated. Other than that, systemic manifestations are lacking. Deformities such as ankylosis of the DIP joints, flexion contractures of the PIP joints and unstable subluxation of the first MCP or CMC joints are frequent. Lateral deviations at both the distal and proximal interphalangeal joints, particularly when radiad at one digit and ulnad at another, are more suggestive of osteoarthritis than they are of rheumatoid arthritis. Although extensive deformations may occur, disability is usually not great. Diagnostic images will show characteristic subchondral sclerosis, marginal spur formation, joint space narrowing, and cystic changes at the involved joint.

With a pathologic condition such as arthritis, there is usually an inflammatory lesion in the muscles, the cell elements of which include lymphocytes, plasma cells, epithelioid cells, and occasionally mononuclear, eosinophile, and polymorphonuclear cells. These cells usually have a nodular arrangement in the tissue but occasionally are scattered. Muscles demonstrate degeneration as evidenced by enlargement, increase in number, and vacuolization of the nuclei. Muscle fibers shrink and break into small elements, and many of the fibers are replaced by fatty and fibrous connective tissue. The blood vessels thicken with collagen and periadventitial or paraadventitial round-cell infiltration. These changes involve the extensor mechanism, subcutaneous tissue, joint capsule, connective tissue septa, and the intrinsic muscles. The PIP joints usually demonstrate limitation of motion so the patient cannot oppose the fingertip to the thumb tip. When the patient tries to grasp an object with the fingers, the thumb opposes the PIP joint. This pressure will eventually lead to a thumb that pushes the fingers in an ulnar direction.

Procedure

The MCP joint is held slightly extended while the examiner moves the PIP joint into flexion, if possible. A positive test, which is indicated by a PIP joint that cannot be flexed, means there is a tight intrinsic muscle or contracture of the joint capsule. If the intrinsic muscles are tight, then when the MCP joints are slightly flexed, the PIP joint will fully flex. This joint will not flex fully if the capsule is tight. The patient remains passive during the test and performs no active movements.

Confirmation Procedures

Cascade sign, test for tight retinacular ligaments, clinical laboratory tests, diagnostic imaging

---

Reporting Statement

Bunnell–Littler test is positive for the right hand at the index finger. This result suggests capsular contracture consistent with osteoarthritis.

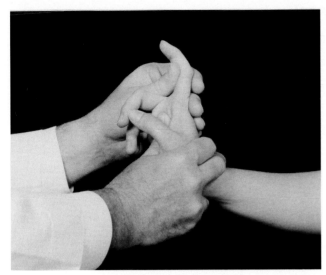

Fig. 6-17 The patient is seated with the elbow flexed and the forearm pronated. The examiner slightly extends the metacarpophalangeal joint of the digit under examination.

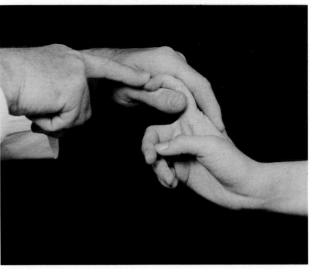

Fig. 6-18 After extending the metacarpophalangeal joint, the examiner tries to move the proximal interphalangeal joint into flexion. The test is positive if the proximal interphalangeal joint cannot be flexed. This result indicates tight intrinsic musculature or contracture of the joint capsule.

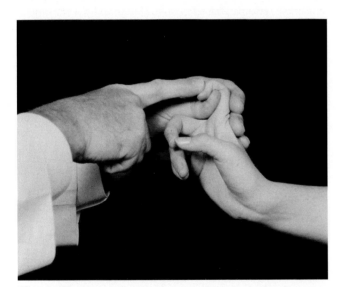

Fig. 6-19 From the position attained in Fig. 6-18, the examiner then slightly extends the proximal interphalangeal joint of the digit, and tries to move the distal interphalangeal joint into flexion.

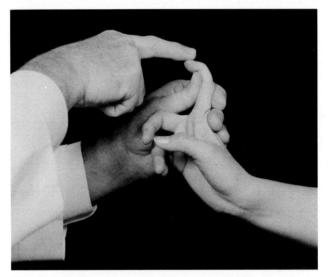

Fig. 6-20 The test is positive if the distal interphalangeal joint cannot be flexed. This indicates tight intrinsic musculature or contracture of the joint capsule.

Comment

Because a sprain is a ligament injury, by definition, it is uncommon in the wrist. Most of the so-called *sprains* that are frequently diagnosed are not sprains at all but are strains of tendon attachments or injuries to the bone. The ligaments of the wrist permit a large amount of motion in the radiocarpal joint but very little motion in the intercarpal joints. The massive ligaments on the volar aspect of the wrist are so strong that a hyperextension injury is more likely to produce an incomplete fracture of the carpal bones, a contusion of the articular surfaces, or possibly a chondral fracture rather than a tearing of the ligaments. With hyperextension there may actually be slipping of one row of carpals on the other. It is this slipping that permits damage to the dorsal carpal ligaments, but it is rather difficult to demonstrate. Suffice it to say that with the common dorsiflexion injury of the wrist, the damage is usually on the dorsal aspect. Therefore, the examiner should be very wary of the diagnosis of sprain of the wrist with a common dorsiflexion injury. During dorsiflexion of the wrist, pain is more frequent over the back of the wrist and forearm than over the front. However, stress on the ligament would appear to have been on the volar side. If there is tenderness over the carpus, careful x-ray study should be made and the carpal bones should be closely studied regarding their position and condition.

The most common carpal fracture is through the navicular at its midpoint. The navicular takes a good deal of stress on the wrist, whether it is in dorsiflexion or palmar flexion, because of its position bridging the two rows of carpals.

Subluxation and dislocation may accompany ligament injury and may have peculiar characteristics when they occur in the wrist. Dislocation of the radiocarpal joint is extremely uncommon even though it occurs as the result of violent action. A complete carpal dislocation is also uncommon and is obviously a serious injury. Both conditions are accompanied by deformity and disability, are readily diagnosed, and usually receive good treatment. Diagnosing the exact dislocation through the carpus is difficult, but careful

x-ray study of the normal as well as the injured wrist in several positions will cut down the margin of error. It is particularly important for these conditions to be diagnosed early because, as with most dislocations, the longer the dislocation remains unreduced, the greater the likelihood that it will recur and permanent residual impairment will result.

The outer layer of the deep fascia of the dorsum of the hand is continuous with the antebrachial fascia. The deep fascia is modified over the wrist to form the dorsal carpal ligament. On either side of the hand the deep fascia becomes fused with the second and fifth metacarpals, with the inner layer forming a compartment through which the extensor tendons can move freely. Distally the deep fascia fuses with the capsules of the MCP joints and adjacent periosteum. The inner layers invest the underlying carpal and metacarpal bones and interosseous muscles.

Procedure

While fixing the other fingers to the exam table, the examiner applies pressure to the dorsum of the digit being examined. The patient attempts to lift or extend the finger off the table. The sign is present if this action causes pain at the dorsum of the wrist. The presence of this sign indicates carpal fracture or sprain.

Confirmation Procedures

Finsterer's sign, Maisonneuve's sign, Finkelstein's test, diagnostic imaging

---

Reporting Statement

Carpal lift sign is present for the right wrist. This result suggests fracture in the proximal or distal row of carpals or in the base of a metacarpal.

∼ Clinical Pearl ∼

Carpal lift is accomplished when the finger is extended against resistance. The earliest sign of carpal fracture or degeneration, before using imaging, is the pain elicited with this test. With a carpal fracture, the carpal lift shifts the bony fragments and produces the corresponding discomfort.

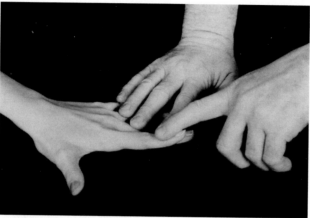

Fig. 6–21   The patient is seated with the elbow flexed. The arm is pronated and the affected hand and wrist are resting flat on the examining table. While fixing the other fingers to the exam table, the examiner applies pressure to the dorsum of the digit under examination. The patient attempts to lift or extend the finger from the table. The sign is present if this action causes pain at the dorsum of the wrist. Such pain indicates carpal fracture or sprain. The pain may be emanating from the proximal or distal row of carpals or from the base of a metacarpal. The examiner should test each digit.

Comment

In the normal wrist and hand the digits are medially deviated slightly in relation to the carpal bones. As well, the metacarpals are at an angle to each other. These positions increase the dexterity of the hand and oblique flexion of the medial four digits and contribute to deformities seen in conditions such as rheumatoid arthritis.

Rheumatoid arthritis is a connective tissue disease characterized by chronic inflammatory changes in the synovial membranes and other structures and by migratory swelling and stiffness of the joints in the early stage. Rheumatoid arthritis is also characterized by a variable degree of deformity, ankylosis, and invalidism in its late stage.

The cause of rheumatoid arthritis has not been determined, but a slight familial tendency has been demonstrated. Hypotheses of the etiologic factors have included infection, abnormality of peripheral circulation, endocrine imbalance, metabolic disturbance, allergic phenomenon, faulty adaptation to physical or psychic stress, and many other concepts. Evidence suggests that infection by slow viruses or organisms of the mycoplasma group may play a role, but proof is lacking. The autoimmune mechanisms may be the underlying cause and proteolytic enzymes released from disrupted lysosomes within the joint may play a part in the chronic synovial inflammation and the destruction of articular cartilage.

Rheumatoid arthritis is currently regarded as one of a group of connective tissue diseases that exhibit somewhat similar clinical and pathologic changes. Other members of the group include systemic lupus erythematosus, polyarteritis nodosa, dermatomyositis, progressive systemic sclerosis, and rheumatic fever.

In the hand and wrist the lesions of rheumatoid arthritis are characteristic and progressively disabling. The thumb is often drawn into adduction, the fingers deviate toward the ulnar side, and individual digits may develop grotesque deformities and severe restriction of function. Arthritic destruction at the wrist may result in dorsal subluxation of the distal end of the ulna, medial subluxation of the carpus on the radius and radial deviation of the hand. The inflammatory synovial reaction damages the joints and involves the tendon sheaths and tendon in producing a variety of deformities.

Procedure

In oblique flexion of the last four digits only the index ray flexes toward the median axis. Thus when the last four digits are flexed separately at the MCP and PIP joints, their axes converge toward the scaphoid tubercle.

Confirmation Procedures

Bunnell-Littler test, test for tight retinacular ligaments, clinical laboratory, diagnostic imaging

---

Reporting Statement

Cascade sign is present. This result suggests rheumatoid arthritis in the carpals of the right wrist.

Cascade sign is present in the right hand. This result suggests internal derangement of the wrist and hand.

∾ Clinical Pearl ∾

A faulty cascade of the fingers, indicating internal derangement of the wrist and hand, is an impediment of the hand grasp in daily activities. Patients usually have adopted accommodating grips. Pain or grip weakness is what precipitates the need for professional care.

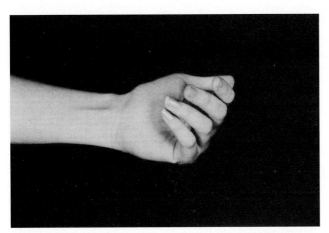

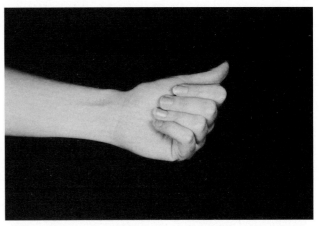

Fig. 6—22   The patient is seated, elbow flexed and the forearm supinated. The patient flexes the fingers at the metacarpophalangeal and proximal interphalangeal joints, as if the hand is gripping a golf club. A complete fist should not be made.

Fig. 6—23   In the normal hand, the longitudinal axis of the four fingers converges over or near the scaphoid tubercle.

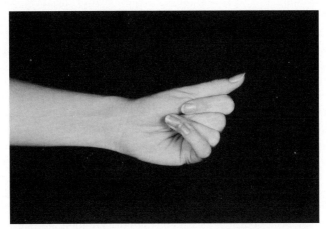

Fig. 6—24   The sign is present if any of the fingers are askew, which indicates internal derangement of the metacarpals or carpals or both.

Dellon's Moving Two-Point Discrimination Test

Comment

Sensation is the acceptance and activation of impulses in the afferents of the nervous system. There are four primary modes of sensation that are determined by the peripheral terminal endings of the sensory axons. These modes are the mechanoreceptors (touch-pressure), nociceptors (pain), and thermoreceptors (cold and warmth). Determination of the electrical conduction velocity of sensory nerves is the only objective way to measure sensation.

Sensibility is the cutaneous appreciation and precise interpretation of sensation. For example, two-point discrimination is a judgment, not a primary sensation. There is no correlation between sensory nerve conduction velocity and two-point discrimination values after repair of peripheral nerves.

Normal cutaneous sensation provides normal quality sensibility that has been termed *tactile gnosia*. All current testing to examine the degree of loss of sensibility is related to cutaneous touch-pressure sensation. The sensation of touch is mediated through myelinated axons that are termed *quickly adapting* and *slowly adapting* in relation to their peripheral receptors. Touch-pressure can be divided into moving touch and constant (static) pressure, in relation to the receptors that are stimulated. Moving touch can be demonstrated with a 30 cycles per second (cps) tuning fork for flutter, which will affect the Meissner corpuscles, or a 256 cps tuning fork for vibration, which will affect the Pacini corpuscles. Static pressure, which will affect the Merkel discs, is evaluated by the Weber two-point discrimination test (Merkel discs) and the von Frey test. Moving touch is evaluated by the moving two-point discrimination test or using the ridge sensimeter. Functional tests, such as a picking-up test or coin test, evaluate both receptor populations. The tests are subjective and related to factors other than sensation, such as comprehension, motor strength, and coordination or concentration.

Procedure

This test is used to predict recovery of function and measures the quickly adapting fibers/receptor system. The examiner moves two blunt points proximally and distally along the long axis of the limb or digit. One or two points are randomly used as the examiner moves distally. The distance between the two points is decreased until the two points can no longer be distinguished.

The object is to determine if the patient can discriminate between being touched with one or two points and the minimum distance at which two points touching the skin are recognized. Clinical testing techniques are for the hand. The test should be demonstrated while the patient is watching the procedure. Several areas on the uninvolved hand should be checked because some patients have congenitally abnormal two-point discrimination.

The testing instrument can be a Boley gauge, a blunt-eye caliper, or paper clip. Testing is begun distally and proceeds proximally. The points of the caliper are set at 10 mm and are brought progressively closer together after each accurate response is obtained. The pressure from the testing instrument should not produce an ischemic area on the skin. When the two points are applied, they make contact simultaneously, and the line between the points is in the longitudinal axis of the finger. The patient closes the eyes for this test and indicates immediately if one or two points are felt. Three to five seconds should be allowed between application of the points. A series of one or two points is applied with varied sequence in each finger zone, and the procedure is performed three times. If the patient does not report two of the three correctly, the result is considered a failure at that distance. If the patient correctly identifies the number of points applied, the testing distance is decreased by 5 mm. There are 10 applications of two points and 10 applications of one point both of which occur randomly. The total incorrect one-point applications are subtracted from the total of correct two-point applications. A score of five or more is considered passing.

The normal threshold for two-point discrimination distance for the volar surface of the hand varies according to the zone being tested. Between the fingertip and the distal interphalangeal (DIP) joint, two-point discrimination is normal between 3 to 5 mm, diminished if between 6 to 10 mm, and absent if greater than 10 mm. Between the DIP joint and the PIP joint, normal is 3 to 6 mm, diminished is 7 to 10 mm, and absent is greater than 10 mm. Between the PIP joint and the finger web, normal is 4 to 7 mm, diminished is 9 to 10 mm, and absent is greater than 10 mm. Between the web and the distal palmar crease, normal is 5 to 8 mm, diminished is 9 to 20 mm, and absent is greater than 20 mm. Between the distal crease and the central palm, normal is 6 to 9 mm, diminished is 10 to 20 mm, and absent is greater than 20 mm. At the base of the palm and wrist normal is 7 to 10 mm, diminished is 11 to 20 mm, and absent is greater than 20 mm. The threshold for the dorsal surface is higher in all zones: normal is 7 to 12 mm, diminished is 13 to 20 mm, and absent is greater than 20 mm.

Below elbow but above the wrist and below knee two-point discrimination distance is normal if between 40 to 50 mm, diminished if between 55 and 80 mm, and absent if greater than 80 mm. Above the elbow and above the knee, two-point discrimination distance is normal if between 65 to 75 mm, diminished if between 80 and 100 mm, and absent if above 100 mm.

Abnormal skin texture, such as heavy scales or calluses, has a marked influence on the test results. Testing can be done in the presence of edema or infection, but the results demonstrate the sensibilities present, which may not reflect the true status of the nerve.

Confirmation Procedures

Interphalangeal neuroma testing, shrivel test, Weber's two-point discrimination test, electrodiagnosis

Reporting Statement

Dellon's moving two-point discrimination test is positive in the index finger on the right hand. This result suggests a pathologic condition of the median nerve.

∾ Clinical Pearl ∾

A Janet's test can be performed simultaneously with Dellon's test. If the patient's responses are bizarre and do not follow anatomic distributions, psychogenic anesthesia is suspected. The patient is instructed to say "yes" when the stimulus is felt and "no" when the stimulus is not felt. The patient will say "no" if functional anesthesia exists.

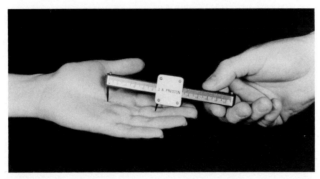

Fig. 6–25 The patient is seated with the elbow flexed. The hand is supinated and is resting on the examining table. The Boley gauge is set at 10 mm of distance or greater. The gauge is applied to the proximal axis of the digit under investigation. The two points must make contact simultaneously and with equal pressure. The patient's eyes should be closed.

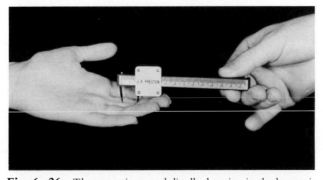

Fig. 6–26 The gauge is moved distally, keeping in the long axis of the finger. The gauge distance is decreased in increments of 5 mm. The test is positive for loss of sensibility if the gauge cannot be perceived as two points at the expected threshold distances for the area tested.

Comment

Stenosing tenosynovitis of the tendon sheath of the abductor pollicis longus and the extensor pollicis brevis was first clearly recognized by de Quervain (1895). In this process an additional etiologic agent may be the presence of accessory tendons in the sheath.

As the tendons to the thumb cross over the lower end of the radius on its radial aspect, they pass through tunnels of grooves on the lower end of the radius. A fibrous retinaculum forms the roof of these tunnels. In particular, the long abductor and short extensor of the thumb pass directly over the styloid process of the radius. Multiple tendons of the abductor may pass through the same sheath, which is subcutaneous. Tenosynovitis in this area is common, usually as a result of overuse of the wrist and thumb. These tendons slide through the tunnel not only during movements of the thumb but also during movements of the wrist while the thumb is fixed. As the condition progresses, the tendons swell, the sheath thickens, and a situation arises that is analogous to *trigger finger.* While one tendon slides through the groove, another one hangs and doubles up. In the early stages the tendon may then slip through the constriction with a palpable click.

During the early stage of this condition, use of the wrist is increasingly painful, and swelling appears over the styloid of the radius, which feels very firm and tender when palpated. At this stage the tendons will slide through the tunnel with discomfort. The condition may progress until it is no longer possible for these tendons to move through the tunnel.

Procedure

Finkelstein's test is used for determining the presence of de Quervain's or Hoffman's diseases, which indicate tenosynovitis of the thumb. Finkelstein's test requires the patient to make a fist with the thumb inside the fingers. The examiner stabilizes the forearm and deviates the wrist in an ulnar direction. This deviation will cause sharp pain in the area of the constriction. During this maneuver all the tendons are forced through the tunnel at the same time. The test is positive if it produces pain over the abductor pollicis longus and the extensor pollicis brevis tendons at the wrist. Pain indicates tenosynovitis in these two tendons. Because the test may cause some discomfort in normal individuals, the examiner should perform the test on the normal side and ask the patient to compare the pain experienced on each side.

Confirmation Procedures

Carpal lift sign, Finsterer's sign, Maisonneuve's sign, clinical laboratory testing, diagnostic imaging

---

Reporting Statement

Finkelstein's test is positive for the right wrist. This result indicates stenosing tenosynovitis of the extensor pollicis longus.

~ **Clinical Pearl** ~

Finkelstein's test produces an exquisitely painful response when stenosing tenosynovitis is present. Initially it is somewhat easier to determine the severity of the condition when the patient actively tucks the thumb in and then deviates the hand and wrist in an ulnar direction. Depending on the response this produces, the passive test can then be performed. The pain elicited by this test is discrete and can be long lasting once excited.

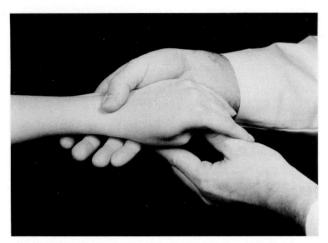

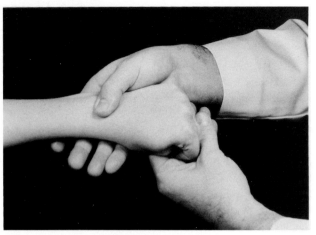

Fig. 6−27 The patient is seated with the elbow flexed and the forearm pronated. The examiner tucks the affected thumb into the palm of the patient's hand.

Fig. 6−28 The patient makes a fist over the thumb, and the examiner helps maintain the fist.

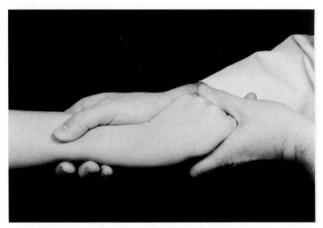

Fig. 6−29 The examiner moves the hand and wrist into sharp ulnar deviation. Pain elicited at the abductor pollicis longus and the extensor pollicis brevis tendons indicates stenosing tenosynovitis.

Comment

Following trauma, whether severe or trivial, the carpal bones may undergo aseptic necrosis. However, often no history of trauma is obtainable. Most commonly the semi-lunar bone is affected (Kienböck's disease), less often the navicular bone is affected (Preiser's disease), and rarely are the other hand bones affected. The amount of aseptic necrosis varies in degree. Regardless, the necrotic trabeculae are slowly resorbed and replaced by creeping substitution. Frequently resorption is incomplete and cyst-like areas form that are filled with fibrous tissue or amorphous debris. The articular cartilage degenerates and is replaced by fibrocartilage. The carpal bones become irregular and the inevitable result is degenerative arthritis of the entire wrist joint.

Symptoms that occur even before roentgenographic evidence appears include wrist pain that radiates up the forearm, tenderness over the affected bone, swelling of the wrist, and limitation of motion, usually dorsiflexion. By passively dorsiflexing either the long finger, if the semilunar bone is involved, or the thumb and index finger, if the navicular bone is involved, pain is reproduced.

A prominent feature of Kienböck's disease is its insidious onset, which frequently occurs without known prior injury. There has been a considerable difference of opinion about the events leading up to this initial complex of findings. Of the possibilities, the occurrence of a simple transverse fracture, resulting from a single episode of trauma, or numerous compression fractures, resulting from repeated compression strains, and lunate or perilunate dislocation, leading to avascular necrosis in anatomically at-risk individuals, are the most popular. These theories have not been supported by well-conceived studies. On the other hand, it is clear that once the process of lunate necrosis has begun, a consistent and progressive sequence of events follows.

Procedure

The sign is present when grasping an object hard, clenching the hand, or making a fist fails to show the normal prominence of the third metacarpal on the dorsal surface, and percussion of the third metacarpal elicits tenderness just distal to the center of the wrist joint. The test is significant for Kienböck's disease (aseptic necrosis of the lunate).

Confirmation Procedures

Carpal lift sign, Maisonneuve's sign, Finkelstein's test, diagnostic imaging

---

Reporting Statement

Finsterer's sign is present in the right wrist. This result suggests lunate carpal aseptic necrosis.

∽ Clinical Pearl ∽

For this sign all the metacarpal heads are percussed. This gross, low-frequency vibration will localize any cortical defect.

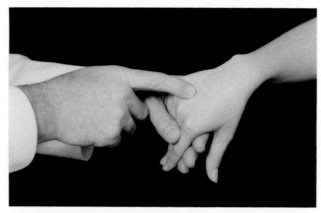

Fig. 6–30 The patient is seated with the elbow flexed and the arm pronated. The examiner locates the proximal head of the third metacarpal. This may be a site of discomfort and abnormal bony contour.

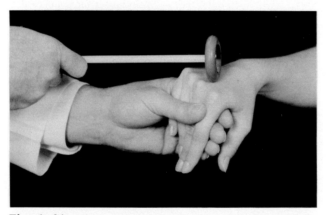

Fig. 6–31 The examiner percusses the proximal head of the third metacarpal with a reflex hammer or tuning fork. Pain elicited distal to the center of the wrist indicates Kienböck's disease (aseptic necrosis of the carpal lunate).

Froment's Paper Sign

Comment

Testing the function of the median and ulnar nerves is the important first step in the evaluation of injuries of the volar aspect of the wrist.

Severance of the median nerve at the wrist results in inability to oppose the thumb and anesthesia of the volar surface of the thumb, and index, and the long, radial half of the ring finger. When this occurs, sensation is the most important function lost. In adults the recovery of sensation is rarely complete following repair of the median nerve. Although a casual examination may show that the patient appreciates pin prick and light touch in a normal manner, a careful examination reveals loss or diminution of two-point discrimination. The patient thereby loses a measure of tactile gnosia, which is essential for rapid and precise manipulation of small objects and for the tactile differentiation of objects.

Severance of the ulnar nerve at the wrist results in the loss of function of the dorsal and volar interossei, the adductor pollicis, and the hypothenar muscles as well as the lumbricales to the ring and little fingers. The patient exhibits anesthesia over the volar surface of the little finger and over the ulnar half of the volar surface of the ring finger. The key function lost is the use of the adductor pollicis and the first dorsal interosseous. The adductor is essential for strong pinching by the thumb. The first dorsal interosseous stabilizes the index finger against the thumb during pinching. The strength of the ulnar-innervated intrinsic muscles fails to return to functional levels in 75% of all ulnar nerve injuries in adults.

Procedure

The patient attempts to grasp a piece of paper between the thumb and index finger. When the examiner attempts to pull the paper away, the terminal phalanx of the thumb will flex because of paralysis of the adductor pollicis muscle. This result indicates a positive test. The test indicates ulnar nerve paralysis.

Confirmation Procedures

Pinch grip test, Wartenberg's sign, electrodiagnosis

Reporting Statement

Froment's test is positive for the right hand, which indicates ulnar nerve palsy.

∾ Clinical Pearl ∾

A change from a tip-to-tip pinch grip position to a pulp-to-pulp position is the earliest sign of ulnar entrapment (anterior interosseous nerve lesions must be differentiated). An EMG requires more gross muscle deficiency for conclusive findings, and the nerve conduction velocity (NCV) may be equivocal in the early stages of nerve degeneration.

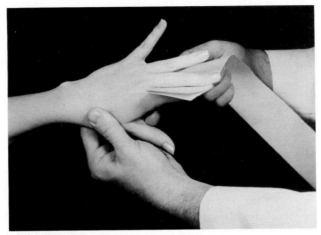

Fig. 6–32   The patient's elbow is flexed, and the forearm is pronated. The patient abducts the fingers from each other. The examiner places a sheet of paper between any two fingers, and the patient adducts the fingers, gripping the paper. Failure to maintain this grip as the examiner tugs on the paper suggests ulnar nerve paralysis.

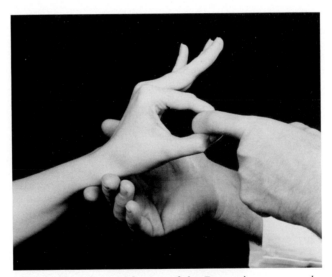

Fig. 6–33   In a modification of the Froment's paper test, the patient adducts and flexes the tip of the finger to the tip of the thumb. The examiner tries to pull the digits apart. Failure of the fingers to maintain sufficient strength to resist this motion suggests ulnar nerve paralysis (anterior interosseous nerve lesions must be differentiated).

Comment

Neuromas can form at the cut end of an injured nerve. A neuroma in continuity may develop along the pathway of an injured nerve. When stimulated, the neuromas may cause exquisite discomfort in the extremity. This usually consists of a pins-and-needles sensation or a shooting pain that radiates from a localized area. Sometimes the pain may become so severe and diffuse that it spreads up the entire extremity. This spread of pain from a neuroma to the point where it involves the entire extremity may be explained by the fiber interaction in injured nerves. Another theory is that the painful nerve impulse stimulates or excites the internuncial pool of the spinal cord so much that normal impulses reaching this area from the periphery are interpreted as painful. This pain also could occur in higher regions of the central nervous system.

Such painful neuromas often are confused with the phantom-limb syndrome. This does not imply that the phantom-limb syndrome is due to a painful neuroma. The point is that the painful neuroma so excites and stimulates certain areas of the central nervous system that the phantom sensation becomes painful.

Painful neuromas should not be confused with causalgia. Pain produced by neuromas should not be called *minor causalgia* because this only adds to the confusion.

Procedure

Neuromas should be carefully sought out by examination of the area using a slender instrument for palpating, such as the blunt end of a reflex hammer. A localized spot in a scar will cause severe pain and is associated with paresthesia. The neuroma itself may be felt as a discrete mass.

Confirmation Procedures

Dellon's moving two-point discrimination test, shrivel test, Weber's two-point discrimination test, electrodiagnosis

Reporting Statement

Interdigital probing reveals the presence of a neuroma in continuity in the median nerve at the base of the first phalanx of the right hand.

∾ Clinical Pearl ∾

Although neuromas in continuity develop more frequently in the lower extremity and near amputations, they do develop elsewhere. Neuromas in continuity are observed at the bifurcation of nerve branches near the base of digits. This may result from the chronic mechanical irritation caused by malalignment of the digit structures.

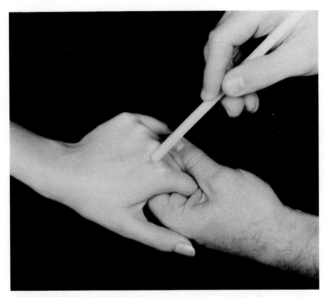

Fig. 6–34 The patient's forearm is pronated. The metacarpophalangeal interdigital tissues are probed with the blunt end of a reflex hammer. If a neuroma is present, severe pain and paresthesia will be elicited. The neuroma may be palpated as a discrete mass.

Comment

A fracture through the flared distal metaphysis of the radius, also known as the *Colles' fracture,* is a common fracture in adults older than age 50. This type of fracture occurs more frequently in women than in men and has the same age and sex incidence as fractures of the neck of the femur. Both fractures occur through bone that has become markedly weakened by a combination of senile and post-menopausal osteoporosis.

The incidence of Colles' fracture is particularly high when walking conditions are slippery because the typical mechanism of injury is as follows: the patient either slips or trips, and in an attempt to break the fall, the patient lands on the open hand with the forearm pronated. This pressure breaks the wrist. Therefore the forces that fracture the distal end of the radius involve not only dorsiflexion and radial deviation but also supination, all of which account for the typical fracture deformity.

The fracture pattern is constant, the main fracture line being transverse within the distal 2 cm of the radius. There may be only two major fragments but comminution of the thin cortex is common, especially in the osteoporotic bone of the elderly. The ulnar styloid is frequently avulsed. The distal end of an intact radius extends beyond the distal end of the ulna. The joint surface is angulated 15 degrees toward the anterior (palmar) aspect of the wrist. After a Colles' fracture these relationships are reversed, and there is always some degree of subluxation of the distal radioulnar joint.

The clinical deformity, frequently called a *dinner fork deformity,* is typical. In addition to the swelling there is an obvious jog just proximal to the wrist, due to the posterior displacement and posterior tilt of the distal radial fragment. The hand is radially deviated, and although it is often less obvious clinically, the wrist appears supinated in relation to the forearm.

Two main types of Colles' fractures can be identified. With the stable type of fracture, there is one main transverse fracture line with little cortical comminution. In the unstable type there is gross comminution, particularly of the dorsal cortex, and marked crushing of the cancellous bone. The intact periosteal hinge is on the dorsal aspect of the fracture in both types.

Median nerve injury occurring coincident with a Colles' fracture (laceration or contusion) is quite rare but should be considered when the fracture is compound. Most early-median nerve problems are related to the progressive edema and hematoma that follow injury and to reduction of the fracture. During the healing phase exuberant fracture callus, especially in the presence of persistent bony deformity, can result in median nerve symptoms. The residual scarring and thickening that follow healing can eventually result in carpal tunnel syndrome, or tardy median nerve palsy, at a much later date.

Procedure

A positive Maissonneuve's sign is characterized by marked hyperextensibility (dorsiflexion) of the hand. The sign is present in Colles' fracture.

Confirmation Procedures

Carpal lift sign, Finsterer's sign, Finkelstein's test, diagnostic imaging

---

Reporting Statement

Maisonneuve's sign is present in the right wrist. This sign indicates a Colles' fracture of the radius.

∽ Clinical Pearl ∽

Maisonneuve's sign remains a finding long after the fracture healing process is completed. A marked hyperextension of the wrist, with or without complaint, warrants imaging.

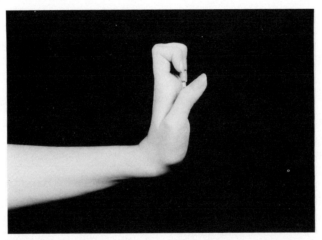

Fig. 6–35 The patient's arm is pronated with the elbow flexed. The hand and wrist are actively dorsiflexed. The sign is present if marked hyperextension of the wrist is apparent. The sign is present in Colles' fracture.

～ Phalen's Sign ～

PHELAN'S SIGN
PRAYER SIGN

Comment

In the distal forearm, the median and ulnar nerves are surrounded by soft tissues and untethered by bone or dense ligamentous tissues. Distal to the sublimis muscle belly, the median nerve lies just beneath the fascia and is protected only by the palmaris longus tendon. Within the carpal tunnel, the median nerve is in the most volar layer of structures and is easily compressed by the volar carpal ligament. The four unyielding walls of the carpal tunnel fix the volume of the tunnel and guarantee compression of the contained structures if edema or bone fragments occupy part of the available space.

The median nerve may be compressed in the carpal tunnel producing carpal tunnel syndrome. Usually there is pain over the median nerve distribution, and as the disease progresses, a definite pattern of hypesthesia or anesthesia will appear over this area. Opposition of the thumb may disappear before there are definite sensory changes in the hand. The large fibers (motor) in the nerves are damaged more than the smaller fibers (sensory) in such types of indirect trauma. Percussion of the median nerve at the flexor crease of the wrist may produce paresthesia along the median nerve. As the disease progresses, the pain may reach the forearm and even the shoulder. The symptoms may be more prominent at night.

The symptoms are aggravated by temporarily occluding the circulation of the arm above the elbow. A partially injured nerve is more susceptible to ischemia than a normal one. Therefore paresthesia and numbness will appear first along the median nerve distribution rather than in the ulnar nerve.

Procedure

The patient flexes the patient's wrists maximally and holds this position for 1 minute by pushing both the wrists together. A positive test is indicated by a tingling sensation that radiates into the thumb, the index finger, and the middle and lateral half of the ring finger. The presence of this sensation indicates carpal tunnel syndrome caused by pressure on the median nerve.

Confirmation Procedures

Tinel's sign at the wrist, wringing test, electrodiagnosis, diagnostic imaging (MRI)

Reporting Statement

Phalen's sign is present in the right wrist. This sign indicates carpal tunnel syndrome and median nerve palsy.

～ Clinical Pearl ～

Phalen's sign duplicates the wrist flexion/extension maneuvers that irritate the median nerve. The presence of Phalen's sign is a good indicator that wrist splints will be useful in the management of the carpal tunnel syndrome. As a screening test, a reverse Phalen's maneuver can be performed. The patient is asked to press the hands together in the vertical plane and raise the elbows until they are horizontal. Loss of any dorsiflexion should be obvious. The most common cause of lost dorsiflexion is stiffness after a Colles' fracture.

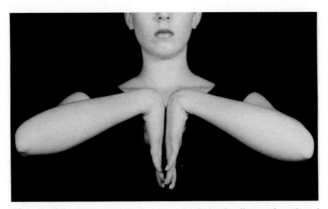

Fig. 6−36 The patient is seated with both elbows flexed and the arms pronated. The wrists are flexed and the dorsal surfaces of the hands are approximated to each other. The position is maintained for at least 60 seconds. Additionally, the elbows can be dropped slightly to increase the wrist flexion angle. Median nerve paresthesia indicates carpal tunnel syndrome. In the flexed wrist position the syndrome is due to neural ischemia.

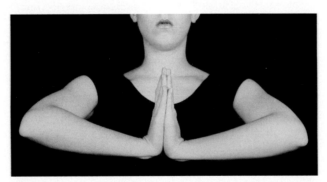

Fig. 6−37 A reversed position for this test is with the patient's wrists extended and the palms of the hands approximated to each other. The patient maintains this position for at least 60 seconds. Median nerve paresthesia indicates carpal tunnel syndrome that is due to neural stretch.

Comment

In the anterior interosseous nerve syndrome, the pronator quadratus is nonfunctioning and pronation is accomplished entirely by the pronator teres, and selective pronation tests are positive in varying degrees. The pronator teres muscle is strongest while the elbow joint is in extension and weaker while the elbow is flexed to 145 degrees. The patient pronates the arm against resistance if the pronator quadratus is nonfunctioning. The patient will have more pronation power while the arm is extended, when the pronator teres is at its maximum advantage, than while the elbow is flexed, when the pronator quadratus contributes its force in pronation.

After supplying the pronator teres, flexor carpi radialis, palmaris longus, and flexor digitorum sublimis muscles, the median nerve divides into two branches. The main trunk continues into the hand, and the anterior interosseous branch supplies the flexor pollicis longus, the flexor digitorum profundus to the index and middle fingers, and the pronator quadratus. Compression of the anterior interosseous branch of the median nerve in the forearm, usually secondary to anomalous muscle and tendon origins, produces the anterior interosseous syndrome. The characteristic physical finding of this compression is paralysis of the muscles that this section of the nerve supplies. During physical examination, there is weakness of grip and a characteristic pinch grip in which the index finger is extended at the distal interphalangeal joint with hyperflexion of the proximal interphalangeal joint. The metacarpophalangeal joint of the thumb has increased flexion and the interphalangeal joint is hyperextended. Thenar muscle function and sensory function in the median nerve distribution are normal.

Procedure

The patient pinches the tips of the index finger and thumb together. Normally this is a tip-to-tip pinch. However, if after attempting this test, the patient is unable to pinch tip to tip and instead has a pulp-to-pulp pinch of the index finger and thumb, this result is considered a positive sign for a pathologic condition in the anterior interosseous nerve, a branch of the median nerve. This sign may indicate entrapment of the anterior interosseous nerve as it passes between the two heads of the pronator teres muscle.

Confirmation Procedures

Froment's paper sign, Wartenberg's sign, electrodiagnosis

Reporting Statement

Pinch grip testing on the right is positive. This result indicates anterior interosseous nerve syndrome in the forearm.

~ **Clinical Pearl** ~

Even minor irritation of the anterior interosseous nerve produces this sign. The inability to pinch grip tip-to-tip influences the patient's ability to pick up small objects, which is the dysfunction that usually causes the patient to seek professional care.

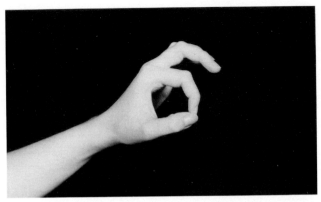

Fig. 6–38 The patient's elbow is flexed and the forearm is pronated. The patient pinches the tip of the index finger to the tip of the thumb. Normally, the pinch grip is tip to tip.

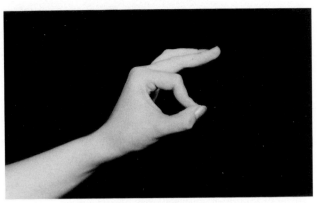

Fig. 6–39 If the pinch grip is tip to pulp or pulp to pulp, the test is positive. A positive test indicates involvement of the anterior interosseous nerve.

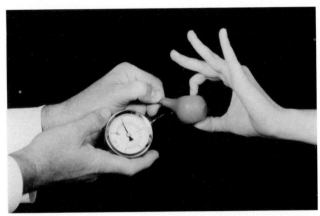

Fig. 6–40 The pinch grip also can be determined with pinch dynamometers. Again, the normal grip is tip to tip. The grip strength of each digit is recorded.

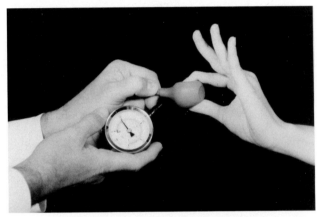

Fig. 6–41 The abnormal grip is tip to pulp or pulp to pulp, both of which produce a corresponding loss of pinch-grip strength.

∼ Shrivel Test ∼

O'RIAIN'S SIGN

Comment

O'Riain has recorded a common but unappreciated observation. The skin of denervated fingers does not wrinkle or shrivel as normal skin does when immersed in warm water. This objective test can be performed without the patient's concentration or cooperation, and is particularly indicated for use with small children. Shriveling of the skin returns progressively with recovery of nerve function. O'Riain recommends immersion in water at approximately 40°C for a period of 30 minutes. Smooth skin indicates a loss of sensibility.

Procedure

The patient's fingers are placed in warm (40° C) water for approximately 30 minutes. The examiner then removes the patient's fingers from the water and observes whether the skin over the pulp is wrinkled. Normal fingers will show wrinkling, and denervated ones will not. The test is valid only in the first few months after injury.

Confirmation Procedures

Dellon's moving two-point discrimination test, interphalangeal neuroma test, Weber's two-point discrimination test, electrodiagnosis

Reporting Statement

O'Riain's sign is present on the second and third digits of the right hand. The presence of this sign indicates denervation.

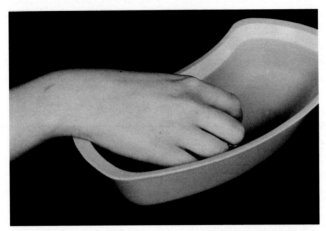

Fig. 6–42   The patient's fingers are immersed in warm (40°C) water for approximately 30 minutes.

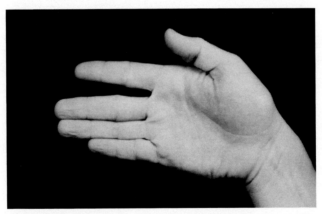

Fig. 6–43   After removing the digits from the water, skin wrinkling is noted. If the skin of the pulp of a finger is not wrinkled, the test is positive. A positive shrivel test indicates denervation of that area. This sign usually is not elicited after 90 to 120 days following injury.

Comment

A study of the structure and function of the dorsal aponeurosis is essential for understanding the forces that are active during flexion and extension of the finger. The dorsal aponeurosis is the main structural basis for the integration and coordination of the extensor and intrinsic muscles.

An important portion of the terminal tendon is the retinacular ligament. This ligament is composed of two parts, a transverse layer that is spread over both lateral tendons and a very slender but strong band that merges with the most lateral fibers of the terminal tendon. The first or broad thin ligament passes proximally across the proximal interphalangeal joint. Some of the ligament's fibers reach as far as the flexor tendon sheath over the first phalanx, to which they adhere. The fibers of the second or oblique ligament pass underneath the transverse part of the retinacular ligament and insert into the lateral border of the first phalanx. Therefore the lateral aspect of the proximal interphalangeal joint is crossed by two structures, the lateral tendon and the retinacular ligament. At the level of the proximal interphalangeal joint, the dorsal aponeurosis forms a hood that is drawn over the joint, further reinforcing the joint at its sides.

The position of the lateral tendon and the retinacular ligament is important, especially the oblique part of the ligament in relation to the axis of motion of the proximal interphalangeal joint. In the fully extended joint, the lateral tendon passes dorsally, and the oblique band passes ventrally to the axis. This relation changes as the joint is flexed, until both structures become displaced ventrally.

On the dorsal side of the second phalanx, a triangular lamina of connective tissue that joins the two lateral tendons with each other, prevents both tendons from sliding off the base of the second phalanx. According to Bunnell, a fascial sheet extending from the lateral band to the collateral ligament and to the base of the second phalanx causes the volar shift of the lateral bands during flexion.

Procedure

The proximal interphalangeal joint is held in a neutral position while the distal interphalangeal joint is flexed by the examiner. If the distal interphalangeal joint does not flex, the retinacular (collateral) ligaments or capsule are tight. If the proximal interphalangeal joint flexes easily, the retinacular ligaments are tight and the capsule is normal. The patient remains passive during the test and does no active movements.

Confirmation Procedures

Bunnell-Littler test, Cascade sign, clinical laboratory testing, diagnostic imaging.

Reporting Statement

The test for tight retinacular ligaments is positive at the distal interphalangeal joint of the index finger of the right hand. This indicates fixation of the ligaments.

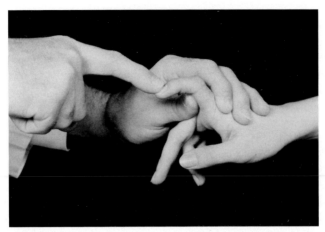

Fig. 6–44 The patient's elbow is flexed and the forearm is pronated. The examiner fixes the proximal interphalangeal joint in the neutral position. The examiner tries to flex the distal interphalangeal joint. If the joint does not flex, the collateral ligaments and the joint capsule are tight. If the joint flexes freely, the collateral ligaments are tight, and the joint capsule is normal.

∼ Tinel's Sign at the Wrist ∼
FORMICATION SIGN
DISTAL TINGLING ON PERCUSSION (DTP) SIGN
HOFFMAN-TINEL SIGN

Comment

Pressure applied to an injured nerve trunk frequently produces a tingling sensation that is transmitted to the periphery of the nerve and localized to a precise cutaneous region. Pain is a sign of nerve irritation; tingling is a sign of regeneration. More precisely, tingling reveals the presence of regenerating axons.

The point of nerve irritation is present as a localized pain that is felt at the point where pressure is applied. If this pain extends along the nerve trunk, it is most intense at the point of pressure. This type of pain is associated with pain produced by pressure of the muscles, and most frequently the muscular pain is more pronounced than the pain along the nerve trunk.

Although the tingling of regeneration is not a painful sensation, it is a vaguely disagreeable feeling. The patient may compare the sensation with that of an electrical shock. This sensation may be felt at the point of compression but is felt most frequently in the skin along the corresponding nerve distribution. The patient does not experience pain in the muscles adjacent to the nerve where tingling is found.

The two types of sensation, pain and tingling, produced by pressure on the nerve are easily differentiated in all cases. The two sensations rarely exist simultaneously in the same nerve or more exactly, at the same point during examination of a nerve. The sensations may follow one another along the same nerve trunk. The two different signs produced by pressure applied to the nerve are similar to the symptoms that are revealed by examination of the skin sensation. Regeneration of the nerve is manifested by paresthesia of a more constant type such as that associated with hypoesthesia produced by touch, by puncture, and especially by slight friction of the skin.

However, in all cases the symptoms produced by pressure of the nerve—pain that indicates the irritation of the axons or tingling that indicates their regeneration—are much easier to differentiate than the signs of cutaneous sensibility. The symptoms also are more constant and appear much earlier. They furnish more precise, more localized, and more important information.

In total nerve interruption along the course of the nerve trunk, a definite zone can be found where pressure produces tingling in the cutaneous distribution of the nerve. This zone of tingling is not extended. It does not exceed 2 or 3 cm. This zone indicates that at this precise point the suddenly interrupted axons have undergone local degeneration.

With complete interruptions of the nerve produced by very tight entrapment, the same characteristics of fixation, prominence, and precise limitation are found, but the zone of tingling is more extended.

It is possible in certain instances to find along the course of the same nerve two different sites of tingling corresponding to two different lesion levels.

Incomplete interruption of a nerve or, more exactly, lesions permitting the passage of regenerating axons, are characterized by progressive extension of the tingling.

The same progressive extension of the tingling zone is found in incomplete interruption with nerve irritability.

Tingling induced by pressure of the nerve does not appear before the fourth or even the sixth week after trauma. Also, the tingling disappears as soon as the nerve returns to its normal structure and the newly formed axons become mature. After 8 or 10 months the tingling stops. Tingling may be absent in certain, rare cases.

The first clinical manifestation of regeneration of a nerve is the occurrence of paresthesia while percussing the nerve. As this is done, beginning distally and proceeding proximally, a point will be reached at which the patient feels a tingling or buzzing sensation accompanied by radiation of sensation down to the involved area. The advancing edge of this sensitive area in the nerve is measured at monthly intervals using some bony prominence as a guide. The steady progress of this sensation down the nerve is a rough test of recovery.

Procedure

The examiner taps over the carpal tunnel at the wrist. A positive test causes tingling in the thumb, index finger, forefinger, and the middle and lateral half of the ring finger (along the median nerve distribution). The tingling and paresthesia must be felt distal to the point of pressure for a positive test. The test is an indication of the rate of regeneration of the sensory fibers of the median nerve. The most distal point at which the abnormal sensation is felt represents the limit of nerve regeneration.

Confirmation Procedures

Phalen's sign, Wartenberg's sign, electrodiagnosis, diagnostic imaging (MRI)

Reporting Statement

Tinel's sign is present at the right wrist, producing paresthesia along the median nerve distribution.

∾ **Clinical Pearl** ∾

Tinel's sign is extremely useful in identifying (1) the most proximal point of nerve regeneration or (2) the most distal point of nerve degeneration. These points are one in the same. Tinel's is most evidenced at the Valleix points (tender points) along the course of the peripheral nerve (as in a neuralgia/neuritis). The examiner also may slide the tip of the index finger across the palm, noting frictional resistance and temperature. Increased thenar resistance from lack of sweating and temperature rise (vasodilation) may occur with median involvement.

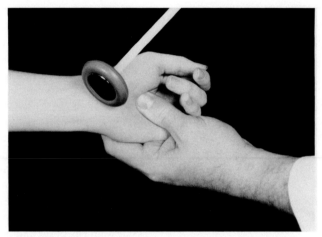

Fig. 6–45 The patient's elbow is flexed and the forearm supinated. The wrist and hand are slightly dorsiflexed by the examiner. The examiner percusses the volar surface of the wrist over the carpal tunnel with a reflex hammer or tuning fork. Tingling that is along the median nerve distribution and distal to the point of percussion indicates regeneration of the nerve. Pain following the same distribution, above and below the point of percussion, indicates neural inflammation and degeneration. Percussion at the Tunnel of Guyon reveals the condition of the ulnar nerve as it passes into the hand.

Comment

Significant diminution of blood flow to individual digits or to an entire hand results in pale nail beds, slow capillary recovery after skin compression, diminished bleeding after skin puncture, lowering of the skin temperature, and pain of varying intensity. Symptoms and signs of pain, pulselessness, pallor, paresthesia, and paralysis indicate arterial insufficiency or inadequate capillary perfusion. The coexistence of pallor with cyanosis and rubor is consistent with vasoconstriction and subsequent vasodilation.

The occurrence of pallor and a significant drop in skin temperature will cause pain that is moderately severe and described as a deep, dull, aching sensation. As the ischemia state persists, pain becomes more intense.

The term Raynaud's disease is used to describe the occurrence of vasospasm without an underlying primary disease. If vasospasm is associated with a known connective tissue disease, then Raynaud's phenomenon is implied. Recognition of a Raynaud's syndrome and the patient's response to this condition is important in explaining pain and cold tolerance associated with a known pathologic condition. When the symptoms of pain occur in a digit of the hand or on the entire extremity, the existence of adequate blood flow in the large and small vessels must be determined.

In patients known to have a nerve lesion—such as ulnar nerve compression at the elbow, posterior interosseous nerve compression in the supinator muscle, or median nerve compression at the wrist—diminished blood flow will cause abnormal sensory changes to occur earlier than would happen in the normal patient, and motor weakness occurs more quickly when partial or complete ischemia occurs.

Various conditions—such as atherosclerotic stenosis, thromboembolism, or compression of major arteries in the thoracic outlet—cause pain, claudication, paresthesia, and intermittent episodes of pallor. The lesions may be partial or complete, and the clinical symptoms vary according to the degree of ischemia.

Acute occlusion of the ulnar artery is associated with unrelenting pain, pallor, and later, rubor and cyanosis. Cold tolerance is diminished, and intrinsic muscle weakness occurs.

Obliteration of the brachial artery due to trauma causes the occurrence of an anterior compartment compression of the forearm muscles, vessels, and nerve and causes pallor of the hand, diminished pulse volume, and severe pain. The effect of diminished arterial inflow and lessened venous outflow on pain has been calibrated by analyzing the effects of traumatic lesions at various levels of the extremity. Decompression of a tight compartment anterior to the elbow and in the forearm will diminish pain almost immediately. Elimination of nerve compression syndromes at the wrist and elbow will provide measurable relief of pain.

Causalgia is a mixed nerve lesion with accompanying or secondary vascular insufficiency.

Sympathetic dystrophy is a part of the spectrum that may occur although no particular nerve injury is demonstrated. There is, however, a vasospastic element that occurs secondary to a major or minor insult of the extremity or an adjacent organ.

Procedure

Application of a pneumatic tourniquet to a normal extremity with pressure elevated to 20 mm of mercury above the patient's resting diastolic blood pressure will obliterate arterial inflow and venous outflow, slow motor nerve conduction, decrease sensory conduction, and cause severe pain in the hand and forearm, all of which occur at the site of tourniquet compression. Anoxia and nerve compression occur simultaneously, and muscle weakness is evident within 3 to 5 minutes. Digital paresthesia occurs and sensation diminishes gradually to anesthesia in about 30 minutes. These painful sensations are a combination of muscle and nerve ischemia as well as nerve compression.

The appearance of symptoms at less than 300 mm of pressure or sooner than 3 to 5 minutes is a positive test result. A positive test indicates neural instability as a result of posterior interosseous nerve or median nerve compression syndromes.

Confirmation Procedures

Allen's test, vascular assessment

Reporting Statement

The tourniquet test is positive in the right forearm. This result indicates neural irritability as a result of posterior interosseous or median nerve compression.

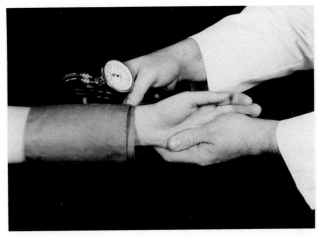

Fig. 6–46 The patient's elbow is flexed and the arm is supinated and resting on the examination table. A blood pressure cuff is applied to the forearm at a spot above the area of complaint. The cuff is inflated to 20 mm above the patient's resting, diastolic blood pressure. Pressure may be increased to reach blanching of the distal extremity. Arm and hand pain, paresthesia, and muscle weakness appearing in less than 5 minutes indicate arterial insufficiency.

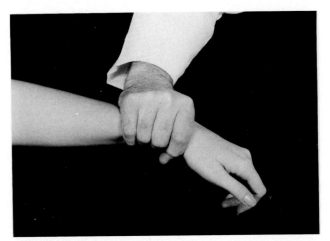

Fig. 6–47 A modified tourniquet test is performed with the examiner occluding the circulation of the extremity manually instead of using a blood pressure cuff. The same principles apply, but this modification does not rely on the accuracy of the pressure to establish occlusion of the arteries.

Comment

The ulnar nerve descends from the medial cord of the brachial plexus on the medial side of the arm and pierces the medial intramuscular septum. The nerve continues in a groove behind the medial humeral epicondyle into the forearm. A branch to the flexor carpi ulnaris is given off in the region of the elbow and distal to this, a branch to the medial half of the flexor digitorum profundus. The nerve trunk enters the forearm posteriorly between the two heads of the flexor carpi ulnaris. The nerve is constricted by a fibrous band between the muscle and the ulna, and it is here that the nerve trunk is vulnerable to compression. The nerve, which lies to the medial side of the ulnar artery in the distal half of the forearm and proximal to wrist, emerges from under the flexor carpi ulnaris to enter the canal of Guyon, the roof of which is the volar carpal ligament. From here the nerve passes between the pisiform and hamate bones, and at this point the nerve divides into a deep motor branch to the ulnar innervated intrinsic muscles and a superficial sensory branch. The latter supplies both the dorsal and volar aspects of the ulnar side of the hand, all of the small fingers, and the ulnar half of the ring finger. The deep motor branch swings across the mid-palm, dorsal to the flexor tendons, as it gives off branches to the palmaris brevis and the three hypothenar muscles: the abductor, opponens, and flexor digiti quinti. The nerve then supplies the four dorsal and three volar interossei, the lumbricales of the small and ring fingers, the adductor pollicis, and the deep head of the flexor pollicis brevis. Proximal to the wrist the palmar and dorsal cutaneous nerves of the hand are given off.

The ulnar nerve is the most commonly injured nerve of the upper extremity. Open wounds, especially at the wrist, are the most common cause of injury, but compression or irritation of the nerve at either the wrist or the elbow is not rare. The major functional loss in low median nerve palsy is a sensory loss. Loss of ulnar nerve function, as with radial nerve function, is a motor loss. Anesthesia in the ulnar distribution of the hand, at its worst, is an inconvenience, but loss of all the interossei and the adductor pollicis interferes seriously with the strength and effectiveness of the patient's grasp.

Ulnar clawhand, *main en griffe,* is primarily due to loss of the interossei, the major function of which is to flex the metacarpophalangeal joints. With the loss of the interossei, the action of the extrinsic finger extensors is unopposed, and a hyperextension deformity of the metacarpophalangeal joints begins. As the volar capsule of these joints stretches, the deformity, which may be barely present in the recently injured extremity, progresses. Lumbricales one and two are most commonly median innervated. Therefore the index and middle fingers usually do not develop the deformity. The interossei and lumbricales also act as interphalangeal joint extensors, and with their paralysis these joints are held in flexion by the now-unopposed flexor digitorum profundi and flexor digitorum sublimis. These flexors are overactive in their attempt to compensate for the lack of the interossei as metacarpophalangeal flexors. Thus a vicious cycle is started. The more the patient attempts to correct the deformity actively, the more exaggerated it will become. The degree of clawing is usually less apparent in the high ulnar palsy than when the ulnar half of the flexor digitorum profundus is spared. The degree of clawing also will depend on other factors, such as the degree of ligamentous laxity in an individual patient's joints and the functions for which the hand is regularly used.

Most obvious in the ulnar clawhand is the apparent deformity of clawing, which is a loss of the transverse arch of the hand, and visible atrophy of the interossei, particularly the first dorsal interosseous muscle mass. Hypothenar atrophy also occurs. The next most apparent condition is the clumsy grip and the marked weakness of grasp. Normal grip strength in the adult male is approximately 90 pounds. In the ulnar palsied hand the grip strength will only be one quarter to one third of that. It is this weakness that is most disabling for gross dysfunction of the hand, such as grasping a shovel or a suitcase handle.

More disabling for fine sophisticated use of the hand is the interference with normal pinch or prehension. The average strength of pinch in the adult male is 20 to 25 pounds, but with ulnar palsy, the strength is only 10% to 20% of that. This loss in strength is due to paralysis of the adductor pollicis, half of the flexor pollicis brevis, and the first dorsal interosseous muscles. The paralysis of these muscles leads not only to weakness but also to gross deformity of pinch, manifested by hyperextension of the thumb metacarpophalangeal joint and hyperflexion of the thumb interphalangeal joint. A good test of adductor pollicis and first dorsal interosseous function is to observe the position of pinch, test its strength, and palpate the first dorsal interosseous muscle on the radial side of the second metacarpal and the adductor pollicis deep in the thumb web while the patient attempts maximum strength of pinch.

The ulnar pinch deformity represents a reversal of the normal longitudinal arch of the first metacarpal and thumb, the integrity of which is dependent on the presence of the adductor pollicis and normal metacarpophalangeal flexion. Many variations of classic ulnar-palsied pinch are possible and are caused by variations in median and ulnar innervation of the intrinsics, whether or not the patient has loose or tight joints.

Ulnar palsy is usually due to trauma of the ulnar nerve as it passes behind the medial humeral epicondyle. The most common causes are old fractures of the elbow and arthritis. Paresthesia or hypesthesia develop in the ulnar nerve distribution with increasing weakness of the intrinsic muscles. Percussion of the nerve in the epicondylar groove will produce paresthesia along its course.

Procedure

The patient performs a hard grasp strength test with a dynamometer. The examiner observes the position and function of the digits in the action. If the position of abduction is assumed by the little finger, the sign is present. The sign is present in ulnar palsy.

Confirmation Procedures

Froment's paper sign, pinch grip test, electrodiagnosis

Reporting Statement

Wartenberg's sign is present in the right hand. The presence of this sign suggests ulnar palsy.

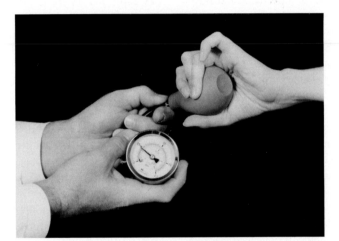

Fig. 6–48 The patient grasps a dynamometer for grip-strength testing. The sign is present if the fifth digit remains abducted and does not contribute to the grip strength. The presence of the sign indicates ulnar nerve paralysis.

~ Weber's Two-Point Discrimination Test ~

Comment

The human nervous system is bombarded by a simultaneous multitude of stimuli. The afferent input is limited by the inconstant threshold of the peripheral nerve endings and the specialized receptor organs associated with them. Sensation is the acceptance and activation of impulses in the afferent nerve fibers of the nervous system.

The brain receives and elaborates a continuously changing flood of sensations. Varied sensations are synthesized into three-dimensional experiences. Central neural mechanisms, such as memory storage and introspection, influence the conscious perception of the external and internal environment. Sensibility is the conscious appreciation and interpretation of the stimulus that produced sensation.

A sensory unit is a single first-order afferent neuron including all peripheral and central branches. Five elementary qualities of sensibility can be evoked: (1) touch-pressure, (2) warmth, (3) cold, (4) pain, and (5) movement and position. Sensation for these qualities depends on many factors. Some involving the sensory unit are (1) the diameter of the first-order afferent neuron, (2) the properties of the sensory receptors, (3) the size and population of the receptive field, and (4) the threshold for the entire sensory unit.

Procedure

Weber's two-point discrimination test was introduced by Weber in 1835. The object is to determine if the patient can discriminate between being touched by one or two points and the minimum distance at which two points that are touching the skin are recognized. The test should be demonstrated while the patient is watching the procedure. Several areas on the uninvolved hand should be checked because some patients have congenitally abnormal two-point discrimination.

The testing instrument can be a Boley gauge, a blunt-eye caliper, or an ordinary paper clip. Testing is begun distally and proceeds proximally. The points of the caliper are set at 10 mm and are brought together progressively as accurate responses are obtained. The pressure from the testing instrument should not produce an ischemic area on the skin. When two points are applied, they make contact simultaneously. The patient closes the eyes. The patient indicates immediately if one or two points are felt. An interval of 3 to 5 seconds should be allowed between application of the points. A series of one or two points is applied with varied sequence in each finger zone. The procedure is done three times; if the patient does not record two of the three correctly, the result is considered a failure at that test distance. If the patient correctly identifies the number of points applied, the testing distance is decreased in varying increments. There are 10 applications of two-points and 10 applications of one point at random. The total incorrect, one-point applications are subtracted from the total of correct, two-point applications. An answer of five or more is considered passing.

The normal threshold for two-point discrimination distance for the volar surface of the hand varies according to the zone being tested. Between the fingertip and DIP joint, normal is 3 to 5 mm, diminished is 6 to 10 mm, and absent is greater than 10 mm. Between the DIP joint and the PIP joint, normal is 3 to 6 mm, diminished is 7 to 10 mm, and absent is greater than 10 mm. Between the PIP joint and the finger web, normal is 4 to 7 mm, diminished is 9 to 10 mm, and absent is greater than 10 mm. Between the web and the distal palmar crease, normal is 5 to 8 mm, diminished is 9 to 20 mm, and absent is greater than 20 mm. Between the distal crease and the central palm, normal is 6 to 9 mm, diminished is 10 to 20 mm, and absent is greater than 20 mm. At the base of the palm and wrist, normal is 7 to 10 mm, diminished is 11 to 20 mm, and absent is greater than 20 mm. The threshold for the dorsal surface is higher in all zones: normal is 7 to 12 mm, diminished is 13 to 20 mm, and absent is greater than 20 mm.

Below the elbow but above the wrist, any two-point discrimination distance is considered normal if between 40 to 50 mm, diminished between 55 and 80 mm, and absent above 80 mm. Above the elbow, two-point discrimination distance is normal between 65 to 75 mm, diminished between 80 and 100 mm, and absent above 100 mm.

Abnormal skin texture, such as heavy scales or calluses, has a marked influence on the test results. Testing can be done in the presence of edema or infection, but the results demonstrate the sensibilities present, which may not reflect the true status of the nerve.

Confirmation Procedures

Dellon's moving two-point discrimination test, interphalangeal neuroma test, shrivel test, electrodiagnosis

Reporting Statement

Weber's two-point discrimination testing demonstrates diminished sensibility (13 to 20 mm) at the dorsal surface of the index finger. This result suggests nerve receptor or impulse transmission deficits.

∽ Clinical Pearl ∽

As with Dellon's moving two-point discrimination test, bizarre responses are reason for suspicion as to the origin of the symptoms. Janet's test can help identify psychogenic anesthesia.

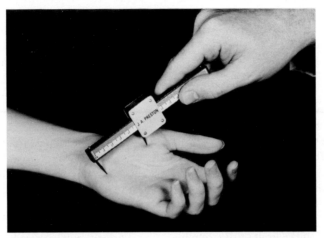

Fig. 6–49 The patient is seated with the elbow flexed. The arm is supinated and resting on the examination table. The hand is relaxed. The Boley gauge is set for 10 mm or more distance. The contact points are made randomly, beginning at the distal portions of the hand. The contacts must touch simultaneously and with equal pressure. The patient's eyes are closed.

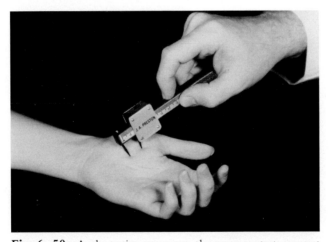

Fig. 6–50 As the testing progresses, the gauge contacts are reset closer together in 5 mm increments. If the patient cannot detect the points in two out of three attempts, the test is positive. A positive test indicates diminished sensibility for the area tested, according to established norms.

Comment

The median nerve enters the hand through the carpal tunnel—a bony trough covered with a stout fibrous roof, called the flexor retinaculum—which it shares with nine tendons, each covered with two layers of synovium. There is no room for the tissues to expand and any swelling of the tendons or the synovium around them compresses the median nerve.

The most common overall cause of carpal tunnel syndrome is fluid retention, of which the most common cause is pregnancy. However, overuse of the tendons from repeated forceful movements of the wrist, either at work or recreation, is probably the most common cause of carpal tunnel syndrome referred to orthopedic and neurosurgical clinics. Any condition that causes synovial thickening, including rheumatoid arthritis and Colles' fracture, can also be responsible.

Median nerve compression causes paresthesia in the median nerve distribution, which is the front of the thumb, index finger, middle finger and the radial half of the ring finger. The palm is not involved because the palmar branch of the median nerve arises above the wrist.

The symptoms are worse at night and the patient will wake and fling the hand up and down to try and relieve the symptoms. In time, the paresthesia is replaced by pain, which can be felt as far up as the elbow, and eventually by numbness in the median distribution.

Most patients notice the little finger is not affected and those who report that all the fingers are involved, should be treated with suspicion.

The differential diagnosis includes peripheral neuropathy, mononeuritis, cervical spondylosis, and tumors of the thoracic outlet that involve the brachial plexus, but these are often forgotten because carpal tunnel syndrome is such a common condition. If there is any doubt, the diagnosis can be confirmed by nerve conduction studies.

Procedure

The patient, using both hands, wrings a towel. Paresthesia in the hand indicates carpal tunnel syndrome. Pain elicited at the elbow indicates epicondylitis. Wrist discomfort indicates arthropathy or carpal derangement.

Confirmation Procedures

Phalen's sign, electrodiagnosis, diagnostic imaging, further testing based upon the area of localized complaint

---

Reporting Statement

Wringing test is positive for the right wrist and hand and elicits paresthesia of the right hand. This result indicates carpal tunnel syndrome.

∽ Clinical Pearl ∽

The wringing test is useful to determine the area for primary investigation. The patient also may be asked to hold both wrists in a fully flexed position for 1 to 2 minutes. The appearance or exacerbation of paresthesia suggests carpal tunnel syndrome. This test is the most sensitive clinical test for carpal tunnel syndrome.

Advanced carpal tunnel syndrome can produce thenar atrophy and distal phalangeal acroasphyxia. The wringing test is particularly useful in eliciting responses in more subtle afflictions of the median nerve.

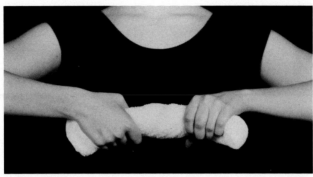

Fig. 6–51 The patient, using both hands, wrings a towel. Maximum effort is applied. The test will localize the discomfort to the primary site of origin. If the test elicits pain at the elbow, epicondylitis is suspected. If the discomfort is felt at the wrist, arthropathy or carpal derangement is suspected. Paresthesia in the hand indicates carpal tunnel syndrome.

Bibliography

American Medical Association: *Guides to the evaluation of permanent impairment*, ed. 3, 1990, Chicago.

American Society for Surgery of the Hand: *The hand-examination and diagnosis*, 1978, Aurora, Co.

Apley AG, Solomon L: *Concise system of orthopaedics and fractures*, London, 1988, Butterworth-Heinemann.

Beckenbaugh RD, Shives TC, Dobyns JH et al: Kienböck's disease: The natural history of Kienböck's disease and consideration of lunate fractures, *Clin Orthop*, 149:98–106, 1980.

Bell JA: Sensibility evaluation, In Hunter JM, Schneider LH, Makin EJ, et al (eds): *Rehabilitation of the hand*, St. Louis, 1978, Mosby.

Bourne G: *The structure and function of nervous tissue*, New York, 1968, Academic Press.

Brashear HR Jr, Raney RB: *Shands' handbook of orthopaedic surgery*, St. Louis, 1978, Mosby.

Bunnell S: Surgery of the rheumatic hand, *J Bone Joint Surg*, 27:759–766, 1955.

Cailliet R: *Hand pain and impairment*, ed. 2, Philadelphia, 1975, FA Davis.

Chusid JG, McDonald JJ: *Correlative neuroanatomy and functional neurology*, Los Altos, 1962, Lange Medical Publications.

Cipriano JJ: *Photographic manual of regional orthopaedic and neurological tests*, ed. 2, Baltimore, 1991, Williams & Wilkins.

Cooney III WP, Dobyns JH, Linscheid RL: Complications of Colles' fracture, *J Bone Joint Surg*, 62A:613, 1980.

Cooney III WP, Linscheid RL, Dobyns JH: External pin fixation for unstable Colles' fracture, *J Bone Joint Surg*, 61A:840, 1979.

D'Ambrosia RD: *Musculoskeletal disorders regional examination and differential diagnosis*, Philadelphia, 1977, JB Lippincott.

Dandy DJ: *Essential orthopaedics and trauma*, Edinburgh, 1989, Churchill Livingstone.

Dellon AL, Curtis RM, Edgerton MT: Evaluating recovery of sensation in the hand following nerve injury, *Johns Hopkins Med J*, 130:235, 1972.

Dellon AL, Curtis RM, Edgerton MT: Reeducation of sensation in the hand after nerve injury and repair, *Plast Reconstr Surg*, 53:297, 1974.

Doherty M, Doherty J: *Clinical examination in rheumatology*, London, 1992, Wolfe Publishing.

Duchenne GB: *Physiology of motion*, (Translated by Emanuel B. Kaplan) Philadelphia, 1975, WB Saunders.

Finkelstein H: Stenosing tendovaginitis at the radial styloid process, *J Bone Joint Surg*, 12:509, 1930.

Finneson BE: *Diagnosis and management of pain syndromes*, Philadelphia, 1969, WB Saunders.

Flatt AE: *The care of minor hand injuries*, St. Louis, 1972, Mosby.

Frykman G: Fracture of the distal radius including sequelae-shoulder-hand-finger syndrome, disturbance in the distal radioulnar joint and impairment of nerve function: A clinical and experimental study, *Acta Orthop Scand Suppl*, 108:1–153, 1967.

Frykman GK: The orthopedic clinics of North America, vol 12 (2), Philadelphia, April 1981 and April 1984, WB Saunders.

Gelberman RH, Bauman TD, Menon J et al: The vascularity of the lunate bone and Kienbock's disease, *J Hand Surg [AM]*, 5:272, 1980.

Goldner JL: Volkmann's ischemic contracture, In Flynn JE ed: *Hand surgery*, ed 2, Baltimore, 1975, Williams & Wilkins.

Goldner JL, Gould JS, Urbaniak JR, McCollum DE: Metacarpophalangeal joint arthroplasty with silicone-dacron prosthesis, Niebauer type, six and a half years experience, *J Bone Joint Surg*, 2(3):200, 1977.

Hoppenfeld S: *Physical examination of the spine and extremities*, New York, 1976, Appleton-Century-Crofts.

Johnson MK: *The hand book*, Springfield, IL, 1973, Charles C. Thomas.

Katz, WA: *Rheumatic diseases diagnosis and management*, Philadelphia, 1977, JB Lippincott.

Kendall HO, Kendall FP, Wadsworth GE: *Muscles testing and function*, ed 2, Baltimore, 1971, Williams & Wilkins.

Landsmeer JMF: *Atlas of anatomy of the hand*, Edinburgh, 1976, Churchill Livingstone.

Lee MLH: The intraosseous arterial pattern of the carpal lunate bone and its relation to avascular necrosis, *Acta Orthop Scand*, 33:43–55, 1963.

Lewis MH: Median nerve decompression after Colles' fracture, *J Bone Joint Surg*, 60B:195–196, 1978.

Linscheid RL et al: Instability patterns of the wrist, *J Hand Surg [AM]*, 8:682, 1983.

Linscheid RL et al: Traumatic instability of the wrist, *J Bone Joint Surg*, 54A:1612, 1972.

Linscheid RL, Dobyns JH: Rheumatoid arthritis of the wrist, *Ortho Clin North Am*, 2:649–665, 1971.

Lister G: *The hand: Diagnosis and indications*, Edinburgh, 1977, Churchill Livingstone.

Lynch AC, Lipscomb PR: The carpal-tunnel syndrome and Colles' fractures, *JAMA*, 185:363–366, 1963.

Magee DJ: *Orthopedic physical assessment*, Philadelphia, 1987, WB Saunders.

Mayfield JK, Williams WJ, Erdman AG et al: Biomechanical properties of human carpal ligaments, *Orthop Trans*, 3:143, 1979.

Mayfield JK: Mechanism of carpal injuries, *Clin Orthop* 149:45–54, 1980.

Mayfield JK, Johnson RP, Kilcoyne RF: Carpal dislocations: Pathomechanics and progressive perilunar instability, *J Hand Surg*, 5:226–241, 1980.

Mayo Clinic: *Clinical examinations in neurology*, ed 3, Philadelphia, 1971, WB Saunders.

Mazion JM: *Illustrated manual of neurological reflexes/signs/tests, Part I, Orthopedic signs/tests/maneuvers for office procedure, Part II*, Orlando, 1980, Daniels Publishing.

McRae R: *Clinical orthopaedic examination*, ed 3, Edinburgh, 1990, Churchill Livingstone.

McNurty RY, Youm Y, Flatt A AE et al: Kinematics of the wrist, II, Clinical applications, *J Bone Joint Surg*, 600:955–961, 1978.

Medical Economics Books: *Patient care flow chart manual*, ed 3, Oradell, NJ, 1982, Medical Economics Books.

Millender LH, Nalebuff EA, Feldon PG: Rheumatoid arthritis, In Green, D ed: *Operative hand surgery*, New York, Churchill Livingstone, 1982.

Mino DE, Palmer AK, Levinsohn EM: The role of radiography and computerized tomography in the diagnosis of subluxation and dislocation of the distal radioulnar joint, *J Hand Surg [AM]*, 8:23, 1983.

Moberg E: Criticism and study of methods for examining sensibility of the hand, *Neurology* 12:8, 1962.

Moberg E: Relation of touch and deep sensation to hand reconstruction, *Am J Surg*, 109:353, 1965.

Moldaver J: Tinel's sign-its characteristics and significance, *J Bone Joint Surg,* 60A:412, 1978.

O'Donoghue DH: *Treatment of injuries to athletes,* ed 3, Philadelphia, 1976, WB Saunders.

Omer GE Jr: Evaluation and reconstruction of the forearm and hand after acute traumatic peripheral nerve injuries, *J Bone Joint Surg,* 50A:1454, 1968.

Omer GE Jr: The assessment of peripheral nerve injuries, In Cramer LM, Chase RA: Symposium of the hand, *Plast Reconstr Surg,* 3(1) St. Louis, 1971, Mosby.

Omer GE Jr: Sensation and sensibility in the upper extremity, *Clin Orthop,* 104:30, 1974.

Omer GE, Spinner M: *Management of peripheral nerve problems,* Philadelphia, 1980, WB Saunders.

Omer GE Jr, Vogel JA: Determination of physiological length of a reconstructed muscle tendon unit through muscle stimulation, *J Bone Joint Surg,* 47A:304, 1965.

Omer GE Jr, Day DJ, Ratliff H, Lambert P: The neurovascular cutaneous island pedicles for deficient median nerve sensibility, new technique and results of serial functional tests, *J Bone Joint Surg,* 52A:1181, 1970.

O'Riain S: Shrivel Test: A new and simple test of nerve function in the hand, *BMJ,* 3:615, 1973.

O'Riain S: New and simple test nerve function in the hand, *BRJ,* 3:615, 1973.

Pahle JA, Raunio P: The influence of wrist position on finger deviation in the rheumatoid hand a clinical and radiological study, *J Bone Joint Surg,* 51B:664−676, 1969.

Palmer AK, Glisson RR, Werner FW: Ulnar variance determination, *J Hand Surg,* 7:376, 1982.

Palmer AK, Livensohn EM, Kuzma GR: Arthrography of the wrist, *J Hand Surg,* 8:15−23, 1983.

Phalen GS: The carpal-tunnel syndrome: Seventeen years' experience in diagnosis and treatment of six hundred fifty-four hands, *J Bone Joint Surg,* 48A:211−228, 1966.

Porter JN: Raynaud's syndrome, In Sabiston DC Jr., ed: *Davis-Christopher textbook of surgery,* Philadelphia, 1977, WB Saunders.

Protas JM, Jackson WT: Evaluating carpal instabilities with fluoroscopy, AJR *Am J Roentgenol,* 135:137, 1980.

Resnick D, Niwayama G: *Diagnosis of bone and joint disorders,* Philadelphia, 1981, WB Saunders.

Scheck M: Long-term follow-up of treatment of comminuted fractures of the distal end of the radius by transfixation with kirschner wires and cast, *J Bone Joint Surg,* 44A:337, 1962.

Silver D: Circulatory problems of the upper extremity, In Sabiston DC Jr., ed: *Davis-Christopher textbook of surgery,* Philadelphia, 1985, WB Saunders.

Southmayd WW, Millender LH, Nalebuff EA: Rupture of the flexor tendons in the index finger after Colles' fracture case report, *J Bone Joint Surg,* 57A:562, 1975.

Spencer PS: The traumatic neuroma and proximal stump, *Bull Hosp Jt Dis Orthop Inst,* 35:85, 1974.

Spinner M: *Injuries of the major branches of peripheral nerves of the forearm,* Philadelphia, 1972, WB Saunders.

Sunderland S: *Nerves and nerve injuries,* Baltimore, 1968, Williams & Wilkins.

Swanson AB, DeGroot GA, Hehl RW, Waller TJ, Boeve NR: Pathogensis of rheumatoid deformities in the hand, In Cruess RL, Mitchell NS: *Surgery of rheumatoid arthritis,* Philadelphia, 1971, JB Lippincott.

Taleisnik J: The ligaments of the wrist, *J Hand Surg [AM],* 1:110, 1976.

Taleisnik J: Rheumatoid arthritis of the wrist, In Strickland JW, Steichen JB, eds: *Difficult problems in hand surgery,* St. Louis, 1982, Mosby.

Thurston SE: *The little black book of neurology,* Chicago, 1987, Mosby.

Tinel J: Nerve wounds: *Symptomatology of peripheral nerve lesions caused by war wounds,* (Translated by F Rothwell; edited by CA Joll), New York, 1918, William Wood.

Tubiana R: *The hand,* Philadelphia, 1981, WB Saunders.

Turek SL: Orthopaedics principles and their application, ed 3, Philadelphia, 1977, JB Lippincott.

Vance RM, Gelberman RH: Acute ulnar neuropathy with fractures at the wrist, *J Bone Joint Surg,* 60A:962, 1978.

von Prince K: Occupational therapy's interest in function following peripheral nerve injury, *Med Bull US Army,* Europe, 23:143−147, 1966.

von Prince K, Butler B: Measuring sensory function of the hand in peripheral nerve injuries, *Am J Occup Ther,* 21:385−396, 1967.

Warwick R, Williams PL: *Gray's anatomy,* Philadelphia, 1973, WB Saunders.

Weber EH: Veber den tastsinn, *Arch Anat Physiol Wissensch Med,* 152, 1835.

Weinstein S: Tactile sensitivity of the phalanges, *Percept Mot Skills,* 14:351−354, 1962.

Werner JL, Omer GE Jr: Evaluating cutaneous pressure sensation of the hand, *Am J Occup Ther,* 24:247, 1970.

Wynn-Parry CB: Rehabilitation of the hand, ed 3, London, 1973, Butterworths.

Younger CP, DeFiore JC: Rupture of the flexor tendons to the fingers after a Colles' fracture a case report, *J Bone Joint Surg,* 59A:828, 1977.

Zoega H: Fracture of the lower end of the radius with ulnar nerve palsy, *J Bone Joint Surg,* 48V:514, 1966.

CHAPTER

~ 7 ~

The Thoracic Spine

*T*horacic spinal pain and dysfunction present a particularly challenging clinical dilemma. Thoracic spinal pain may arise from somatic as well as visceral origins. Pain felt along the thoracic spine may arise from the ribs, the abdomen, or from the vertebral column.

The thoracic spine is the part of the vertebral column that is most rigid because of the rib cage. The rib cage, in turn, provides protection for the heart and lungs.

Thoracic pain occurs as a referred visceral symptom from the chest and abdomen or as a symptom of a problem of musculoskeletal origin. Sudden pain in the thoracic region occurs less frequently than in the more mobile cervical and lumbar spines.

The structure of the thorax as a whole is such that overall motion of this portion of the spine is limited.

The stabilizing influences of the thoracic spine include four elements. The first element is the vertebral articular process. The interlocking arrangement of the thoracic facets prevents anterior displacement of the vertebra and forms the imbrication of the thoracic spine.

The second primary stabilizing influence of the thoracic spine is the vertebral body. At the posterior of the vertebral bodies the height of the body is greater than in the anterior. This contributes to the thoracic spine kyphosis.

The third stabilizing influence is the structure of the ribs and their attachments to the spine. The ribs help to stiffen the thoracic spine.

The fourth primary stabilizing influence for the thoracic spine is the structure of the intervertebral disc. The thoracic spine intervertebral discs are more narrow and thin than in the cervical or lumbar spines. They are also less elastic than all the other disc tissues of the spine.

Added to the bony and discal stabilizing influences of the thoracic spine are the muscles supporting the spinal column.

The thoracic spinal column serves as the attachment for many of the muscles of the trunk, shoulder, and arm.

Among these muscles are the trapezius and latissimus dorsi. The deeper muscles of the trunk include the levator scapulae, rhomboid major, and rhomboid minor. Still deeper are the sacrospinalis muscle groups, which include the spinalis dorsi, longissimus dorsi, and the iliocostalis lumborum.

During an examination of the thorax and thoracic spine, the assessment is primarily of the thoracic spine. The examination is extensive. Without a history of specific trauma or injury to the thoracic spine, the examiner must be prepared to assess the other implicated tissues. If a problem is suspected superior to the thoracic spine, a thorough examination of the cervical spine and upper limb should be accomplished. If a problem is suspected inferior to the thoracic spine, the examination of the lumbar spine and lower limb is completed.

Index of Tests

Adam's positions
Amoss' sign
Anghelescu's sign
Beevor's sign
Chest expansion test
First thoracic nerve root test
Forestier's bowstring sign
Passive scapular approximation test
Rib motion test
Schepelmann's sign
Spinal percussion test
Sponge test
Sternal compression test

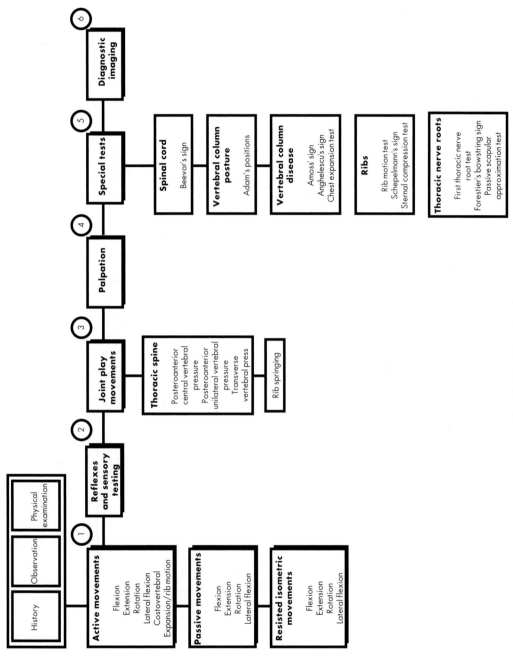

Fig. 7-1 Thoracic spine assessment.

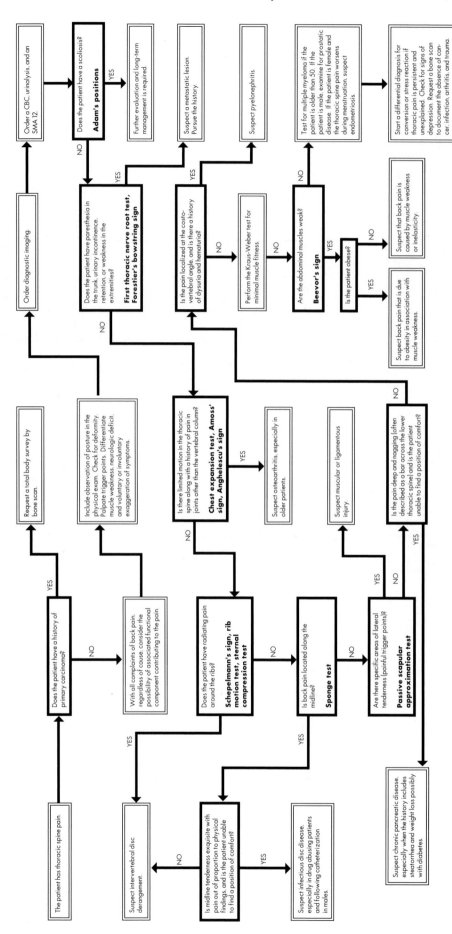

Fig. 7–2 Assessment of thoracic spine pain.

RANGE OF MOTION

Determination of the active range of motion of the thoracic spine is accomplished while the patient is standing. Movement is limited by the rib cage and the long spinous processes of the thoracic spine. An individual can touch the toes with a completely rigid spine if sufficient range of motion in the hip joints exists. Conversely, tight hamstrings may alter movement significantly. Range of motion studies may be done while the patient is seated. In the seated position the effect of hip movement will be eliminated or decreased. The most painful movements are completed last.

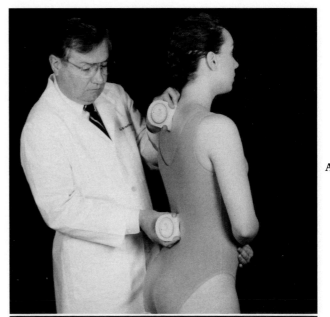

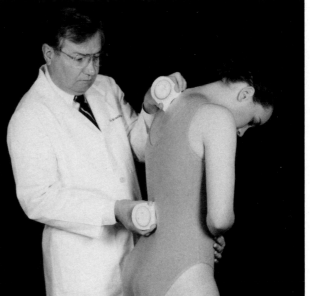

A

B

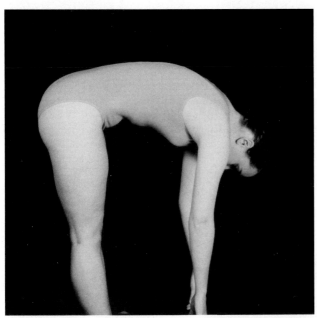

Fig. 7–3   Normal flexion range of motion in the thoracic spine is 20 to 45 degrees. The range of motion at each vertebra is difficult to measure. The examiner can use a measuring tape to determine overall movement. This is an indirect measurement. The examiner first measures the length of the spine from the C7 spinous process to the T12 spinous process. The patient bends forward, and the spine is again measured. A minimum of 2.7 cm difference in tape measure length is considered normal.

The spine also may be measured from the C7 spinous process to S1. The patient bends forward, and the spine is again measured. A minimum 10 cm difference in tape measure length is considered normal. In this instance the examiner is measuring motion in the thoracolumbar spine. The most movement, 7.5 cm, occurs between T12 and S1.

In a third method, the patient bends forward and tries to touch the toes while keeping the knees straight. The examiner measures the distance from the patient's fingertips to the floor.

Fig. 7–4   For testing flexion with an inclinometer, the patient is seated or standing. One inclinometer is placed in the sagittal plane at the T1 level and the other at the T12 level, also in the saggital plane (**A**). Both instruments are zeroed. If seated, the patient places the hands on the hips, and if standing, the patient crosses the arms in front of the chest. The thoracic spine is flexed forward so as not to involve lumbar spine motion (**B**). Both instrument readings are recorded. The T12 value is subtracted from the T1 value to arrive at the thoracic flexion angle.

Retained flexion of the thoracic spine of 30 degrees or less is an impairment of the thoracic spine in the activities of daily living.

Continued.

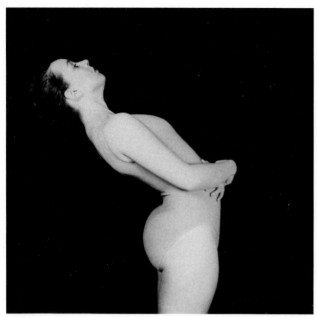

Fig. 7–5 Extension in the thoracic spine is normally 25 to 35 degrees. As extension occurs, the movement between the individual spinous processes is difficult to detect. As with flexion, a tape measure will determine the distance between C7 and T12 spinous processes. A minimum 2.5 cm difference in tape measure length between standing and extension is normal.

As the patient extends, the thoracic spine should curve backward or at least straighten in a smooth, even manner.

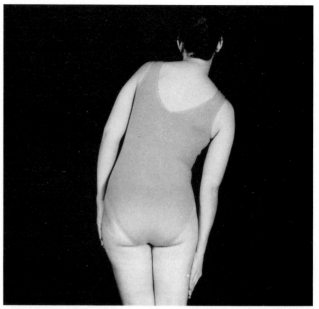

Fig. 7–6 Lateral flexion is approximately 20 to 40 degrees to the right and left. It is tested as the patient runs a hand down the side of the leg, without bending forward or backward. A tape measure can be used to determine the distance from the fingertips to the floor. The examiner compares the measurements bilaterally. The distances should be equal. This procedure measures movement in the lumbar spine as well as the thoracic spine.

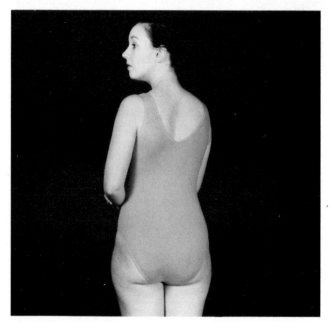

Fig. 7–7 Rotation in the thoracic spine is approximately 35 to 50 degrees. The patient crosses the arms in front, or places the hands on opposite shoulders, and rotates to the right or the left. The examiner assesses the amount of rotation, comparing both ways.

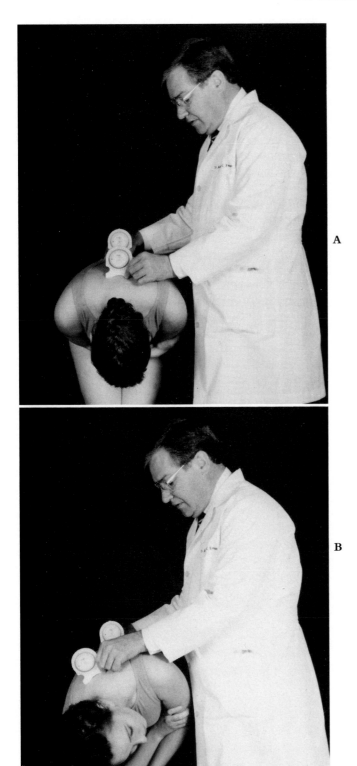

Fig. 7–8 When an inclinometer is used to assess thoracic spinal rotation, the patient is standing. The patient is flexed forward. The patient may brace the position with the arms. One inclinometer is placed at the T1 level in the coronal plane and the other at the T12 level also in the coronal plane **(A)**. Both instruments are zeroed. The patient rotates to one side and the angles indicated on both instruments are recorded **(B)**. The T12 measurement is subtracted from the T1 measurement to arrive at the thoracic rotation angle. The measurements are repeated for rotation to the opposite side.

Retained active rotation of the thoracic spine of 20 degrees or less is an impairment of the function of the thoracic spine in the activities of daily living.

MUSCLE TESTING

In addition to the bony and discal stabilizing influences of the thoracic spine, there are also muscles supporting the spinal column. The thoracic spinal column serves as the attachment for many of the muscles of the trunk, shoulder, and arm.

Among these muscles are the trapezius and latissimus dorsi. The deeper muscles of the trunk include the levator scapulae, rhomboid major, and rhomboid minor. Still deeper are the sacrospinalis muscle groups. These include the spinalis dorsi, longissimus dorsi, and the iliocostalis lumborum.

The trapezius muscle attaches to the spinous processes from the upper cervicals to the lower thoracic spine. In the lower part the muscle overlaps the long attachment of the latissimus dorsi muscle.

The latissimus dorsi muscle attaches to the spinous processes, beginning in the midthoracic region, and extends to the pelvis. The trapezius and latissimus dorsi are the two most superficial muscles of the back. In addition to movement, these muscles also serve to enclose the deeper muscle layers.

The deeper muscles are broad and flat and are not as frequently subjected to injury. These muscles are the levator scapulae, rhomboid major, and the rhomboid minor, and they lie under the trapezius, in the upper portion of the dorsal spine. The muscles extend down toward the level of the upper limit of the latissimus dorsi.

Still deeper are the muscles that run from the spine to the pelvis and form the sacrospinalis group. This group is a combination of many muscles, whose course parallels the spinal column. The sacrospinalis group of muscles includes the spinalis dorsi, the longissimus dorsi, and the iliocostalis lumborum.

The sacrospinalis group fills the sulcus between the spinous processes, the bodies of the vertebrae, and the arc of the ribs. This group of muscles interdigitates in such a manner that each supports the other. These muscles make up the lumbar mass of muscles that extends from the occiput to the sacrum and laterally to the spinous processes.

These muscles have multiple actions depending upon the relationship between them. One muscle may serve to stabilize the spine, while another muscle member moves.

The back extensors may be considered the most important of all the trunk muscles. There are several reasons why abdominal muscles are discussed in detail in literature and back extensors are given little emphasis. Lower back muscle weakness is seldom encountered except in paralytic cases. The incidence among nonparalytic, or so-called *normal* individuals is probably less than 1%.

On the other hand, abdominal muscle weakness is frequently encountered. Parts of the abdominal muscles can be tested separately, while the back extensors can be tested only as a group.

During the trunk extension test, back extensors are assisted by the latissimus dorsi, quadratus lumborum, and the trapezius.

The head and neck extensor muscles and the hip extensors should be tested before the back extensors are tested.

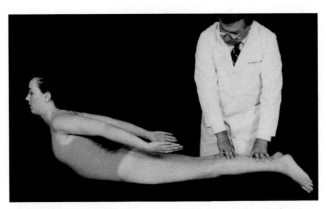

Fig. 7–9   The patient is prone. The hip extensors must be given fixation of the pelvis to the thighs and the examiner must stabilize the legs firmly on the examining table. The patient then attempts trunk extension. The ability to complete spine extension and hold against strong pressure with hands clasped behind the head is normal. The ability to perform this only with the hands behind the back is good. If performed only with the hands clasped behind the back, the ability to lift the thorax, so the xiphoid process of the sternum is raised slightly from the table, is fair.

When marked weakness is present, usually such weakness extends throughout the back. If cervical extensors can lift the head, a head-raising movement can furnish slight resistance against other back extensors.

When the lower back is strong and the upper back is weak, an attempt to raise the thorax will result in the back extensors extending the lower back by anteriorly tilting the pelvis, but the thorax will not be lifted from the table.

Comment

Kyphosis is a condition that is most prevalent in the thoracic spine. The examiner must determine that a kyphosis is actually present.

A slight kyphosis or posterior curvature is normal and is found in every individual. In addition, some individuals have a flat scapula, that gives the appearance of an excessive kyphosis. With pathologic kyphosis, it is actually the spine that has the excessive curve.

There are four types of kyphotic deformities. These deformities are (1) decreased pelvic inclination (20 degrees) with a thoracolumbar or thoracic kyphosis (round back); (2) localized, sharp, posterior angulation that is called a *gibbus* (or *hump back*); (3) decreased pelvic inclination (20 degrees) with a mobile spine (flat back); (4) Dowager's hump, which results from postmenopausal osteoporosis.

There are few conditions that produce decreased kyphosis. The lordotic interscapular thoracic spine (Pottenger's saucering) involves the T2 to T6 vertebra. This type of flattened thoracic spine may have its beginning in the juvenile years, ages 2 through 5. The etiology of this flattened spine may be a congenital fixation of the thoracic spine.

The examiner should also be aware that if a thoracolumbar kyphosis exists, the kyphosis is due to a postural deficit, resulting from poor postural habits. This etiology of kyphosis is most prevalent in adolescents. A patient with this condition is not round shouldered but round backed. Thoracolumbar kyphosis is classified as a round back type I or type II. Type I results from postural habitus and type II from structural abnormalities. Among etiologies for the thoracolumbar kyphosis are juvenile osteochondrosis (Scheuermann's disease) and vertebra plana (Calve's disease).

The lower the thoracolumbar kyphosis occurs in the thoracic spine, the more it is a fixed and unyielding kyphosis. The patient may have normal and supple flexion in the areas of the spine above the thoracolumbar kyphosis.

In regard to the thoracic kyphosis, the examiner must observe for gibbus deformity. The gibbus deformity is associated with spinal tuberculosis and involves only two or three vertebral elements. The gibbus is a short, sharply angled, and acute kyphosis.

Often, with the dramatic and adverse changes of thoracic kyphosis, there is a parallel development of lateral curvature (scoliosis).

The presence of scoliosis needs to be determined. Nonstructural scoliosis is associated with poor postural habits. When the patient with nonstructural or postural scoliosis is placed in proper standing or seated attitudes, the scoliosis disappears. Poor posture, hysteria, nerve root irritation, inflammation in the spine area, leg length discrepancy, or hip contracture can cause nonstructural scoliosis.

An idiopathic structural scoliosis does not have any specific etiology. Structural changes may be due to a congenital problem, such as wedge vertebrae, hemivertebra, or failure of segmentation. The increase or decrease of kyphosis in a juvenile will alert the examiner to other postural deficits that may indicate the onset of scoliosis.

Senile scoliosis is the result of spinal column changes associated with aging of the adult thoracic spine. A scoliotic curve develops but does not have all the characteristics demonstrable in adolescent scoliosis. Upon a more thorough examination, senile scoliosis might actually be a mild or moderate, adolescent, structural scoliosis that was previously undetected. Changes or increases in curvature are usually due to the effects of gravity or injury to the thoracic spine. These patients often present with thoracic pain and are surprised to learn that scoliosis exists.

Once scoliosis is identified the degree of curvature has to be determined. Accurate techniques of measurement must be employed. Once a particular method of curvature measurement is established, all further studies must be measured the same way.

Scoliosis is a deformity in which there are one or more lateral curvatures of the thoracic or lumbar spine. The curvature may occur in the thoracic spine alone, in the thoracolumbar area, or in the lumbar spine alone.

Several curve patterns may form in scoliosis. These curve patterns are described according to the level of the apex of the curve. A right thoracic curve has a convexity toward the right and the apex of the curve is in the thoracic spine. For a thoracic curve, the apex is between T2 and T11. The thoracolumbar curve has its apex at T12 or L1. The scoliotic involvement of the thoracic spine results in a poor cosmetic appearance or defect. This is due to deformation of the ribs and spine.

With structural scoliosis, the vertebral bodies rotate toward the convexity of the curve and become distorted. This rotation causes the ribs on the convex side of the curve to push posterior. A rib hump and narrowing of the thoracic cage on the convex side results. As the vertebral body rotates to the convex side of the curve, the spinous process deviates toward the concave side. The ribs on the concave side move anterior, resulting in hollowing and widening of the thoracic cage on the concave side.

With idiopathic scoliosis, the rib contours are not normal and there is asymmetry of the ribs.

Procedure

If the patient has an *S* or *C* scoliosis, the curvature may straighten when the spine is flexed forward. If it does, it is a negative sign and evidence of functional scoliosis. A positive sign is noted when the scoliosis is not improved after flexing forward. A positive sign is evidence of pathologic or structural scoliosis, and it indicates altered morphology, pathology, trauma, and subluxation.

An anterior Adam's position requires the examiner to be positioned in front of the patient. A posterior Adam's position requires the examiner to be positioned behind the patient.

Confirmation Procedures

Postural assessment, diagnostic imaging

Reporting Statement

An anterior Adam's position reveals a mild left convex cervicothoracic scoliosis, without the rib humping sign.

A posterior Adam's position reveals a moderate right convex thoracolumbar scoliosis, with a marked rib humping sign.

∼ Clinical Pearl ∼

When the scoliotic curvature disappears in the Adam's position, the curves are mild to moderate, or less than 25 degrees. These curves have more of a functional component than a structural component and are amenable to conservative management.

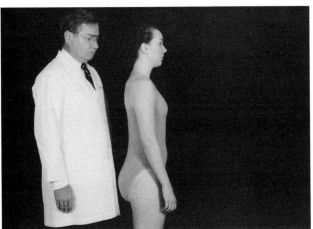

Fig. 7–10 The patient is standing. The examiner notes any spinal asymmetry, scapular winging, chest rotational deformity, etc.

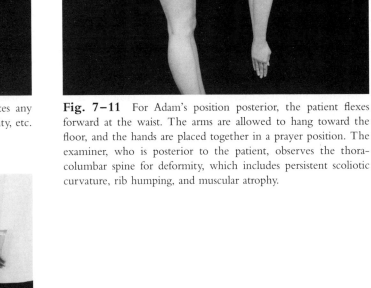

Fig. 7–11 For Adam's position posterior, the patient flexes forward at the waist. The arms are allowed to hang toward the floor, and the hands are placed together in a prayer position. The examiner, who is posterior to the patient, observes the thoracolumbar spine for deformity, which includes persistent scoliotic curvature, rib humping, and muscular atrophy.

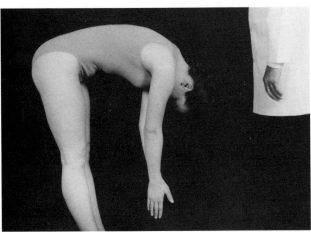

Fig. 7–12, left. In Adam's position anterior, the patient assumes the Adam's position by flexing the spine at the waist and additionally flexing the cervical spine. The examiner, who is anterior to the patient, observes for upper thoracic scoliosis defects.

Comment

Ankylosing spondylitis, an ascending disease, affects the thoracic region after the lumbar. Patients with this condition do experience back pain, but the anterolateral chest pain and the limited chest expansion are what bother them the most. In some, these symptoms may occur rather early in the life of the disease, but they usually become bothersome after 6 years of illness. Chest pain, which usually occurs during inspiration, and the limited chest expansion are primarily caused by involvement of costovertebral and manubriosternal joints, as well as the costochondral junctions and the clavicular joints. The girdlelike restriction may cause a sense of anxiety and dyspnea, particularly upon exertion. However, respiratory problems are surprisingly uncommon, even though restricted ventilatory volumes are detected by pulmonary function studies. Of course, should concomitant disease result in impaired diaphragmatic breathing, then a problem is likely to develop.

Tenderness is elicited over the manubriosternal joint, the costochondral junctions, and the entire dorsal spine. With more advanced disease a dorsal kyphosis is evident and the thoracic cage remains in the expiratory position. Chest expansion, normally no less than 1 inch in females and 1.5 inches in males, may be diminished by 50% or more. A football abdomen, a spherical protrusion, may result from abdominal breathing.

The posture of the hang-dog cervical spine, dorsal kyphosis with the chest cage fixed in expiration, straightening of the lumbar spine, marked flexion contractures of the hips and knees, and a gaze that is fixed on the floor are highly characteristic of the terminal stage of ankylosing spondylitis and should offer no problems with diagnosis.

Ankylosing spondylitis may be primarily or secondarily associated with a variety of conditions. Most of these disorders follow manifestation of spondylitis, but some may precede the actual onset of musculoskeletal symptoms by several months and occasionally by years. In some instances these allied conditions may overlap one another. Aortitis may be found in both idiopathic ankylosing spondylitis and in Reiter's syndrome. Heel pain is common to psoriatic arthritis, Reiter's syndrome, and enteropathic arthropathy, whether or not there is associated inflammation of the spine. The detection of HLA-B27 antigen, not only in ankylosing spondylitis but also in Reiter's disease and psoriatic arthritis, creates an even closer relationship between these conditions.

Procedure

The recumbent patient places the hands far behind the body and tries to arise from the supine position to the seated position. The patient can also be side-lying. The examiner should note the patient's position of comfort and any spinal complaints that the patient presents. The patient arises from the side-lying position to a sitting position. The sign is present when either action elicits a localized thoracic or thoracolumbar spinal pain. The sign suggests ankylosing spondylitis, severe sprain, or intervertebral disc syndrome.

Confirmation Procedures

Chest expansion test, Forestier's bowstring sign, clinical laboratory testing, diagnostic imaging

---

Reporting Statement

Amoss' sign is present and suggests the presence of ankylosing spondylitis. Further laboratory testing is warranted.

~ **Clinical Pearl** ~

It is occasionally observed that the patient defers to a side-lying posture when trying to stand after lying supine. This is Amoss' Sign. Amoss' sign may not produce pain, but it reveals stiffness and lack of mobility and is still useful for detecting chronic spondylitis, which, at the least, requires imaging of the thoracolumbar spine.

The Thoracic Spine

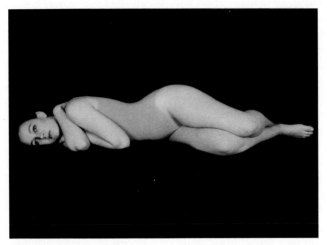

Fig. 7–13 The patient is in a side-lying posture on the examining table. The examiner notes the position of comfort, and any spinal complaints that the patient presents.

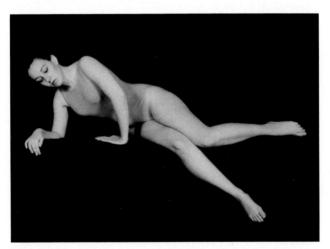

Fig. 7–14 The patient arises from the side-lying position to a seated position. The sign is present when this action elicits a localized thoracic or thoracolumbar spinal pain. The sign suggests ankylosing spondylitis, severe sprain, or intervertebral disc syndrome.

Comment

With tuberculous spondylitis any single vertebra or several vertebrae may be involved. The disease most often involves the lower thoracic and the lumbar spine. The infection starts in the cancellous bone area of the vertebral body. Most commonly an exudative reaction with marked hyperemia produces severe generalized osteoporosis. The body is softened and easily yields to compression forces. In the thoracic spine the normal kyphotic curve increases the pressure on the vertebrae anteriorly, so anterior wedging is severe. An angular kyphosis results if the vertebral body is crushed.

The infection advances and destroys the epiphyseal cortex, the intervertebral disc, and the adjacent vertebrae. The infective exudate may spread anteriorly beneath the anterior longitudinal ligament to reach the neighboring vertebrae.

Infection of the posterior bony arch and the transverse processes is unusual. More commonly, granulation tissue develops and compresses the spinal cord and the nerve roots. Pressure on nerve structures is more likely in the thoracic spine where the caliber of the spinal canal is small. Sequestra and bone fragments are rarely extruded into the canal, being limited by the strong posterior longitudinal ligament.

The most common vertebral infection is an exudative type that constitutes a severe hypergic reaction. This causes an extreme degree of osteoporosis that spreads rapidly. Abscess formation is frequent and constitutional symptoms are pronounced.

Procedure

Anghelescu's sign is for identifying tuberculosis of the vertebrae or other destructive process of the spine. In the supine position the patient places weight on the head and heels while lifting the body upward. Inability to hyperextend the spine indicates a disease process.

Confirmation Procedures

Chest expansion test, Forestier's bowstring sign, clinical laboratory testing, diagnostic imaging

---

Reporting Statement

Anghelescu's sign is present and strongly suggests tuberculous spondylitis. Further laboratory testing and diagnostic imaging are warranted.

∾ Clinical Pearl ∾

When testing for Anghelescu's sign, the loss of the ability to achieve a near opisthotonos posture is significant. While the true opisthotonos posture involves the cervical spine, very few patients normally have enough strength in the neck to accomplish this.

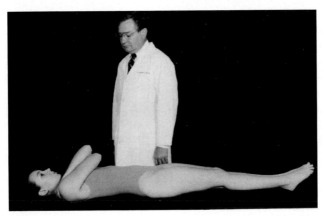

Fig. 7–15   The patient is supine on the examining table. The examiner observes for postural symmetry and notes any positions of antalgia.

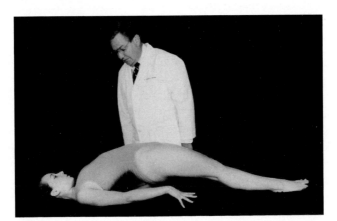

Fig. 7–16   From the supine position, the patient attempts to extend the thoracic spine sufficiently to raise it from the table. Without thoracic spinal pathology, the patient will be able to rest the weight of the body on the heels and the shoulders (a near opisthotonos posture). This position cannot be achieved in tuber-culous spondylitis.

Comment

Within the thoracic spine there is overlap of dermatomes. The dermatomes follow the ribs, and the absence of only one dermatome may lead to no loss in sensation at all.

Absence of the abdominal reflexes may be an early sign of corticospinal disease, which is regarded as a common sign of multiple sclerosis but is by no means pathognomonic of this disease. When the abdominal reflexes are absent, hyperreflexia of the lower extremities and the Babinski sign are present.

The fifth thoracic (T5) segment is at the level of the nipple, T10 at the umbilicus, and T12 at the groin.

The motor and sensory roots become progressively longer as they proceed from their respective cord segments to their points of exit.

Acute postinfectious polyneuropathy (Guillain-Barré syndrome), an acute idiopathic polyneuritis, is a disease of unknown origin characterized by rapid onset of ascending weakness with associated sensory disturbance. All races, all age groups, and both sexes are susceptible to this disease. The pathologic picture is characterized by peripheral nerve demyelination and frequently a mononuclear inflammatory reaction. There are numerous theories as to causation of this disease. One theory is that the disease results from an autoimmune reaction against a peripheral nerve antigen, specifically myelin. Other theories postulate that the disease is secondary to a bacterial, viral, or neurotoxic substance. It is known that about one half of the cases of acute postinfectious polyneuropathy will occur after an upper respiratory or gastrointestinal infection.

The typical medical history includes an acute upper respiratory illness followed by a few days of pins-and-needles paresthesia, followed by lower extremity weakness, which is characteristically a symmetrically ascending motor weakness accompanied by minimal sensory changes and intact sphincter control. Aching or tenderness may be present but neither is a prominent feature. A minority of patients exhibit profound sensory losses. Temporary bowel or bladder paralysis may occur but is always affected to a lesser degree than the lower extremities. The disease may ascend to involve the bulbar muscles, resulting in respiratory paralysis and death. The course of the disease ranges from several days to a week. If the patient survives the first 2 weeks, the prognosis is good. Motor power returns gradually over the course of a year.

Procedure

Beevor's sign, though not an abdominal reflex, can be observed during an examination. In this test the recumbent patient lifts the head off the examining table. Normally the upper and lower abdominal muscles contract equally and the umbilicus does not move or drift. When the lower abdominal muscles alone are weakened, the umbilicus will be drawn upward by the contraction of the intact upper musculature. This effect is associated with a spinal cord lesion at the T10 level.

Confirmation Procedures

Sensory assessment, reflex testing, electrodiagnosis, diagnostic imaging (MRI)

Reporting Statement

Beevor's sign is present, as demonstrated by cephalad umbilical drift. This sign reveals lower abdominal muscular weakness and suggests myelopathy associated with the T10 spinal level.

~ **Clinical Pearl** ~

In the presence of prolonged illness followed by lower extremity paresthesia (regardless of how minor), this test needs to be performed. Beevor's sign affords an early, noninvasive indicator of the existence of thoracic spinal cord myelopathy.

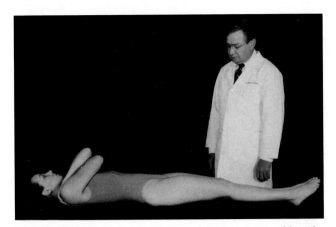

Fig. 7—17 The patient is supine on the examining table. The abdominal muscles are palpated and the position of the umbilicus established.

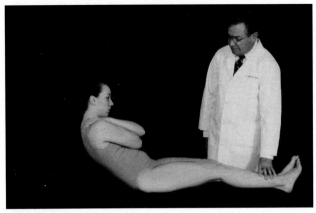

Fig. 7—18 The examiner fixes the patient's legs to the table with mild downward pressure. The patient performs a partial sit-up, with the arms folded across the chest. The examiner notes any drift of the umbilicus. During a sit-up the uppermost fibers of the abdominal musculature are primarily the ones tested. Drift occurs toward the stronger or uninvolved musculature. Cephalad drift implicates lower thoracic spine involvement. Caudad drift implicates upper thoracic spine involvement but not above T7.

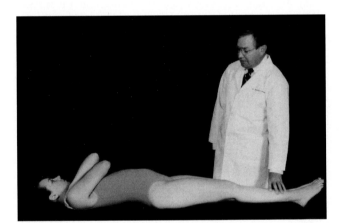

Fig. 7—19 If extensive abdominal muscle weakness or paresis exists, the back will arch from the table as the patient attempts the partial sit-up. The thorax may pull away from the pelvis until it is firmly fixed by extension of the thoracic spine. The arching of the back stretches the abdominal muscles and they may appear firm under tension. The examiner needs to be careful not to mistake this tautness for firmness due to actual contraction of the muscles.

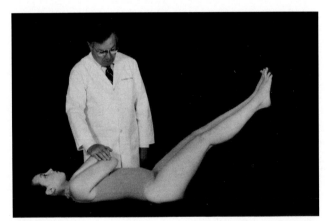

Fig. 7—20 As an alternative, the patient can perform a partial bilateral leg lift to test the abdominal musculature. In this procedure the examiner can apply a mild downward pressure to the patient's thorax, fixing it to the examining table for stability. Umbilical drift is noted. Leg-lifting primarily tests the lowermost fibers of the abdominal musculature.

Chest Expansion Test

Comment

Children breathe abdominally. Women perform upper thoracic breathing. Men are upper and lower thoracic breathers. In the aged, the breathing is in the lower thoracic and abdominal regions. Chest wall movement that occurs during breathing displaces the pleural surfaces, thorax musculature, nerves, and ribs. Pain is accentuated by breathing and coughing, if any of these structures are injured.

With pectus carinatum (pigeon chest) the sternum projects anterior and inferior, increasing the anteroposterior dimension of the chest. The sternal deformity impairs the effectiveness of breathing by restricting the ventilation volume.

The pectus excavatum (funnel chest) deformity occurs after the sternum is pushed posteriorly by an overgrowth of the ribs. The anteroposterior dimension of the chest is decreased, and the heart may be displaced. During inspiration this deformity causes depression of the sternum, which affects respiration and may result in kyphosis.

With emphysema (barrel chest) the sternum projects anterior and superior so that anteroposterior diameter is increased.

Ankylosing spondylitis is a disease of the spine that occurs in late adolescence or early adulthood and is characterized pathologically by progressive inflammation of the spine, sacroiliac joints, and the larger joints of the extremities—particularly the hips, knees, and shoulders—leading to fibrous or bony ankylosis and deformity. Other conditions that may sometimes be associated with similar ankylosing disease of the spine need to be differentiated by their own unique clinical, pathologic, and laboratory characteristics.

Ankylosing spondylitis starts insidiously in a young adult. Symptoms at first are vague and poorly localized. Aching and stiffness around both sacroiliac joints occur as a morning backache that subsides with activity but returns after sitting in one position for prolonged periods. The pain and stiffness become progressively worse and spread slowly, within 6 months to a year, to the rest of the spine. Limitation of motion is first detected in the lower spine, but is finally notable throughout the spine. Chest expansion is restricted because of disease of the costovertebral joints.

Procedure

Costovertebral joint movement is determined by measuring chest expansion. The tape measure is placed around the chest at the level of the fourth intercostal space. The patient exhales deeply, and the measurement is taken. The patient then inhales with maximum effort and the second measurement is taken. The normal difference between inspiration and expiration is 5.75 cm to 7.62 cm (1.5 to 3 inches).

A second method of determining chest expansion is with measurements at three different levels. The levels for measurement under the axillae are, at the nipple line and at the T10 rib level. The measurements are taken during expiration and inspiration.

Following measurement of chest expansion, the patient takes a deep breath and coughs. The examiner can determine whether this action causes or alters any pain. A positive test would be less than 3 cm (1.25 inches) of difference. A positive test indicates spinal ankylosis.

Confirmation Procedures

Amoss' sign, Forestier's bowstring sign, clinical laboratory testing, range of motion testing, spirometer testing, diagnostic imaging of the pelvis and sacroiliac joints

---

Reporting Statement

Chest expansion in this female patient is 1.91 cm (0.75 inches), which suggests thoracic involvement by ankylosing spondylitis.

Chest expansion in this male patient is 2.54 cm (1 inch), which suggests the existence of ankylosing spondylitis that affects the thoracic spine.

∽ Clinical Pearl ∽

Chest expansion measurements are sensitive indicators of early involvement of the costovertebral joints in ankylosing spondylitis. The chest expansion test is often positive before the patient realizes a change in chest comfort.

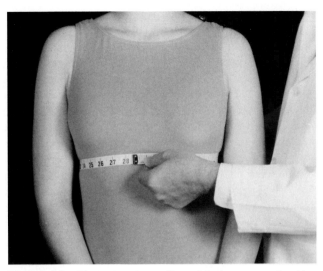

Fig. 7–21 The patient is standing with the arms at the sides. The examiner places a tape around the patient's chest at any of the following points. (1) At the fourth intercostal space, (2) at the axillary level, (3) at the level of the nipples, or (4) at the T10 rib level. The patient exhales deeply. The examiner records the measurement.

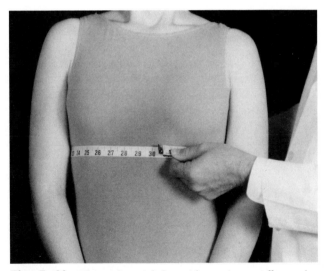

Fig. 7–22 The patient inhales with maximum effort and a second measurement is taken. The normal difference between inspiration and expiration is 5.75 to 7.62 cm (1.5 to 3 inches).

Comment

There are four physical components of the nervous system that refer pain or discomfort. These tissues include the spinal cord, the dural sleeve of a nerve root, the nerve trunk, and a peripheral or cutaneous nerve. The symptoms from each vary and may be clinically differentiated.

Compression of the spinal cord does not result in pain. Paresthesia (pins and needles) are bilateral and disregard segmentation of the body. Other associated neural structures, compressed simultaneously, cause pain that follows dermatome patterns.

At the point of emergence from the dura, the nerve roots are invested with a dural sleeve. Pressure on the dural sleeve will produce discomfort. Pain is felt in all or any part of the dermatome. Paresthesia, a compression phenomenon, is felt at the distal end of the dermatome. Paresthesia often conspicuously occupies an area that is not supplied by any one nerve root. The paresthesia has no edge or depth, and numbness displaces paresthesia. Pressure on a nerve root causes analgesia, and minimal pressure evokes paresthesia.

Weakness results from compression of the nerve root within the parenchyma. Weakness is discernible during resisted movements.

Compression of a nerve root does not cause pain, a pressure on the surrounding dural sleeve, at the transverse process, will hurt. Impaired conduction along a nerve leads to muscle weakness, manifested during resisted movements. Paresthesia rather than numbness, are brought on as a release phenomenon. The lesion always lies proximal to the upper edge of the paresthetic area.

Compression of a peripheral or cutaneous nerve does not cause pain. Furthermore, no weakness is manifested because the efferent fibers have left the body of the nerve proximally. Numbness rather than paresthesia, occupies the cutaneous area supplied by the nerve. The edge is well defined and toward the center of the area full anesthesia is often demonstrable.

The dura mater does not conform to the rules of segmental reference. The dura mater descends from the foramen magnum of the skull to the inferior edge of the first or second sacral vertebra. The dura mater keeps the spinal cord buffered in cerebrospinal fluid. From the dura mater protrude 30 pairs of nerve roots covered by the dural sheath.

Compression or stretching of the dura mater causes extrasegmentally referred pain. The dura mater is adjacent to the intervertebral discs and vulnerable to posterior pressure exerted by the posterior longitudinal ligament.

Dura mater pain often pervades many dermatomes simultaneously. This pain is a frequent cause of scapular pain, and the symptoms are usually central or unilateral.

Pressure on the dura mater at thoracic levels may radiate pain to the base of the neck, and this pain also may radiate to the posterior or anterior aspect of the trunk. The pain will spread over many dermatomes simultaneously. The symptoms are usually central or unilateral.

Pressure on the dura mater at lumbar levels may cause pain that reaches the lower thorax in the posterior, the lower abdomen, the upper buttocks, sacrum, and coccyx. Again, many dermatomes may be occupied simultaneously.

Pain perceived elsewhere in places other than its true site is called *referred pain*. Nearly all pain is referred. The examiner's task is to determine the origin of the pain.

The site where symptoms are referred is determined by the sensory cortex. The sensory cortex attributes the impulses it receives to the appropriate areas of the body. With stimuli to the skin the sensory cortex achieves a high degree of accuracy. Over time a stimulus reaching certain cells in the cortex is interpreted as damage in a specific area of the skin.

A painful stimulus arising from deep-seated structure is received by the same cortical cells. The sensory cortex interprets this new impulse based upon experience. Pain is referred to the area of skin served by those particular cortical cells.

The area of skin associated with sensory cells is the dermatome. The dermatome corresponds to the embryologic neural segment from which the structure was derived. Thus a pain in tissue of T5 segmental origin will be referred by the sensory cortex to the T5 dermatome and from the T8 structure to the T8 dermatome.

The 40 dermatome segments of a month-old fetus are distributed horizontally. At this stage the dermatomes are superimposed directly over the segments from which they are derived. The growth of the four limbs draws the dermatomes down the arms and the legs. However, in the trunk, the original arrangement of circular dermatome bands remains intact.

Pain is referred in compliance with certain rules. These rules define the tissues from which pain could and could not arise.

1. Pain is referred segmentally. A T5 tissue refers pain to the T5 dermatome. Pain can occupy all or any part of the dermatome.

If the patient describes symptoms straddling more than one dermatome, or if the pain migrates from one dermatome to another, four possibilities arise. (a) The patient is describing a nonorganic pain. (b) The lesion itself is shifting, which often happens with vertebral element displacements. (c) The lesion is spreading, as in metastasis. (d) The pain stems from a tissue that cannot refer pain segmentally. An exception of importance is the dura mater, which refers pain extrasegmentally.

2. Pain is referred distally. The source of symptoms must be sought locally or proximally.

3. Referred pain does not cross the midline. A T5 left rib will not cause discomfort on the right side of the body. A pain felt centrally must originate from a central structure. Pain that cannot be accounted for by a unilateral structure must be sought centrally. A pain alternating from one side of the body to the other must have a central source. That central source must be able to shift from one side to the other, such as during an intervertebral disc displacement.

4. The extent of pain reference is controlled. The referred pain is controlled by the size of the dermatome and the position in the dermatome of the tissue lesion. A large dermatome permits greater reference than a small one. A lesion in the proximal part of the dermatome refers pain further than a lesion in the distal part.

5. The more intense the pain the greater the number of cortical cells excited. The spread to adjacent cells in the sensory cortex is interpreted as an enlargement of the painful area.

6. The deeper a soft-tissue lesion lies, the larger the reference to be expected. However, bone lesions produce minimal pain radiation.

Procedure

Pain from stretching the first thoracic nerve root via the ulnar nerve identifies the T1 or T2 roots. Disc lesions at either level are rarities and are not accompanied by easily identifiable neurologic signs. If weakness is present, the possibility of serious disease should be considered.

The patient abducts the arm to 90 degrees and flexes the pronated forearm to 90 degrees. Symptoms should not appear in this position. The patient fully flexes the elbow, and places the hand behind the neck. This action stretches the ulnar nerve and the T1 nerve root. Pain in the scapular area is a positive test.

Confirmation Procedures

Cervical range of motion, thoracic spinal range of motion, reflex testing, sensory assessment, electrodiagnosis, Roos' test, diagnostic imaging

---

Reporting Statement

Stretch of the first thoracic nerve root is positive on the right because scapular pain is produced. This result indicates nerve root compression at T1.

∽ Clinical Pearl ∽

The first thoracic nerve root stretch indicates nerve root compression. This stretch can also indicate the existence of an inflammation of the lower two branches of the brachial plexus, a nonvascular thoracic outlet syndrome. This diagnosis is further confirmed by Roos' test.

Continued.

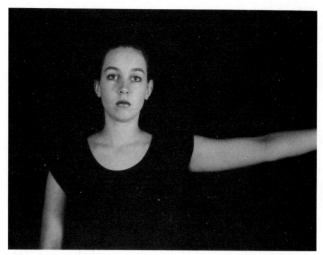

Fig. 7–23   The patient is seated and abducts the shoulder to 90 degrees. The arm is pronated.

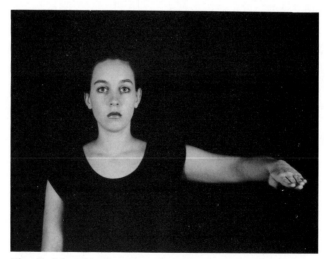

Fig. 7–24   The elbow is flexed to 90 degrees.

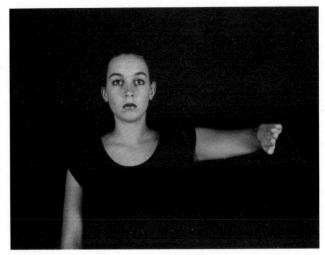

Fig. 7–25 The forearm is pronated fully to a 90-degree position, which should not be uncomfortable at this point.

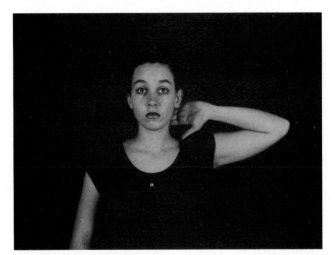

Fig. 7–26 The elbow is fully flexed and the pronated hand is placed behind the head. Pain elicited in the scapular region suggests T1 nerve root involvement.

Comment

Ankylosing spondylitis is an inflammation of the joints of the spine that often results in bony ankylosis. The process is chronic, usually low grade, and begins mainly in young men. Early symptoms include pain and stiffness of the back; later there is disability because of the so-called *poker spine*.

On the one hand, ankylosing spondylitis is a disease of the cartilaginous and fibrocartilaginous joints of the spine. On the other hand, the disease affects the diarthrodial articulations, such as the sacroiliac joint, the hips, and the shoulders. Ankylosing spondylitis is primarily an axial disease. However, in approximately 35% of the patients, peripheral involvement of the hands, knees, ankles, and other joints does occur and is sometimes the very first manifestation of the disease. However, it is rare that peripheral arthritis results in significant deformity. All axial joints—including the manubriosternal, costovertebral, and symphysis pubis—may be affected.

Although ankylosing spondylitis is an entity distinct from rheumatoid arthritis, the early pathologic changes are similar. Like rheumatoid arthritis, ankylosing spondylitis is a synovial disease characterized grossly by proliferative granulation tissue, adhesions of the joint, and probably a greater tendency for fibrous and bony ankylosis. The earliest findings of the disease are found in the sacroiliac joint and typify those also seen in the apophyseal joints of the lumbar, dorsal, and cervical spine as well as the shoulders, hips, costovertebral, manubriosternal, and symphysis pubis articulations. Joint spaces are initially widened because of proliferative synovitis that gives way to erosive changes of the articular margins, narrowing, and then fusion. There may be no semblance of a joint. The histologic counterpart of these findings is synovial membrane thickening with plasma cell and lymphocyte infiltration that are arranged in nests surrounding the smaller synovial blood vessels. Foci of chronic inflammation also may be found in adjacent bone, usually independent of the synovial process.

Most of the patient's discomfort and disability are caused by involvement of the dorsolumbar spine, albeit the sacroiliacs are concomitantly affected. Muscle pains, initially diffuse, may become increasingly concentrated in the dorsolumbar region. Stiffness is profound at times. Bending, lifting, and turning become formidable chores. Examination usually shows mild to severe direct tenderness of the dorsolumbar apophyseal joints, marked paravertebral muscle spasm, straightening of the lumbar spine, and sometimes an ironed-out appearance caused by muscle atrophy. Limitation of motion can be marked even if symptoms are minimal or absent. The normal arching of the spine during flexion is lost, but this may not be fully appreciated because of the compensatory flexion at the hips. Lateral flexion of the dorsolumbar spine cannot be disguised so well. It is sometimes lost. Minor limitations of motion can be confirmed by marking a point 10 cm above the fifth lumbar process and measuring the linear distance between the fifth lumbar spinous process and this point during flexion and extension. The distance should normally increase by 5 cm (2 inches) or more (Schober test). Spondylitis of the dorsolumbar area, even if a fixed ankylosis ensues, usually does not pose a serious threat of disability.

Procedure

The standing patient performs side bending and reveals ipsilateral tightening and contracture of the paraspinal musculature. Normally the contralateral musculature demonstrates tightening. The test is significant for ankylosing spondylitis.

Confirmation Procedures

Amoss' sign, Anghelescu's sign, chest expansion test, clinical laboratory testing, diagnostic imaging

---

Reporting Statement

Forestier's bowstring sign is present on the right. This sign suggests the presence of ankylosing spondylitis in the thoracolumbar spine.

~ Clinical Pearl ~

Although the presence of Forestier's bowstring sign suggests spondylitis, this test also indicates strain and intervertebral disc involvement. Any loss of symmetrical motion must be examined further.

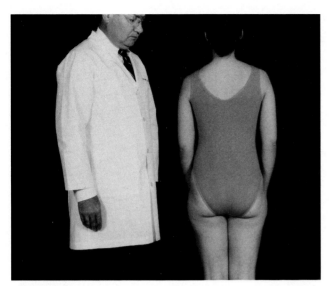

Fig. 7–27   The patient is standing with the arms at the side. The examiner notes any loss of symmetry of the spinal musculature and notes the posture.

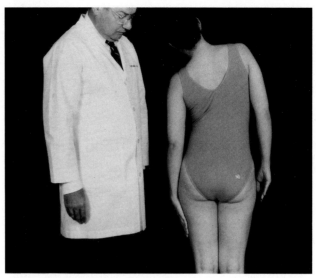

Fig. 7–28   The patient flexes the thoracic spine laterally. The sign is present when there is tightening or contracture of the musculature on the same side as flexion. This suggests ankylosing spondylitis.

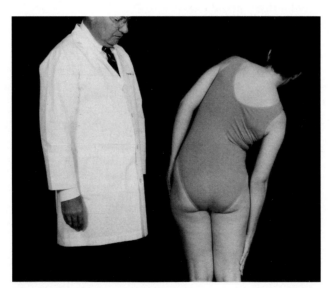

Fig. 7–29   The lateral flexion is compared bilaterally. Motion toward the opposite side is expected to produce normal tightening on the contralateral side. Overall, this tightening represents asymmetrical motion of the thoracic spine.

Comment

The scapular reflex is a contraction of the scapular muscles upon stimulation of the interscapular region. This reflex demonstrates the integrity of the cord between the upper two or three dorsal and lower two or three cervical nerves. However, only a third of the patients exhibit a good reflex response. The examiner should observe the quality of the skin's vascular response following the reflex stimulus. Each side should be equally hyperemic.

The dorsal (erector spinae) reflex is a local contraction of the erector spinae musculature that follows stimulation of the skin along the border of the muscle. This reflex demonstrates integrity of the dorsal region of cord.

These reflexes are carried out by stimulating the respective area with a Wartenberg pinwheel or a reflex hammer. Reflexes are examined bilaterally.

In acute intervertebral disc herniation, sequestered disc fragments are forced into the spinal canal. Although compression of the theca may be slight, impingement of the anterior median longitudinal artery, an end artery, produces ischemia of the spinal cord over several segments.

The critical zone of the spinal cord is that portion of the cord that lies within the portion of the spinal canal extending from the vertebral segments T4 to T9. This portion of the spinal canal is the narrowest zone of the canal and corresponds to that part of the cord possessing the least amount of vascular supply. Therefore the spinal cord may be compromised by two factors—compression and interruption of the vascular supply. Ischemia produces edema and central necrosis of the cord.

Injury to the long thoracic nerve frequently occurs along with sprain or other injury at the base of the neck. The long thoracic nerve comes directly off the nerve roots and does not participate in the brachial plexus. The nerve passes down and supplies the various serrations of the serratus anterior. Bruising or damage to this nerve may occur and pass unrecognized until distressing winging of the scapula is noted. The cause of this winging may be a sharp blow at the base of the neck that laterally impinges the nerve against the lower cervical vertebrae. Because the long thoracic nerve is primarily a motor nerve, there is usually little pain or discomfort to guide the examiner. There may be weakness or complete paralysis of the nerve, resulting in loss of fixation of the scapula to the chest wall.

Procedure

The patient may stand or lie prone as the examiner passively approximates the scapulae. This approximation is accomplished by lifting the shoulder tips up and back. Pain in the scapular area indicates a T1 or T2 nerve root problem on the side where the pain is being experienced.

Confirmation Procedures

First thoracic nerve root test, Roos' test, electrodiagnosis, diagnostic imaging

---

Reporting Statement

Passive scapular approximation test is positive on the right. This result suggests a compression syndrome at the T1 or T2 nerve root.

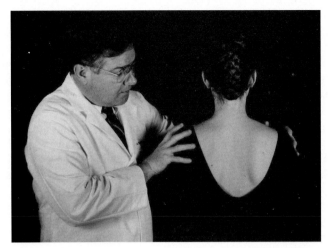

Fig. 7-30 The patient is standing, with the arms at the sides. The examiner observes for thoracic spinal symmetry and posture.

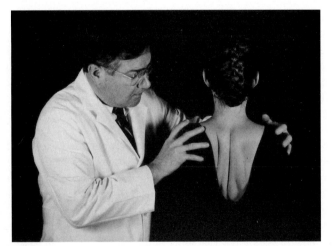

Fig. 7-31 The examiner approximates the scapulae by pulling the shoulder tips backward. Pain in the scapular area indicates a T1 or T2 nerve root involvement.

Comment

The costovertebral joints are synovial joints that are found between the ribs and the vertebral body. There are 24 of these joints, and they are divided into two parts. Ribs 1, 10, 11, and 12 form joints with a single vertebrae. Ribs 2 through 9 have an intraarticular ligament. The intraarticular ligament divides the joint into two parts so each rib forms a joint with two adjacent vertebrae. Ribs 2 through 9 also articulate with the intervening intervertebral disc.

The costotransverse joints are synovial joints found between the ribs and the transverse processes of the vertebrae for ribs 1 through 10. Ribs 11 and 12 do not form a joint with the transverse processes. Therefore this joint does not exist at these two levels.

The costochondral joints are formed between the ribs and the costal cartilage. The sternocostal joints are found between the costal cartilage and the sternum. The costochondral joints of ribs 2 through 6 are synovial. The first rib costal cartilage is united with the sternum by a synchondrosis and is not synovial. Ribs form joints with an adjacent rib or costal cartilage. At each of these articulations a synovial interchondral joint exists.

The ribs help to stiffen the thoracic spine. The ribs articulate with the demifacets on vertebrae T2 to T9. For T1 and T10 vertebrae, there is a complete facet for ribs 1 and 10, respectively. The first rib forms a joint with T1 only; the second rib with T1 and T2 and so on.

Ribs 1 through 7 articulate with the sternum directly and are classified as true ribs. Ribs 8, 9, and 10 join with the costocartilage of the rib above and are classified as false ribs. Ribs 11 and 12 are classified as floating ribs because they do not attach to the sternum or costal cartilages at their distal ends.

Ribs 11 and 12 form joints only with the bodies of T11 and T12 vertebrae. These ribs do not have a joint with the transverse processes of the vertebrae or with the costocartilage of the rib above. The ribs are held by ligaments to the body of the vertebrae and to the transverse processes of the same vertebra. Some of these ligaments also bind the ribs to the vertebra above.

At the top of the rib cage, the ribs are horizontal. As the rib cage descends, the ribs become more and more oblique. Rib 12 is more vertical than horizontal. During inspiration, the ribs are pulled up and forward. The first six ribs increase the anteroposterior dimension of the chest, mainly by rotating around their long axes. Rotation downward of the rib neck is associated with depression of the chest. Rotation upward of the same portion of the ribs is associated with chest elevation. Collectively, these motions are known as the pump handle action. These movements are accompanied by elevation of the manubrium and sternum, superior and anterior.

Ribs 7 through 10 mainly increase lateral, or transverse, dimension. The ribs move superior, posterior, and medially to increase the infrasternal angle, or inferiorly, anteriorly, and laterally to decrease the angle. These movements are known as the bucket handle action.

Ribs 8 through 12 move laterally in a caliper action that increases the lateral dimension.

The ribs are elastic in children but become increasingly brittle with age. In the anterior half of the chest the ribs are subcutaneous. In the posterior half the ribs are covered by muscles.

Procedure

While the patient is lying supine the examiner's hands are placed over the upper chest. As the patient inhales and exhales, the examiner feels for the anteroposterior movement of the ribs. Any restriction or difference in motion is noted.

If a rib stops moving in relation to the other ribs during exhalation, it is classified as an elevated rib. If a rib stops moving in relation to the other ribs during inhalation, it is classified as a depressed rib. A depressed rib is usually the uppermost rib. An elevated rib is usually the lowest rib. The examiner moves the hands down the chest, testing the movement of the ribs in the middle and lower thoracic areas.

In testing lateral movement the examiner's hands are placed around the sides of the rib cage. The examiner's hands are at 45 degrees to the vertical axis of the patient's body. Beginning at the level of the axilla the examiner feels the movement of the ribs during inspiration and expiration.

For springing the ribs the patient is prone or on a side as the examiner's hands are placed around the posterolateral aspect of the patient's rib cage. The examiner's hands are at 45 degrees to the vertical axis of the patient's body. The examination involves springing of the ribs by pushing inward with the hands. The amount and quality of movement occurring on both sides should be noted. If a rib appears hypomobile or hypermobile compared to the others being tested, it is tested individually.

Confirmation Procedures

Chest expansion test, sternal compression test, diagnostic imaging

Reporting Statement

Rib motion for ribs 5 to 7 on the right is inhibited during inhalation. This result suggests a depressed fifth rib.

Rib motion for ribs 5 to 7 on the right is inhibited during exhalation. This inhibition of movement suggests an elevated seventh rib.

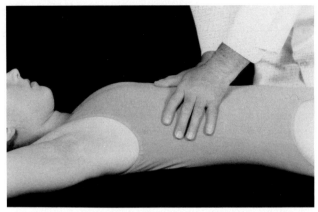

Fig. 7–32 With the patient supine, the examiner's hands are placed over the chest. The examiner feels for the anteroposterior movement of the ribs as the patient inhales and exhales. Any restriction or difference in motion is noted.

If a rib stops moving in relation to the other ribs during exhalation, it is classified as an elevated rib. If a rib stops moving in relation to the other ribs during inhalation, it is classified as a depressed rib. A depressed rib is usually the uppermost rib. An elevated rib is usually the lowest rib. The examiner moves the hands down the chest, testing the movement of the ribs in the middle and lower thoracic areas.

Comment

Because a multitude of muscles attach to the chest, almost any manifestation of strain may occur. Strain may be caused by violent exertion or by overstretching of the muscles. The symptoms will depend entirely on the area involved. In the long muscles of the back of the thorax, this condition may be indistinguishable from or may be a part of a lumbar strain. In the front of the chest the strain may involve the muscles of the abdominal wall, where the muscles attach to the lower ribs. Strain also may involve the intercostal muscles, although this is infrequent because the muscles are well protected by other muscle structures. These muscles do not act forcibly enough to rupture their fibers. A strain is much more likely to involve an area connecting to the chest than the chest itself. This is particularly true of the scapular muscles. Strain of the rhomboids will occur either at the scapular attachment or along the spine much more frequently than at the costal attachment. Similarly the serrati may be more likely to get injured in their substance than in their costal origins. Careful analysis of the active motion that causes pain will usually determine the proper muscle group.

Strain of the muscle at its attachment to the rib is likely to be more painful than it is disabling. However, there may be considerable attendant muscle spasms that will splint the chest and interfere with deep breathing. These spasms actually may prevent certain types of activity. A strain of the abdominal recti attached to the lower ribs may interdict undertaking of certain sports, such as rowing or wrestling, where forcible use of the abdominal muscles is required. Similarly a spasm of the shoulder muscles may interdict throwing.

Procedure

Schepelmann's sign identifies rib integrity. The patient raises the arms while in the seated position and then bends laterally. If pain is created on the concave side, it is due to intercostal neuritis. If pain is created on the convex side, the diagnosis is intercostal myofascitis. Intercostal myofascitis must be differentiated from the fibrous inflammation of pleurisy.

Confirmation Procedures

Rib motion testing, chest expansion test, Amoss' sign, Forestier's bowstring sign, sternal compression test, diagnostic imaging

---

Reporting Statement

Schepelmann's sign is present on the right, concave side. The presence of this sign suggests intercostal neuritis.

Schepelmann's sign is present on the right, convex side. The presence of this sign suggests intercostal myofascitis.

~ Clinical Pearl ~

Schepelmann's test provides an efficient method for localizing rib injury. The patient moves actively and can limit the motion according to the pain.

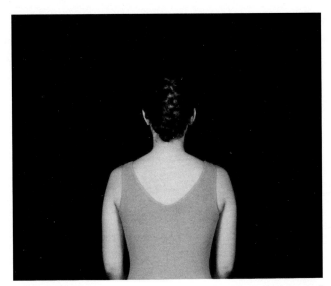

Fig. 7–33 The patient is seated comfortably and the spinal contours are noted.

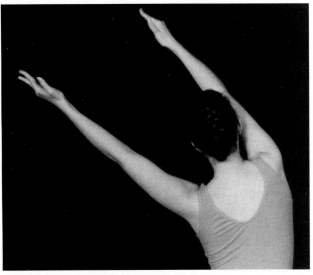

Fig. 7–34 The patient fully abducts the shoulders, bringing the hands overhead. The patient flexes the thoracic spine laterally. Pain elicited on the side of flexion (concave) indicates intercostal neuritis. Pain elicited on the convex side indicates intercostal myofascitis.

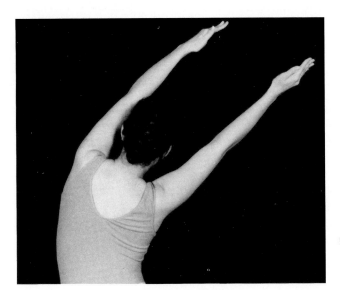

Fig. 7–35 The test is performed bilaterally.

Comment

There is a significantly increased incidence of fractures of the spine because of osteoporosis in the later years of life. Even after relatively minor trauma, compression fractures with vertebral collapse are common in older people. After age 70 in the asymptomatic population, the incidence of such fractures is 20%. In the aging spine, the etiology of such fractures may be spontaneous and obscure without a major traumatic event. The fractures may occur because of sneezing, raising windows, or lifting weights. The patient can experience severe pain in the spine, although absence of discomfort is common. Minor falls may also produce such fractures. In addition to having back pain these patients may have local tenderness and may be reluctant to move while in bed in order to avoid further pain. Some patients have root pain, and a very small minority have injury to the spinal cord. About 15% of such patients may develop paralytic ileus, particularly in association with fractures of T12 and L1. It is generally considered that retroperitoneal hemorrhage is the underlying factor in the production of the ileus either by the size of the hemorrhage or by irritation of the celiac plexus.

Procedure

While the patient is seated or standing and the thoracic spine is slightly flexed, the examiner percusses the spinous processes and the associated musculature of each of the thoracic vertebra with a neurologic reflex hammer. Evidence of localized pain indicates a possible fractured vertebra. Evidence of radicular pain indicates a possible disc lesion. Due to the nonspecific nature of this test, other conditions also will elicit a positive pain response. If a ligamentous sprain exists, then percussion of the spinous processes will elicit pain. Percussion of the paraspinal musculature will elicit a positive sign for strain.

Confirmation Procedures

Soto-Hall sign, Dejerine sign, Valsalva maneuver, Lhermitte's sign, diagnostic imaging

---

Reporting Statement

Spinal percussion elicits pain on the spinous process of T4. This pain suggests osseous injury at that level.

Spinal percussion elicits pain at the paraspinals on the right of T5. This pain suggests soft-tissue injury at that level.

∾ Clinical Pearl ∾

When soft-tissue percussion reproduces the complaint, the examiner may expect the same phenomenon from applications of ultrasound to the tissue. The uses of such therapies may be delayed until the soft tissue is no longer reactive to percussion.

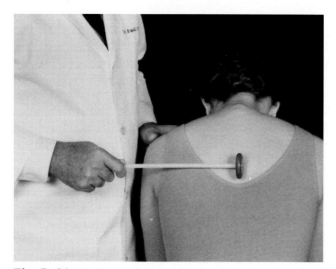

Fig. 7–36 In the seated or standing position, the patient flexes the thoracic spine, exposing the spinous processes as much as p6ossible. The examiner percusses the spinous processes of each vertebra. Localized pain is evidence of a fracture or severe sprain. Radiating pain suggests intervertebral disc syndrome.

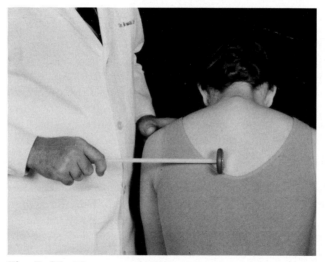

Fig. 7–37 The paravertebral tissues are percussed. Pain elicited in the soft tissues suggests muscular strain and highly sensitive myofascial trigger points.

Comment

Minor injuries of the soft tissue are due to mild overuse or overstretching. Severe thoracic soft-tissue injuries are characterized by traumatic effusion, pain, and loss of function. Traumatic effusion is composed of four types of physiologic tissue reactions.

Tissue tearing or crushing with rupture of the blood vessels causes bleeding into the tissue. The capillaries are constricted in the injury area or site. Resultant clotting seals the damaged vessels. Fibroblasts begin the repair process, and lymphatic drainage takes place.

Local inflammation causes the undamaged capillaries to dilate and become more permeable, allowing inflammatory exudates to form. The exudates stimulate fibroblast repair and white blood cell activity with resultant local heat, redness, swelling, and pain.

There is formation of tissue thickening or tissue adhesions from the blood and exudates, especially if any of the lymphatica are damaged or if the circulation is impaired.

If a thoracic spinal joint is involved in the soft-tissue injury, synovial effusion may result.

With muscle strain the interstitial exudates and fluids gel when the muscle is at rest. The patient experiences a stiffening of the muscle upon resting the injured part. This stiffening is followed by the onset of a cramp or spasm of the injured muscle, and associated pain and ache occurs in the part. This pain is all relieved by movement. As the exudates are forced out of the tissue, through mechanical action of muscle contraction, the part is no longer stiff or sore. However, after excessive movement the strained muscle fibers are once again aggravated and become uncomfortable. The patient is forced to rest the part, the cycle begins again.

Myofascial fibrositis is an inflammatory nonsuppurative condition affecting the interstitial tissues of the body and is an established clinical syndrome. Previous terms applied to this condition often caused confusion. These terms are *nonarticular rheumatism, fibromyositis, myositis,* and *muscular rheumatism.* Other commonly used terms include *wry neck* and *lumbago.*

Primary myofascial fibrositis occurs independent of pathologic causes elsewhere in the body. Secondary myofascial fibrositis is myofascial inflammation that is secondary to the development of another pathologic condition and is associated with conditions such as rheumatoid arthritis, osteoarthritis, hypertrophic or degenerative arthritis, spondylosis, septic foci, rheumatic fever, diabetes, and influenza. Secondary myofascial fibrositis may also be the residual effect of traumatic injuries.

When the tissues involved fail to heal completely following injury, the condition of myofascial inflammation is called a *residual complication.*

Older patients who develop clinical cases of myofascial fibrositis experience a gradual onset of their symptoms (senile myofascial fibrositis). The etiology of this type of myofascial fibrositis is one that is mixed and complex and is probably associated with a combination of factors that include endocrine imbalances, dietary deficiencies, and degenerative tissue changes.

Normal fibrous tissue is composed of bands of collagen, fibroblasts, elastic tissue fibrils, fluid spaces, reticuloendothelial cells, capillaries, and nerves.

The inflammatory reaction of these tissues includes the swelling and fragmentation of the bands of collagen and the proliferation of fibroblasts. If the fibroblasts proliferate, it causes contractures and blocks the free flow of tissue fluids. This blockage results in difficulty moving the joints and produces pressure on the vessels and nerves in the immediate vicinity. Although small nodules form, they are often too small to be palpated. The nodules are discovered because of tenderness produced by pressure or other means.

The onset of the clinical symptoms may be sudden or insidious. The limitation of joint movement in acute cases is caused by muscle spasm. In chronic cases the spasm may be mixed with contractures. Postinertial dyskinesia, which is the gelling stiffness that results from movement of a part that has been rested, is a consistent complaint.

Swelling of the tissues is sometimes found by the examiner. However, many times the swelling sensation is subjective. The nodules that have been described are located by palpation. Especially when the nodules form over a firm undersurface, such as bone. By carefully searching the area, the examiner can discern acutely tender areas of myofascial fibrositis, which are called *trigger points.*

Sensitive areas in the soft tissues throughout the body have been described for years. Pressure upon these areas causes local and referred pain into distal areas of the body. These tender areas are often identified as symptoms of the following conditions: myofascial pain syndrome, myalgia, myositis, fibrositis, fibromyositis, fibromyalgia fascitis, myofascitis, muscular rheumatism, strain, and sprain.

The small hypersensitive area that makes up a trigger site may be stimulated by pressure, goading, needling, excessive heat, local icing, and motion.

Trigger points are characterized as hard nodules of fibrous connective tissue that surrounds sparse muscle fibers. There also are infiltrations of lymphocytes.

Myofascial fibrositis is classified as acute, subacute, or chronic, depending on the pain, pressure sensitivity, reflex spasm, swelling, impaired mobility, and increased temperature in the area.

Diagnostic criteria for myofascial fibrositis include exquisite pain and tenderness, circumscribed painful tissue hardening, and pressure on the trigger point, which causes pain referral.

Predisposing factors for myofascial fibrositis include chronic muscular strain, repeated excessive muscular activity, direct trauma, chilling of fatigued muscles, arthritis, nerve root injury, and psychogenic anxiety.

Procedure

A hot sponge is passed up and down the spine several times. If any lesion of the spine is present, pain is felt as the sponge passes over the lesion. The test is positive for acute inflammatory lesions of the spine.

Confirmation Procedures

Palpation, thoracic spinal range of motion, thoracic spinal muscle testing

Reporting Statement

The sponge test is positive at the midthoracic spine and reveals focal areas of tenderness. This result suggests local tissue inflammation.

∾ Clinical Pearl ∾

As with spinal percussion, the focal areas of tenderness found with the sponge test may be hypersensitive to mechanical stimulation. This sensitivity represents spasmophilia and must be absent before aggressive physical therapy can commence.

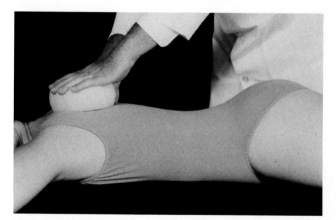

Fig. 7–38 The patient is prone. The examiner notes spinal symmetry and any muscular induration. A hot sponge is placed at the superior aspect of the thoracic spine.

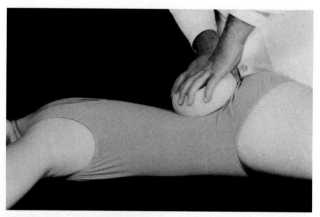

Fig. 7–39 The sponge is passed down the spinal column to the lumbosacral area. This is repeated several times. Pain is felt in locally inflamed areas, as the sponge passes over them. This pain indicates local acute inflammation.

Comment

Fractures of the ribs are common, and they usually are caused by a direct blow from a blunt object. In this instance there is likely to be a fracture of one or, at most, two ribs. Forceful compression of the chest in one of its diameters may produce single or multiple fractures. In the first instance, the patient will relate a history of a blow to the chest that may have been forceful enough to knock the wind out of the person and cause severe localized pain. As the patient tries to breathe deeply, there is severe pain. Muscle spasm splints the chest and prevents deep breathing. The result is rapid, shallow respiration due to the combination of air hunger plus pain during inspiration. In the second instance, the patient may relate a history of being crushed in a pileup or of falling forcibly onto a side with an object between the chest and the ground. Here again the patient will experience labored breathing accompanied by severe pain. Careful examination at the time of injury will elicit tenderness directly over the rib or ribs, and pain occurs in this same area during deep breathing. Although direct pressure on the involved rib is avoided, compression of the chest will cause pain. If the sixth rib is broken at the anterior axillary line, pressure made directly backward on the sternum will cause pain in the area of the fracture, and deep inspiration will be painful. Any attempt at coughing or sneezing is disastrous. A patient who tries to do so will grab the chest and attempt to restrict the motion manually. There may be a palpable defect in the rib if the fracture is complete, and it is possible to elicit crepitus. Manipulation to elicit such an effect is not justifiable. Fracture can be differentiated from a simple contusion because contusion does not usually cause pain during motion of the rib.

Procedure

While the patient is in the supine position, the examiner exerts downward pressure on the sternum. Localized pain at the lateral border of the ribs indicates a rib fracture.

Confirmation Procedures

Chest expansion test, Schepelmann's test, diagnostic imaging

Reporting Statement

The sternal compression test is positive and elicits pain at the lateral border of the sixth rib on the right. This result suggests rib fracture.

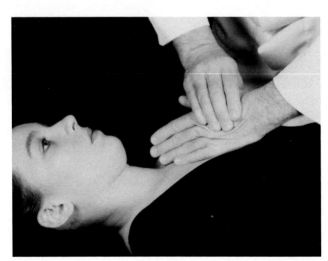

Fig. 7–40 The patient is supine with the arms at the side or crossed low over the abdomen. The examiner places the ulnar aspect of one hand in the vertical axis of the sternum. The other hand is placed on top of it. The examiner exerts a downward pressure on the sternum. Localized pain in the ribs indicates fracture.

Bibliography

Adams JC: *Outline of orthopaedics,* London, 1968, E & S Livingstone.

Adams RD, Victor M: *Principles of neurology,* ed 3, New York, 1985, McGraw Hill.

American Medical Association: *Guides to the evaluation of permanent impairment,* ed 3, Chicago, 1990, The Association.

American Orthopaedic Association: *Manual of orthopaedic surgery,* Chicago, 1972, The Association.

Aminoff MJ: *Electrodiagnosis in clinical neurology,* ed 2, New York, 1986, Churchill Livingstone.

Ansel BM: Rheumatic disorders in childhood, *Clin Rheum Dis,* 2:303, 1976.

Apley AG, Solomon L: Concise system of orthopaedics and fractures, London, 1988, Butterworth-Heinemann.

Appelrouth D, Gottlieb NL: Pulmonary manifestations of ankylosing spondylitis, *J Rheumatol,* 2:446, 1975.

Asbury AK, McKhann GM, McDonald WI: Disease of the nervous system, Philadelphia, 1986, WB Saunders.

Avioli LV: Osteoporosis, pathogenesis and therapy, In Avioli LV, Vrane SM (eds). *Metabolic bone disease,* New York, 1977, Academic Press.

Avioli LV: Senile and post-menopausal osteoporosis, *Adv Intern Med,* 21:391, 1976.

Baker AB, Joynt RJ: *Clinical neurology,* New York, 1985, Harper & Row.

Beetham WP, Polley HF, Slocumb CH, Weaver WF: *Physical examination of the joints,* Philadelphia, 1965, WB Saunders.

Benson MKD, Byrnes DP: The clinical syndromes and surgical treatment of thoracic intervertebral disc prolapse, *J Bone Joint Surg [BR],* 57:471, 1975.

Bernat JL: A dangerous backache, *Hosp Pract [Off],* 12:36, 1977.

Blount WP, Moe JH: The Milwaukee brace, Baltimore, 1973, Williams & Wilkins.

Bondilla KK: Back pain: Osteoarthritis, *J Am Geriatr Soc,* 25:62, 1977.

Bourdillon JR: *Spinal manipulation,* ed 3, New York, 1982, Appleton-Century-Crofts.

Bradford DS: Juvenile kyphosis, *Clin Orthop,* 128:45, 1977.

Bradford DS et al: Scheuermann's kyphosis and roundback deformity: Results of Milwaukee brace treatment, *J Bone Joint Surg [AM],* 56:740, 1974.

Bradford DS et al: Scheuermann's kyphosis: Results of surgical treatment by posterior spine arthrodesis in 22 patients, *J Bone Joint Surg [Am],* 57:439, 1975.

Brashear HR, Raney RB: *Shand's handbook of orthopaedic surgery,* St. Louis, 1978, Mosby.

Brown MD: Diagnosis of pain syndromes of the spine, *Orthop Clin North Am,* 6:233, 1975.

Bunnell WP: Treatment of idiopathic scoliosis, *Orthop Clin North Am,* 10:813, 1979.

Cailliet R: Scoliosis: *Diagnosis and management,* Philadelphia, 1975, FA Davis.

Carman DL et al: Measurement of scoliosis and kyphosis radiographs. Intraobserver and interobserver variation, *J Bone Joint Surg [AM],* 72:328, 1990.

Cipriano JJ: *Photographic manual of regional orthopaedic and neurological tests,* ed 2, Baltimore, 1991, Williams & Wilkins.

Crosby EC, Humphrey T, Lauer EW: *Correlative anatomy of the nervous system,* New York, 1962, MacMillan Publishing.

Cyriax J: *Textbook of orthopaedic medicine, vol 1: Diagnosis of soft tissue lesions,* London, 1982, Bailliere Tindall.

Cyriax JH, Cyriax PJ: *Illustrated manual of orthopaedic medicine,* London, 1983, CM Publications.

D'Ambrosia, RD: *Musculoskeletal disorders regional examination and differential diagnosis,* Philadelphia, 1977, JB Lippincott.

Dandy DJ: *Essential orthopaedics and trauma,* Edinburgh, 1989, Churchill Livingstone.

Dawson DM, Hallett M, Millender LH: *Entrapment neuropathies,* Boston, 1983, Little Brown & Co.

DeJong RN: *The neurologic examination,* ed 4, New York, 1978, Harper & Row.

Dickson RA: Conservative treatment for idiopathic scoliosis, *J Bone Joint Surg [Br],* 67:176, 1985.

Doherty M, Doherty J: Clinical examination in rheumatology, London, 1992, Wolfe Publishing.

Engelman EG, Engleman EP: Ankylosing spondylitis: Recent advances in diagnosis and treatment, *Med Clin North Am,* 61:347, 1977.

Evans RC: *Differential diagnosis of conditions presenting neck and arm pain,* Minneapolis, 1979, Northwestern College of Chiropractic.

Ferris B, Edgar M, Leyshon A: Screening for scoliosis, *Acta Orthop Scand,* 1988; 59:417, 1988.

Gartland JJ: *Fundamentals of orthopaedics,* London, 1968, E & S Livingstone.

Goldstein LA, Waugh TR: Classification and terminology of scoliosis, *Clin Orthop,* 93:10, 1973.

Gregersen GG, Lucas DB: An in vivo study of the axial rotation of the human thoracolumbar spine, *J Bone Joint Surg,* 49A:247, 1967.

Grieve GP: *Common vertebral joint problems,* New York, 1981, Churchill Livingstone.

Harvey MA, James B: *Differential diagnosis,* Philadelphia, 1972, WB Saunders.

Heim HA: Scoliosis, *Clin Symp,* 25:1–32, 1973.

Hollingshead WH, Jenkins DR: *Functional anatomy of the limbs and back,* Philadelphia, 1981, WB Saunders.

James JP: The etiology of scoliosis, *J Bone Joint Surg,* 52B:410, 1970.

Judge RD, Zuidema GD, Fitzgerald FT: *Clinical diagnosis: A physiologic approach,* Boston, 1982, Little, Brown & Co.

Kapandji IA: *The physiology of the joints: The trunk and vertebral column,* vol 3, New York, 1974, Churchill Livingstone.

Katz WA: *Rheumatic diseases diagnosis and management,* Philadelphia, 1977, JB Lippincott.

Keim HA: *The adolescent spine,* New York, 1982, Springer-Verlag.

Kendall HO, Kendall FP, Wadsworth GE: *Muscles testing and function,* ed 2, Baltimore, 1971, Williams & Wilkins.

Kimura J: *Electrodiagnosis in disease of nerve and muscle: Principles and practice,* Philadelphia, 1983, FA Davis.

Krupp MA, Chatton MJ: *Current diagnosis and treatment,* Los Altos, CA, 1972, Lange Medical Publications.

Levene DL: Chest pain: An integrated diagnostic approach, Philadelphia, 1977, Lea & Febiger.

MacConaill, MA Basmajian JV: *Muscles and movements: A basis for human kinesiology,* Baltimore, 1969, Williams and Wilkins.

Macnab I: *Backache,* Baltimore, 1977, Williams & Wilkins.

Magee DJ: *Orthopedic physical assessment,* Philadelphia, 1987, WB Saunders.

Maigne R: *Orthopaedic medicine: A new approach to vertebral manipulation,* Springfield, 1972, Charles C. Thomas.

Maitland GD: *Vertebral manipulation,* London, 1973, Butterworths.

Manniche C et al: Clinical trial of intensive muscle training for chronic low back pain, *Lancet,* 24:1473, 1988.

Mazion JM: *Illustrated manual of neurological reflexes/Signs/Tests, Part I, orthopedic signs/tests/maneuvers for office procedure, Part II,* Orlando, 1980, Daniels Publishing.

McKenzie RA: *The lumbar spine: Mechanical diagnosis and therapy,* Wikanae, New Zealand, 1981, Spinal Publications.

McRae R: *Clinical orthopaedic examination,* ed 3, Edinburgh, 1990, Churchill Livingstone.

Medical Economics Books: *Patient care flow chart manual,* ed 3, Oradell, NJ, 1982, Medical Economics Books.

Medical Research Council: *Aids to the investigation of peripheral nerve injuries,* ed 4, London, 1982, Her Majesty's Stationery Office.

Mercer LR: *Practical orthopedics,* ed 3, St. Louis, 1991, Mosby.

Mitchell FL, Moran PS, Pruzzo NA: *An evaluation and treatment manual of osteopathic muscle energy procedures,* Valley Park, MO, 1979, Mitchell, Moran and Pruzzo.

Moe JH, Kettleson DN: Idiopathic scoliosis, *J Bone Joint Surg [AM],* 52:1509, 1970.

Moe JH, Winter RB, Bradford DS, Lonstein JF: *Scoliosis and other spinal deformities,* Philadelphia, 1978, WB Saunders.

Moll JH, Wright V: Measurement of spinal movement, In Jayson M (ed), *Lumbar spine and back pain,* New York, 1976, Grune & Stratton.

Moll JMH, Wright V: An objective clinical study of chest expansion, *Ann Rheum Dis,* 31:1–8, 1972.

Montgomery SP, Erwin WE: Scheuermann's kyphosis: Long-term results of Milwaukee brace treatment, *Spine,* 6:5, 1981.

Morrisey RT et al: Measurement of Cobb angle on radiographs of patients who have scoliosis. Evaluation of intrinsic error, *J Bone Joint Surg [Am],* 72:320, 1990.

Nash CL: Scoliosis bracing, *J Bone Joint Surg [AM],* 62:848, 1980.

Nash CL, Moe JH: A study of vertebral rotation, *J Bone Joint Surg,* 52A:223, 1969.

O'Donoghue, DH: *Treatment of injuries to athletes,* ed 4, Philadelphia, 1984, WB Saunders.

Omer GE, Spinner M: *Management of peripheral nerve problems,* Philadelphia, 1980, WB Saunders.

Papaioannu T, Stokes I, Kenwright J: Scoliosis associated with limb length inequality, *J Bone Joint Surg,* 64A:59, 1982.

Ramsey RG: *Neuroradiology,* Philadelphia, 1987, WB Saunders.

Resnick NW, Greenspan SL: Senile osteoporosis reconsidered, *JAMA,* 261:1025, 1989.

Riggs R et al: Short- and long-term effects of estrogen and synthetic anabolic hormone in post-menopausal osteoporosis, *J Clin Invest,* 51:1659, 1972.

Riggs BL, Melton LJ III: *Osteoporosis: Etiology, diagnosis and management,* New York, 1988, Raven Press.

Rodnitzky RL: *Van Allen's pictorial manual of neurologic tests,* Chicago, 1988, Mosby.

Rothman RH, Simeone FA: *The spine,* Philadelphia, 1982, WB Saunders.

Rowland LP: *Merritt's textbook of neurology,* ed 7, Philadelphia, 1984, Lea & Febiger.

Ruge D, Wiltse LL: *Spinal disorders: Diagnosis and treatment,* Philadelphia, 1977, Lea & Febiger.

Simons GW, Sty JR, Storkshak RJ: Retroperitoneal and retrofascial abscesses, *J Bone Joint Surg [AM],* 65:1041, 1983.

Simmons EH: Kyphotic deformity of the spine in ankylosing spondylitis, *Clin Orthop,* 128.65, 1977.

Sunderland S: *Nerves and nerve injuries,* ed 2, New York, 1979, Churchill Livingston.

Thurston SE: *The little black book of neurology,* Chicago, 1987, Mosby.

Tsou PM: Embryology of congenital kyphosis, *Clin Orthop,* 128:18, 1977.

Tsou PM, Yau A, Hodgson AR: Embryogenesis and prenatal development of congenital vertebral anomalies and their classification, *Clin Orthop,* 152:211, 1980.

Turek SL: *Orthopaedics principles and their application,* ed 3, Philadelphia, 1977, JB Lippincott.

Turner PG, Green JH, Galasko CS: Back pain in childhood, *Spine,* 14:812, 1989.

Wedgewood RJ, Schaller JG: The pediatric arthritides, *Hosp Pract [Off]* 12:83, 1977.

Weinstein SL: Adolescent idiopathic scoliosis: Prevalence and natural history, *Am Acad Orthop Surg Lect,* 38:115, 1989.

White AA: Kinematics of the normal spine as related to scoliosis, *J Biomech,* 4:405, 1971.

Whiteside TE: Traumatic kyphosis of the thoracolumbar spine, *Clin Orthop,* 128:78, 1977.

Wiles P, Sweetnam R: *Essentials of orthopaedics,* London, 1965, JA Churchill.

Williams P, Warwick R: *Gray's anatomy,* ed 36 [BR], Philadelphia, 1980, WB Saunders.

Wyke B: Morphological and functional features of the innervation of the costovertebral joints, *Folia Morphol,* 23:296, 1975.

CHAPTER

~ *8* ~

The Lumbar Spine

Other than the common cold, back pain is the most prevalent human affliction. Physicians with busy practices see many patients with this symptom. Most patients have a mechanical cause (muscle strain or annular tear) for their back pain and do not have an underlying, serious, systemic medical illness.

Even if treatment involves only a localized part of the lumbar spine, in each case the lumbar spine has to be considered as a functional unit consisting of bones, ligaments, intervertebral discs, muscles, and all other soft tissues. Because of their central location spinal elements represent the focal point for the equilibrium of the body. Because of the many connections and relations, spinal changes influence some organs directly and the functional equilibrium of the spine depends upon the efficient performance of other organs.

The spine contributes to many mutual relationships within the total body. With its equilibrium (statics), the spine exerts, influences, and receives forces (dynamics), all of which are interwoven with the far-reaching chain of motion (kinetics). In addition, the spine is able to exercise considerable influence upon neighboring structures as well as upon remote organs. This is its action upon nerves and blood vessels. To a considerable degree this complicated system depends on the metabolism, the mineral metabolism of the bones, the nutrition of the bradytrophic ligamentous and disc tissues. Improper function of the endocrine glands also affects the spine. During fetal development, the spine may be exposed to many influences, such as drug-induced malformations, lack of oxygen, or radiation. Occupational and daily living stresses, as well as traumatic influences, may combine to have an unfavorable effect when coupled with the aging process, which has a marked effect on the disc apparatus and the bony substance. More resources for the diagnosis and treatment of spinal diseases are available today than previously. Degeneration of the posture during the younger years and a lack of exercise along with physical weakness and degenerative changes in later life have taken on a serious social significance.

The spine is an intricate and interesting mechanical structure. The spine's functions are mechanical, and it is well suited for serving its basic mechanical roles. The materials used to execute the design are appropriate for enhancing these functions. The spine must transfer loads from the trunk to the pelvis, must allow for physiologic motion, and must protect the spinal cord from damage. When a proper appreciation of normal anatomy and mechanics has been gained, the pathophysiology of the diseased or deformed spine becomes clear.

The lumbar spine is designed to withstand loading and to provide truncal mobility. The primary plane of motion is during flexion-extension, although there is significant axial rotation at the L5 level. This rotation in the lower lumbar spine is particularly important, considering that the annulus fails and tears with torsional forces. Coupling in the lumbar spine is the opposite of cervical and thoracic spine coupling. The spinous processes move toward the concavity of the curve in physiologic lateral flexion.

Optimum spinal mobility in relation to age is difficult to pin down. The only generalization it is possible to make is that spinal mobility is probably greatest during adolescence and early adulthood. This tendency is significant when planning treatment and in determining prognoses.

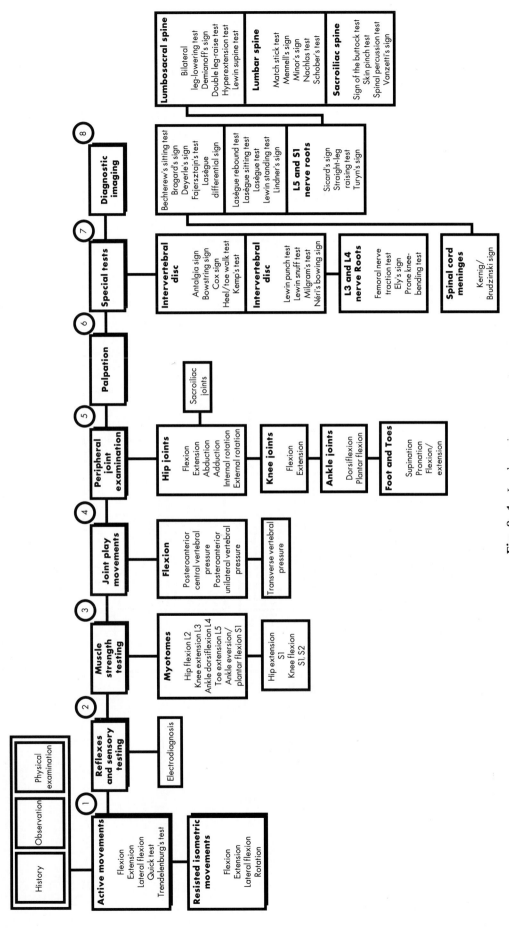

Fig. 8–1 Lumbar spine assessment.

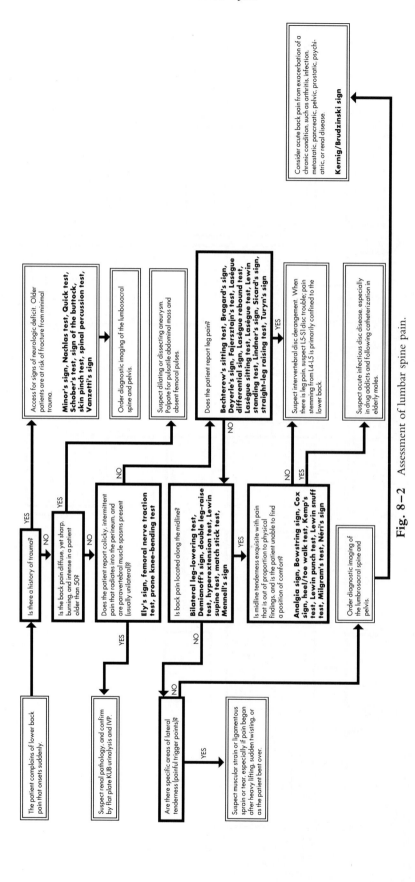

Fig. 8–2 Assessment of lumbar spine pain.

RANGE OF MOTION

The spine is more flexible during youth and moves less as a person gets older. This difference occurs because the soft tissues that connect the vertebral bodies in a young person are more elastic than they are in an older person.

As with the cervical spine, the lumbar spine ranges of motion are flexion-extension, right and left lateral flexion, and right and left rotation. Combinations of these motions allow the patient to move into numerous positions. In general, motions of the lumbar spine occur in combinations. As degenerative changes progress in the discs and facets, there is a corresponding decrease in normal motion.

Rotation in the lumbar spine ranges from 3 to 18 degrees, and it is accomplished by a shearing movement of the lumbar vertebrae on each other.

Although the examination is usually done in the standing position, if it is done while sitting, then pelvic and hip movement can be eliminated. If the patient stands, the examiner watches for the accessory movement and tries to eliminate this movement as much as possible by stabilizing the pelvis. It is not possible to quantify lumbar spinal rotation with an inclinometer. The loss of lumbar spinal rotation is not identified as an impairment of the lumbar spine in the activities of daily living.

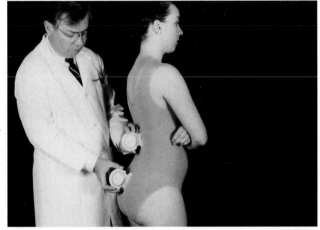

A

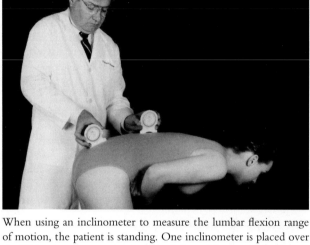

B

Fig. 8–3   For flexion, 80 degrees of movement is normal. The examiner must ensure that the movement is occurring in the lumbar spine and not in the hips or thoracic spine. An individual can touch the toes, even if no movement occurs in the spine. During flexion the lumbar curve goes from its normal lordotic curvature to a straight, or even to a slightly kyphotic, curve. If the spine does not do this, there is hypomobility in the lumbar spine. The examiner should note how far forward the patient is able to bend and compare this finding with the straight-leg raising tests.

Continued.

When using an inclinometer to measure the lumbar flexion range of motion, the patient is standing. One inclinometer is placed over the T12 spinous process in the sagittal plane. The second inclinometer is placed at the level of the sacrum, also in the sagittal plane (**A**). Both inclinometers are zeroed at these positions. The patient flexes forward and the angle of both inclinometers is recorded (**B**). The sacral inclination is subtracted from the T12 inclination to obtain the lumbar flexion angle. Flexion movement of 60 degrees or less is an impairment to the lumbar spine in the activities of daily living.

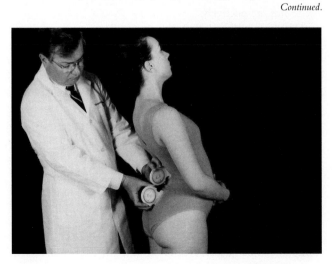

Fig. 8–4, left.   Extension is limited to 35 degrees in the lumbar spine. While performing extension, the patient can be allowed to place the hands in the small of the back to help stabilize the back. Extension, as measured with an inclinometer, is performed with the patient standing. One inclinometer is placed over the T12 spinous process, in the sagittal plane. The second inclinometer is placed at the sacrum, also in the sagittal plane. Both instruments are zeroed in this position. The patient extends the lumbar spine and the angles of both instruments are recorded. The sacral inclination angle is subtracted from the T12 inclination angle to obtain the lumbar extension angle. Lumbar extension range of motion that is 20 degrees or less is an impairment to the lumbar spine in the activities of daily living.

Continued.

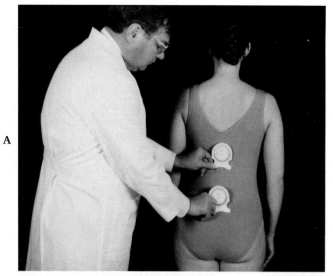

A

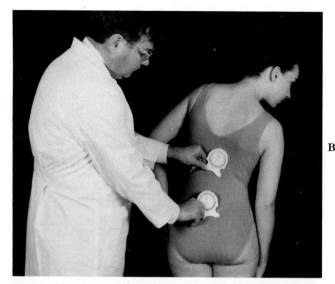

B

Fig. 8–5 Lateral flexion is approximately 25 degrees in the lumbar spine. The patient is instructed to slide a hand down the side of the leg, and not to bend forward or backward during the movement. The examiner can assess the movement and compare it to the opposite side. The lumbar curve should form a smooth curve on the side of flexion. There should be no obvious angulation at only one level. If angulation does occur, it may indicate hypomobility or hypermobility at one level of the lumbar spine.

If the movement of lateral flexion toward the painful side intensifies the symptoms, the lesion is intraarticular because the muscles and ligaments on that side are relaxed. If a disc protrusion is present, it is lateral to the nerve root, which increases the pain during ipsilateral flexion. If lateral flexion away from the painful side

Continued.

side intensifies the symptoms, the lesion may be articular or muscular in origin, or a disc protrusion medial to the nerve root may exist.

To use an inclinometer to measure the lateral lumbar flexion, the patient is standing and the lumbar spine is in neutral position. One inclinometer is placed at the T12 spinous process, in the coronal plane. The second inclinometer is placed at the superior aspect of the sacrum, in the coronal plane. Both instruments are zeroed to this position (**A**). The patient laterally flexes the lumbar spine to one side, and the inclinations of both instruments are recorded (**B**). The sacral angle is subtracted from the T12 angle to obtain the lumbar lateral flexion angle. The procedure is repeated for the range of motion to the opposite side. Lateral flexion, of 20 degrees or less, to either side is an impairment of the lumbar spine in the activities of daily living.

MUSCLE TESTING

The most superficial layer of tissue, below the subcutaneous layer, contains the thoracolumbar fascia. This tissue attaches medially to the thoracic spinous processes and inferiorly to the iliac crest and lateral crest of the sacrum. Laterally, the tissue serves as the origin of the latissimus dorsi and transversus abdominis muscle. Superiorly, the tissue attaches to the angles of the ribs in the thoracic region. Below the fascia lie the superficial multisegmental muscles, collectively named the erector spinae muscles. Their origin is a thick tendon attached to the posterior aspect of the sacrum, iliac crest, lumbar spinous processes, and supraspinous ligament. The muscle fibers split into three columns at the level of the lumbar spine. These columns are the lateral iliocostalis, the intermediate longissimus, and the more medial spinalis. The action of this group of muscles is to extend the spine. With unilateral action the muscle group flexes the spine to one side.

Deep to the erector spinae, lie the transversospinal muscles, including the multifidus and rotators. The multifidus originates at the posterior surface of the sacrum, the aponeurosis of the sacrospinalis, the posterior superior iliac spine, and the posterior sacroiliac ligament. The multifidus inserts two to four segments above its origin, into the

spinous processes. The multifidus extends the spine and rotates it toward the opposite side. The rotators have similar attachments and action, but they ascend only one or two segments. Additional deep muscles include the interspinalis, which connects pairs of adjacent lumbar spinous processes, and the intertransversarii (medial, dorsal lateral, and ventral lateral groups), which connect pairs of adjacent transverse processes. These muscles extend and bend the column to the same side, respectively.

The forward and lateral flexor muscles of the lumbar spine are located anterior and lateral to the vertebral bodies and transverse processes. The iliopsoas consists of two separate muscular heads, the iliacus and psoas major. The origins of the psoas major arise from the invertebral disc by five slips, each of which starts from adjacent upper and lower margins of two vertebrae, and membranous arches that emanate from the bodies of the four upper lumbar vertebrae. These arches permit the lumbar arteries and veins and the sympathetic rami communicantes to pass beneath them. The iliacus arises from the iliac fossa and joins the psoas under the inguinal ligament. The iliacus then crossses the hip joint capsule and inserts into the lesser trochanter of the femur. These muscles flex the lumbar spine and bend it toward the same side. The quadratus lumborum, which lies lateral to the vertebral column, arises from the posterior part of the iliac crest and iliolumbar ligament and inserts into the twelfth rib and the tips of the transverse processes of the upper four lumbar vertebrae. This muscle fixes the diaphragm during inspiration and bends the trunk toward the same side when it acts alone.

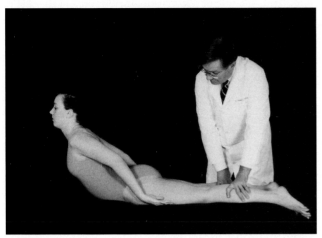

Fig. 8–6   During trunk extension, back extensors are assisted by the latissimus dorsi, quadratus lumborum, and trapezius. The patient is lying prone on the examination table. Hip extensors must give fixation of the pelvis to the thighs, and the examiner must stabilize the legs firmly on the table. The patient then extends the trunk.

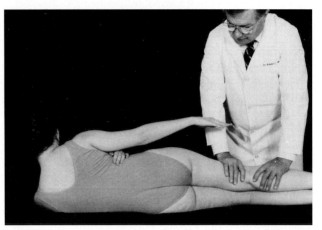

Fig. 8–7   Lateral flexion of the trunk requires a combination of lateral flexion and hip abduction. The latter is produced by downward tilting of the pelvis on the thigh. The lateral trunk muscles that enter into the movement are the lateral fibers of the external and internal obliques, the quadratus lumborum, the latissimus dorsi, and the rectus abdominis.

The patient is side-lying, with the head, upper trunk, pelvis, and lower extremities in a straight line. The top arm is extended down along the side. The patient is not allowed to hold on to the pelvis and attempt to pull up with the hand. The under arm is forward, across the chest. This rules out assistance by pushing up with the elbow.

The hip abductors must fix the pelvis to the thigh. The opposite adductors also help stabilize the pelvis. The legs must be held down by the examiner to counterbalance the weight of the trunk. The legs must not be held so firmly as to prevent the upper leg from moving slightly downward to accommodate for downward displacement of the pelvis on that side. If the pelvis is pushed upward or not allowed to tilt downward, there may be an inability to raise the trunk laterally, but this inability is not due to weakness of the lateral abdominals. During the test the patient laterally flexes the trunk away from the examination table.

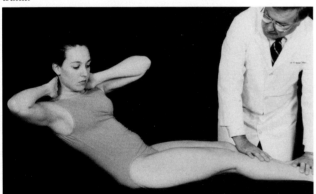

Fig. 8–8   To raise the trunk obliquely forward combines trunk flexion and rotation. It is accomplished by the combined actions of the external oblique on one side, the internal oblique on the opposite side, and the rectus abdominis.

The patient is supine on the examination table, and the legs are supported by the examiner. The patient clasps the hands behind the head. The patient flexes, rotates the trunk, and holds the position. If the muscles are weak, the trunk will derotate, or extend. Flexion of the pelvis may occur as the patient attempts to hold the hyperextended trunk up from the table. Although not anatomically part of the lower back, anterior abdominal muscles, such as the rectus abdominis, external abdominal oblique, internal abdominal oblique, transversales (flexors of the lumbar spine), gluteal muscles (extensors of the hip and trunk), hamstrings (extensors of the knee), quadriceps (extensor of the knee), and gastrocnemius and soleus (plantar flexors of the foot) are important support structures of the lumbosacral spine.

Abnormalities in these muscles (shortening or increased muscle tone) may result in abnormal kinetics of the lumbosacral spine and lower back pain.

Comment

Two terms, *contained disc* and *noncontained disc,* are used to describe disc degenerative changes that allow nuclear herniation. These terms refer to the state of the annulus fibrosus. A contained disc indicates that the annulus fibrosus is intact and is restraining the nucleus pulposus. A noncontained disc indicates that the annulus fibrosus is completely radially torn and is allowing the nuclear material to sequester or free a fragment into the vertebral canal.

Disc protrusion is an extension of nuclear material through the annulus into the spinal canal, with no loss of continuity of the extruded material. The annulus fibrosus is stretched, thinned, and pressurized. Protrusion and herniation are synonymous.

Disc prolapse exists when the extruded material loses continuity with the existing nuclear material and forms a free fragment in the spinal canal. Disc prolapse is the most common indication for disc surgery.

The usual pressure in the nucleus pulposus is 30 pounds per square inch (psi). This pressure is 30% less in the standing position than in the seated position, and is 50% less in the reclining position than in the seated position. Cerebrospinal fluid pressure is 100 to 200 mm of water in the recumbent position, and 400 mm in the seated posture.

A disc may protrude either lateral to a nerve root, medial to a nerve root, under a nerve root, or central to the nerve root.

About 90% or more of the lumbar lesions occur at either the L4-L5 or L5-S1 disc level. The L4-L5 disc usually compresses the fifth lumbar nerve root, resulting in pain sensations down the lower extremity in the L5 dermatome. The L5-S1 disc usually compresses the first sacral nerve root, resulting in pain distribution down the S1 dermatome. Of these patients, 60% will have an antalgic lean. Two facts are important, the side of sciatic pain distribution and the side of antalgic inclination. By evaluating the antalgic posture the examiner may determine whether the problem is a medial, central, or lateral disc protrusion.

Procedure

When the disc protrudes lateral to the nerve root, the patient assumes an antalgic lean away from the side of the disc lesion or pain. When the disc protrudes medial to the nerve root, the patient assumes an antalgic lean into the side of the disc lesion or pain. With a central disc lesion, the patient assumes a flexed posture of the lumbar spine, with or without leaning to either side. With protrusion under the nerve root, the patient may not lean at all.

Confirmation Procedures

Bowstring sign, Cox sign, heel/toe walk test, Kemp's test, Lewin punch test, Lewin snuff test, Milgram's test, Néri's sign

Reporting Statement

The patient demonstrates antalgic positioning toward the right, away from the left side sciatica. This suggests a left side lateral disc protrusion.

The patient demonstrates a right side antalgic posturing toward the side of pain. This posture suggests a right side medial disc protrusion.

The patient demonstrates a fixed and slightly flexed antalgic posture with no lateral flexion component. This posture suggests a central disc protrusion.

∾ Clinical Pearl ∾

If the antalgia is not readily apparent in a static posture, it will appear with forward flexion of the trunk. If a disc protrusion exists, even in the mildest degree, trunk flexion exerts enough pressure to irritate the inflamed muscle or to stretch neural structures over the bulging disc. The antalgia is manifested at this point.

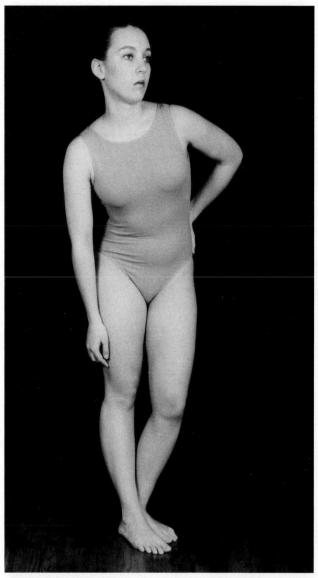

Fig. 8–9 When the disc protrudes lateral to the nerve root, the patient assumes an antalgic lean away from the side of the disc lesion or pain. In this illustration the patient is experiencing left leg sciatica.

Continued.

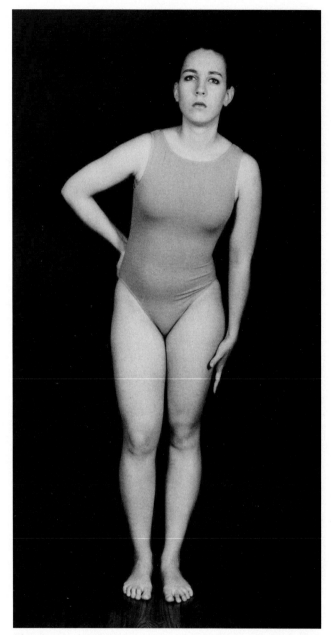

Fig. 8–10 When the disc protrudes medial to the nerve root, the patient assumes an antalgic lean into the side of the disc lesion or pain. In this illustration the patient is experiencing left leg sciatica.

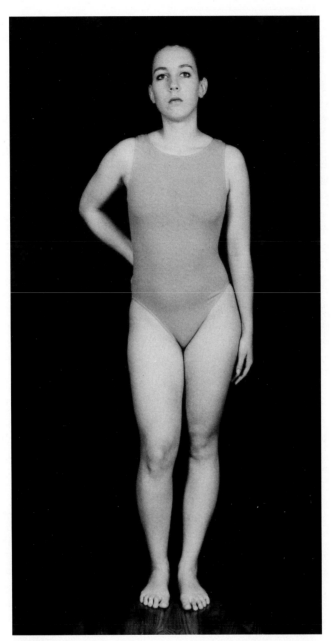

Fig. 8–11 With a central disc lesion, the patient assumes a flexed posture of the lumbar spine, with or without leaning to either side.

Comment

Lumbar disc protrusions are a common cause of lower back pain with sciatica. This protrusion usually occurs against a background of degenerative joint disease. The disc protrusion of a young adult is likely to be traumatic and should not be classified as osteoarthritis.

The precipitating trauma of an intervertebral disc syndrome is usually slight. The annulus fibrosus ruptures posteriorly, and a fragment of the nucleus is extruded into the vertebral canal. In other instances, there may be a frank prolapse of the nucleus pulposus through the tear. If there is concomitant rupture of the posterior longitudinal ligament, the protrusion may be in the midline, posteriorly. This is instead of a usual posterolateral position. The fibrocartilage or nucleus pulposus may impinge on the related nerve root and compress it against the lamina and ligamentum flavum. Because the rupture is usually to one side of the midline, only one nerve root is affected in its extrathecal course. Because the roots of the cauda equina run vertically within the theca, one or more of these passing caudal nerves also may be compressed. If the rupture is in the midline, roots on both sides may be involved. If it is large enough, the protrusion also may compress the cauda equina. The majority of disc lesions are at the L4–L5 or L5–S1 level. It is only here that a disc lesion produces the syndrome of lower backache with sciatica. Unlike the situation in the cervical spine, cord compression is not a feature of lumbar disc lesions, because the spinal cord ends opposite the lower border of L1. However, cauda equina compression can occur at these levels.

The apophyseal joints are usually involved pari passu with disc degeneration. They are also part of the pattern of joint involvement in multiple osteoarthritis and are likely to contribute to the symptomatology.

Pain is aggravated by movement of the spine, such as rolling over in bed, and by any maneuver that causes elevation of the cerebrospinal fluid pressure within the theca. Pain is more constantly aggravated by maneuvers that stretch sciatic nerve. Forward flexion of the lumbar spine or straight leg raising with the patient supine produces pain. The back is usually held rigid and movements are limited by muscle spasm, which results in antalgia to one side or the other and flattening of the lumbar lordosis. Forward flexion is more limited than lateral flexion.

Procedure

While in a seated position, the patient attempts to extend each leg, one at a time. The examiner resists the patient's attempts at hip flexion with downward pressure on the thigh. This extension is followed by an attempt to extend both legs. The test is positive if backache or sciatic pain is increased or the maneuver is impossible. In disc involvements, extending both legs will usually increase the spinal and sciatic discomfort. A positive test indicates sciatica, a disc lesion, exostoses, adhesions, spasm, or subluxation.

Confirmation Procedures

Bragard's sign, Deyerle's sign, Fajersztajn's test, Lasègue differential sign, Lasègue rebound test, Lasègue sitting test, Lasègue test, Lewin standing test, Lindner's sign, Sicard's sign, straight-leg raising test, Turyn's sign

---

Reporting Statement

Bechterew's sitting test is positive on the right and elicits pain that begins in the lumbar spine and radiates down the right leg. This result suggests a disc lesion in the lumbar spine and nerve root irritation on the right.

∼ **Clinical Pearl** ∼

Simple flattening or even reversal of the lumbar curve is frequently not associated with radicular pain. The pain is localized in the lower lumbar spine, and any movement of the spine accentuates the pain. In these instances the prime pathologic feature is sprain of an intervertebral joint rather than root irritation.

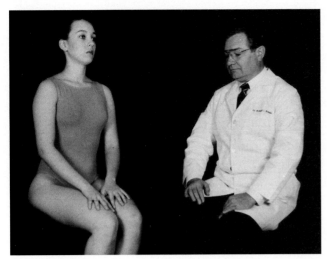

Fig. 8–12   The patient is in the seated position.

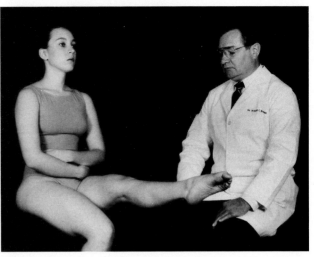

Fig. 8–13   The patient attempts to extend each leg one at a time.

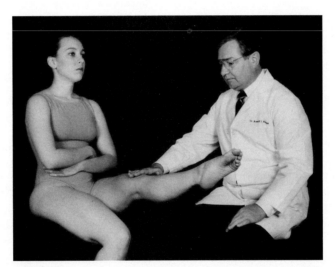

Fig. 8–14   The examiner resists the patient's attempts at hip flexion with downward pressure on the thigh. The test is positive if the maneuver increases backache or sciatic pain or if the maneuver is impossible. Unileteral leg testing is followed by the patient's attempt to extend both legs siumltaneously. With disc involvements, extending both legs will usually increase the spinal and sciatic discomfort. A positive test indicates sciatica, disc lesion, exostoses, adhesions, spasm, or subluxation.

Comment

The legs, as they are raised or lowered, exert a strong, downward pull on the pelvis. This pull is in opposition to the upward pull of the abdominal muscles. If the patient can tilt the pelvis posteriorly to flex the spine and hold the low back flat on an examining table as the legs are raised or lowered, the abdominal muscles must act to hold that position.

If the abdominal muscles are weak and the hip flexor muscles are strong, the back cannot be held flat while the legs are raised or lowered. The lower back will appear hyperextended as the legs are raised, and the abdominal muscles will be put on stretch.

The actions of various segments of the abdominal muscles are so closely allied with and interdependent on other parts that no specific functions can be ascribed to any single segment.

From a mechanical standpoint, the pelvis can be tilted toward the posterior rib cage by an upward pull on the pubis, by a downward pull on the ischium, and by an oblique pull from the anterior iliac crest. The muscle or muscle fibers that lie in these lines of pull are the rectus abdominis, the hip extensors, and the lateral fibers of the external oblique. These muscles act to tilt the pelvis posteriorly, whether the subject is standing or lying supine. During double leg raising from a supine position, the hip extensors cease to actively assist in tilting the pelvis posteriorly. The rectus abdominis and the external oblique muscles assume the major roles if an effort is made to flex the lumbar spine and keep the lower back flat on the examination table, while the thoracic spine remains extended. Without the resistance of the lower extremities, the pelvis can be tilted posteriorly by the external oblique without assistance from the rectus abdominis. Against resistance, as occurs during double leg raising, the rectus abdominis must come into strong action.

The abdominal muscles elongate and the back starts to arch if the patient's strength is not sufficient enough to maintain the pelvis in posterior tilt.

At the initiation of double leg raising or leg lowering, the thorax will show a tendency for the ribs to pull inward, decreasing the infrasternal angle. This movement is compatible with the line of pull and the action of the external oblique.

Procedure

The patient lowers the straightened legs from a 90 degree angle to a 45 degree angle. The test is positive if the legs drop or if the move produces pain. A positive test indicates lumbosacral involvement, disc lesions, or exostoses.

Confirmation Procedures

Demianoff's sign, double leg-raise test, hyperflexion test, Lewin supine test, match stick test, Mennell's sign, Minor's sign, Nachlas test, Quick test, Schober's test, sign of the buttock, skin pinch test, spinal percussion test, Vanzetti's sign

---

Reporting Statement

The bilateral leg-lowering test is positive and elicits lower back pain. This result indicates mechanical lumbosacral involvement.

∽ **Clinical Pearl** ∽

Because of the presence of the nociceptive nerve ending within the annulus fibrosus of the disc, annular tears can cause pain in the lower back, buttocks, sacroiliac region, and lower extremity. This pain can occur without nerve compression by a disc protrusion. Disc protrusion that does not compress the nerve root can cause an inflammatory response and secondary radiculitis by chemically induced inflammatory neural pain.

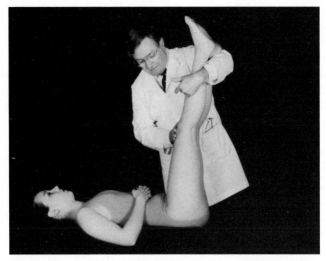

Fig. 8–15   The patient is supine with both legs fully extended. The examiner lifts both legs, simultaneously, to a near 90-degree, hip-flexion angle.

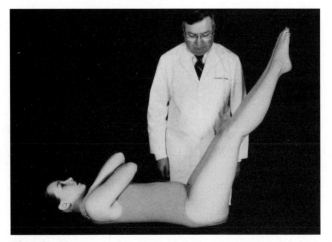

Fig. 8–16   From this elevated leg position, the patient is instructed to lower the legs, from a 90-degree angle to a 45-degree angle. The test is positive if the legs drop or if lower back pain is produced. A positive test indicates lumbosacral involvement, disc lesions, or exostoses.

Comment

Lower back pain is frequently associated with sciatica and can be elicited in the posterior part of a degenerated disc because the posterior longitudinal ligament in this region contains sensible nerve fibers. However, lower back pain is not the direct result of nerve root compression. Disc degenerations do not elicit a referred radiating pain that can be confused with the pain of lumbosacral nerve root compression. Lower back pain is present in most cases of sciatica and often appears earlier than does the radiating pain. In some cases the pain has its onset with the onset of the radiating pain. The lower back pain is not as important in the diagnosis as the levels and sites of nerve root compression.

In adult individuals the cord ends near the caudal end of the first lumbar vertebra. In its caudal extension the dural sac encloses the lumbosacral nerve roots. At each segment, a pair of nerve roots, symmetrically enclosed by dural nerve root sleeves, leaves the dural sac and departs from the spinal canal through the intervertebral foramina at that level.

In the lower lumbar region the point of departure of the nerve roots from the dural sac is more cranial than the point at which the nerve roots depart from the spinal canal through their respective intervertebral foramina. The difference in height amounts to about one segment. The fourth lumbar root (L4) leaves the dural sac a little caudal of the intervertebral disc between the third and fourth lumbar vertebrae (third lumbar disc). The fifth lumbar root (L5) leaves the dural sac near the level of the fourth lumbar disc. The first sacral root (S1) leaves the dural sac medial of S1 and a little below the level of the L5 disc.

All the lower sacral nerve roots depart from the tapering end cone of the dural sac, which is caudal to the level of the L5 disc. This end cone varies in how far it reaches into the sacral canal. The levels at which the lower sacral nerve roots depart from the dural sac are different in individual cases.

After leaving the dural sac, the lumbosacral nerve roots run caudally and laterally in the direction that they depart from the spinal canal. The fourth lumbar (L4) nerve root leaves the spinal canal through the intervertebral foramen at the cranial border of the L4 disc, the caudal border of the fifth intervertebral foramen, and S1 and S2 through the first and second sacral foramina respectively.

The neurologic symptoms caused by disc protrusions bulging from different lumbar discs depend on the nerve root that is closest to the site of the disc protrusion, and therefore is the first one compressed. At their point of departure from the dural sac, the nerve roots are firmly fixed to the dural sac and cannot, at this point, be easily pushed aside by disc protrusions. This firmness contributes to the occurrence of typical nerve root syndromes caused by disc protrusions located near the point from which the nerve roots depart.

Procedure

With the patient in the supine position, the examiner moves the patient's leg until it is above the examiner's shoulder. At this point, firm pressure should be exerted on the hamstring muscles. If pain is not elicited, pressure is applied to the popliteal fossa. Pain in the lumbar region or radiculopathy is a positive sign for nerve root compression.

Confirmation Procedures

Antalgia sign, Cox sign, heel/toe walk test, Kemp's test, Lewin punch test, Lewin snuff test, Milgram's test, Néri's sign

---

Reporting Statement

Bowstring sign is present on the right. The presence of this sign indicates lumbosacral nerve root compression.

⤳ Clinical Pearl ⤳

Nerve roots must change their lengths depending on the degree of flexion, extension, lateral flexion, and rotation of the lumbar spine. Lumbar nerve roots that are limited in motion by fibrosis of either intraspinal or extraspinal origin will create traction on the nerve root complex, causing ischemia and secondary neural dysfunction.

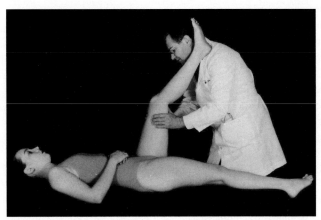

Fig. 8–17   The patient is in the supine position with both legs fully extended. The examiner places the patient's affected leg atop a shoulder. The examiner exerts firm pressure near the insertion of the hamstring muscles. If this maneuver is painlful, firm pressure is applied to the popliteal fossa. Pain in the lumbar region or radiculopathy is a positive sign for nerve root compression.

Comment

Pain in the segmental distribution of a root is the hallmark of root compression syndrome. Pain in the spine and restriction of spinal movement are common and are the result of local involvement of the sensitive tissues and the root. Herniated disc, metastatic malignancy, a primary neoplasm, recent trauma, or inflammation may be responsible.

Pain that radiates down the leg follows the primary anterior division of the nerve and may be localized by the patient anywhere in the distribution of the root. This root pain is aggravated by spinal movement, by local pressure over the nerve, or by straining the nerve. Pressure over the muscle in the area of pain usually produces discomfort.

Paresthesia in root distribution is common and is usually experienced distally, in the foot. This paresthesia may be aggravated or relieved by the same factors that influence the pain, but the paresthesia is constant.

Weakness and atrophy in the corresponding myotomic distribution result from prolonged or severe root compression and stretch reflexes, with arcs that are largely or entirely incorporated in the involved root, will be diminished or lost.

Suspicion of a single nerve root compression syndrome should be prompted by the combination of a history of pain and the presence of paresthesia in the appropriate distribution of one nerve only. Findings necessary to confirm the diagnosis are those that relate spinal movement to the radiating pain, those that demonstrate muscular weakness and tenderness in the myotome, and those that localize sensory and reflex deficits to the dermatome and myotome.

A herniated intervertebral disc produces a persistent, unilateral, isolated syndrome. Bilateral and multiple nerve root involvement can be due to extensive degenerative joint disease. When nerve root involvement is progressive and acute or subacute, then metastatic malignancy or inflammation is suggested.

Nerve root compression may herald an intraspinal mass that later will impinge on the spinal cord or cauda equina. The examiner must always look closely for motor, sensory, and reflex changes below the affected root because these changes may indicate involvement of the cord or cauda equina.

A herniated intervertebral disc is the most common cause of frank root compression syndromes affecting the extremities.

Procedure

If the Lasègue or straight leg raising tests are positive, the leg is lowered below the point of discomfort, and the foot is sharply dorsiflexed. The sign is present if pain is increased. The presence of the sign is a finding associated with sciatic neuritis, spinal cord tumors, intervertebral disc (IVD) lesions, and spinal nerve irritations.

Confirmation Procedures

Bechterew's sitting test, Deyerle's sign, Fajersztajn's test, Lasègue differential sign, Lasègue rebound test, Lasègue sitting test, Lasègue test, Lewin standing test, Lindner's sign, Sicard's sign, straight-leg raising test, Turyn's sign

> **Reporting Statement**
>
> Bragard's sign is present and indicates sciatic neuritis on the right.

∽ Clinical Pearl ∽

Either the Bragard's sign or Hyndman's sign (for neck flexion movement) must be accomplished as a finishing maneuver in any positive straight leg raising test. Pain that increases during neck flexion, ankle dorsiflexion, or both indicates an inflamed nerve root. Pain that does not increase with these maneuvers may indicate a problem in the hamstring area or in the lumbosacral or sacroiliac joints.

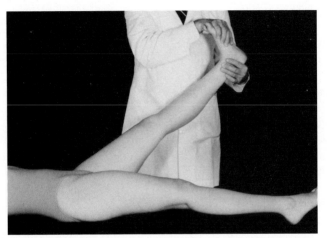

Fig. 8–18 If a straight-leg raising test is positive, the affected leg is lowered just below the angle of pain production and is held by the examiner. The examiner sharply dorsiflexes the foot. The sign is present if the pain is duplicated or increased. The presence of the sign indicates sciatic neuritis, spinal cord tumors, intervertebral disc (IVD) lesions, and spinal nerve irritations.

Comment

There are several maneuvers that tighten the sciatic nerve and compress an inflamed nerve root against a herniated lumbar disc. With the straight-leg raising tests the L5 and S1 nerve roots move several millimeters at the level of the foramen. The L4 nerve root moves a smaller distance, and the proximal roots show little motion. The straight-leg raising tests are most important and valuable for detecting lesions of the L5 and S1 nerve roots. Young patients with herniated discs have marked propensities for positive straight-leg raising tests. Although the test itself is not pathognomonic, a negative test rules out the possibility of a herniated disc. After age 30, a negative straight-leg raising test no longer precludes this diagnosis.

The straight-leg raising tests are performed while the patient is supine. The examiner raises the affected leg slowly. Only when leg pain or radicular symptoms are reproduced is the straight-leg raising test considered positive. Back pain alone is not a positive finding for straight-leg raising.

Many variations of the straight-leg raising test have been developed. Contralateral straight-leg raising is performed in a way similar to the straight-leg raising test except that with the former test the examiner raises the *unaffected* leg. If this movement reproduces the patient's sciatica in the affected extremity, the test is positive. This result suggests a herniated disc and is an indication that the prolapse, although it may be large, is medial to the nerve root, in the axilla.

When the roots of the femoral nerve are involved, they are tensed, not by the straight-leg raising test but by the reverse of straight-leg raising, such as hip extension and knee flexion.

Procedure

Cox sign occurs during straight-leg raising when the pelvis rises from the table instead of the hip flexing. Cox sign is present when patients have a prolapse of the nucleus into the intervertebral foramen.

Confirmation Procedures

Antalgia sign, bowstring sign, heel/toe walk test, Kemp's test, Lewin punch test, Lewin snuff test, Milgram's test, Néri's sign

> ### Reporting Statement
>
> Cox sign is present during straight-leg raising on the right. This sign indicates a prolapse of nuclear material into the neural foramen.

∿ Clinical Pearl ∿

Cox sign is a consistent finding associated with disc prolapse. The sign is often overlooked in the patient's pain presentation. A false negative may occur if the examiner does not observe the movements of the buttocks on the affected side. The sign is present the moment hip flexion motion is locked and the buttock rises from the examination table.

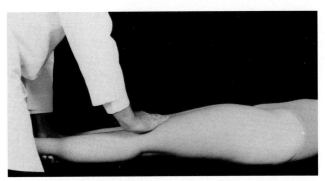

Fig. 8–19 The patient is supine with the legs fully extended. The examiner places one hand under the ankle of the affected leg and the other hand on the knee.

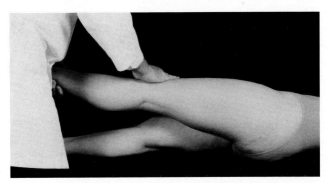

Fig. 8–20 The examiner performs a straight-leg raising test on the affected leg. Cox sign is present if during the straight-leg raising the pelvis rises from the table rather than the hip flexing. The sign is present in patients with prolapse of the nucleus into the intervertebral foramen.

Comment

Back strain can be defined as nonradiating lower back pain associated with mechanical stress to the lumbosacral spine. The exact number of patients with back strain is difficult to determine. Most patients with back pain (90 percent) have it for a mechanical reason. Of patients with mechanical lower back pain, back strain may account for 60% to 70%.

The cause of back strain is not always clear, but it may be related to muscular strain that is secondary to either a specific traumatic episode or continuous mechanical stress. The lumbosacral spine has two major biomechanical functions. The first function is to support the upper body in a balanced, upright position while allowing the second function—locomotion. In a static, upright position, maintenance of erect posture is achieved through a balance among the expansile pressure of the intervertebral discs, the stretch placed on the anterior and posterior longitudinal and facet joint ligaments, and the sustained involuntary tone of the surrounding lumbosacral and abdominal muscles. The balance of the spine is also related to the reciprocal physiologic curves in the cervical, thoracic, and lumbosacral areas of the vertebral column. The balance in curvature results in an individual's posture. Proper alignment is also influenced by structures in the pelvis and lower extremities, including the hip joint capsule and the hamstring and gluteus maximus muscles.

Movement of the lumbar spine is associated with a lumbar pelvic rhythm that results in the simultaneous reversal of the lumbar lordosis and rotation of the hips. During flexion and extension of the lumbar spine, tension is produced in the paraspinous, hamstring, and gluteal muscles; the fascia that surrounds the muscles; and the ligaments that support the vertebral bodies and discs. In addition to the normal stresses placed on these structures during lowering and raising of the torso, the stresses on these anatomic structures are increased to an even greater degree when an individual must lift a heavy object. During lateral flexion paraspinous muscle activity increases on both sides of the spine, but it primarily increases on the side toward the lateral flexion. During axial rotation of the spine the erector spinae muscles on the ipsilateral side and the rotator and multifidus muscles on the contralateral side are active. Lateral flexion is accomplished by contraction of the abdominal wall oblique muscles with the ipsilateral quadratus lumborum and psoas major muscles.

Lower back pain that is associated with back strain may be related to anatomic structures that are tonically contracted while in the resting position. Lower back pain also may occur during motion, if the stress is greater than the supporting structures can sustain or if the components of the lumbosacral spine are structurally abnormal.

Procedure

While the patient is in a supine position, the examiner performs a straight-leg raising test. The sign is present when this action produces a pain in the lumbar region. This pain prevents the patient from raising the leg high enough to form an angle, between the examination table and the leg, of 15 degrees or more. The sign differentiates pain that originates in the sacrolumbalis muscles from lumbar pain of any other origin. When the test is positive, it demonstrates that the pain is due to the stretching of the sacrolumbalis (iliocostalis lumborum).

Confirmation Procedures

Bilateral leg-lowering test, double leg-raise test, hyperextension test, Lewin supine test, match stick test, Mennell's sign, Minor's sign, Nachlas test, Quick test, Schober's test, sign of the buttock, skin pinch test, spinal percussion test, Vanzetti's sign

---

Reporting Statement

Demianoff's sign is present. This sign indicates strain of the sacrolumbalis musculature.

~ Clinical Pearl ~

Demianoff's sign is clearly separate from Cox sign. Demianoff's sign involves production of lower back pain, which prevents further raising of the leg. Sciatica is absent. Cox sign is present when the pelvis is locked, which prevents further elevation of the leg because of increasing sciatica.

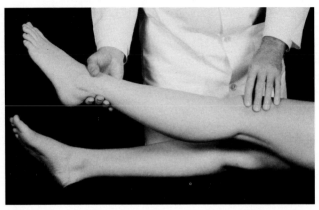

Fig. 8–21   The patient is in a supine position. The examiner performs a straight-leg raising test on the affected leg. The sign is present when this action produces a pain in the lumbar region. The pain prevents the examiner from raising the leg high enough to form an angle of 15 degrees or more with the examination table. When the sign is present, it demonstrates that pain is due to the stretching of the sacrolumbalis (iliocostalis lumborum) musculature.

Comment

The pain pattern that is associated with nerve root irritation due to a movable lamina arch or neural arch (spondylolisthesis) resembles the pain caused by compression of the nerve root by an intervertebral disc or by compression of the nerve root by other mechanical means. Pain usually occurs when the spine is extended or when the spinous process is compressed or manipulated, causing secondary irritation of the dura. Pain may radiate along the course of the femoral or sciatic nerve, depending on the site of the bone abnormality.

Degenerative arthritis in the hip, alteration of the hip joint capsule or of the surrounding osseous structures, may cause pain anteriorly, laterally, and posteriorly in the groin. Pain radiation may be associated with this through the lateral femoral cutaneous nerve, through the obturator nerve along the medial aspect of the thigh, or through branches of the sciatic nerve along the posterior thigh.

Destructive lesions of the sacrum, pelvis, pubis, or ischium cause pain along the femoral, obturator, or sciatic nerves. The onset of this pain may be vague and gradual, and the distribution of the pain may be deep with few cutaneous changes. The radiculopathy may resemble a primary nerve root irritation.

Procedure

While the patient is seated, the affected leg is passively extended at the knee until pain is reproduced. The knee is then slightly flexed while strong pressure is applied by the examiner into the popliteal fossa. The sign is present if this pressure increases radiculitis symptoms. The sign demonstrates irritation of the sciatic nerve above the knee. This irritation is caused by stretching the nerve over an abnormal mechanical obstruction.

Confirmation Procedures

Bechterew's sitting test, Bragard's sign, Fajersztajn's test, Lasègue differential sign, Lasègue rebound test, Lasègue sitting test, Lasègue test, Lewin standing test, Lindner's sign, Sicard's sign, straight-leg raising test, Turyn's sign

---

Reporting Statement

Deyerle's sign is present on the right. This sign indicates irritation of the sciatic nerve above the knee.

∽ Clinical Pearl ∽

Deyerle's sign is a variation of the Lasègue sitting test. The sign demonstrates the effects of inflammation or partial denervation (neural compression) in the sciatic distribution. The pain response may be due to myalgic hyperalgesia as a response to denervation hypersensitivity.

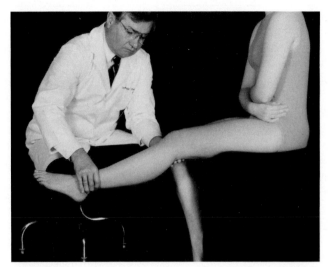

Fig. 8–22 The patient is seated. The examiner extends the patient's affected leg to the point at which pain is reproduced.

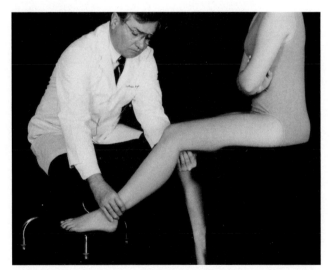

Fig. 8–23 The knee is slightly flexed while strong pressure into the popliteal fossa is applied by the examiner. The sign is present if radicular symptoms are increased.

Double Leg-Raise Test
BILATERAL STRAIGHT-LEG RAISING TEST

Comment

Sprain is frequent in the mobile lumbar spine, which has many ligaments giving support to the various joints. The supraspinous ligament, which extends along the tips of the spinous processes, is particularly susceptible. A sprain involving this ligament can be diagnosed by tenderness over the ligament or over the tip of the spinous process, where the ligament attaches. Active contraction of the muscles to pull the spine into hyperextension is pain free, as is passive extension. Active flexion of the back, which occurs during an attempt to sit up from the supine position, is pain free until tension is put on the spinous process by forcing the head toward the knees. Passive hyperflexion of the spine will cause pain.

Injury to other ligaments of the back is much more difficult to diagnose. The interspinous ligament is damaged infrequently, because it has elastic fibers and is not readily overstretched. However, the articular ligaments around the apophyseal joints are frequently damaged, as are the anterior spinal and the lateral spinal ligaments. Whether or not the ligamentum flavum is damaged by hyperflexion is problematic because it is also an elastic structure and probably will allow as much motion without damage as the range of flexion of the back will permit. Diagnosis of these sprains depends on whether tests that bring stress upon certain areas are used. With a sprain, passive movements that put stress on the involved ligament will cause pain. For example, sprain of the capsule on the left will cause pain during lateral flexion to the right or during flexion of the trunk.

Procedure

While the patient is supine, the examiner performs a straight-leg raising test on each of the lower extremities, noting the angle at which the pain is produced. Next, both lower limbs are raised together. If pain is produced at an earlier angle by raising both legs together, then the test is positive. In the presence of disc disease with resulting vertebral instability, the double leg raising movement will cause pain in the lumbar area. The test is specific and highly accurate for lumbosacral joint involvement.

Confirmation Procedures

Bilateral leg-lowering test, Demianoff's sign, hyperextension test, Lewin supine test, match stick test, Mennell's sign, Minor's sign, Nachlas test, Quick test, Schober's test, sign of the buttock, skin pinch test, spinal percussion test, Vanzetti's sign

Reporting Statement

The double leg-raise test is positive and elicits pain in the lumbosacral spine. This result indicates lumbosacral joint involvement and implies a ligamentous sprain.

Clinical Pearl

Atypical cases of disc prolapse are common. A definite history of injury or strain is often lacking. The pain may begin gradually rather than suddenly, and the symptoms may be confined to the back and never radiate down the leg. On the other hand, the pain is sometimes felt predominantly in the limb and is scarcely perceptible in the back.

The Lumbar Spine

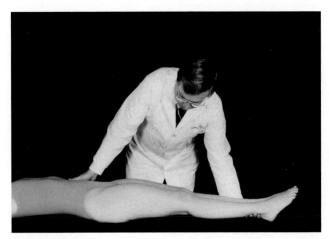

Fig. 8–24   The patient is supine with both legs fully extended. The examiner performs a straight-leg raising test on each of the lower extremities and notes the angle at which the pain is produced. The examiner then raises both lower limbs together.

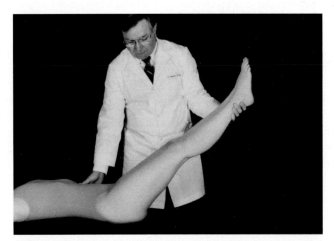

Fig. 8–25   If raising both legs together produces pain at an earlier angle than raising each leg singly, then the sign is positive. The test is specific and highly accurate for lumbosacral joint involvement.

Ely's Sign
ELY'S HEEL-TO-BUTTOCK TEST

Comment

In sequestration of nuclear tissue adjacent to or under a nerve, adhesions may form within and without the nerve root sheath, binding the root firmly to the floor of the spinal canal. During movements of the trunk and legs the nerve roots are no longer freely movable or capable of moving in and out of the intervertebral foramina without tension. When fixed to the floor or the spinal canal or within the foramina, the nerve roots are subjected to abnormal tension during movement of the trunk and legs, particularly those movements that require the extended leg to flex at the hip. Tension on the nerve roots causes radicular pain.

The condition is characterized by the localization of the pain in the dermatome supplied by the affected nerve root. The pain, although often widely distributed throughout the dermatome, occasionally is limited to a small area within it. Although dermatomal in distribution, nerve root pain in the leg seldom extends beyond the ankle. However, any associated dermatomal paresthesia or dysesthesia is usually most prominent distally and may be described in the foot. Pain is present in the spinal column and is temporarily associated with pain in the leg, with paresthesia, or both.

Root pain is frequently produced or aggravated by coughing, sneezing, and straining (such as during defecation) or by any other measures that suddenly increase intrathoracic and intraabdominal pressure. Such increases in pressure block venous flow from the epidural space through the intervertebral veins. Because the intervertebral veins do not contain valves, such increases in pressure may also permit a return of blood with consequent distention of the veins in the epidural space. This condition in turn forces the dura, which envelops the nerve roots, toward the spinal cord. Because the nerve roots are affixed to the spinal cord proximally and peripherally at the intervertebral foramen, the displacement of the dura results in stretching of the involved nerve root. This stretching results in pain if the root is diseased. In addition, distention of the intervertebral vein may result in direct compression of the nerve root.

Root pain may awaken the patient at night after several hours of sleep and may be relieved 15 to 30 minutes after the patient assumes an upright position. The patient may learn to prevent the pain by sleeping in a chair. However, in contrast to peripheral neuritis, the position is the important determining factor. If the patient lies down in a similar position during the day, the pain occurs as it does at night. This feature of root pain has its basis in the lengthening of the spinal column that takes place when the horizontal position is assumed, and the shortening that takes place when the patient is in the upright position. Because the length of the spinal cord remains the same regardless of the position assumed by the patient, the lengthening of the spinal column results in a tensing of, or traction on, the nerve roots that emerge from the lumbar and sacral segments of the cord. From these segments, the roots course downward and outward to emerge from their respective intervertebral foramina.

Procedure

The patient is prone, with the toes hanging over the edge of the table, legs relaxed. One or the other heel is approximated to the opposite buttock. After flexion of the knee, the thigh is hyperextended. With any significant hip lesion it will be impossible to do this test normally. With irritation of the iliopsoas muscle or its sheath it will be impossible to extend the thigh to any normal degree. This test will aggravate inflammation of the lumbar nerve roots and will be accompanied by production of femoral radicular pain. The test will also stretch lumbar nerve root adhesions, which will be accompanied by upper lumbar discomfort.

Confirmation Procedures

Femoral nerve traction test, prone knee-bending test

> ### Reporting Statement
> Ely's sign is present on the right. This sign indicates femoral nerve, or radicular, inflammation.

Clinical Pearl

In the uncommon cases of high lumbar and midlumbar disc prolapse, the pain radiates toward the groin and front of the thigh rather than to the back of the thigh and leg.

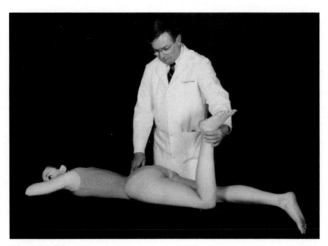

Fig. 8–26 The patient is prone. The legs are fully extended, with the toes hanging over the edge of the table. The examiner flexes the knee of the affected leg to 90 degrees.

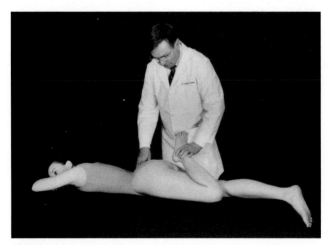

Fig. 8–27 The heel of the affected leg is approximated to the opposite buttock. After flexion of the knee, the thigh can be hyperextended. With irritation of the iliopsoas muscle or its sheath, it will be impossible to extend the thigh to any degree. Pain in the anterior thigh is a positive finding and indicates inflammation of the lumbar nerve roots.

～ Fajersztajn's Test ～
WELL-LEG-RAISING TEST OF FAJERSZTAJN
PROSTRATE LEG-RAISING TEST
SCIATIC PHENOMENON
CROSS-OVER SIGN

Comment

Limitation of motion is usually noted during the symptomatic phase of disc disease. The range of motion should be noted, not only in flexion and extension but also in rotation. The examiner must not equate flexion of the hips with flexion of the lumbar spine, and attention should be directed to whether reversal of the normal lumbar lordosis occurs. Even in patients who have only sciatica, marked restriction of motion may be present in the lumbar spine.

When acute sciatica is present, the patient usually lists away from the side of the sciatica, producing the sciatic scoliosis. When the disc herniation is lateral to the nerve root, the patient will incline away from the side of the irritated nerve root, in an attempt to draw the nerve root away from the disc fragment. On the contrary, when the herniation is in an axillary position, medial to the nerve root, the patient will list toward the side of the lesion to decompress the nerve root.

When doing a unilateral straight-leg raising test, 80 to 90 degrees of hip flexion is normal. If one leg is lifted and the patient complains of pain on the opposite side, it is an indication of a space-occupying lesion (herniated disc). This finding indicates a rather large intervertebral disc protrusion usually medial to the nerve root. The test causes stretching of the ipsilateral as well as the contralateral nerve root, pulling laterally on the dural sac.

Procedure

Straight-leg raising and dorsiflexion of the foot are performed on the asymptomatic side of a sciatic patient. When this test causes pain on the symptomatic side, Fajersztajn's sign is present. The sign indicates sciatic nerve root involvement, such as a disc syndrome or dural root sleeve adhesions.

Confirmation Procedures

Bechterew's sitting test, Bragard's sign, Deyerle's sign, Lasègue differential sign, Lasègue rebound test, Lasègue sitting test, Lasègue test, Lewin standing test, Lindner's sign, Sicard's sign, straight-leg raising test, Turyn's sign

---

Reporting Statement

Fajersztajn's test is positive on the left at 30 degrees of elevation. This result indicates nerve root compression by a space-occupying mass in or near the axilla of the nerve root.

～ Clinical Pearl ～

There are several causes of pain in the back or lower extremities. Some of these causes are (1) tumors of the spinal cord or cauda equina, (2) tumors of the spinal column, (3) tuberculosis of the spine, (4) osteoarthritis, (5) tumors of the ilium or sacrum, (6) spondylolisthesis, (7) prolapsed intervertebral disc, (8) ankylosing spondylitis, (9) vascular occlusion, (10) intrapelvic mass, and (11) arthritis of the hip. All of these possible causes must be considered in differential diagnosis.

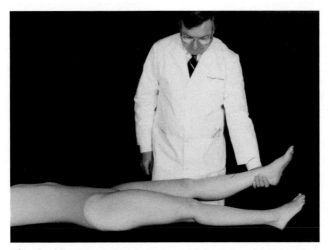

Fig. 8–28 The patient is supine with both legs fully extended. The examiner performs a straight-leg raising test on the unaffected leg.

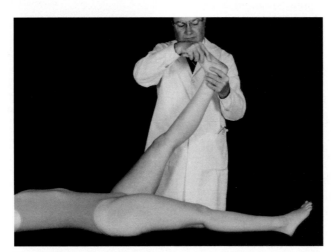

Fig. 8–29 The leg is lowered to a point just below that which produces sciatic symptoms in the affected leg. The examiner sharply dorsiflexes the foot (Bragard's sign). If this maneuver causes pain on the symptomatic side, the test is positive. A positive test indicates sciatic nerve root involvement, such as medial disc protrusion syndrome or dural root sleeve adhesions.

Femoral Nerve Traction Test

Comment

When a herniated annulus fibrosus compresses a nerve root, the irritation produces pain as well as motor and sensory loss of the lower extremities. As the nerve root becomes irritated, it becomes inflamed and even more sensitive to pressures. The patient will notice a lancinating pain that begins in the thigh and progresses distally in a pattern typical of a dermatome. The onset of pain may be gradual or extremely sudden and may be associated with a popping or tearing in the spine. This may represent the extrusion of disc material against the nerve root. When this occurs, the back pain frequently resolves and the patient is left with the radicular symptoms.

Usually the disc rupture is lateral to the nerve root, and the patient lists or leans away from the side of the sciatica to release the pressure. Occasionally the disc presents medially or in the axilla of the nerve root, and the patient will list toward the side of the sciatica. The pain is increased by any maneuver that suddenly increases intraspinal pressures, such as a Valsalva maneuver or the triad of Dejerine (coughing, sneezing or bearing down with defecation). The pain may be so severe as to paralyze the patient in a fixed position.

It is rare that the major presenting symptom is motor weakness, particularly if the fourth or fifth lumbar nerve is affected. Weakness of the quadriceps with later buckling of the knee (fourth lumbar) or a complete foot drop (fifth lumbar), without pain, may present a confusing picture.

A large, midline disc herniation can compress several nerve roots of the cauda equina and can mimic an intraspinal tumor. Usually lower back and perineal symptoms predominate with radicular symptoms being masked. Difficulty with urination, such as frequency or overflow incontinence, may develop early. In male patients, a recent history of sexual impotence may be elicited. The patients will experience pain down the posterior thighs to the soles of the feet accompanied by weakness of the legs and feet.

Procedure

The patient lies on the unaffected side, with the unaffected limb slightly flexed at the hip and knee. The patient's back should be straight and not hyperextended. The patient's head should be slightly flexed. The examiner grasps the patient's affected or painful limb and extends the knee, while gently extending the hip approximately 15 degrees. The patient's knee on the affected side is then flexed. This further stretches the femoral nerve. Pain will radiate down the anterior thigh if the test is positive.

This is a traction test for the nerve roots at the midlumbar area (L2, L3, and L4). As with the straight-leg raising test, there may be a contralateral positive test as well. Pain in the groin and hip that radiates along the anterior medial thigh, indicates an L3 nerve root problem. Pain extending to the midtibia indicates an L4 nerve root problem.

Confirmation Procedures

Ely's sign, prone knee-bending test

Reporting Statement

Femoral nerve traction testing on the right is positive and accompanied by radiating pain to the groin. This positive result indicates an L3 nerve root radiculopathy.

Femoral nerve traction testing on the right is positive, with pain extending to the midtibia. This positive result indicates an L4 nerve root radiculopathy.

∾ Clinical Pearl ∾

With upper lumbar disc disturbances, there may be weakness of the quadriceps muscle and a diminished or absent patellar reflex. The straight-leg raising tests and signs may be negative. Pinwheel examination usually reveals hyperesthesia or hypoesthesia of the L4 dermatome.

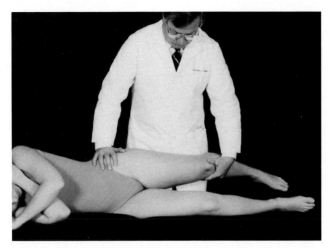

Fig. 8–30   The patient is lying on the unaffected side. The unaffected limb is slightly flexed at the hip and knee. The patient's back should be straight and not hyperextended. The patient's head should also be slightly flexed. The examiner grasps the patient's affected, or painful, leg and extends the knee while gently extending the hip approximately 15 degrees.

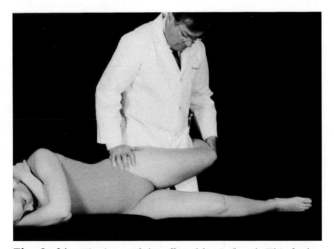

Fig. 8–31   The knee of the affected leg is flexed. This further stretches the femoral nerve. The test is positive if pain radiates down the anterior thigh. A positive test indicates a radiculopathy that involves L2, L3, and L4.

Comment

When lower extremity weakness is apparent, atrophy may signify a lower motor neuron lesion or muscular disorder. However, disuse of a muscle from any cause—whether pain, immobilization, or paralysis of central origin—will result in some loss of muscle mass. The quadriceps are prone to disuse atrophy.

The patient who can hop well does not have a serious weakness of the gastrocnemius, which is a strong muscle and is difficult to evaluate through direct testing. The examiner observes the patient walk on the toes, during which the patient's body weight is completely supported on one foot and then the other. If weakness exists the heel will drop while the patient is walking. The contours of the musculature may demonstrate atrophy or hypertrophy. A patient who has suffered a stroke and who has a moderate degree of spasticity and increased tone in antigravity muscles may still be able to rise on the toes. When weakness is evident while attempting this maneuver, the disorder is usually a primary lesion of the nerve root, peripheral nerve, or muscle.

Having the patient walk on the heels is an especially valuable screening test, because dorsiflexion of the ankles and toes is weakened in many muscular and neural disorders. If necessary the examiner may help the patient maintain balance in this maneuver. A normal patient can hold the foot and toes anteriorly off the floor, while strongly dorsiflexing the great toe, during walking on the heels. If the patient can do this, foot drop does not exist. However, the patient could still have minor weakness of the muscles of the anterior compartment, and these should be tested directly. Foot drop may be of either central or peripheral origin. Severe foot drop of peripheral origin is clearly revealed by the abnormal nature of the gait and by an observable loss of dorsiflexion of the ankle and toes. If foot drop of a peripheral origin (lower motor neuron) has been present for several weeks, shrinkage and softness of the anterior compartment also will be apparent. When the leg is shaken, such as during the test for alternating motion rate, the foot will be unstable and flop about. The foot is less floppy with central disorders (upper motor neuron lesions) and may be fixed in plantar flexion. When dorsiflexion of the ankles and toes is weak, the toes of the spastic leg are dragged during walking. Before the examiner concludes there is weakness of dorsiflexion, the foot should be passively dorsiflexed to be certain that previous weakness, now healed, did not permanently shorten the gastrocnemius.

Procedure

The examiner observes the patient walking on the toes, which requires each foot, one at a time, to completely support the patient's body weight. If weakness exists, the heel will drop while the patient is walking. The contours of the musculature may demonstrate atrophy or hypertrophy.

Having the patient walk on the heels is an especially valuable screening test because many muscular and neural disorders result in weakened dorsiflexion of the ankles and toes. The patient may need help maintaining balance during this maneuver. The normal patient can hold the foot and toes anteriorly off the floor, while strongly dorsiflexing the great toe during walking on the heels. If the patient can do this, foot drop does not exist.

Confirmation Procedures

Antalgia sign, bowstring sign, Cox sign, Kemp's test, Lewin punch test, Lewin snuff test, Milgram's test, Néri's sign

---

Reporting Statement

The toe walk test is positive on the right and demonstrates weakness in the S1 dermatome.

The heel walk test is positive on the right and demonstrates weakness in the L5 dermatome.

∿ Clinical Pearl ∿

The inability to walk on the toes indicates an L5-S1 disc problem based upon weakness of the calf muscles supplied by the tibial nerve. The inability to walk on the heels indicates an L4-L5 disc problem based upon weakness of the anterior leg muscles supplied by the common peroneal nerve.

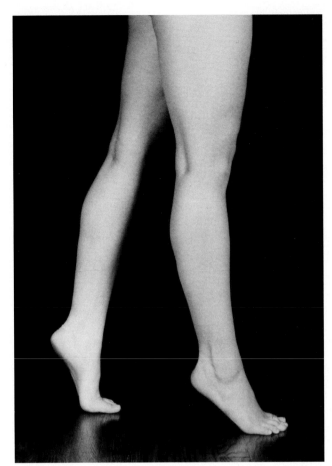

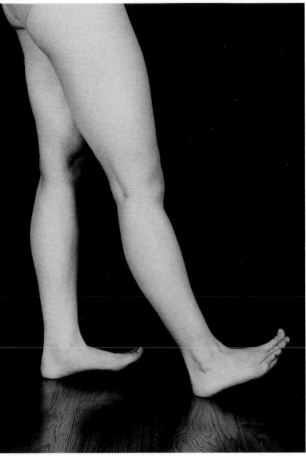

Fig. 8—32 The patient is standing and is instructed to walk on the toes. Weakness is evident if the heel drops while walking.

Fig. 8—33 The patient then walks on the heels. If necessary the examiner may help the patient maintain balance during this maneuver. If the patient cannot walk on the heels, foot drop exists.

Comment

During the third through the fifth decades of life, changes that occur in the lumbar spine can be quite pronounced, with the first manifestations of aging being reflected in the intervertebral disc. Biochemical changes can be produced by one of three different phenomena: (1) degeneration of the annulus with disc nuclear herniation through posterolateral annular rents, (2) nuclear degeneration with intact annulus, or (3) simultaneous degeneration of both the annulus and the nucleus. The biomechanical insufficiency of the involved disc compels the posterior elements, or the facets and capsules, to assume a more compressive, tensile, and shear load, resulting in capsular strain, hypermobility, and articular cartilage degeneration. The hypermobility can produce traction spurs. The ligamentum flavum also will be compelled to assume more tensile loads while becoming redundant as the total spine length decreases with disc degeneration. The vertebrae themselves tend toward a lowering and broadening in the superior, inferior, and midbody transverse breadth, a total change that, in static terms, begins to acutely or insidiously affect the neural elements.

If a disc lesion occurs in a spinal canal that is small, compression of the neural elements will result, and the patient will experience symptoms. In pure terms this can be thought of as a relative spinal stenosis. The stenosis occurs secondarily to the herniated nucleus pulposus occupying space in a small spinal canal. On the other hand, a similarly sized disc herniation in a large spinal canal will cause no symptoms because the neural elements have enough room to escape the pressure. Thus symptoms in persons of this age group are not only a result of a disc herniation itself but also the size of the spinal canal with which the individual is born.

Patients in the fifth decade of life and older can manifest the hypermobile end-stage changes of the aging process. Degeneration of both facet joints and the intervertebral disc leads to a narrowing of the spinal canal. The canal is rimmed by large osteophytes, which develop to diminish the load on the now incompetent intervertebral disc. The facets are hypertrophic and deformed by the osteophytic spurs that are encased within the thickened joint capsule. The ligamentum flavum becomes redundant and, in combination with the changes just mentioned, the spinal canal and foramina are affected. Changes in the lumbar spinal canal occur to some degree in all active people as they age. However, not everyone suffers from significant impairment. The symptoms a person will have depend upon the original size of the spinal canal. If the individual's spinal canal is small, the changes that are caused by aging and occur in the disc and facet joints will lead to an absolute spinal stenosis with compression of the neural elements. If the spinal canal is large, the normal changes of aging will lead to a relative spinal stenosis with no neural compression.

Procedure

The patient is prone, and the legs are fully extended. The examiner anchors the patient's lumbosacral spine with one hand. With the other hand the examiner slowly extends the hip of the affected leg. The test is positive if the patient experiences radiating pain in the anterior thigh. A positive test indicates inflammation of the L3 and L4 nerve roots.

Confirmation Procedures

Bilateral leg-lowering test, Demianoff's sign, double leg-raise test, Lewin supine test, match stick test, Mennell's sign, Minor's sign, Nachlas test, Quick test, Schober's test, sign of the buttock, skin pinch test, spinal percussion test, Vanzetti's sign

---

Reporting Statement

The hyperextension test is positive on the right and elicits anterior thigh pain. This pain suggests inflammation of the L3 and L4 nerve roots.

∾ **Clinical Pearl** ∾

There are five criteria for diagnosis of sciatica due to a herniated intervertebral disc. (1) Leg pain is the dominant symptom when compared with back pain, and it affects only one leg and follows a typical sciatic or femoral nerve distribution. (2) Paresthesia is localized to a dermatomal distribution. (3) Straight-leg raising is reduced to 50% of what is considered normal and pain is elicited in the symptomatic leg when the unaffected leg is elevated. This pain radiates proximally or distally with digital pressure on the tibial nerve in the popliteal fossa. (4) Two of four neurologic signs (atrophy, motor weakness, diminished sensory appreciation, and diminution of reflex activity) are present. (5) A contrast study or other diagnostic imaging is positive and corresponds to the clinical level.

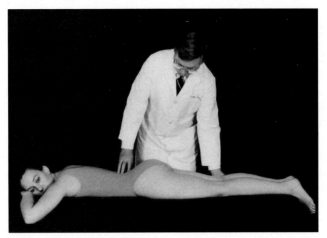

Fig. 8–34 The patient is prone and the legs are fully extended. The examiner anchors the patient's lumbosacral spine with one hand.

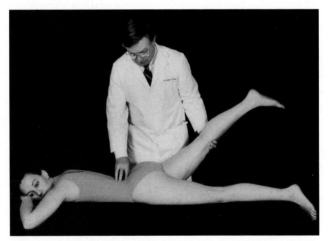

Fig. 8–35 With the other hand the examiner slowly extends the hip of the affected leg. The test is positive if the patient experiences radiating pain in the anterior thigh. A positive test indicates inflammation of the L3 and L4 nerve roots.

Comment

Disc prolapse occurs in three stages, and it only occurs if the disc has deteriorated as a result of repeated microtrauma and if the annulus fibers have started to degenerate. Disc prolapse usually follows lifting of a weight while the trunk is in flexion. During the first stage trunk flexion flattens the discs anteriorly and opens out the intervertebral space posteriorly. During the second stage, as soon as the weight is lifted, the increased axial compression force crushes the whole disc and violently drives the nuclear substance posteriorly until it reaches the deep surface of the posterior longitudinal ligament. During the third stage, when the trunk is nearly straight, the path taken by the herniating mass is closed by the pressure of the vertebral plateaus and a hernia remains trapped under the posterior longitudinal ligament. This hernia causes acute pain, which is felt in the lower back. This occurrence corresponds to the initial phase of the lumbar sciatica complex. This initial acute lower back pain can regress spontaneously or with treatment but, as a result of repeated trauma, the hernia grows in size and protrudes more and more into the vertebral canal. Once this protrusion occurs, the hernia meets with a nerve root, often one of the roots of the sciatic nerve. In fact, the hernia progressively pushes on the nerve root until the latter is jammed against the posterior wall of the intervertebral foramen. The posterior wall is formed by the joint between the articular processes, its anterior capsular ligament and the lateral border of the ligamentum flavum. The compressed nerve root causes pain in the spinal segment that corresponds to the root and, finally, impairs reflexes and creates motor disturbances, such as those that occur in sciatica with paralysis.

The clinical picture depends on the spinal level of disc prolapse and nerve root compression. If prolapse occurs at L4-L5, the root of L5 is compressed and pain is felt in the posterolateral aspect of the thigh, the knee, the lateral border of the calf, the lateral border of the instep of the foot, and the dorsal surface of the foot to the great toe. If the prolapse lies at L5-S1, S1 is compressed and pain is referred to the posterior aspect of the thigh, knee, and calf; the heel; and the lateral border of the foot to the fifth toe. However, this correlation of clinical picture and lesion level is not absolute. A hernia at L4-L5 may lie closer to the midline and compress L5 and S1 simultaneously, or even, occasionally, S1 alone. Surgical exploration at L5-S1, performed on the strength of the S1 root pain, may fail to recognize that this lesion lies one level above.

Procedure

While in a seated position, the patient is supported by the examiner, who reaches around the patient's shoulders and upper chest from behind. The patient is directed to lean forward to one side and then around until the patient is eventually bending obliquely backward. The maneuver is similar to that used for cervical compression. If this compression causes or aggravates a pattern of radicular pain in the thigh and leg, the sign is positive and indicates nerve root compression. Local back pain should be noted, but it does not constitute a positive test. However, this pain may indicate a strain or sprain and thus be present when the patient leans obliquely forward or at any point in motion.

Because the elderly are less prone to an actual herniation of a disc because of lessened elasticity involved in the aging process, other reasons for nerve root compression are usually the cause. Degenerative joint disease, exostoses, inflammatory or fibrotic residues, narrowing from disc degeneration and tumors must all be considered.

This test must elicit a more positive finding when the patient is standing than when sitting.

Confirmation Procedures

Antalgia sign, bowstring sign, Cox sign, heel/toe walk test, Lewin punch test, Lewin snuff test, Milgram's test, Néri's sign

---

Reporting Statement

Kemp's test (seated) is positive on the right and results in pain that radiates into the right side S1 dermatome. This pain indicates S1 nerve root compression syndrome.

Kemp's test (standing) is positive on the right and elicits pain that radiates into the right side L5 dermatome. This result indicates L5 nerve root compression syndrome.

Kemp's test is inconclusive on the right and elicits nonradiating pain at the L5-S1 area. This result suggests facet or pericapsular inflammation.

~ **Clinical Pearl** ~

Kemp's test can be performed when the patient is either in the standing or the seated position. Sitting increases intradiscal pressure and therefore maximizes stress on the disc. Standing increases weight bearing and maximizes stress to the facets. The test should be performed in both positions.

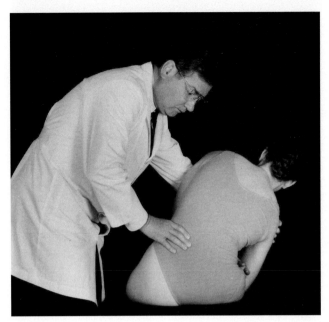

Fig. 8–36 While in a seated position, the patient is supported by the examiner, who reaches around the patient's shoulders and upper chest, from behind. The patient is directed to lean obliquely forward and away from the affected side.

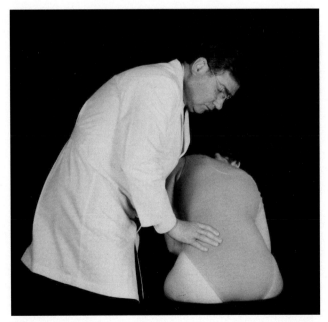

Fig. 8–37 The examiner actively rotates the patient's trunk from the original position and circumducts the trunk toward the affected side.

Continued.

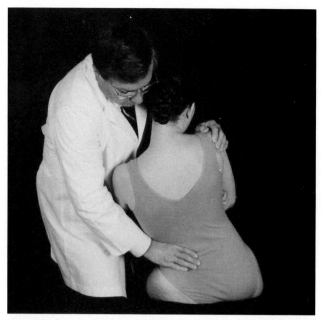

Fig. 8–38 Circumduction of the trunk toward the affected side occurs to the point at which the spine is posterolaterally extended. If this compression causes or aggravates a pattern of radicular pain in the thigh and leg, the test is positive and indicates nerve root compression. Local pain should be noted, but it does not constitute a positive test. Degenerative joint disease, exostoses, inflammatory or fibrotic residues, narrowing from disc degeneration, and tumors must be evaluated.

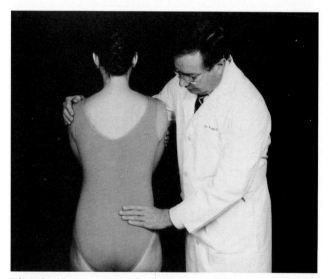

Fig. 8–39 An alternative is to have the patient assume a standing position. The examiner anchors the pelvis, on the affected side, with one hand. With the other hand the examiner grasps the patient's opposite shoulder.

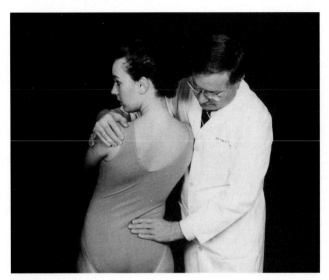

Fig. 8–40   While fixing the pelvis, the examiner firmly moves the patient's opposite shoulder obliquely backward, toward the affected side. This maneuver rotates the trunk, extends it, and exerts downward pressure over the affected lumbosacral area. The test is positive if this compression causes or aggravates a pattern of radicular pain in the thigh and leg. A positive test indicates nerve root compression. In the standing position the test position must elicit a more positive finding than is elicited in the seated position.

∼ Kernig/Brudzinski Sign ∼

Comment

With treatment the fatality rate of adult bacterial meningitis is usually less than 10%, but severe neurologic sequelae are possible. The two leading causes of these sequelae in the adult are pneumococci (*Streptococcus pneumoniae*) and meningococci (*Neisseria meningitidis*).

Pneumococcal meningitis is usually preceded by pneumonia and is often associated with alcoholism, debilitation, and old age. This type of meningitis usually occurs sporadically, except in developing countries.

Meningococcal meningitis occurs in epidemics (serogroups A or C) in the pediatric age group and may be acquired by susceptible adults.

Meningitis caused by Gram-negative enteric bacteria is always a disease of the hospitalized or nursing home patient and often follows bacteremia from other foci, such as cellulitis or urinary tract infection.

Consider the possibility of bacterial meningitis must be considered in any patient with fever and even minimal mental or neurologic symptoms.

Whenever the diagnosis is suspected, a lumbar puncture must be performed and bacterial cultures obtained. When the cerebrospinal fluid (CSF) is abnormal, tuberculous and fungal cultures should be obtained.

Prognosis depends on the interval between the onset of the illness and the institution of therapy.

If severe backache, stiff neck, and the Kernig/Brudzinski sign are absent, but mental symptoms are prominent, and the CSF shows normal sugar, a low number of cells, or a mononuclear pleocytosis (lymphocytosis), then encephalitis must be suspected. Patients with herpes simplex encephalitis classically present with an acute onset of mental and behavioral symptoms and often with an amnestic syndrome. The patients may have lateralized findings, such as hemiparesis or aphasia.

Procedure

For the Brudzinski part of the sign, the patient is in the supine position, and the examiner passively flexes the patient's head. The sign is present if flexion of both knees occurs. The sign is frequently accompanied by flexion of both hips and is present with meningitis.

For the Kernig part of the sign, the patient is supine. The examiner flexes the hip and knee of either leg to 90 degrees, respectively.

The examiner attempts to completely extend the leg. If pain prevents this, the sign is present. The sign is often accompanied by involuntary flexion of the opposite knee and hip and is present in meningitis.

Confirmation Procedure

Cerebrospinal fluid examination

Reporting Statement

The Kernig/Brudzinski sign is present. This sign indicates meningeal irritation or inflammation.

∼ Clinical Pearl ∼

Following myelography, a percentage of patients suffer from general malaise, headache, nausea, pain, and stiffness for a week or longer, and the symptoms are strikingly aggravated by the erect position or activity. These conditions may be signs of arachnoiditis. Subarachnoid fibrosis typically affects the lowermost segment of the thecal sac. This whole process represents meningismus or the apparent irritation of the spinal cord, in which the symptoms simulate a meningitis. However, no actual infectious agent—such as bacteria, fungi, or viruses—can be found.

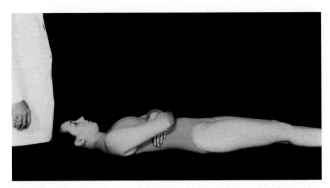

Fig. 8—41   For the Brudzinski sign the patient is in the supine position.

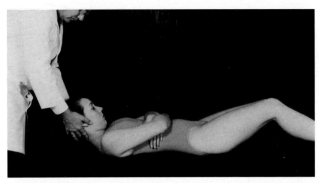

Fig. 8—42   The patient's head is passively flexed by the examiner. The sign is present if flexion of both knees occurs. The sign is frequently accompanied by flexion of both hips. The sign is present in meningitis.

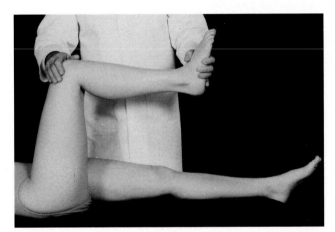

Fig. 8—43   For the Kernig sign, the patient is supine. The examiner flexes the hip and knee of either leg to 90 degrees, respectively.

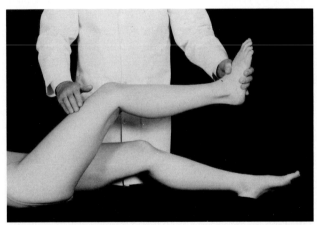

Fig. 8—44   The examiner attempts to completely extend the leg. If pain prevents this extension, the sign is present. The sign is often accompanied by involuntary flexion of the opposite knee and hip. The sign is present in meningitis.

Comment

Lower lumbar root compression syndromes secondary to degenerating and herniating intervertebral discs produce lower back pain and radiating pain (sciatica) in the buttock, posterior thigh, lateral leg, calf, or ankle. This is a common affliction that is often preceded by months or years of intermittent back pain. A typical posture is demonstrated by stiffness and deviation of the lumbar spine. In most cases the L4 or L5 intervertebral disc is involved, causing compression of the L5 and S1 nerve roots, respectively. The spinal cord does not descend to this level, but a large disc herniation, especially one that is located centrally, may impinge on other roots in the cauda equina, including those subserving bowel and bladder function.

With lower lumbar compression, attempted forward bending is limited by pain and inflexibility of the lumbar spine, and percussion by a fist or reflex hammer over the lower segments may aggravate the complaint in the thigh or leg (doorbell sign). The motor deficits that ensue from paresis of these roots are most apparent below the knee. Seldom is weakness of the calf so severe that the patient cannot walk on the toes, but atrophy of the gastrocnemius may be seen. Heel walking is especially revealing. Severe foot drop is unlikely, but toe drop is common with some atrophy of the anterior compartment. Nevertheless, dorsiflexion of the foot and toes should be tested directly for minor weakness. The test of straight-leg raising frequently demonstrates marked limitation in range of thigh flexion on the painful side. Squeeze tenderness of the calf is common. The ankle jerk reflex is a stretch reflex of the gastrocnemius-soleus. It is commonly diminished or absent when S1 root impingement occurs but may be normal in L5 root syndromes.

Neoplasms or inflammation of the spine or cauda equina may produce a syndrome similar to that produced by compression of the lower lumbar root, as may a retroperitoneal tumor and invasive neoplasm in the pelvis.

Procedure

If the examiner flexes the hip of a patient with sciatica while the knee is extended and this movement elicits pain but flexing the thigh on the pelvis while the knee is flexed produces no sciatic pain, then the sign is present. This sign rules out hip joint disease.

Confirmation Procedures

Bechterew's sitting test, Bragard's sign, Deyerle's sign, Fajersztajn's test, Lasègue rebound test, Lasègue sitting test, Lasègue test, Lewin standing test, Lindner's sign, Sicard's sign, straight-leg raising test, Turyn's sign

Reporting Statement

The Lasègue differential sign is present on the right. This result indicates radiculopathy rather than hip articular disease.

∼ Clinical Pearl ∼

Lasègue described how painful it is for patients with sciatica when the sciatic nerve is stretched by extending the knee while the hip is flexed. He also described the pain relief that occurs when the knee was then flexed. This is the classic leg-raising sign. Variations of this sign, with interpretations of its meaning, lend much more knowledge to the examining physician than merely noting at what degree of leg raise the patient experiences either back pain, leg pain, or both.

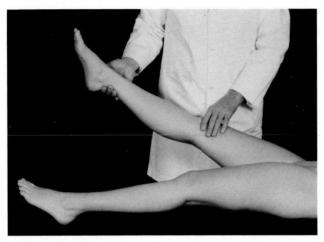

Fig. 8–45 The patient is supine with the legs fully extended. The examiner performs a straight-leg raising test on the affected leg and notes the angle at which sciatic pain is produced.

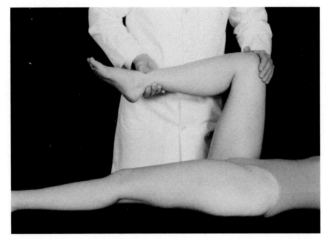

Fig. 8–46 The examiner flexes the thigh and the knee, relieving the stretch on the sciatic nerve. The sign is present if the pain is relieved. The presence of the sign indicates neural pain rather than hip articular pain.

Comment

Spasm of the posterior trunk muscles, sometimes accompanied by functional scoliosis and often by pain, usually indicates an underlying strain of the posterior joints, disc, or both. Unilateral spasm suggests a unilateral posterior joint strain. Lesions involving both disc and posterior joints are often accompanied by spasm of the spinal flexors, producing a straight or slightly kyphotic lumbar spine. Psoas spasm produces flexion deformity at the hip, and this may be missed at the initial examination. Spasm of the piriformis muscle, a common cause of buttock pain, can be diagnosed by palpation medial to the lower part of the neck of the femur.

Sciatic nerve entrapment usually occurs at the sciatic notch as the nerve exits from the pelvis. The nerve is compressed against the bony edge as it traverses the belly of the piriformis muscle. The syndrome is characterized by pain that is behind the greater trochanter and is referred down the thigh, the outer side of the leg, and the sole of the foot. Diagnostic findings include a positive Lasègue test, hypoesthesia of the lateral half of the sole of the foot, and pain behind the greater trochanter when the hip and knee joints are flexed to a right angle and the thigh is forced into adduction and internal rotation.

Pain during hip movement is emphasized as the diagnostic feature that differentiates sciatica because of a disc (when only straight-leg raising is painful) from peripheral entrapment of the nerve as it traverses the sciatic notch. When the nerve is stretched by straight-leg raising, pain is aggravated by internal rotation and relieved by external rotation.

Sensory changes, when present, are below the buttock and in the sole of the foot. Pressure on the nerve roots by a disc may involve the peroneal distribution above the ankle and the buttock itself. The condition is not common and may coexist with a prolapsed disc. The diagnosis of nerve entrapment is frequently missed initially and recognized only when sciatica persists after excision of the disc.

Procedure

To continue a differential after the straight-leg raising test, the examiner fixes the pelvis on the same side by pressing heavily with a hand on the region of the ipsilateral anterosuperior iliac spine and repeats that straight-leg raising test. Any undue pain experienced is associated with sciatic involvement due to a nerve root disorder, piriform spasm, or ischiotrochanteric groove adhesions. Differentiation of piriform spasm from other causes can be accomplished by reproducing the pain during internal rotation of the femur when it is at a lower level than the original point of pain. After a positive Lasègue test, the examiner may permit the leg to drop to the examination table without warning the patient. If this Lasègue rebound test causes a marked increase in the back pain, sciatic neuralgia, and muscle spasm, then disc involvement is suspected.

Confirmation Procedures

Bechterew's sitting test, Bragard's sign, Deyerle's sign, Fajersztajn's sign, Lasègue differential sign, Lasègue sitting test, Lasègue test, Lewin standing test, Lindner's sign, Sicard's sign, straight-leg raising test, Turyn's sign

---

Reporting Statement

Lasègue rebound testing is positive on the right and indicates lumbar disc involvement.

~ **Clinical Pearl** ~

The relationship of the lumbar roots and the lumbar discs is of major clinical importance. A massive posterior extrusion of one of the lumbar discs may severely injure the cauda equina (both intrathecal and extrathecal roots). Although these lesions are rare, they do occur. In these instances, the size and shape of the spinal canal and the size of the extruded mass are major factors in the severity of the clinical syndrome.

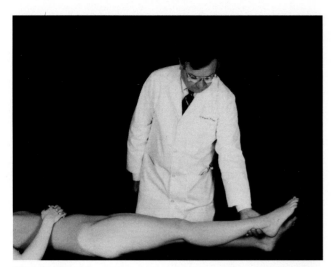

Fig. 8–47 The patient is in a supine position with both legs fully extended. The examiner performs a straight-leg raising test on the affected leg.

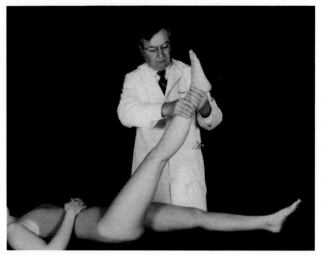

Fig. 8–48 The leg is elevated to the point at which pain is produced.

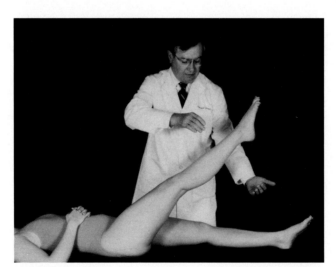

Fig. 8–49 Without warning the examiner removes support from the elevated leg, allowing it to drop to the examination table. If the test causes marked increase in back pain, sciatic neuralgia, and muscle spasm, the test is positive. A positive test indicates disc involvement.

Comment

Traumatic lumbar intervertebral disc prolapse is found in young adults who are most often male and usually employed in work that involves the lifting of heavy weights. Furniture movers, dockers, miners, truck drivers (who have to load their own trucks), and medical and nursing workers are particularly vulnerable.

The patient develops acute pain in the back immediately after lifting a weight or unexpectedly bearing a heavy load, such as when the worker slips or helpers release their grip prematurely. The sudden force is taken by the flexed and rotated spine. The patient develops immediate, midline lumbar pain that is severe enough to stop motion. The patient is afraid to move and feels as if the back is locked by the pain.

The pain may extend into the leg in the sciatic distribution, and there may be a loss of nerve root function. The pain is severe enough to drive the sufferer to bed after the first attack. Recumbency relieves the symptoms.

Procedure

The patient, whose legs are dangling, is seated upright on the edge of a table or chair that has no backrest. The examiner faces the patient and—under the guise of checking the circulation, feeling the skin, or checking for flat foot—extends the patient's leg at the knee. The lower extremity from the hip to the foot, is made parallel with the floor. When radiculoneuropathy is not present, the patient should not experience discomfort from this action.

Initially the significance of the test is the same as the Lasègue test. However, the modification of performing the straight-leg raise while the patient is in the seated position provides several advantages.

In the supine position, straight-leg raising may be difficult because the patient may squirm and shift the pelvis, making the leg abduct and rotate.

The apprehensive patient may attempt to ward off anticipated pain and make the test positive sooner than is warranted.

When the test is performed in the seated position, the patient faces the examiner, feels more secure and at ease, and is less likely to even know the part is being tested.

The test has excellent objective values when the examiner is able to determine immediately the slightest attempt on the part of the patient to withdraw by leaning back from the induced pain.

Confirmation Procedures

Bechterew's sitting test, Bragard's sign, Deyerle's sign, Fajersztajn's test, Lasègue differential sign, Lasègue rebound test, Lasègue test, Lewin standing test, Lindner's sign, Sicard's sign, straight-leg raising test, Turyn's sign

---

Reporting Statement

Lasègue sitting test is positive on the right. This result indicates sciatic nerve inflammation.

~ **Clinical Pearl** ~

By raising the foot, the examiner has performed a modified straight-leg raising test. Because the thigh is already flexed to 90 degrees in this position, straightening the knee to the horizontal places stretching forces on the nerve roots. The results of this seated tension should correspond to the results obtained from the tests done in the supine position.

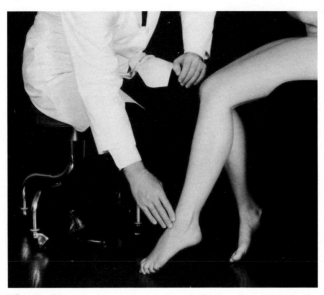

Fig. 8–50   The patient is seated with the legs hanging over the edge of the examination table.

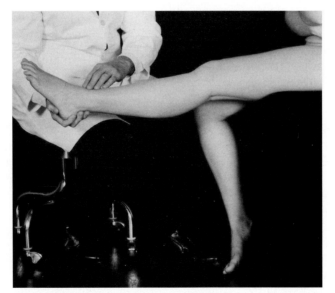

Fig. 8–51   The examiner faces the patient and, under the guise of checking the circulation, feeling the skin, or checking for flat foot, the examiner extends the patient's affected leg at the knee. The lower extremity, from the hip to the foot, is brought up until parallel with the floor. Pain in the sciatic distribution is a positive finding. A positive test indicates radiculoneuropathy.

Lasègue Test

LASÈGUE SIGN

Comment

The Lasègue test is the pain induced by stretching the sciatic nerve or one of its roots. The sign is elicited by gradual and slow extension of the knee of the elevated lower limb, which is performed while the patient is supine. The pain that is induced is similar to that felt spontaneously by the patient, such as pain in the same area of distribution.

The nerve root glides freely through the intervertebral foramen and during extension of the knee, the nerve roots are pulled out of the foramen for several millimeters at the L5 level.

The following interpretations can be made when the Lasègue test is present.

(1) When the patient is supine and the lower limbs are resting on the examination table, the sciatic nerve and its roots are under no tension.

(2) When the lower limb is raised while the knees are flexed, the sciatic nerve and its roots are still under no tension.

(3) If the knee is extended while the leg is elevated, the sciatic nerve—which must cover a longer distance—is subjected to increasing tension.

In the normal patient, the nerve roots slide freely through the intervertebral foramina and no pain results. When the lower limb is nearly vertical for people with diminished flexibility, pain is felt on the posterior aspect of the thigh as a result of stretching the hamstrings. However, this pain does not constitute a positive Lasègue sign.

(4) On the other hand, when one nerve root is trapped in the foramen or when the root must cover a longer distance because of a prolapsed disc, any stretching of the nerve will become painful with moderate elevation of the lower limb. This result constitutes a positive Lasègue sign, which is evident before 60 degrees of flexion is attained. Pain may be elicited at 10, 15, or 20 degrees of flexion, which allows a rough quantification of the severity of the lesion.

One point deserves emphasis. During extension of the knee while the leg is elevated, the force of the traction on the nerve roots can reach 3 kg. The resistance to traction of the nerve roots is 3.2 kg. If a root is trapped or shortened by a prolapsed disc, any rough manipulation of the leg can cause rupture of some axons and may result in paralysis. This is usually short lived, but occasionally may take a long time to disappear. Therefore two precautions must be observed. (1) The examiner must always elicit the Lasègue sign cautiously and stop when the patient feels pain. (2) The examiner must never attempt to elicit the Lasègue sign when the patient is under general anesthesia because the protective pain reflex is absent. The reflex can occur when the patient is being placed prone on an operating table and the hips are allowed to flex while the knees are extended. Hip flexion must always be associated with knee flexion, which relaxes the sciatic nerve and the trapped root.

Procedure

The patient lies supine with legs extended. The examiner places one hand under the heel of the affected leg and the other hand on the knee, and flexes the thigh on the pelvis while the knee is flexed. The examiner then slowly extends the knee, while the leg is elevated. If this maneuver is markedly limited due to pain, the test is positive and suggests sciatica from lumbosacral or sacroiliac lesions, subluxation syndrome, disc lesions, spondylolisthesis, adhesions, or interventricular foramen (IVF) occlusion.

Confirmation Procedures

Bechterew's test, Bragard's sign, Deyerle's sign, Fajersztajn's test, Lasègue differential sign, Lasègue rebound test, Lasègue sitting test, Lewin standing test, Lindner's sign, Sicard's sign, straight-leg raising test, Turyn's sign

> ### Reporting Statement
>
> Lasègue test is positive on the right. This result indicates sciatica associated with nerve root inflammation or compression.

∼ Clinical Pearl ∼

Whenever the presence of the Lasègue sign is questionable, combine it with flexion of the cervical spine (Lindner's sign). This combination places the greatest pull and stretch on the nerve roots behind the intervertebral discs and often elicits pain.

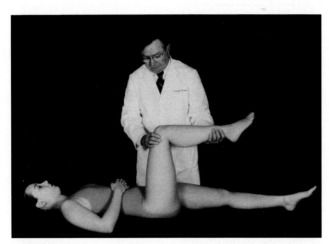

Fig. 8–52   The patient is supine, with both legs fully extended. The examiner places one hand under the ankle of the affected leg and the other hand at the knee. The hip and knee are flexed to 90 degrees, respectively. The nerve roots are under no tension and pain should not be elicited.

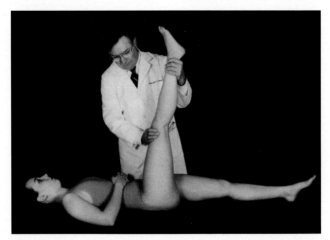

Fig. 8–53   The knee is extended by the examiner. If this maneuver is limited by pain, the Lasègue test is positive. The test suggests sciatica from lumbosacral or sacroiliac lesions, subluxation syndrome, disc lesions, spondylolisthesis, adhesions, or interventricular foramen (IVF) occlusion.

Comment

When compressed axially, the substance of the nucleus pulposus can stream out in various directions. If the annulus is still strong, the increase in pressure within the disc can cause the vertebral plateaus to give way. This corresponds to intravertebral prolapse.

The annulus fibers begin to degenerate after 25 years of age, allowing the tearing of fibers within each of its layers. Therefore under axial stress the nuclear material can stream out through the torn annulus. This streaming of nuclear material can be concentric but is more often radial. Anterior prolapse is the rarest. Posterior prolapse is the most frequent, especially posterolateral prolapse. Thus when the disc is crushed, part of the nuclear substance may stream out anteriorly but more often it streams out posteriorly and can thus reach the posterior edge of the disc to touch the posterior longitudinal ligament. At first the streamer, which is still attached to the nucleus, gets trapped under the posterior longitudinal ligament. When this happens it is still possible to bring the streamer back into its fibrous casing by using vertebral traction. Very often the streamer breaks through the posterior longitudinal ligament and may lie within the vertebral canal, which produces the so-called *free* type of disc prolapse. In other cases the nuclear streamer is trapped under the posterior longitudinal ligament and gets nipped off by the annulus fibers, which preclude any restoration to normal because the fibers snap back into position. In some cases the streamer, after reaching the deep aspect of the posterior longitudinal ligament, slides either superiorly or inferiorly. This is a case of subligamentous prolapse.

It is only when the herniating nucleus presses against the deep surface of the posterior longitudinal ligament that the nerve endings of the ligament are stretched, which causes lower back pain. Finally, compression of the nerve roots by the herniating disc causes nerve root pain, or sciatica.

Procedure

Punching the buttock produces a referred pain in the back. While the patient is in the standing position, the examiner punches the side of the buttock with the lesion. If this punch elicits pain, the test is positive. Punching the opposite buttock should not elicit pain. The test is significant for a spinal lesion, usually involving a protruded disc.

Confirmation Procedures

Antalgia sign, bowstring sign, Cox sign, heel/toe walk test, Kemp's test, Lewin snuff test, Milgram's test, Néri's sign

---

Reporting Statement

Lewin punch test is positive on the right. This result suggests an intervertebral disc protrusion.

~ Clinical Pearl ~

In some instances of an acute attack, even light fist percussion over the lumbar spine, in the midline, will produce such severe accentuation of the local and radiating pain that the patient's knees may buckle. There may be some evidence of a vasovagal response.

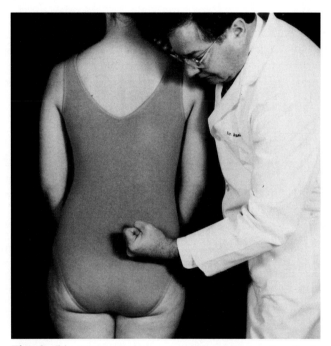

Fig. 8–54 While the patient is standing, the examiner firmly percusses the patient's buttock, on the affected side. If the "punch" produces a referred pain in the back, the test is positive. Punching the opposite buttock does not produce pain. The positive test indicates a spinal lesion, usually a protruded disc.

Comment

The intervertebral discs are not solid lumps of inert gristle, as patients often think, but living structures that flatten during the day and reexpand at night. The discs consist of a firm nucleus pulposus surrounded by the annulus fibrosus, a ring of fibrocartilage, and fibrous tissue that links two vertebrae together. The disc is a symphysis between each pair of vertebrae and, with the two posterior facet joints, allows movement between the vertebrae.

The tension within the disc is maintained by fluid imbibition at the cellular level. If imbibition fails, the pressure within the disc falls, and the disc collapses. Increased movement occurs between the adjacent vertebrae, and the annulus fibrosus is exposed to increased stress. This condition is accompanied by vague lower back pain.

As the degeneration proceeds, the annulus fibrosus softens and the degenerative disc bulges the annular ligament backwards, usually just lateral to the midline. If this bulge occurs in a tight spinal canal opposite a nerve root, the function of the root is affected.

Of all lumbar disc protrusions 90% involve the lowest two spaces, L4-L5 or L5-S1. Lesions that press on the L5 nerve root cause altered sensibility on the outer side of the calf and weakness of the peronei and ankle extensors, while those lesions affecting the S1 nerve root produce altered sensibility on the foot or back of the calf, weak ankle flexors, and a depressed ankle jerk. The resting muscle tone of the glutei, hamstrings, calf muscles, and other posterior muscle groups also may be reduced and these muscles may atrophy.

Unless there are neurologic symptoms and signs below the knee, the patient probably does not have a true prolapsed intervertebral disc. If the disc presses on a nerve root, the postural reflexes work to diminish the pressure on the root. The spine is held curved to produce a sciatic scoliosis and straight leg raising, which stretches the nerve, is restricted by pain.

Procedure

An aromatic substance is introduced, and the patient is instructed to sniff it up the nostril in order to induce sneezing. The test is positive when sneezing elicits an exacerbation of well-localized spinal and radicular pain. The test is significant for intervertebral disc rupture.

Confirmation Procedures

Antalgia sign, bowstring sign, Cox sign, heel/toe walk test, Kemp's test, Lewin punch test, Milgram's test, Néri's sign

---

Reporting Statement

Lewin snuff test is positive and reproduces the radiating pain. This positive test indicates an intervertebral disc rupture.

∿ Clinical Pearl ∿

The sneeze produces a sudden Valsalva maneuver. If it is assumed that motion of an irritated nerve root over a disc bulge is one of the causes of pain, any production of a Valsalva effect abruptly increases the patient's pain as the defect appears and disappears and thereby moves the nerve root over the disc.

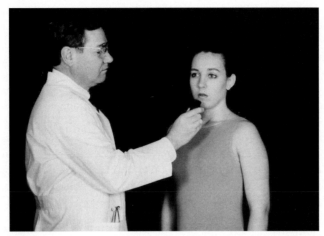

Fig. 8–55 The patient is introduced to a pungent, aromatic substance and instructed to inhale it through a nostril to induce sneezing.

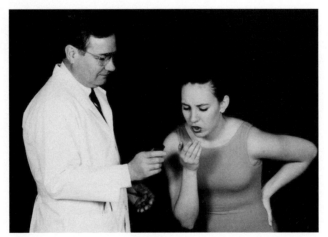

Fig. 8–56 The test is positive when sneezing elicits an exacerbation of well-localized, spinal and radicular pain. The test indicates intervertebral disc rupture.

Comment

Rupture of a muscle is felt as a tearing sensation. Swelling and tenderness at the site of the rupture follow within hours, and bruising appears about 24 hours later. The bruising, which is caused by bleeding from the ends of the ruptured muscle, can be dramatic and even alarming.

During examination, a defect can be felt in the muscle belly, and the belly becomes prominent as the muscle contracts. The swelling can occasionally be mistaken for a soft-tissue mass. The rectus femoris and hamstrings are the muscles most often affected.

A hematoma in a muscle is a serious lesion that is sometimes called a charley horse. The lesion usually follows direct trauma or, more rarely, a tear of the central fibers of the muscle.

As the blood in the hematoma becomes organized, it interferes with normal muscle function. In some patients the hematoma becomes ossified, which restricts muscle movement severely.

If a child has tight hamstrings that prevent flexion of the trunk or hip, suspect spondylolisthesis. Radiographs of the lumbosacral spine are essential in any child with tight hamstrings or calf muscles.

The sciatic nerve is considered to supply the posterior aspect of the hip and thigh.

The innervation to the short muscles of the hip and thigh (the obturator, sciatic, and sacral plexuses) also supply the sensory branches from the hip joint capsule. The cutaneous branches around the hip originate at a higher level than the motor and capsular nerves. The lateral femoral cutaneous nerve that covers the anterolateral thigh is L2. The anterior of the thigh is covered by the continuation of the femoral nerve by L2 to L4, the upper portion of the thigh is covered by the iliohypogastric, and the buttocks is covered by the posterior primary division of T12 to L3. Superficial cutaneous abnormality is referred from higher spinal levels.

Procedure

The patient is standing. From behind the examiner stabilizes the pelvis with one hand while sharply pulling the knee on that side into extension. The examiner then repeats this move on the opposite side and braces a shoulder against the patient's sacrum and sharply pulls both of the patient's knees into extension. The test is positive when pulling one or both knees into extension elicits pain that is followed by one or both knees snapping back into flexion. This positive finding represents unilateral or bilateral hamstring spasm.

Confirmation Procedures

Bechterew's sitting test, Bragard's sign, Deyerle's sign, Fajersztajn's test, Lasègue differential sign, Lasègue rebound test, Lasègue sitting test, Lasègue test, Lindner's sign, Sicard's sign, straight-leg raising test, Turyn's sign

---

Reporting Statement

Lewin standing test is positive on the right. This result indicates a hamstring spasm.

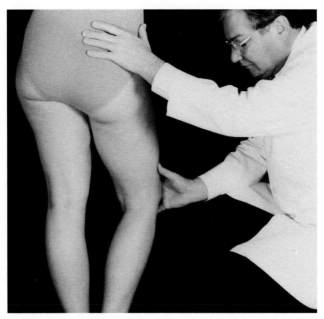

Fig. 8–57 While the patient is standing, the examiner stabilizes the patient's pelvis on the affected side with one hand.

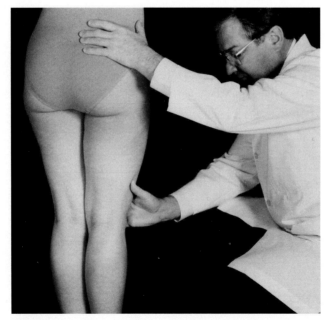

Fig. 8–58 The examiner then sharply pulls the knee of the affected leg into extension. This maneuver is repeated on the unaffected side. Next, the examiner braces a shoulder against the patient's sacrum and pulls both knees sharply into extension. The test is positive if pulling the knee into extension causes pain and is followed by a snapping back, of either knee, into flexion. This positive finding represents unilateral or bilateral hamstring spasm, as seen in sciatic radiculopathy.

Comment

Lumbar spondylosis is a condition in which there is progressive degeneration of the intervertebral discs leading to changes of the adjacent vertebrae, ligaments and osteoarthritis.

Most patients with lumbar spondylosis are older than those with primary disc lesions. A chief symptom is lower back pain, which is often described as both generalized and specific aching, involving certain areas of point tenderness. Activity increases the discomfort, and rest eases it. Sciatic pain is rare. When present, sciatic pain is generalized, it involves one or both lower extremities, and it often reflects root compression at several levels.

Examination reveals moderate paraspinal muscle spasm in the lumbar region with some limitation of the lumbar spine mobility in most movements. Extension is usually a bit more restricted than flexion. There is some flattening of the normal lumbar lordosis. Usually a moderate paraspinal muscle spasm is present. Straight leg raising is not as painful with spondylosis as with a herniated lumbar disc. Deep tendon reflex changes are elicited but are somewhat vague, which reflects nerve root compression at several levels.

The patient with lumbar spondylosis and a stenotic canal has a long history of intermittent lower back pain that is often related to specific positions and activities. The patient is frequently unable to sleep in a prone position (which tends to increase the lumbar lordosis). The patient finds it necessary to sleep on a side with the hips and knees flexed to maintain a strong lumbar flexion.

With lumbar spondylosis accompanied by a stenotic lumbar spinal canal, the physical examination is unrevealing despite intermittent symptoms that are often severe. Flexion and straight-leg raising are often performed without difficulty. Severe pain during lumbar extension may be the only positive result.

Procedure

While the patient is supine, the examiner supports the patient's legs on the table. The patient is directed to sit up without using the hands. The test is positive if the patient is unable to do this. A positive test is frequently associated with lumbar arthritis, lumbar fibrosis, degenerative disc thinning with protrusion, sacroiliac or lumbosacral arthritis, and sciatica. The patient is frequently able to localize the site of the complaint.

Confirmation Procedures

Bilateral leg-lowering test, Demianoff's sign, double leg-raise test, hyperextension test, match stick test, Mennell's sign, Minor's sign, Nachlas test, Quick test, Schober's test, sign of the buttock, skin pinch test, spinal percussion test, Vanzetti's sign

---

Reporting Statement

Lewin supine test is positive. This result indicates a pathologic condition of lumbosacral origin, which precludes the patient from completing the test.

∼ Clinical Pearl ∼

The security and comfort of the back depend not only on the lumbar muscles and ligaments but also on the strength of the abdominal wall and prevertebral muscles. The abdomen should be palpated to determine if divarication of the rectus abdominis muscle is present. The clinical test for diagnosis of rectus divarication involves instructing the supine patient to raise the head from the examination table. The examining hand can easily feel the gap between the contracted pillars of the rectus, and the fingers will sink into the soft abdominal wall. The width of the gap may vary from 1 cm to a hand's breadth.

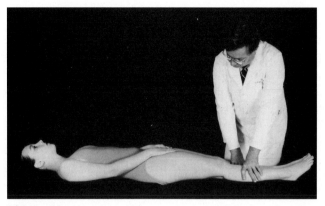

Fig. 8–59 The patient is supine, with both legs fully extended. The examiner firmly applies downward pressure to the patient's legs.

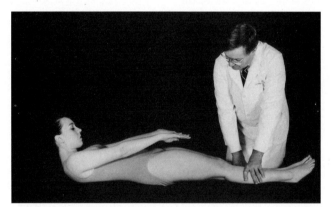

Fig. 8–60 The patient is directed to sit up without using the hands. The test is positive if the patient is unable to do this. A positive test indicates lumbar arthritis, lumbar fibrosis, a degenerative disc with protrusion, sacroiliac or lumbosacral arthritis, or sciatica. The patient is frequently able to localize the site, or origin, of the pain.

Comment

Before the development of signs and symptoms compatible with a diagnosis of a herniated lumbar disc, most patients have previously experienced lower back pain and other symptoms, which in retrospect can be related to the ensuing disc syndrome. Frequently the preexisting lower back pain is not severe and does not cause impairment. When the back pain becomes associated with pain radiating down the course of the sciatic nerve, the possibility of lumbar disc disease should be seriously considered. Position is usually a factor in intensifying or decreasing the pain. Most patients report that weight bearing, prolonged standing, walking, and sometimes sitting aggravate the pain. Resting in bed eases the pain. Symptoms may be aggravated by coughing, sneezing, or straining at the stool. Physical activity aggravates the pain.

The various nerve roots, when compressed by the protruding disc, produce characteristic signs and symptoms.

Whenever the straight-leg raising test produces a questionable result of pain, it should be combined with flexion of the cervical spine (Lindner's sign). This combination places pull and stretch on the nerve roots behind the intervertebral disc and often elicits pain. The simultaneous flexion of the neck and elevation of the contralateral leg can produce pain in the ipsilateral sciatic notch in patients with either free fragments or herniated discs. Raising the contralateral leg alone might not elicit pain in either leg.

Procedure

Passive flexion of the patient's head onto the chest can be accomplished in either a supine, seated, or standing position. If pain occurs in the lumbar spine and along the sciatic nerve distribution, the test is positive and, according to Lindner, is an indication of root sciatica.

Confirmation Procedures

Bechterew's sitting test, Bragard's sign, Deyerle's sign, Fajersztajn's test, Lasègue differential sign, Lasègue rebound test, Lasègue sitting test, Lasègue test, Lewin standing test, Sicard's sign, straight-leg raising test, Turyn's sign

---

Reporting Statement

Lindner's sign is present and reproduces radiating leg pain on the right in the L5 dermatome. This result indicates L5 nerve root irritation or inflammation.

∾ Clinical Pearl ∾

Flexion of the head upon the chest increases the traction of the nerve root against the disc bulge. When the disc is a contained disc, in which the annulus is not ruptured, the flexion or maintenance of a flexed position of the trunk obliterates the disc bulge. Motion of an irritated nerve root over a bulging disc is often the source of the patient's back and leg pain. Relief of pain with trunk flexion occurs only because the disc bulge has disappeared.

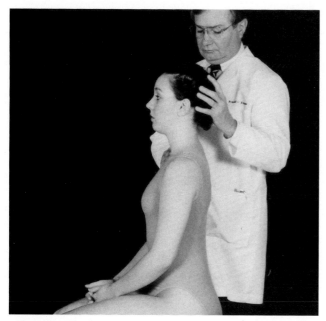

Fig. 8–61 The patient is seated with the arms in a comfortable position.

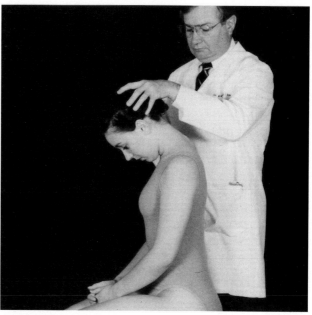

Fig. 8–62 The examiner passively flexes the patient's head onto the chest. If pain occurs in the lumbar spine and the sciatic nerve distribution, the test is positive. A positive test is an indication of root sciatica.

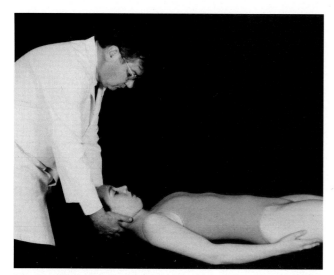

Fig. 8–63 A supine version of this test can also be performed.

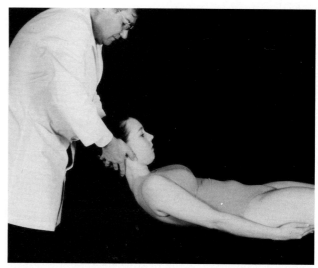

Fig. 8–64 For the supine version the head is passively flexed toward the chest. If pain occurs in the lumbar spine and the sciatic nerve distribution, the test is positive. A positive test is an indication of root sciatica. This result should be differentiated from Brudzinski's sign and the Soto-Hall maneuver. These tests are similar but have slightly different significances.

Comment

The sensory distribution of each nerve root, or dermatome, varies from person to person, and there is often overlap. A *dermatome* is defined as the area of skin supplied by a single nerve root.

The examiner must also be aware of the sensory, motor, and sympathetic distribution of peripheral nerves to be able to differentiate between lesions of the nerve roots and peripheral nerves. The effects of a mixed motor (motor, sensory, and sympathetic) peripheral nerve lesion include: (1) flaccid paralysis (motor), (2) loss of reflexes (motor), (3) muscle wasting and atrophy (motor), (4) loss of sensation (sensory), (5) trophic changes in the skin (sensory), loss of secretions from sweat glands (sympathetic), and loss of pilomotor response (sympathetic).

Pressure on a peripheral nerve resulting in a neurapraxia leads to temporary nonfunctioning of the nerve. With this type of injury, there is primarily motor involvement. Pressure on a nerve root leads to a loss of tone and muscle mass. Spinal nerve roots have a poorly developed epineurium and lack a perineurium. This makes the nerve root more susceptible to compressive forces, tensile deformations, chemical irritants (such as alcohol, lead, and arsenic), or metabolic abnormalities. For example, diabetes may cause a metabolic peripheral neuropathy of one or more nerves.

In peripheral nerves, the epineurium consists of loose areolar connective tissue matrix surrounding the nerve fiber and allows changes in growth length of the bundled nerve fibers (funiculi) without allowing the bundles to be strained. The perineurium protects the nerve bundles by acting as a diffusion barrier to irritants and provides tensile strength and elasticity to a nerve.

In the past there have been many names given to the condition now known universally as *reflex sympathetic dystrophy* (RSD). Because this condition may follow trauma, it is called posttraumatic pain syndrome.

The most important clinical finding in reflex sympathetic dystrophy is pain. However, the distinguishing feature of the pain in RSD is its severity. The degree of pain is completely out of proportion to the inciting trauma. The nature of the pain varies widely, but early in the condition the pain is usually described as burning or stinging. Later, the pain is often described as a pressure or cutting pain that becomes constant and unrelenting. Motion severely aggravates the pain, and there is almost a complete cessation of voluntary movement of the involved part. Although the pain may start in one area, it rapidly spreads to adjacent sites, and eventually involves the entire extremity. In untreated, severe cases the pain progresses to the point that the patient may request amputation of the affected part or even consider suicide. The pain is made markedly worse by attempting active or passive movement of the joints. Severe and excruciating paresthesia may be produced by lightly stroking the skin, even in uninjured areas. Tenderness is always present and is much more severe than one would normally expect.

Although pain is the most prominent symptom, swelling is the most common physical finding. The swelling usually starts in the area of greatest involvement, but it soon spreads proximally and distally to the immediate adjacent areas of the extremity. The swelling is soft initially, but turns to brawny edema if the condition persists. The brawny edema often gets so severe that it acts as a mechanical block to motion. This fixed edema eventually gives way to periarticular thickening and to fibrous tendon adhesions. Elevation of the extremity is most effective in reducing swelling when used early in the disease, but this elevation is beneficial any time.

Metabolic changes form an important part of any neurologic disorder and may occur in the skin, nails, subcutaneous tissues, muscles, bones, and joints. In addition to a neurologic basis, factors such as activity, blood supply, and lymph drainage are involved in the causation of trophic changes. When a peripheral nerve is completely interrupted, the skin loses its delicate indentations, becomes inelastic, smooth, and shiny. When interruption is partial, trophedema occurs. There is gradual fibrosis of the subcutaneous tissue and the overlying skin becomes fissured and prone to heavy folds. This alteration in the quality of the skin produces a peau d'orange affect similar to that described for malignant lumps in the female breast. This is accentuated when the skin is gently squeezed together or when the back is fully extended.

Procedure

Trophedema is nonpitting to digital pressure, but when a blunt instrument, such as the end of a match stick or cotton tip applicator is used, the indentation produced is clear cut and persists for several minutes, which is distinctly longer than such an indentation would persist in normal skin. The match stick test may be positive and yield deep indentations over an extensive area (commonly over the lower back and hamstrings) or in mild cases, the test may only yield slight indentations of skin overlying a tender motor point or the neurovascular hilus.

Confirmation Procedures

Bilateral leg-lowering test, Demianoff's sign, double leg-raise test, hyperextension test, Lewin supine test, Mennell's sign, Minor's sign, Nachlas test, Quick test, Schober's test, sign of the buttock, skin pinch test, spinal percussion test, Vanzetti's sign

Reporting Statement

Match stick testing reveals localized trophedema. This result suggests denervation supersensitivity, such as that seen in lumbar sprain.

∼ Clinical Pearl ∼

Reflex sympathetic dystrophy can occur in any disease that produces pain. This type of dystrophy is a likely secondary condition after 4 months of unrelenting pain from the primary disorder. The earliest sign, other than the symptoms of burning or stinging pain, is localized trophedema. The match stick test can be applied to any cutaneous area of pain because the test is sensitive to the earliest changes in fluid management in the skin by the sympathetically operated cutaneous vascularity. The result of this test becomes the earliest warning sign of the advancing reflex sympathetic dystrophy. An intervertebral disc syndrome with protracted nerve root compression is a common onset mechanism.

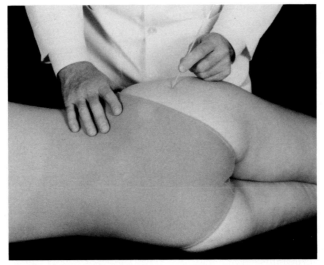

Fig. 8–65 The patient may be in either the prone or side-lying positions. The examiner applies the blunt end of a cotton tip applicator to the affected area of skin. The indentations produced are clear cut and persist for several minutes, which is distinctly longer than when performed on normal skin. The match stick test is positive if it yields deep indentations over an extensive area (commonly over the lower back and hamstrings) or, in mild cases, if it yields slight indentations of skin overlying a tender motor point or the neurovascular hilus. A positive test is associated with denervation supersensitivity, as seen with a lumbar sprain.

Comment

Fat nodules, located on the fascia over muscle or bone, may be painful when direct pressure is applied or trunk bending occurs. The aching and radicular sensation that occurs when the nodule is palpated is readily identified with the painful mass. All pain is temporarily relieved with topical anesthesia of the mass. The radicular component is referred pain similar to that associated with: (1) the painful tendon attachment, (2) periosteal pain, (3) the deep aching associated with compression of a small blood vessel, and (4) the irritation of a sensory nerve penetrating the fascia. Straight-leg raising may be uncomfortable, but it is not radicular.

The findings obtained are different from those associated with nerve root radiculopathy, but they are easy to confuse. All tender areas in the buttock are not fat nodules. Many tender areas may represent pain referral from an irritated nerve root. For example, a nerve root ganglion or cyst may cause pain, in the buttock, that is similar to that which occurs with a painful fat nodule that is more proximal.

There are 14 local areas in which tenderness during palpation is very constant in certain conditions. There are five areas on each side of the back to be examined, one in each buttock, and one in the back of each thigh. These local areas are as follows.

(1) Medial to the posterior superior iliac spine is the most superficial posterior ligament of the sacroiliac joint. Tenderness here suggests a pathologic condition involving the sacroiliac joint.

(2) Lateral to the posterior superior iliac spine is the puny part of the gluteal muscle origin that may be torn by minor trauma. Tenderness here suggests a pathologic condition resulting from a muscle tear.

(3) Above the posterior superior iliac spine is where the sacrospinalis muscle joins its tendon. Muscle fiber tears frequently occur at this junction during minor lifting trauma.

(4) Above and medial to the posterior superior iliac spine is the area over the interlaminar facet joint, where tenderness may be felt if dysfunction is present.

(5) Medial and inferior to the posterior superior iliac spine is the area where local tenderness may be felt from a pathologic condition involving a disc.

(6) Tenderness lateral to the ischial tuberosity, where the sciatic trunk emerges from beneath the piriformis muscle, suggests either tightness of the muscle or a pathologic condition of a radicular origin.

(7) Tenderness elicited by deeply rolling with the fingers over the sciatic trunk in the back of the thigh indicates neuritis.

Procedure

The examiner places a thumb over the posterior superior iliac spine (PSIS), exerts pressure, slides the thumb outward, and then slides it inward. The sign is positive if tenderness is increased. This result is significant if, when sliding outward, sensitive deposits in structures on the gluteal aspect of the PSIS are noted. If, when sliding inward, tenderness is increased, this is a significant result for strain of the superior sacroiliac ligaments. Confirmation can be made if tenderness is increased when the examiner posteriorly pulls the anterior superior iliac spine (ASIS) while standing behind the patient or when the examiner pulls the PSIS forward while standing in front of the patient. This test is helpful in determining that tenderness is due to strained superior sacroiliac ligaments. A positive result indicates deposits in the structure or adjacent to the structure of the sacroiliac joint. These deposits are the result of ligamentous strain or sprain.

Confirmation Procedures

Bilateral leg-lowering test, Demianoff's sign, double leg-raise test, hyperextension test, Lewin supine test, match stick test, Minor's sign, Nachlas test, Quick test, Schober's test, sign of the buttock, skin pinch test, spinal percussion test, Vanzetti's sign

---

Reporting Statement

Mennell's sign is positive on the right. The presence of this sign indicates a pathologic condition involving the sacroiliac joint structures.

∼ Clinical Pearl ∼

This method of tissue examination provides pertinent information, providing the results are accurately interpreted. Palpation of the lumbosacral region, with the patient in either the erect or the prone position, may evoke tender areas in the midline, at the level of the disc lesion, and in the paravertebral area on the side of the nuclear extrusion. It is not uncommon to be able to elicit tenderness along the iliac crest or even over the posterior aspect of the sacroiliac joint, on the side of an irritated nerve root.

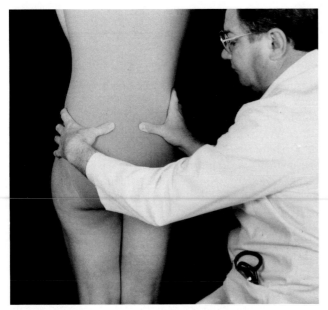

Fig. 8–66 The patient is standing. The examiner places a thumb over the PSIS on the affected side and exerts pressure.

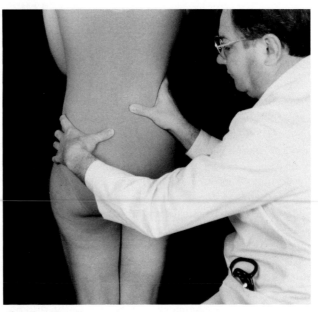

Fig. 8–67 The examiner then slides the thumb upward and inward.

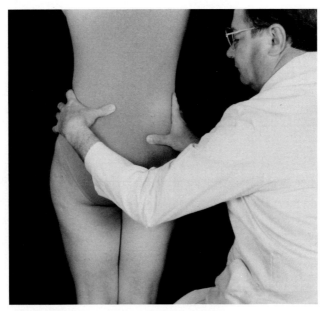

Fig. 8–68 While maintaining the pressure, the examiner moves the thumb downward and outward. The sign is positive if tenderness is increased in either direction. This sign is significant if when sliding outward, sensitive deposits in structures on the gluteal aspect of the PSIS are noted. If tenderness is increased when sliding inward, it indicates inflammation or strain in the superior sacroiliac ligaments. A positive sign indicates involvement of the structure or something adjacent to it, involvement of the sacroiliac joint, or a ligamentous sprain.

Comment

The weakest portion of the posterior annulus in the lumbar spine is either side of the midline, where the annulus lacks the reinforcement of the strong central fibers of the posterior longitudinal ligament. Either side of the midline is also the most common site of nuclear protrusions in the lumbar spine. Having penetrated the annulus, the protrusion lodges under the posterior longitudinal ligament. The ligament is stretched commensurate with the size of the fragment and the degree of internal pressure within the disc. In this position the protrusion is a firm, smooth mound. To accommodate the sequestered fragment, the posterior ligament is lifted off the vertebral bodies. As the nuclear mass increases in size, further stripping of the ligament occurs. The mass may migrate in any direction—cephalad, caudad, medially, or laterally. The mass commonly moves in a lateral direction close to and parallel to a nerve root, and it may even extend into the intervertebral foramen. Under the ligament, the mass lies tightly compressed and folded upon itself. The mass can be completely free or it may still be attached to material in the nucleus by strands of irregular, stringy, fibrous tissue. This type of protrusion is, by far, the most common lesion encountered.

Occasionally, a dissecting protrusion may erode through the posterior ligament at a distance from its site of exit from the annulus. More commonly the fragment is extruded through the annulus and the ligament. These free sequestra, regardless of their mode of origin, may move in any direction in the spinal canal. The usual course for these sequestra is along one of the extrathecal nerve roots, and they may lodge in the intervertebral foramen.

It becomes apparent that both the dissecting and the extruded nuclear materials can make contact with one of the nerve roots anywhere from the point of exit at the dura to the intervertebral foramen. In most instances the nuclear material lodges directly under or slightly to either side of the root, putting it in tension. Because of the lack of elasticity of the roots outside the dura, even a small protrusion is capable of putting tension on the root. In this position, local secondary inflammatory changes bind the root tightly to the underlying nuclear mound, so it is very difficult for the root to be displaced to one side or the other of the mass. In cases of long standing the root may actually become embedded in the heap of local fibrotic tissue that is formed. The root also responds to the abnormal situation by becoming injected, edematous, and cordlike. Within the nerve sheath, granulation tissue appears that, with maturation, is converted to dense fibrous tissue that binds the nerve fasciculi together and in some instances actually destroys the fibers. The neurologic deficits resulting from this process may be permanent.

Procedure

The patient is lying supine with both lower limbs straight out and is directed to raise the limbs until the heels are 6 inches off the table. The patient holds the position for as long as possible. The test is positive if the patient experiences lower back pain. Because this maneuver increases the subarachnoid pressure, if the patient can hold the position for 30 seconds without pain, a pathologic condition of intrathecal origin can be ruled out. If the test is positive, there may be pathologic condition, such as a herniated disc, in or outside the spinal cord sheath.

Confirmation Procedures

Antalgia sign, bowstring sign, Cox sign, heel/toe walk test, Kemp's test, Lewin punch test, Lewin snuff test, Néri's sign

---

Reporting Statement

Milgram's test is positive, because the patient is unable to lift the legs as a result of lumbosacral pain. This result suggests a herniated intervertebral disc.

❧ Clinical Pearl ❧

This test increases thecal pressure. The ability to hold this position for any time rules out a pathologic condition of thecal origin.

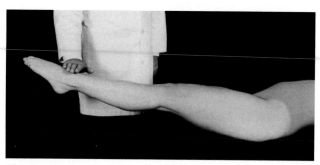

Fig. 8–69 The patient is supine with both legs fully extended. The patient is instructed to raise both legs to a position where the heels are approximately six inches from the examining table.

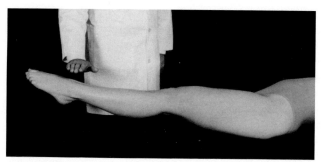

Fig. 8–70 The test is positive if the patient experiences lower back pain that prevents raising of the legs more than two to three inches, if at all. Because this maneuver increases the subarachnoid pressure, if the patient can hold the position for any length of time without pain, pathologic intrathecal process can be ruled out. A positive test indicates a space-occupying pathologic condition, such as a herniated disc.

Comment

The symptom complex of sciatic pain varies widely, and it occurs when a nuclear sequestrum touches one of the nerve roots. In a small percentage of patients the attack comes on suddenly, and the pain radiates the full length of the limb, along the dermatome of the involved nerve root. In a large percentage of patients the pain comes on slowly and is often felt as an ache that is in one side of the buttocks and that spreads gradually and distally. In some patients the pain is localized to the posterior or posterolateral aspects of the thigh, depending on whether S1 or L5 nerve roots are implicated. In some the pain may extend as far as the calf (the lateral aspect of the lower leg), the sole of the foot, or the dorsum of the outer three toes, depending on the nerve root affected. From time to time, the presenting complaint is pain that is limited to a small but specific area, such as the buttocks, the back of the thigh, the calf, or the sole of the foot. In rare instances, the pattern of pain spread may be reversed. For example, the pain may begin in the calf or sole of the foot and gradually spread cephalward.

In a small percentage of patients, back pain and sciatica appear simultaneously. Two clinical types of this syndrome are discernible. In one type the symptoms of back pain and sciatica appear suddenly and simultaneously. In the other type the onset is gradual. The former is associated with some sudden flexion stress that is applied to the lumbar spine and causes rupture of the annulus and retropulsion of the nuclear material. The latter is consistent with gradual extrusion of the nuclear fragments through the annulus fibrosus. The pain in the back and the sciatica may be of almost equal severity, but in most instances the intensity of one overshadows the other. When pain in both the back and the leg is severe, and the onset is sudden, the patient may be incapacitated and may present a dramatic clinical picture. The pain may be so severe that the affected leg is held in the flexed position and the patient avoids any maneuver that might extend the limb. There is severe spasm of the lumbar paravertebral muscles and frequently a severe list of the trunk.

Procedure

Sciatic radiculitis is suggested by how a patient with this condition rises from a seated position. The patient supports the body with the uninvolved side by balancing on the healthy leg, placing one hand on the back, and flexing the knee and hip of the affected limb. The sign is often present with sacroiliac lesions, lumbosacral strains and sprains, fractures, disc syndromes, dystrophies, and myotonia.

Confirmation Procedures

Bilateral leg-lowering test, Demianoff's sign, double leg-raise test, hyperextension test, Lewin supine test, match stick test, Mennell's sign, Nachlas test, Quick test, Schober's test, sign of the buttock, skin pinch test, spinal percussion test, Vanzetti's sign

---

Reporting Statement

Minor's sign is present. This sign indicates a pathologic condition of lumbosacral origin.

∽ Clinical Pearl ∽

With lumbar disc lesions, all movements—extension, flexion, lateral flexion, and rotation—of the spine are affected. With an acute lesion, extension and flexion are seriously restricted, but lateral flexion and rotation are free. The degree of restriction is governed by the phase and severity of the local pathologic process. During an acute attack, the striking feature of the spine is the complete loss of its inherent flexibility. The patient avoids motion in any direction.

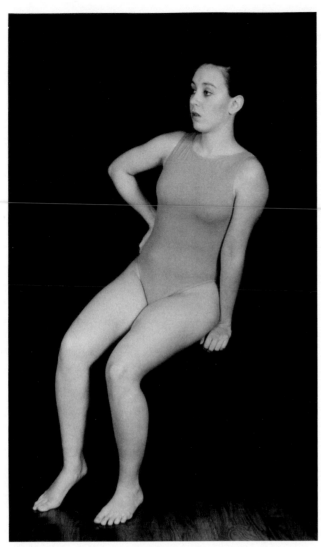

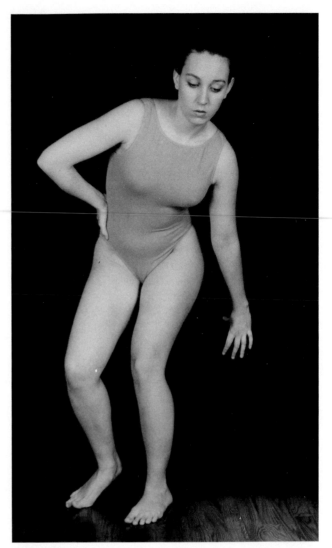

Fig. 8–71 The patient is seated and is asked to stand. The examiner observes how the patient rises from a seated position.

Fig. 8–72 The sign is present if the patient supports weight on the uninvolved side by balancing on the healthy leg, placing one hand on the back, and flexing the knee and hip on the affected side. The sign is often present with sacroiliac lesions, lumbosacral strains and sprains, fractures, disc syndromes, dystrophies, and myotonia.

Comment

Acute lumbosacral strain is the most common cause of acute lower back pain. The lumbosacral joint, because of its position in the skeleton, supports the body weight and acts as a fulcrum for this weight in activities that involve bending and lifting. Mechanical damage to this joint is frequent because of the functional demands placed on the lower back area by everyday activities. In this joint, the traumatic force usually involves lifting of a load when the spine is flexed forward. In this position the lumbosacral joint is functioning as a fulcrum. Acute lumbosacral strain occurs when a load is applied while the spine is twisted or rotated or when a sudden force is applied unexpectedly before the back muscles brace to meet it. The latter instance occurs less frequently than the former.

The resulting pathologic change is a partial tearing or stretching of the overlying paravertebral muscles, lumbar fascia, and interspinous ligaments. If the injury results in more serious damage to the spine, then by definition it cannot be a lumbosacral strain. Injury to the soft parts initiates paravertebral muscle spasm, which accounts for the clinical picture seen with this condition.

Two facts are basic for understanding an acute lumbosacral strain. First the stimulus for normal tone of the paravertebral muscles is the upright position. These muscles are in normal postural tone only in the standing or seated positions and are completely flaccid in the prone or supine positions. Spasm of the paravertebral muscles involves markedly exaggerated tone that is initiated by the stimulus of overload and is maintained by the stimulus of the upright position. If the patient were put to bed immediately after sustaining the injury, it is doubtful whether the symptoms and signs associated with an acute lumbosacral strain could develop. It is this basic physiologic fact that accounts for the extreme duration of pain and the impairment that occurs in patients with paravertebral muscle spasm who are allowed to remain ambulatory. The above explanation also accounts for the rapid subsidence of symptoms that result from absolute bed rest.

Second, in patients with acute lumbosacral strain there is always a lag period between the time the lower back damage was sustained and the onset of the clinical symptoms. This lag period may vary from hours to days and depends on whether the patient remains upright. It is during this lag period that the paravertebral muscle spasm builds to a point of clinical significance.

The severity of the clinical features of acute lumbosacral strain depends directly on the degree of paravertebral muscle spasm present. The patient gives a history of a twisting or lifting injury to the lower back and states that the onset of symptoms occurred either immediately or, more commonly, after a lag period of several hours or days. The patient walks guardedly and slowly because movement of the spine is painful. The back may be held in flexion or may exhibit a list to one side with a tilted pelvis. The paravertebral muscles feel extremely taut and hard, and the normal lumbar lordotic curve is obliterated. Spinal movements are limited in direct proportion to the amount of muscle spasm present and are associated with a sharp, diffuse, catching type of pain in the lower back, with possible radiation to the buttocks and thighs or upward to the neck.

Procedure

To eliminate lumbosacral muscular influence in this test, the patient is placed prone and relaxed on a rigid table. Pain in the lower back and lower extremity is noted during passive flexion of the knee. The test is positive if pain is noted in the sacroiliac area or lumbosacral area, or if the pain radiates down the thigh or leg. A positive test indicates a sacroiliac or lumbosacral disorder.

Confirmation Procedures

Bilateral leg-lowering test, Demianoff's sign, double leg-raise test, hyperextension test, Lewin supine test, match stick test, Mennell's sign, Minor's sign, Quick test, Schober's test, sign of the buttock, skin pinch test, spinal percussion test, Vanzetti's sign

---

Reporting Statement

Nachlas test is positive on the right and elicits pain radiating down the anterior thigh. This positive result indicates inflammation of the upper lumbar nerve roots.

∼ Clinical Pearl ∼

Intermittent prolapse of nuclear material is called a concealed disc. Degenerated nuclear material still within the confines of the annulus, which may be weakened by degenerative process but remains intact, may bulge beyond its normal limits when the spine is subjected to certain stresses. Depending on the stresses the prolapse appears and then disappears. Extension and hyperextension of the spine favor the prolapse, which can produce a defect in the anterior aspect of a myelographic column of dye. When the spine is relieved of stress, such as when the patient is relaxed and lying in the prone position, the defect disappears.

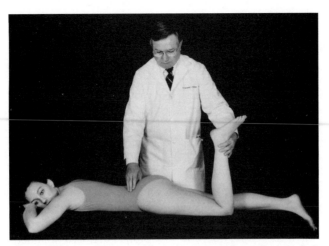

Fig. 8–73 The patient is prone, with both legs fully extended. The examiner flexes the knee of the affected leg to 90 degrees.

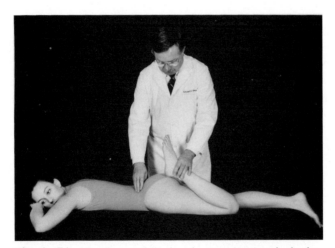

Fig. 8–74 The knee is fully flexed, approximating the heel to the ipsilateral buttock. The test is positive if pain is noted in the sacroiliac area or lumbosacral area, or if pain radiates down the thigh or leg. A positive test indicates a sacroiliac or lumbosacral disorder.

Comment

Abnormal physical stresses placed on a degenerated disc may exceed the mechanical strength of the degenerated disc and annulus, resulting in rupture of the annulus. Herniation of nuclear material (either wholly or in fragments) into the spinal canal causes either compression of or tension on a lumbar or sacral spinal nerve root as the root prepares to exit from the spinal canal and is the essential pathologic lesion of the condition known as *herniated intervertebral disc.* The nuclear material may push the posterior longitudinal ligament ahead of it like a sac, or the material may rupture through the posterior longitudinal ligament to extrude directly into the spinal canal.

The general process of intervertebral disc degeneration may extend over a period of years. The clinical picture characteristic of a herniated intervertebral disc does not arise until some of the nuclear material herniates or ruptures the posterior longitudinal spinal ligament. This rupture causes pressure on the adjacent spinal nerve root as it passes by and exits from the spine. The actual contact between disc material and the nerve root may be sudden and commonly follows an acute rise in intrathecal pressure that is triggered by sneezing, lifting, or straining at the stool.

Back pain is associated with disc degeneration, but the predominant symptom is sciatic pain that begins when the nuclear material protrudes posterolaterally into the spinal canal and compresses the nerve root. In most instances a diagnosis of herniated disc is untenable without sciatic leg pain. Many back conditions may be associated with leg pain, but only nerve root irritation at this level produces pain along the distribution of the sciatic nerve. Pain that follows the distribution of the sciatic nerve is associated with signs of a lumbosacral nerve root compression syndrome.

The patient with a herniated intervertebral disc presents with lower back pain that is accompanied by pain radiating into the posterior buttock and leg or just the leg. When viewed while standing, the patient may exhibit a list of the pelvis or a sciatic scoliosis.

Procedure

While in a standing posture, the patient is directed to bow forward. The sign is present when the patient flexes the knee on the affected side. The trunk flexion action causes pain in the leg. This pain is a common sign with lower disc problems as well as lumbosacral and sacroiliac strain subluxations.

Confirmation Procedures

Antalgia sign, bowstring sign, Cox sign, heel/toe walk test, Kemp's test, Lewin punch test, Lewin snuff test, Milgram's test

---

Reporting Statement

Néri's sign is present on the right. This sign indicates lower lumbar intervertebral disc involvement.

~ **Clinical Pearl** ~

Muscle tenderness may be associated with nerve root irritation. With an acute attack, tenderness of the buttock, thigh, and calf on the affected side is often demonstrable. When pain is localized to a specific area along the course of the sciatic nerve, careful regional examination is essential for ruling out local lesions such as an abscess, neurofibroma, glomus tumor, lipoma, or sterile abscess, that irritate the sciatic nerve.

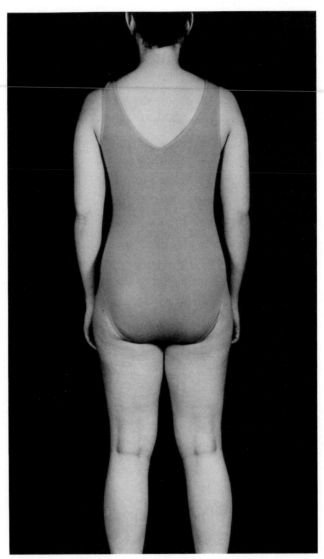

Fig. 8–75 The patient is standing with the arms comfortably at the sides.

Continued.

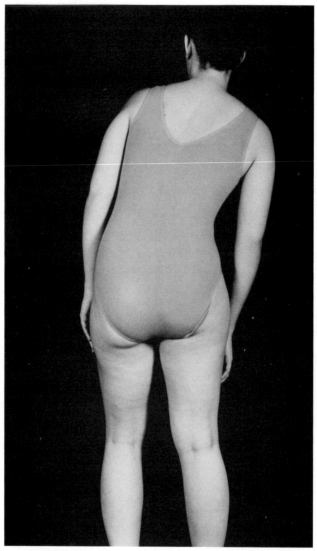

Fig. 8–76 The patient is directed to flex the trunk or bow forward. A lateral antalgic positioning may be noted but does not constitute a positive finding for this test.

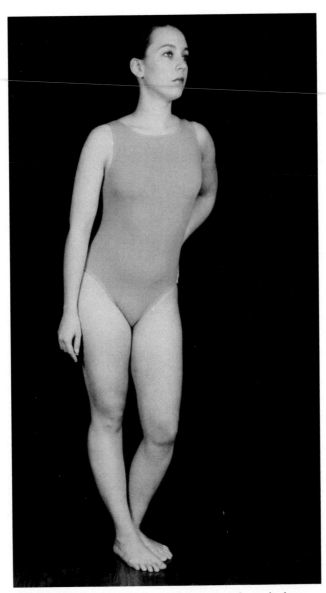

Fig. 8–77   The sign is present if the patient flexes the knee on
the affected side and if trunk flexion causes pain in the leg. The sign
is present for lower lumbar disc involvement as well as lumbosacral
and sacroiliac strains or subluxations.

Prone Knee-Bending Test

Comment

The femoral nerve arises from the L1, L2, L3, and L4 spinal roots and innervates the iliopsoas, sartorius, and quadriceps femoris muscles. Proximal lesions result in weakness of thigh flexion or, more prominently, loss of extension at the knee. The nerve can be injured by pelvic fractures, by surgery, and by direct, penetrating wounds. The nerve can be paralyzed by pressure during childbirth or by arterial aneurysms, retroperitoneal hemorrhage, pelvic neoplasms, or abscesses. Probably the most common syndrome involving the femoral nerve is the painful mononeuritis that occurs with diabetes. The quadriceps muscle atrophies quickly, and the knee jerk is lost early. Weakness while stepping up and the inability to rise from a one-legged squat are reliable motor signs of quadriceps paralysis. Quadriceps strength can be tested directly. Sensory distribution includes the anteromedial thigh and the anteromedial leg to the foot. It is appropriate to seek signs of more widespread deficits before concluding that this nerve alone is paralyzed because similar findings may result from a lesion higher in the lumbar plexus.

Femoral nerve injuries fall into two categories, those distal to the inguinal ligament in the femoral triangle and those proximal and, by definition, intrapelvic. Theoretically, injury to the pelvic portion of the femoral nerve should give, in addition to quadriceps paralysis and hypesthesia over the anteromedial thigh, a loss of sartorius muscle function. The branch to the sartorius is somewhat variable in origin and course. One of the clearly intrapelvic femoral nerve lesions appears to spare this muscle, while several thigh level lesions may have sartorius loss. Preservation or loss of this muscle's function does not indicate the level of the femoral nerve involvement.

Only sensory function is mediated by the lateral femoral cutaneous nerve. This nerve is not a branch of the femoral nerve, and it follows a different peripheral course. Classic entrapment of the lateral femoral cutaneous nerve occurs where it passes under the inguinal ligament medial to the anterior superior iliac spine. This entrapment results in a syndrome of dysesthesia and pain, called meralgia paraesthetica, along the lateral thigh. Some loss of sensitivity to pain and touch is often typical in a small area. The skin may become sensitive to touch and pinching. There is no atrophy and no motor or reflex change. Entrapment of the lateral femoral cutaneous nerve is distinguished by its common occurrence, curability, and tendency to be easily mistaken for symptoms of L2 and L3 nerve root compression syndromes. This type of entrapment is initiated by obesity or local trauma caused by a belt or truss. Like other entrapment neuropathies, lateral femoral cutaneous nerve entrapment is apt to occur with metabolic disorders, which may make the peripheral nerves vulnerable to pressure.

Procedure

The patient lies prone while the examiner passively flexes the knees so that the patient's heels rest against the buttocks. The examiner should ensure that the patient's hips are not rotated. If the examiner is unable to flex the patient's knees past 90 degrees because of a pathologic condition, the test may be done by passive extension of the hips while the knees are flexed. Unilateral pain in the lumbar area may indicate an L2 or L3 nerve root lesion. The test also stretches the femoral nerve. Pain in the anterior thigh indicates tight quadriceps muscles. The flexed-knees position should be maintained for 45 to 60 seconds.

Confirmation Procedures

Ely's sign, femoral nerve traction test

> ### Reporting Statement
>
> Prone knee-bending test is positive and elicits pain in the right anterior thigh. This result indicates L2 or L3 nerve root inflammation.

Clinical Pearl

Prone knee flexion can provide provocative testing for lumbar disc protrusion. The pathophysiology of this test depends on compression of spinal nerves during hyperextension of the lumbar spine. The compression intensifies intervertebral disc protrusion into the spinal canal. The lumbar intervertebral foramina are narrowed and the spinal canal cross-sectional area is decreased by lumbar extension. The presence of a protruded disc that has not produced other physical findings may be detected by this test.

The Lumbar Spine

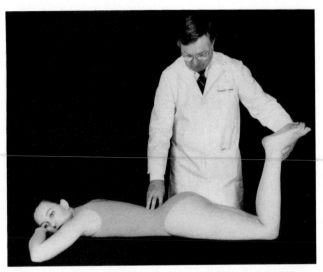

Fig. 8−78   The patient is in the prone position with both knees fully extended. The examiner passively flexes both knees to 90 degrees.

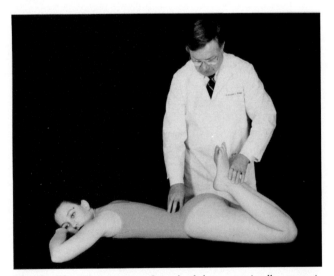

Fig. 8−79   The examiner flexes both knees maximally, approximating the heels to the buttocks. If the examiner is unable to flex the patient's knees past 90 degrees, the test is positive. Unilateral pain in the lumbar area indicates an L2 or L3 nerve root lesion. The test also stretches the femoral nerve. Pain in the anterior thigh indicates tight quadriceps muscles.

Comment

Back pain is the most common and troublesome complaint because its causes are legion and exact diagnosis is often difficult. The impairment, with which back pain is usually associated, is often severe and prolonged. It is helpful to consider the subject under three headings.

(1) Back pain may be associated with a spinal pathologic process, such as vertebral infections, tumors, ankylosing spondylitis, polyarthritis, Paget's disease, and primary neurologic disease.

(2) Back pain may be associated with nerve root pain. The most common causes are intervertebral disc prolapse and compression of nerve roots within the neural canals.

(3) Back pain may be caused by disturbance of the mechanics of the spine (mechanical back pain). This is the largest group of conditions that cause back pain. The mechanical disturbances are clear (osteoporotic spinal fractures, senile kyphosis, spondylolisthesis, Scheuermann's disease [spinal osteochondrosis], and sometimes osteoarthritis). In other cases, although the symptoms may be identical in character, the cause cannot be determined with any accuracy. These cases of mechanical lower back pain formerly attracted many emotive but valueless names, such as lumbago, and lower back strain.

While taking a history and examining a patient suffering from back pain, the possibility of extraspinal causes should be exhausted, then an attempt should be made to place the patient in one of the three groups described above.

Procedure

While the patient is standing, the Quick test may be done. The patient squats down, bouncing two or three times, and returns to the standing position. This action will quickly test the ankles, knees, and hips for any pathologic condition. If the patient can fully squat and bounce, without any signs and symptoms, these joints, in all probability, are free of a pathologic condition related to the complaint. This test should be used with caution and should not be done with patients suspected of having arthritis in the lower limb joints, with pregnant patients, or with older individuals who exhibit weakness and hypomobility. If this test is performed and is negative, there is no need to test the peripheral joints in the supine position.

Confirmation Procedures

Bilateral leg-lowering test, Demianoff's sign, double leg-raise test, hyperextension test, Lewin supine test, match stick test, Mennell's sign, Minor's sign, Nachlas test, Schober's test, sign of the buttock, skin pinch test, spinal percussion test, Vanzetti's sign

---

Reporting Statement

Quick test demonstrates that the ankles, knees, and hips are free of a pathologic condition associated with the patient's lower back or lower extremity complaints.

~ **Clinical Pearl** ~

The Quick test is probably the least demanding screening test for lumbar and lower extremity complaints. In a few, short, and active movements, three major contributors to lower extremity complaints (ankles, knees, and hips) can be ruled in or out of the differential diagnosis process.

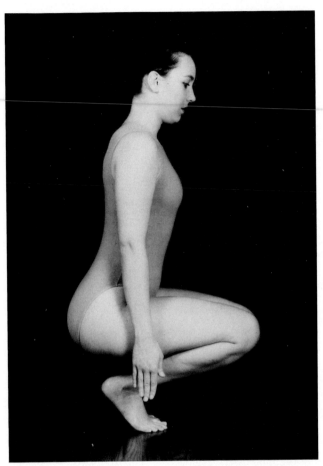

Fig. 8–80 The patient is standing. The patient is instructed to squat down, bounce two or three times, and return to the standing position. If the patient can fully squat and bounce without any signs and symptoms, the ankles, knees, and hips are free of a pathologic condition related to the complaint. This test should be used with caution and should not be performed with patients suspected of having arthritis in the lower limb joints, with pregnant patients, or with older individuals who exhibit weakness and hypomobility.

Comment

Ankylosing spondylitis is frequently seen in young adults, who are usually males. This condition is characterized by an inflammatory process that involves primarily the soft-tissue elements of the spine. The synovial membranes, capsules, and ligaments of the joints of the spine become swollen, edematous and thickened. These changes are followed by calcification and eventually ossification. The result is bony ankylosis of all the affected joints. With ankylosing spondylitis, the pathologic process is confined to the intervertebral joints, the posterior articular joints, the sacroiliac joints, and the surrounding ligaments. The peripheral joints of the extremities are spared.

The proliferative process in the soft tissue in and about the intervertebral foramina (the capsules of the posterior joints, the ligamentum flavum, and the posterior longitudinal ligament) narrows the outlet and may press and irritate the nerve roots that are traversing the bony canals. In addition, the sheaths of the nerves are involved, so the roots are enmeshed and fixed in a mass of fibrous tissue. It becomes apparent that body movements that stretch the roots, such as flexing the leg when extended at the knee, will accentuate the pain in the back and leg.

Lower back pain and sciatica are common complaints in all stages of this disorder, and the incidence of sciatica is greater than formerly realized. In the early stages, diagnostic imaging is not informative, so making the diagnosis is very difficult. At this early stage the clinical picture may mimic that of a disc lesion in the lumbar spine although the early clinical picture does not unequivocally simulate that of a lumbar disc lesion. Lower back pain is the first manifestation. The area involved is not only the lumbosacral region but also the regions of the sacroiliac joints. Pain may be referred to the buttocks and the posterior aspects of the thighs. The syndrome is punctuated by remissions. The pain, which is not of a mechanical nature, is influenced by weather changes. The patient experiences considerable stiffness in the dorsal region and in the thoracic cage. Later, sciatica in one or both legs appears, and all movements of the spine are restricted, especially flexion. As time goes on the lumbar spine is flattened, the patient begins to stoop forward, the cervical curve becomes exaggerated, and flexion contractures of the hips develop. At this point the clinical picture of ankylosing spondylitis is evident and can be confirmed by diagnostic imaging. Imaging reveals characteristic changes in the posterior articulations and the sacroiliac joints.

Some muscle spasm of the dorsolumbar spine can be demonstrated, and some tenderness can be elicited over the spinous processes and a little to each side of the midline. As the process progresses, the excursions of the thorax become smaller and smaller until the thoracic cage becomes completely rigid and fixed. Throughout the active stages of the disease the sedimentation rate is always elevated and is a good index to the activity of the process, but serologic tests for rheumatoid factor are usually negative.

Procedure

Schober's test may be used to measure the amount of flexion occurring in the lumbar spine. To do this, a point is marked at the level of S2. Then points are marked 0.5 cm below and 10 cm above the S2 level. The distance between the inferior and superior points is measured. The patient is asked to flex forward, and the distance is remeasured. The difference between the two measurements is an indication of the amount of flexion occurring in the lumbar spine. The distance should increase at least 5 cm to 8 cm.

Confirmation Procedures

Bilateral leg-lowering test, Demianoff's sign, double leg-raise test, hyperextension test, Lewin supine test, match stick test, Mennell's sign, Minor's sign, Nachlas test, Quick test, sign of the buttock, skin pinch test, spinal percussion test, Vanzetti's sign

---

Reporting Statement

Schober's test demonstrates that no motion occurs in the lumbosacral spine during flexion.

Schober's test demonstrates that motion greater than the base of 10 cm occurs in the lumbosacral spine during flexion.

～ Clinical Pearl ～

For a modification of this test, the patient is placed in a maximal flexion position (seated or standing) and, starting from the upper sacral spinous prominence, three, 10 cm segments are marked up the spine. The distances between the marks are then remeasured while the patient is erect. The lowest segment should shorten by at least 50%, the middle should shorten by 40%, and the upper should shorten by 30%. The shortening effect will be greater in tall subjects.

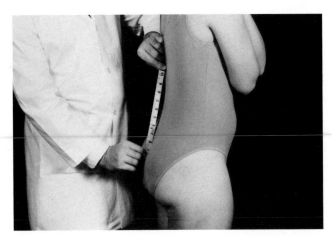

Fig. 8–81   The patient is standing with the arms folded across the chest. The examiner marks a point level with S2. Points 0.5 cm below and 10 cm above the original S2 level line are marked.

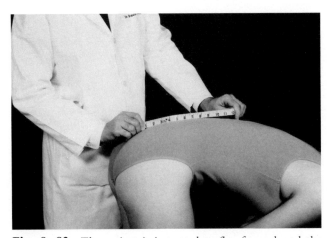

Fig. 8–82   The patient is instructed to flex forward, and the distances between the inferior and superior points are remeasured and compared with the original measurements. The difference between the two sets of measurements indicates the amount of flexion occurring in the lumbar spine. The distance should increase at least 5 cm to 8 cm.

∽ Sicard's Sign ∽

Comment

Characteristic of sciatic pain, increased intraabdominal pressure produced by coughing and sneezing markedly increases the severity of the pain. Patients with a severe attack will walk with the hip and knee slightly flexed and place the foot slowly on the floor. This carefulness is done to prevent any undue traction of the nerve root, which normally occurs when the extended leg is flexed at the hip. On the other hand, some of the patients exhibit no external malfunction. They do not experience back pain or muscle spasm. Back motion is free and unrestricted and the patients are able, in most instances, to carry on their daily activities.

A sudden onset of pain usually occurs when a nuclear extrusion touches a nerve root. This phenomenon may occur either during the stage of nuclear sequestration (the intermediate stage) or toward the end of the pathologic process in the nucleus. Fibrosis of the disc is the predominant feature, but fragments of nuclear material that may be extruded may still be present. The distance that the pain spreads along a dermatome is directly proportional to the amount of tension and compression to which the root is subjected.

An interesting phenomenon is observed in patients with severe sciatica. The pain may suddenly disappear, but the motor and sensory deficits remain, which indicates that the physiologic function of the root is completely interrupted.

This lack of pain must not be misconstrued as evidence that the patient is getting better.

Any of the patterns of sciatica may be initiated simply by contact with a sensitive nerve root and without actual herniation of nuclear material. Slight bulging, without rupture, of the annulus may be sufficient to precipitate a sciatic syndrome merely because the bulge touches the hypersensitive nerve root.

Procedure

While the patient is supine, the extended leg is raised to a point just short of that which produces pain. When the sign is present, dorsiflexion of the great toe reproduces sciatic pain. The test is significant for sciatic radiculopathy.

Confirmation Procedures

Bechterew's sitting test, Bragard's sign, Deyerle's sign, Fajersztajn's test, Lasègue differential sign, Lasègue rebound test, Lasègue's sitting test, Lasègue test, Lewin standing test, Lindner's sign, straight-leg raising test, Turyn's sign

Reporting Statement

Sicard's sign is positive on the right. This sign indicates sciatic radiculopathy.

∽ Clinical Pearl ∽

The second, third, and fourth nerve roots do not have an increase in tension during the straight-leg raising, but they do undergo an increase in tension during the femoral stretch tests.

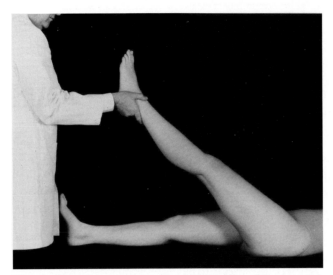

Fig. 8–83   The patient is supine with both legs fully extended. The examiner straight-leg raises the affected leg to the point at which symptoms are reproduced.

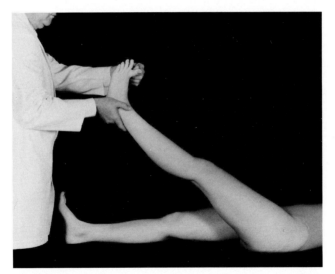

Fig. 8–84   The leg is lowered to a point just below that which produces symptoms, and the examiner sharply dorsiflexes the great toe of the affected foot. The sign is present if toe dorsiflexion reproduces the symptoms. The sign is present with sciatic radiculopathy.

Comment

The most common injury to the buttocks is from a direct blow. This does not usually cause injury to the skin because of the ample underlying padding. Contusion of the muscle is a common occurrence, but usually it is of little consequence. In most of the areas of the buttocks there is a thick muscle mass that is in little danger of being caught between two unyielding objects. As a result, the condition resulting from a blow is diffuse without gross hematoma formation in the muscle. A tender, painful muscle mass results and although it may be uncomfortable, the condition is not disabling. During athletic competition the buttocks are usually not protected by any padding other than that inherent in the athlete's anatomy. Superficial contusion is common, and the examiner should be wary of the condition that is unduly severe or that causes something other than local symptoms.

A contusion of the sciatic nerve may result in pain that begins in the buttock and extends down the back of the thigh into the calf and foot in a way that is similar to sciatic pain from other causes. This pain is nonradicular in character and follows the whole distribution of the sciatic nerve rather than any single nerve root. Straight-leg raising causes pain in the area of the contusion. During the acute period, hypesthesia (hypoesthesia) of the skin may be evident in the lower portion of the extremity. This contusion of the sciatic nerve will require no particular treatment other than protection against stretch.

Another area of the buttocks in which a complication of contusion may arise is over the ischial tuberosity. Here the bone is subcutaneous, although it is protected by a layer of muscle of greater or lesser thickness. A contusion here may cause a fracture of the tuberosity, in which case there will be severe pain. The pain is increased by straight-leg raising or by any local pressure. More commonly, the result of the blow will be periostitis or fibrositis over the roughened surface of the bone. In other cases there will be involvement of the ischial bursa. It is impossible, in the early stages, to distinguish between these conditions.

Procedure

The patient lies supine, and the examiner performs a passive unilateral straight-leg test. If there is unilateral restriction, the examiner flexes the knee to see whether hip flexion increases. If the problem is in the lumbar spine, hip flexion will increase. If hip flexion does not increase when the knee is flexed, it is a positive sign of the buttock. The sign is present in instances of bursitis, tumor, or abscess. The patient also exhibits a noncapsular pattern of the hip.

Confirmation Procedures

Bilateral leg-lowering test, Demianoff's sign, double leg-raise test, hyperextension test, Lewin supine test, match stick test, Mennell's sign, Minor's sign, Nachlas test, Quick test, Schober's test, skin pinch test, spinal percussion test, Vanzetti's sign

---

Reporting Statement

The sign of the buttock is present on the right. The presence of this sign indicates that a condition affecting the hip or buttock is responsible for the patient's pain complaint.

～ Clinical Pearl ～

Trochanteric bursitis causes localized pain and tenderness over the trochanter and occasionally causes pain that radiates down the lateral thigh. The pain is particularly strong when lying on the affected side. Pain from ischiogluteal bursitis is felt posteriorly and is particularly exacerbated by sitting.

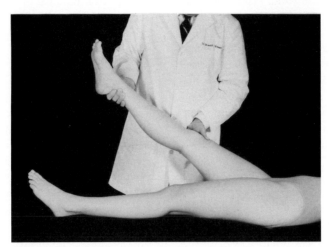

Fig. 8–85   The patient is supine with both legs fully extended. The examiner performs a straight-leg raising test on the affected leg.

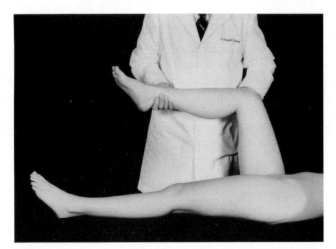

Fig. 8–86   If there is restriction of the leg movement because of pain or myospasm, the examiner flexes the knee. If the problem is in the lumbar spine, hip flexion will increase. If hip flexion does not increase when the knee is flexed, it is a positive sign of the buttock. A positive sign indicates hip or buttock bursitis, tumor, or abscess.

Comment

Fibromyalgia syndrome or fibromyositis syndrome really does not present a formidable differential diagnosis even though it causes symmetrical arthralgia and myalgia, which are usually worse after awakening in the morning. Patients complain of stiffness, but, unlike persons with rheumatoid arthritis, they are not stiff. Joint swelling is absent and tenderness is mild, except over tense muscles. Muscle atrophy is never seen. There are no constitutional symptoms, such as fever and weight loss. The erythrocyte sedimentation rate is normal, and the test for rheumatoid factor is negative. Patients are rarely anemic, and diagnostic imaging of the joints is normal. Most patients with the fibromyalgia syndrome are emotionally tense.

Nonarticular (soft tissue) *rheumatism* is a term that encompasses a large group of miscellaneous conditions with a common denominator of musculoskeletal pain and stiffness. This designation is for convenience only and not because of any common etiologic or clinical characteristics. Although some forms of nonarticular rheumatism, such as bursitis and tendinitis, present well-defined features, the causes of others, including fibrositis and myalgia, are not as clear.

Fibrositis is defined as inflammatory hyperplasia of white connective tissue. It is now a term used rarely in the presence of such real tissue inflammation as arthritis, tendinitis, or myositis. Among rheumatologists, fibrositis indicates aching, stiffness, tenderness, and pain around joints, muscles fibers, and subcutaneous tissues without the presence of an inflammatory pathologic process. Fibrositis is a local and diffuse idiopathic condition. The symptom complex of fibrositis, with or without connective tissue inflammation, may be a prominent manifestation of many rheumatic diseases, including systemic lupus erythematosus, rheumatoid arthritis, and subdeltoid bursitis.

Procedure

The skin pinch test involves smoothly rolling the skin over the spinous process of the vertebrae, by using the forefingers over the advancing thumbs. The skin is picked up before rolling it. Skin rolling is then performed over each side of the back. Fibrositic infiltration and trigger points are demonstrated by tightness and acute tenderness. There will be tightness and tenderness, maximally over the level at which a pathologic bone condition exists or over the vertebra above the level at which a pathologic joint or disc condition exists.

Confirmation Procedures

Bilateral leg-lowering test, Demianoff's sign, double leg-raise test, hyperextension test, Lewin supine test, match stick test, Mennell's sign, Minor's sign, Nachlas test, Quick test, Schober's test, sign of the buttock, spinal percussion test, Vanzetti's sign

---

Reporting Statement

Skin pinch testing over the lumbosacral area demonstrates trophedematous tissue. A positive test indicates fibrositic infiltration and trigger points in the affected tissue.

∾ Clinical Pearl ∾

Trophedematous subcutaneous tissue has a boggy, inelastic texture when rolled between the thumb and finger. This type of tissue is distinguishable from subcutaneous fat. When a patch of skin and subcutaneous tissue a centimeter in diameter is gently squeezed together, instead of immediately forming a fold of flesh, trophedematous tissue does not budge, or it finally yields altogether, with a sudden expanding movement similar to that of inflating a rubber dinghy or air mattress.

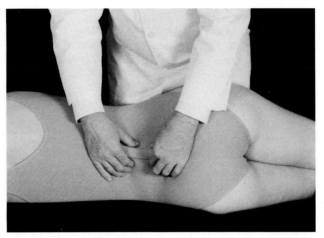

Fig. 8–87 The patient is either in the prone or side-lying positions. The examiner picks up an area of skin overlying the affected level of the spine. The examiner performs smooth rolling of the skin over the spinous process of the vertebrae, moving the forefingers over the advancing thumbs. Skin rolling is then performed over each side of the back. The test is positive if tightness and acute tenderness are elicited. A positive test indicates fibrositic infiltration and trigger points.

Comment

Vehicular accidents are a common source of trauma to the lumbosacral spine and may cause a wide variety of fractures and dislocations. Compression fractures at the anterior edge of the vertebral bodies may be caused by a hyperflexion motion alone or in combination with a vertical compression. The stability of these fractures depends on the degree of vertebral compression and the presence or absence of posterior ligamentous damage.

Traumatic injuries of the lumbosacral spine are among the most common causes of disability following trauma.

Because the question of cord damage is dominant, spine fractures are classified as stable or unstable. In stable fractures the cord is rarely damaged and movement of the spine is safe. In unstable fractures the cord may have been damaged, but if it has escaped damage, it may still be injured by movement.

Stability depends largely on the integrity of the ligaments, and in particular the posterior ligament complex. This complex consists of the supraspinous ligament, the interspinous ligaments, the capsules of the facet joints, and possibly the ligamentum flavum. Fortunately only 10% of the spinal injuries are unstable and less than 5% are associated with cord damage.

Injuries usually occur when the spinal column is compressed and collapsed in its vertical axis. This injury typically occurs during a fall from a height or when the patient gets trapped under a cave-in, the direction of the force at any level of the spine is determined by the position of the vertebral column during impact. The flexible lumbar segments also may be injured by violent, free movements of the trunk. The important types of displacement are (1) hyperextension, (2) flexion, (3) flexion combined with rotation, and (4) axial displacement (compression).

Hyperextension is rare in the thoracolumbar spine. When hyperextension occurs, the anterior ligaments and the disc may be damaged or the neural arch may be fractured. Usually the injury is stable, but fracture of the pedicle is often unstable.

If the posterior ligaments remain intact, forced flexion will crush the vertebral body into a wedge. This is a stable injury and is by far the most common type of vertebral fracture. If the posterior ligaments are torn, the upper vertebral body may tilt forward on the one below. This type of subluxation is often missed because by the time the diagnostic image is made, the vertebrae have fallen back into place.

Most serious injuries of the spine are due to a combination of flexion and rotation. The ligaments and joint capsules, which are strained to the limit, may tear. The facets may fracture, or the top of one vertebra may be sheared off. The result is a forward shift, or dislocation, of the vertebra above, with or without concomitant bone damage. All fracture-dislocations are unstable.

A vertical force acting on a straight segment of the lumbar spine will compress the vertebral body and may cause a comminuted, or burst, fracture. If the vertebra is split, a large fragment may be driven backwards into the spinal canal. It is this fragment that makes these fractures dangerous. Such fractures are associated with a high incidence of neurologic damage.

Compression of a lumbar vertebra may occur with minimal force in osteoporotic or pathologic bone.

Procedure

While the patient is standing and the trunk is slightly flexed, the examiner uses a neurologic hammer to percuss the spinous processes and the associated musculature of each of the lumbar vertebra. Evidence of localized pain indicates a possible vertebra fracture. Evidence of radicular pain indicates a possible disc lesion. Because of the nonspecific nature of this test, other conditions will also elicit a positive pain response. For example, a ligamentous sprain will cause pain when the spinous processes are percussed. Percussing the paraspinal musculature will elicit a positive sign for muscular strain.

Confirmation Procedures

Bilateral leg-lowering test, Demianoff's sign, double leg-raise test, hyperextension test, Lewin supine test, match stick test, Mennell's sign, Minor's sign, Nachlas test, Quick test, Schober's test, sign of the buttock, skin pinch test, Vanzetti's sign

---

Reporting Statement

Spinal percussion elicits pain on the spinous process of L5. This result suggests osseous injury at that level.

Spinal percussion elicits pain at the paraspinals on the right of L5. This result suggests soft-tissue injury at that level.

~ Clinical Pearl ~

When soft-tissue percussion reproduces the complaint, the examiner may expect the same phenomenon from the use of ultrasound on the tissue. The uses of such therapies may be delayed until the soft tissue is no longer reactive to percussion.

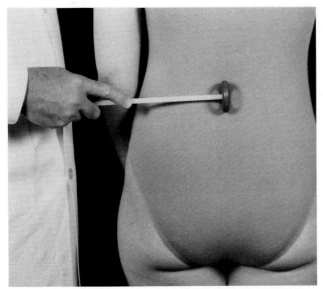

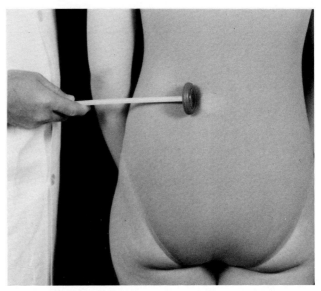

Fig. 8-88 In the standing position the patient flexes the lumbosacral spine, exposing the spinous processes as much as possible. The examiner percusses the spinous processes of each vertebra. Localized pain is evidence of a fracture or severe sprain. Radiating pain suggests an intervertebral disc syndrome.

Fig. 8-89 The paravertebral tissues are percussed similarly. Pain elicited in the soft tissues suggests muscular strain and highly sensitive myofascial trigger points.

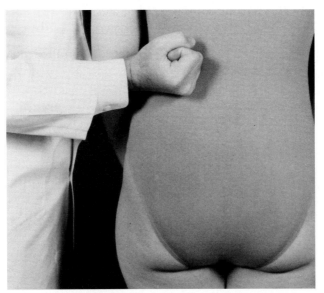

Fig. 8-90 The examiner may perform gross percussion of the lumbar paraspinal tissue. This maneuver is similar to the Lewin punch test. Pain elicited suggests soft-tissue injury.

Comment

During the unilateral straight-leg raising test, tension develops sequentially. It first develops in the greater sciatic foramen, followed by tension over the ala of the sacrum. Next, as the nerve crosses over the pedicle, tension develops in this area. Finally, tension occurs in the intervertebral foramen. The straight-leg raising test will cause traction on the sciatic nerve, lumbosacral nerve roots, and dura mater. Adhesions within these areas may be due to herniation of the intervertebral disc or to extradural or meningeal irritation. Pain that is felt by the patient comes from the dura mater, nerve root, adventitial sheath of the epidural veins, or the synovial facet joints. The test is positive if pain extends from the back, down the leg along the sciatic nerve distribution.

A central protrusion of an intervertebral disc will lead to pain primarily in the back. A protrusion in the intermediate area will cause pain in the posterior aspect of the lower limb and lower back. A lateral protrusion will cause primarily posterior leg pain.

The straight-leg raising test is performed by the examiner while the patient is completely relaxed. It is a passive test, and each leg is tested individually. While the patient is in the supine position, with the hip medially rotated and the knee extended, the examiner flexes the hip until the patient complains of pain or tightness. The examiner drops the leg back slightly until there is no complaint. The patient is then instructed to flex the neck, so the chin is on the chest. In some cases, if the patient has limited neck movement, the examiner may dorsiflex the patient's foot (Bragard's sign). Both actions may be done simultaneously. The neck flexion movement has also been called the Hyndman's sign or Brudzinski's sign. Pain that increases during neck flexion, foot dorsiflexion, or both results from stretching of the dura mater of the spinal cord. Pain that does not increase with neck flexion may indicate tight hamstrings or lumbosacral or sacroiliac joint involvement. Unilateral straight-leg raising is full at 60 to 70 degrees. At this level the nerves are completely stretched, primarily the L5, S1, and S2 nerve roots, having an excursion of several millimeters. Pain after 60 to 70 degrees is probably joint pain from the lumbar area or sacroiliac joints. The examiner compares both legs for any differences.

In the dynamics of unilateral straight-leg raising, the slack in sciatic arborization is taken up from 0 to 35 degrees. There is no dural movement. When approaching 35 degrees, tension is applied to the sciatic nerve roots. In the range of 35 to 70 degrees the sciatic nerve roots tense over the intervertebral disc. The rate of nerve root deformation diminishes as the angle increases. Above 60 to 70 degrees there is practically no further deformation of the root that occurs during further straight-leg raising and the pain probably originates in the joint.

Procedure

The patient lies supine with the legs extended. The examiner places one hand under the heel of the affected leg and the other hand on the knee. With the limb extended the examiner flexes the thigh on the pelvis. If this maneuver is markedly limited due to pain, the test is positive and may suggest sciatica from lumbosacral or sacroiliac lesions, subluxation syndrome, disc lesions, spondylolisthesis, adhesions, or IVF occlusion.

The exacerbation of pain by raising the extended leg is further evidence of the effects of traction on a sensitized nerve root. Normally the leg can be raised 15 to 30 degrees before the nerve root is tractioned through the intervertebral foramen. Pain, duplicating sciatica, that is elicited by this maneuver indicates a space-occupying lesion—such as lumbar disc protrusion, tumor, adhesions, edema, and tissue inflammation—at the nerve root level.

Confirmation Procedures

Bechterew's sitting test, Bragard's sign, Deyerle's sign, Fajersztajn's test, Lasègue differential sign, Lasègue rebound test, Lasègue sitting test, Lasègue test, Lewin standing test, Lindner's sign, Sicard's sign, Turyn's sign

---

Reporting Statement

Straight-leg raising is positive on the right at 30 degrees. This result indicates stretching of the dura mater due to a space-occupying mass in the path of the nerve root.

Straight-leg raising is positive on the right at 45 degrees. This result suggests sciatic irritation because of sacroiliac inflammation.

Straight-leg raising on the right produces pain, at 70 degrees, in the lower back. This result indicates lumbosacral involvement.

~ **Clinical Pearl** ~

As many authors have pointed out, the nerve roots have a narrow range of movement for stretching. Most authors as well conclude that the nerve roots, in the normal conditions, are not stretched by the straight-leg raising test until 35 to 70 degrees of angulation have been reached. However, if the nerve exists with a space-occupying mass (protrusion of disc material) that deflects the nerve's normal pathway, the amount of allowable stretch is already used up by the mass. In this case the positive sign, pain radiating down the sciatic distribution, occurs at a much lower angulation. This pain has been misconstrued by many to indicate the involvement of the sacroiliac joint instead of the sensitive finding that a nerve root compression syndrome exists. Sciatica that is in the leg and produced from 0 to 30 degrees is due to nerve root compression. Sciatica that is in the leg and produced from 30 to 60 degrees is probably due to sacroiliac joint disease. Sciatica that is in the leg and produced above 60 degrees is probably due to lumbosacral disease.

It is a cardinal point that most, if not all, ranges of movement given for the sciatic nerve roots are based on the absence of a space-occupying mass. The angles change dramatically in the presence of disease. This change is the basis of the Cox sign (which reveals the diseased or compressed nerve root) and Deyerle's sign (which reveals the normal nerve root but diseased sacroiliac or lumbosacral musculature).

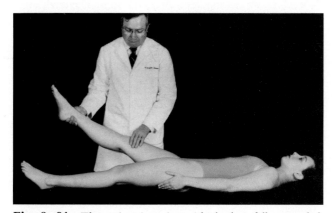

Fig. 8–91 The patient is supine with the legs fully extended. The examiner places one hand under the ankle of the affected leg and the other hand on the knee. The examiner flexes the thigh on the pelvis.

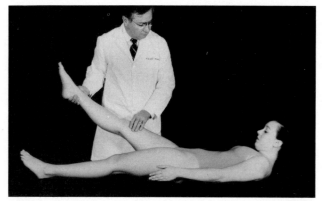

Fig. 8–92 Once the leg reaches the point at which symptoms are reproduced, the patient is instructed to flex the cervical spine and approximate the chin to the chest. If this maneuver is markedly limited because of pain, the test is positive. A positive test suggests sciatica from lumbosacral or sacroiliac lesions, subluxation syndrome, disc lesions, spondylolisthesis, adhesions, or IVF occlusion. The angle at which symptoms were reproduced is recorded for future testing.

Comment

Pain that radiates down the back of the leg is termed sciatica regardless of whether it is associated with lower back pain. The pain can be referred from the back along the thigh to the foot and toe. On the other hand, sciatica also can be caused by referred pain that radiates in the opposite direction from the foot upward. In some cases of sciatica the presence of trigger areas in the lower part of the back can be demonstrated. These trigger areas, when compressed, will set off the pain along the sciatic distribution.

Although herniated intervertebral discs are credited for most cases of sciatica, they do not account for all such symptoms. Diagnosis should be based on careful neurologic evaluation and, when necessary, diagnostic imaging and other tests. The straight-leg raising test is not pathognomonic. There are instances when, although a disc is central and there are no symptoms of pressure on the nerve root, there is sciatic radiation of the pain and the prolapsed disc is credited as the cause of sciatica.

Sciatica has a variety of causes, some of which produce this type of posterior leg pain without seeming to involve the sciatic nerve or its contributory roots. Conditions that should be ruled out include the following: (1) prolapsed intervertebral disc pressure, infection, and traumatic sciatic neuritis, perineural fibrositis, infections, and tumors of the spinal cord; (2) lumbosacral and sacroiliac sprain and strain, degenerating intervertebral discs, fibrositis, osteomyelitis, hip joint disease, and secondary carcinomatous deposits in bone; (3) nephrolithiasis, prostatic, renal, and anal disease; (4) toxic and metabolic disorders, conversion hysteria, and arterial insufficiency.

Procedure

When the patient is in the supine position with both lower limbs resting straight out on the table, dorsiflexion of the great toe elicits pain in the gluteal region. The sign is significant for sciatic radiculopathy.

Confirmation Procedures

Bechterew's sitting test, Bragard's sign, Deyerle's sign, Fajersztajn's sign, Lasègue differential sign, Lasègue rebound test, Lasègue sitting test, Lasègue test, Lewin standing test, Lindner's sign, Sicard's sign, straight-leg raising test

Reporting Statement

Turyn's sign is present on the right. The presence of this sign suggests sciatic radiculopathy.

≈ Clinical Pearl ≈

A straight-leg raising test that is positive under 30 degrees reveals a large disc protrusion. The nerve root is stretched long before it would normally be. The straight-leg raising is most useful for identifying L5-S1 disc lesions because the pressures on the nerve root are highest at this level. During straight-leg raising, L4-L5 is not as apt to give as much pain as the L5-S1 because the pressure between the disc and the nerve root at L4-L5 is half that at L5-S1. Therefore the L5-S1 disc lesion gives more pain in the lower back and leg than does the L4-L5 disc lesion. No movement on the nerve root occurs until straight-leg raising reaches 30 degrees. No movement on L4 occurs during a straight-leg raising test. From this the presence of a Turyn's sign indicates a large disc protrusion at the level of the L5-S1 nerve root.

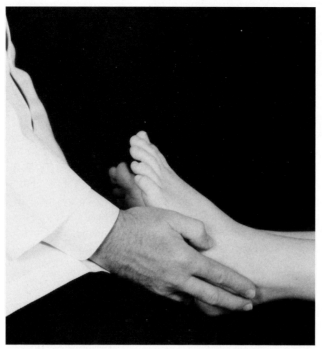

Fig. 8–93 The patient is in the supine position, with both lower limbs fully extended on the examination table.

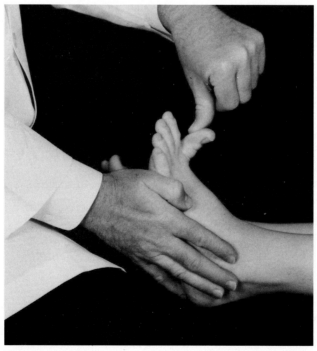

Fig. 8–94 The examiner sharply dorsiflexes the great toe of the affected leg. Pain elicited in the gluteal region is a positive sign. The sign is present in sciatic radiculopathy.

Comment

Scoliosis is a lateral curvature of the spine. For the management of any case the first and most important decision to make is whether there is any deformity of the vertebrae (structural scoliosis). If the vertebrae are normal (nonstructural scoliosis) the deformity is usually one of the following: (1) compensatory, resulting from tilting of the pelvis from real or apparent shortening of one leg, or (2) sciatic, resulting from a unilateral protective muscle spasm, especially accompanying a prolapsed intervertebral disc.

With sciatic scoliosis the underlying cause is a prolapsed intervertebral disc that impinges on a lumbar or sacral nerve. The deformity also may be observed in some cases of acute lower back pain, the pathogenesis of which is not clear. For this type of scoliosis the curve is in the lumbar region. The abnormal posture is assumed involuntarily in an attempt to reduce the painful pressure upon the affected nerve or joint. The predominant feature is severe back pain, or sciatica, that is aggravated by movements of the spine. The onset of this pain is usually sudden. The scoliosis is poorly compensated and the trunk may be tilted markedly to one side. The curvature is not associated with rotation of the vertebrae.

With structural scoliosis there is alteration in vertebral shape and mobility, and the deformity cannot be corrected by alteration of posture. A careful history and examination are required to find a cause and give a prognosis. Structural scoliosis may be congenital and may be due to a hemivertebra, to fused vertebrae, or to absent or fused ribs.

With paralytic scoliosis the deformity is secondary to loss of the supportive action of the trunk and spinal muscles, which is almost always a sequel to anterior poliomyelitis.

Neuropathic scoliosis is seen as a complication of neurofibromatosis, cerebral palsy, spina bifida, syringomyelia, Friedreich's ataxia, and neuropathic conditions. Primary disorders of the supportive musculature (muscular dystrophy, arthrogryposis) are responsible for myopathic scoliosis. Metabolic scoliosis is uncommon but occurs in cystine storage disease, Marfan's syndrome, and rickets. Idiopathic scoliosis is the most common, and by far, the most important of the structural scolioses. The cause of idiopathic scoliosis remains obscure. Several vertebrae at one or, less commonly, two distinct levels are affected and cause a primary curve. In the area of the primary curve there is loss of mobility (the fixed curve) and rotational deformity of the vertebrae (the spinous processes rotate into the concavity, and the bodies, which carry the ribs in the thoracic region, rotate into the convexity). Above and below the fixed primary curves, secondary curves that are mobile develop to maintain the normal position of the head and pelvis. The spinal deformity is accompanied by shortening of the trunk, and there is often impairment of respiratory and cardiac function. In severe cases this may lead to invalidism and a shortened life expectancy.

Procedure

With sciatica the pelvis is always horizontal even though scoliosis exists. When scoliosis is present with other spinal lesions, the pelvis will be tilted.

Confirmation Procedures

Bilateral leg-lowering test, Demianoff's sign, double leg-raise test, hyperextension test, Lewin supine test, match stick test, Mennell's sign, Minor's sign, Nachlas test, Quick test, Schober's test, sign of the buttock, skin pinch test, spinal percussion test

---

Reporting Statement

Vanzetti's sign is present in the presentation of a right-sided antalgia. The presence of this sign suggests a sciatic scoliosis.

~ Clinical Pearl ~

Vanzetti's sign allows quick observation of the patient to determine the source of the patient's antalgia before performing the more aggressive assessments of the lumbosacral spine.

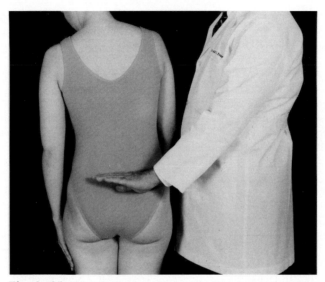

Fig. 8–95   The patient is standing with the arms comfortably at the sides. The examiner assesses the level of the pelvis and sacrum. In spite of the antalgia the pelvis is always horizontal in sciatic conditions. For other spinal lesions, when scoliosis is present, the pelvis is tilted.

Bibliography

American Medical Association: *Guides to the evaluation of permanent impairment,* ed 3, Chicago, 1990, The Association.

Apley AG, Solomon L: *Concise system of orthopaedics and fractures,* London, 1988, Butterworth-Heinemann.

Batson OV: The function of the vertebral veins and their role in the spread of metastasis, *Ann Surg,* 112:138, 1940.

Borenstein DG, Wiesel SW: *Low back pain medical diagnosis and comprehensive management,* Philadelphia, 1989, WB Saunders.

Bradford FK: Low back sprain and ruptured intervertebral disc, *Med Times,* 88:797-808, 1960.

Breig A, Troup JDG: Biomechanical considerations in straight-leg-raising test: Cadaveric and clinical studies of the effects of medial hip rotation, *Spine,* 4:242, 1979.

Brody IA, Williams RH: The signs of Kernig and Brudzinksi, *Arch Neurol,* 21:215, 1969.

Brudzinski J: A new sign of the lower extremities in meningitis of children (neck sign), *Arch Neurol,* 21:216, 1969.

Cailliet R: *Low back pain syndrome,* ed 3, Philadelphia, 1981, FA Davis.

Cailliet R: *Soft tissue pain and disability,* Philadelphia, 1977, FA Davis.

Cipriano JJ: *Photographic manual of regional orthopaedic and neurological tests,* ed 2, Baltimore, 1991, Williams and Wilkins.

Cloward RB: Lesions of the intervertebral disc and their treatment by interbody fusion methods: The painful disc, *Clin Orthop* 27:51, 1963.

Cox JM: *Low back pain mechanism, diagnosis and treatment,* ed 5, Baltimore, 1990, Williams and Wilkins.

Cyriax J: *Textbook for orthopaedic medicine, vol 1: Diagnosis of soft tissue lesions,* London, 1975, Bailliere Tindall.

Cyrias JH: Lesions discals lombaires, *Acta Orthop Belg,* 27:442, 1961.

D'Ambrosia RD: *Musculoskeletal disorders regional examination and differential diagnosis,* Philadelphia, 1977, JB Lippincott.

Dandy DJ: *Essential orthopaedics and trauma,* Edinburgh, 1989, Churchill Livingstone.

Daniels L, Worthingham C: *Muscle testing: Techniques of manual examination,* Philadelphia, 1980, WB Saunders.

DePalma AF, Rothman RH: *The intervertebral disc,* Philadelphia, 1970, WB Saunders.

Deyerle WM, May VR: Sciatic tension test, *South Med J,* 49:999, 1956.

Doherty M, Doherty J: *Clinical examination in rheumatology,* London, 1992, Wolfe Publishing.

Dommisse GF, Grobler L: Arteries and veins of the lumbar nerve roots and cauda equina, *Clin Orthop,* 115:22, 1976.

Dyck P: The femoral nerve traction test with lumbar disc protrusion, *Surg Neurol,* 6:163, 1976.

Dyck P: The stoop-test in lumbar entrapment radiculopathy, *Spine,* 4:89, 1979.

Edgar MA, Ghadially JA: Innervation of the lumbar spine, *Clin Orthop,* 115:35, 1976.

Edgar MS, Park WM: Induced pain patterns on passive straight-leg-raising in lower lumbar disc protrusion, *J Bone Joint Surg,* 56B:658, 1974.

Epstein BS: *The spine, a radiological text and atlas,* ed 3, Philadelphia, 1969, Lea & Febiger.

Ericksen MF: Aging in the lumbar spine, *Am J Phys Anthropol,* 48:241, 1974.

Fahrni WH: Observations on straight-leg raising with special reference to nerve root adhesions, *Can J Surg,* 9:44, 1966.

Farfan HF: *Mechanical disorders of the low back,* Philadelphia, 1973, Lea & Febiger.

Fernstrom U, Goldie I: Does granulation tissue in the intervertebral disc provoke back pain? *Acta Orthop Scand,* 30:202, 1960.

Gartland JJ: *Fundamentals of orthopaedics,* Philadelphia, 1974, WB Saunders.

Gillis L: *Diagnosis in orthopaedics,* London, 1969, Butterworths.

Goddard BS, Reid JD: Movements induced by straight-leg-raising in the Lumbo-sacral roots, nerves, and plexus and in the intra pelvic section of the sciatic nerve, *J Neurol Neurosurg Psychiatry,* 28:12, 1965.

Gunn CC, Milbrandt WE: Early and subtle signs in low-back sprain, *Spine,* 3:267, 1978.

Hansson T, Bigos S, Beecher P, Worthley M: The lumbar lordosis in acute and chronic low-back pain, *Spine,* 10:154, 1985.

Helfet AJ, Gruebel Lee DM: *Disorders of the lumbar spine,* Philadelphia, 1978, JB Lippincott.

Herlin L: *Sciatic and pelvic pain due to lumbosacral nerve root compression,* Springfield, 1966, Charles C. Thomas.

Herron LD, Pheasant HC: Prone knee-flexion provocative testing for lumbar disc protrusion, *Spine,* 5:65, 1980.

Hollinshead WH: *Anatomy for surgeons, vol 3, the back and limbs,* ed 3, Philadelphia, 1982, Harper and Row.

Hudgins WR: The crossed-straight-leg-raising test, *N Engl J Med,* 297:1127, 1977.

Jackson HC, Winkelman KK, Bichel WH: Nerve endings in the human lumbar spine column and related structures, *J Bone Joint Surg,* 48A:1272, 1966.

Kapandji IA: *The physiology of the joints, vol 3, the trunk and the vertebral column,* Edinburgh, 1974, Churchill Livingstone.

Katz WA: *Rheumatic diseases diagnosis and management,* Philadelphia, 1977, JB Lippincott.

Katznelson A, Nerubay J, Level A: Gluteal skyline (G.S.L.): A search for an objective sign in the diagnosis of disc lesions of the lower lumbar spine, *Spine,* 7:74, 1982.

Keim HA: *The adolescent spine,* ed 2, New York, 1976, Springer-Verlag.

Kelsey JL: An epidemiological study of acute herniated lumbar intervertebral disc, *Rheumatol Rehab,* 14:144, 1975.

Kendall HO, Kendall FP, Wadsworth GE: *Muscles testing and function,* ed 2, Baltimore, 1971, Williams and Wilkins.

Kernig W: Concerning a little noted sign of meningitis, *Arch Neurol,* 21:216, 1969.

Koppell HP, Thompson WAL: *Peripheral entrapment neuropathies,* Baltimore, 1963, Williams and Wilkins.

LaFreniere JG: *The low-back patient, procedures for treatment by physical therapy,* New York, 1985, Masson Publishing.

Lecuire J et al: 641 operations for sciatic neuralgia due to discal hernia, a computerized statistical study of the results, *Neurochirugia (Stuttg),* 19:501, 1973.

MacNab I: *Backache,* Baltimore, 1977, Williams and Wilkins.

Magee DJ: *Orthopedic physical assessment,* Philadelphia, 1987, WB Saunders.

Magora A: Investigation of the relation between low back pain and occupation: 4, physical requirements: bending, rotation, reaching and sudden maximal effort, *Scand J Rehab Med,* 5:186, 1973.

Mason M, Currey HLF: *Clinical rheumatology,* Philadelphia, 1970, JB Lippincott.

Mayo Clinic and Mayo Foundation: *Clinical examinations in neurology,* ed 5, Philadelphia, 1981, WB Saunders.

Mazion JM: *Illustrated manual of neurological reflexes/signs/tests, part I, orthopedic signs/tests/maneuvers for office procedure, Part II,* Orlando, 1980, Daniels Publishing.

McRae R: *Clinical orthopaedic examination,* ed 3, Edinburgh, 1990, Churchill Livingstone.

Medical Economics Books: *Patient care flow chart manual,* ed 3, Oradell, NJ, 1982, Medical Economics Books.

Mennell JM: *Back pain,* Boston, 1960, Little, Brown.

Morris JM, Lucas DB, Bresler B: Role of the trunk in stability of the spine, *J Bone Joint Surg,* 43A:327, 1961.

Nachemson A: The lumbar spine-an orthopaedic challenge, *Spine,* 1:59, 1976.

O'Donoghue DH: *Treatment of injuries to athletes,* ed 4, Philadelphia, 1984, WB Saunders.

Olson WH, Brumback RA, Gascon G, Iyer V: *Handbook of symptom oriented neurology,* Chicago, 1989, Mosby.

Omer GE, Spinner M: *Management of peripheral nerve problems,* Philadelphia, 1980, WB Saunders.

Post M: *Physical examination of the musculoskeletal system,* Chicago, 1987, Mosby.

Rodnitzky RL: *Van Allen's pictorial manual of neurologic tests a guide to the performance and interpretation of the neurologic examination,* ed 3, Chicago, 1969, Mosby.

Rothman RH, Simeone FA: *The spine,* vol 2, Philadelphia, 1975, WB Saunders.

Scham SM, Taylor TKF: Tension signs in lumbar disc prolapse, *Clin Orthop,* 75:195, 1971.

Schmorl G: *The human spine in health and disease,* ed 2, New York, 1971, Grune and Stratton.

Spangfort E: Lasegue's sign in patients with lumbar disc herniation, *Acta Orthop,* 42:459, 1971.

Thurston SE: *The little black book of neurology,* Chicago, 1987, Mosby.

Turek SL: *Orthopaedics principles and their application,* ed 3, Philadelphia, 1977, JB Lippincott.

Urban LM: The straight-leg-raising test: A review, *J Orthop Sports Phys Ther,* 2:117, 1981.

Vernon-Roberts B, Perie CJ: Degenerative changes in the intervertebral disc of the lumbar spine and their sequela, *Rheum Rehab,* 16:13, 1977.

Waddell G, McCulloch JA, Kummel E, Venner RM: Nonorganic physical signs in low back pain, *Spine,* 5(2):177, 1980.

White AA III, Panjabi MM: The basic kinematics of the human spine, a review of past and current knowledge, *Spine,* 3:12-20, 1978.

White AA III, Panjabi MM: *Clinical biomechanics of the spine,* Philadelphia, 1978, JB Lippincott.

Wiesel SW, Bernini P, Rothman RH: *The aging lumbar spine,* Philadelphia, 1982, WB Saunders.

Wilkins RH, Brody IA: Laseque's sign, *Arch Neurol,* 21:219, 1969.

Woodhall R, Hayes GJ: The well-leg-raising test, *N Engl J Med,* 297:1127, 1977.

CHAPTER

~ *9* ~

The Pelvis and Sacroiliac Joint

*T*he pelvis is a uniquely devised mechanism that is designed to transfer the body weight from the single weight-bearing axis of the trunk to the bipolar weight-bearing of the lower extremities. The spine attaches to the pelvis by a single connection to the sacrum and is anchored in all four directions by various combinations of muscles and ligaments for stability. Through the bony ring of the pelvis, weight is transferred from the spinal column to the two lower extremities. It is necessary for the pelvic ring to be intact to give stability. The primary function of the pelvis, including the bones, joints, ligaments, and muscles, is the mechanical transfer of weight. A secondary function of the bony pelvis is protection of the viscera. Enclosed within the pelvis, is the bladder, the female genitalia, the rectum, and the great vessels and nerves that extend to the lower extremity.

The sacroiliac articulation is formed by narrow, closely fitted, irregularly shaped and cartilage-covered surfaces of the posterior and internal ilium and the lateral border of the sacrum.

The lumbosacral trunk lies anteriorly in direct relationship to the sacroiliac joint. An inflammatory neuritis is not an uncommon accompaniment of sacroiliac arthritis. The anterior ligaments are thin and easily distended by intraarticular swelling.

The upper two thirds of the joint are covered posteriorly by the posterior end of the ilium. The lower third of the joint is covered by the sacroiliac ligaments but can often be palpated in thin individuals.

The conditions that affect the sacroiliac joints are those that involve any joint. The sacroiliac joint is a favored site for tuberculous infection and is often the starting point for ankylosing spondylitis. Degenerative arthritic changes are often pronounced at this joint.

Index of Tests

Anterior innominate test
Belt test
Erichsen's sign
Gaenslen's test
Gapping test
Goldthwait's sign
Hibb's test
Iliac compression test
Knee-to-shoulder test
Laguerre's test
Lewin-Gaenslen's test
Piedallu's sign
Sacral apex test
Sacroiliac resisted-abduction test
Smith-Petersen test
Squish test
Yeoman's test

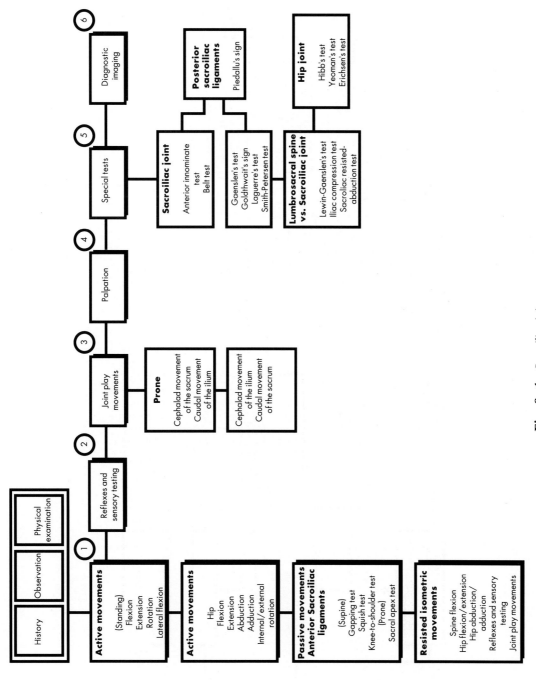

Fig. 9–1 Sacroiliac joint assessment.

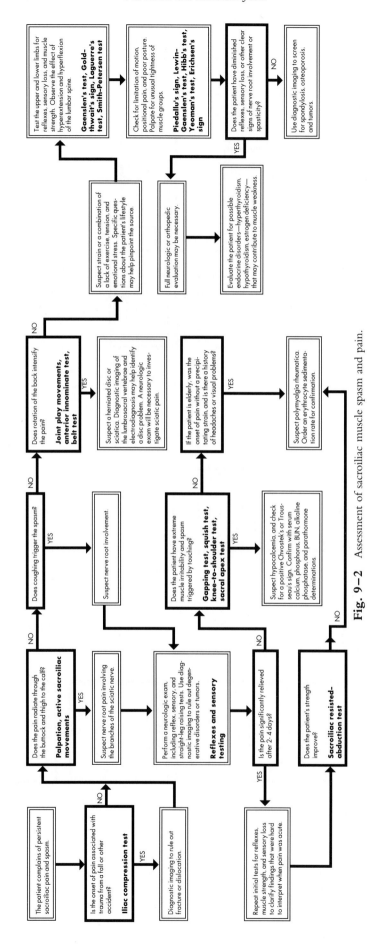

Fig. 9–2 Assessment of sacroiliac muscle spasm and pain.

RANGE OF MOTION

Unlike other peripheral joints the sacroiliac joints do not have muscles directly controlling their movement. However, contraction of the muscles of the other joints may stress these joints or the symphysis pubis. The examiner must be careful during active or resisted isometric movements of the other joints and must ask the patient about the exact location of the pain or discomfort experienced during each movement. Resisted abduction of a hip can cause pain in the sacroiliac joint because the gluteus medius muscle pulls the ilium away from the sacrum when it contracts strongly.

The sacroiliac joints move in a nodding fashion of anteroposterior rotation. The sacrum moves forward on the ilia when the patient changes from a standing to a reclined position or when the trunk is flexed. Normally the posterior superior iliac spines approximate when the patient is standing and separate when the patient is lying prone. When the patient stands on one leg, the pubic bone on the supported side moves forward in relation to the pubic bone on the opposite side. This movement is the result of rotation of the sacroiliac joint.

Comment

A sprain of the iliosacral ligaments is possible. The injury affects the ligament that extends from the posterior projection of the wing of the ilium to the posterior sacrum. The sprain of this ligament also can have an effect within the pelvis. Many of the conditions that used to be called sacroiliac sprains were actually other diseases. The term was a wastebasket nomenclature. The sacroiliac ligaments are so strong that ordinary stresses will cause damage to the lumbosacral ligament before they cause damage to the sacroiliac ligaments.

Following injury of the sacroiliac joint there will be pain localized to the joint. There also may be referred pain to the groin, hamstrings, or back of the thigh. Ordinarily, this pain will not ordinarily be along the sciatic distribution. Many of the tests that will elicit pain in the sacroiliac joint will also be positive in conditions such as ruptured intervertebral disc, sciatic neuritis, and lumbosacral sprain. The fact that the tests cause pain is of little significance. The significance is in the location of the pain. With an acute injury this significance may be extremely difficult to determine accurately. The common tests—such as straight-leg raising, which puts torsion force on the sacroiliac joint, or the similar test of forward flexion of the trunk while the knees are straight—will cause pain when sacroiliac joint involvement exists. These tests will also be positive in many other conditions. Some tests are designed to stress the sacroiliac area specifically. Gaenslen's test involves flexing the opposite thigh onthe abdomen to immobilize the pelvis in forward flexion. Next the involved leg is pushed into hyperextension, which causes rotary stress on the sacroiliac joint. Obviously, this test also would strain other areas. A single positive test, such as this one, is not diagnostic.

Procedure

The patient, with lower-trunk pain, is in the standing position and is instructed to place the lower extremity that is opposite the painful side approximately two or three feet in front of the foot of the other extremity. This position makes it appear as if the patient is taking a big step forward. The patient then bends the upper trunk acutely over the forward extremity, to put all the weight on the front leg. The patient flexes to the point at which the heel of the back foot raises from the floor. The production or aggravation of lower-trunk pain on the side of the posterior leg indicates a positive test. A positive test indicates unilateral forward displacement of the ilia (anterior innominate) in relation to the sacrum.

Confirmation Procedures

Knee-to-shoulder test, Lewin-Gaenslen's test, Piedallu's sign, sacral apex test, sacroiliac resisted-abduction test

Reporting Statement

The anterior innominate test is positive on the right. This result indicates unilateral forward displacement of the ilia on the sacrum.

∿ Clinical Pearl ∿

The sacroiliac joint, most inaccessible to palpation, is difficult to assess clinically. Only florid inflammation or damage to the fibrous portion is likely to result in local posterior tenderness. This tenderness is probably ligamentous.

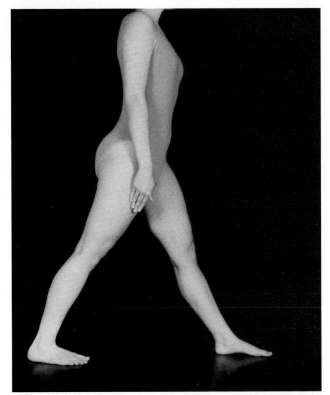

Fig. 9–3 The patient is standing and is instructed to take a big step forward, placing the unaffected leg 2 or 3 feet ahead of the affected leg.

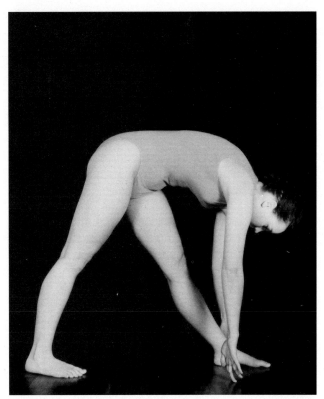

Fig. 9–4 The patient flexes at the waist and tries to touch the floor. This movement places weight onto the forward leg and stretches the affected sacroiliac joint.

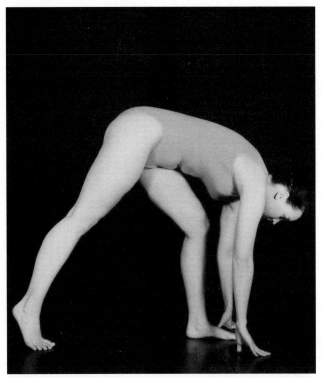

Fig. 9–5 The production of pain in the lower trunk, especially on the affected side, as the heel on the affected side lifts, indicates a positive test. A positive test indicates unilateral forward displacement of the ilium in relation to the sacrum.

Comment

Sacroiliac sprain denotes painful stretching of the ligaments around the joint. The occurrence of this condition is regarded as uncommon because the sacroiliac ligaments are very strong. The movements of bending, lifting, and hyperextension that produce torsion strain of the joint are more likely to cause a sprain of the thinner capsular ligaments surrounding the small lumbosacral joints. However, there can be no question that sacroiliac sprain does occur and can be identified readily by an acute onset during a torsion movement and by tenderness over the joint accentuated by a maneuver that reproduces the sprain.

Certain circumstances favor sprain of the sacroiliac ligaments. The ligaments are softened and elongated by pregnancy, prolonged periods of bending and lifting, or degenerative arthritis. The mechanism of injury usually involves the act of straightening up from a stooped position. It is tempting to suppose that muscular incoordination is at fault. The hip flexors hold the ilium forward while the sacrum is rotated backward, or the hamstrings and the gluteus maximus extend the hip, rotating the ilium backward while the sacrum is held forward by the weight of the trunk. This theory has support because a postural defect of pelvic inclination and excessive lumbar lordosis are associated findings.

Sacroiliac subluxation implies that ligamentous stretching has been sufficient to permit the ilium to slip on the sacrum. An irregular prominence of one of the articular surfaces becomes wedged upon another prominence of the apposed articular surface. The ligaments are taut, reflex muscle spasm is intense, and pain is severe and continuous until reduction is accomplished.

Procedure

The patient with lower back symptomatology is in the standing position. The patient flexes the dorsolumbar spine while the examiner notes the amount of movement necessary to aggravate the pain. While positioned behind the patient, the examiner grasps the patient's iliac crests and braces a hip against the patient's sacrum. The patient is directed to flex the spine again as the examiner immobilizes the patient's pelvis. If the lesion is of a pelvic nature, flexing the spine, with the pelvis immobilized, will not reproduce the discomfort. If the lesion is of a spinal nature, the pain will be aggravated in both instances.

Confirmation Procedures

Gaenslen's test, Goldthwait's sign, Smith-Petersen test

Reporting Statement

The belt test is positive on the right side of the pelvis and results in significant reduction of sacroiliac pain.

This result indicates sprain of the sacroiliac ligaments. The belt test aggravates both spinal and pelvic complaints. This result suggests lumbosacral capsular sprain.

～ Clinical Pearl ～

Because of the stabilizing effect of the very strong ligamentous structures, sprain of the sacroiliac ligaments is usually accompanied by a sacroiliac subluxation and is called a subluxation-sprain. Posterior subluxation results from a flexion-type injury, which occurs with activities such as in lifting or pushing. Anterior subluxation results from extension-type injuries, which occurs when falling forward or extending the leg.

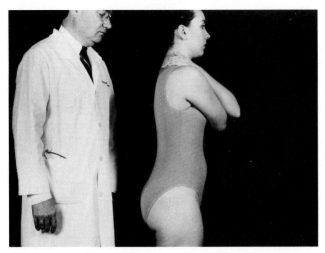

Fig. 9–6 The patient is in the standing position. The examiner, who is positioned behind the patient, notes spinal contours.

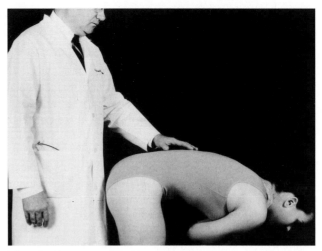

Fig. 9–7 The patient flexes at the waist, as far forward as possible. The examiner notes the amount of flexion necessary to aggravate the lower back or create sacroiliac discomfort.

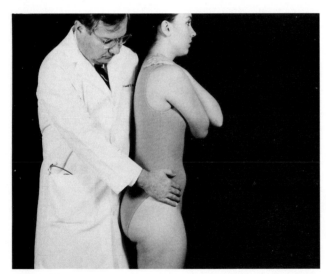

Fig. 9–8 Once the patient stands erect, the examiner grasps the patient's iliac crests and braces a hip against the patient's sacrum.

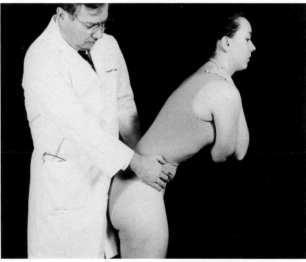

Fig. 9–9 While in this braced position, the patient flexes at the waist. If the source of pain is pelvic, then the move will not reproduce the discomfort because the pelvis is immobilized. Pain of spinal origin will be aggravated in both positions.

Comment

The pelvic curve begins at the lumbosacral joint and ends at the termination of the coccyx. The curve is anteriorly concave and is somewhat tilted downward. The thoracic and pelvic curves are called *primary curves* because they are present in the fetus.

The sacrum is a large triangular bone inserted like a wedge between the two iliac bones. The base of the sacrum articulates with L5, producing the rather acute lumbosacral angle that is formed by increased anterior width of both the body of L5 and the L5-S1 intervertebral disc.

The coccyx is usually a solid bone formed by the fusion of four rudimentary vertebrae. Occasionally the first coccygeal vertebrae exists as a separate segment, and no vertebral canal exists within the coccyx itself.

Articulation of the pelvis with the vertebral column occurs at the interspace between L5 and the sacrum. This articulation is similar in just about all respects to the articulations that connect the vertebrae with each other. In addition, the iliolumbar ligament connects the pelvis with the vertebral column on either side.

The sacroiliac articulation is an amphiarthrodial, or slightly movable, joint. The articular surfaces of the sacrum and ilium are covered with articular cartilaginous plates that are in close contact with each other and bound together by fibrous strands.

The sacrococcygeal articulation is a joint similar to the articulation between vertebral bodies.

The pubic symphysis is an amphiarthrodial joint formed between the two oval symphyseal surfaces of the pubic bones.

Procedure

While the patient is prone, the examiner places his hands over the dorsum of the ilia and proceeds to give a forceful, sharp, bilateral thrust toward the midline. The sign is present when this procedure produces pain over the sacroiliac area. Pain is felt in sacroiliac joint disease but not in hip joint disease.

Confirmation Procedures

Hibb's test, Laguerre's test

Reporting Statement

Erichsen's sign is present on the right and suggests sacroiliac disease instead of pathologic condition involving the hip joint.

~ Clinical Pearl ~

Patients who possess an anomalous relation of the piriformis muscle to the sciatic nerve are particularly susceptible to developing symptoms of sciatic neuritis when the muscle is hypertonic or spastic. About 10% of the population possesses such an anomaly. A reflex spasm of this muscle may occur because of intraarticular sacroiliac subluxation and sacroiliac irritation. Such a spasm is probably the cause of a positive Lasègue test, which occurs in the range of 20 to 45 degrees.

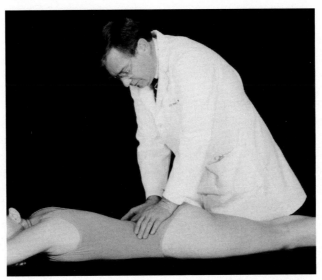

Fig. 9–10   While the patient is lying prone on a firm examining table, the examiner places both hands over the dorsum of the ilia and gives a sharp, forceful thrust toward the midline. The production of pain over the sacroiliac area is a positive sign and indicates sacroiliac joint disease.

Comment

The sacroiliac joints are the key of the arch between the two pelvic bones. With the symphysis pubis, the joints help transfer the weight from the spine to the lower limbs. This triad of joints also acts as a buffer to decrease the force of jarring and bumping, which occurs within the spine and upper body, from the lower limb's contact with the ground. Because of this shock-absorbing function, the structure of the sacroiliac and symphysis pubis joints is different from most joints.

The sacroiliac joints are part synovial and part syndesmosis. A syndesmosis is a type of fibrous joint in which the intervening fibrous connective tissue forms an interosseous membrane or ligament. The synovial portion of the joint is C-shaped with the convex iliac surface of the *C* facing anteriorly and inferiorly. The greater or more acute the angle of the *C,* the more stable the joint and the less likely it is for a lesion of the joint to occur. The sacral surface is slightly concave.

The size, shape, and roughness of the articular surfaces vary among individuals. In the child these surfaces are smooth. In the adult the surfaces become irregular depressions and elevations that fit into one another. By doing so, the articular surfaces restrict movement at the joint and add to strength of the joint for transferring weight from the lower limb to the spine. The articular surface of the ilium is covered with fibrocartilage. The articular surface of the sacrum is covered with hyaline cartilage, which is three times thicker than that of the ilium. In older persons, part of the joint surfaces may be obliterated by adhesions.

The sacroiliac joints, although mobile in young people, become progressively stiffer with age. In some cases, ankylosis results. The movements occurring in the sacroiliac and symphysis pubis are small in relation to the movements in the spinal joints.

The symphysis pubis is a cartilaginous joint. There is a disc of fibrocartilage, called the interpubic disc, between the two joint surfaces.

The sacroiliac joints and symphysis pubis have no muscles that directly control their movements. However, the joints are influenced by the action of the muscles that move the lumbar spine and hip because many of these muscles attach to the sacrum and pelvis.

The sacrococcygeal joint is usually a fused line (symphysis) united by a fibrocartilaginous disc. It is found between the apex of the sacrum and the base of the coccyx. Occasionally the joint is freely movable and synovial. With advanced age the joint may fuse and be obliterated.

Procedure

The patient is lying supine. The examiner acutely flexes the knee and thigh of the unaffected leg, to the patient's abdomen. This move brings the lumbar spine firmly into contact with the table and fixes both the pelvis and lumbar spine. With the examiner standing at a right angle to the patient, the patient is brought well to the side of the table, and the examiner slowly hyperextends the affected thigh. This hyperextension is accomplished by gradually increasing the pressure of one hand on top of the knee, while the examiner's other hand is on the flexed knee. The hyperextension of the affected hip exerts a rotating force on the corresponding half of the pelvis. The pull is made on the ilium, through the *Y* ligament, and the muscles attached to the anterior iliac spine. The test is positive if pain is felt in the sacroiliac area or referred down the thigh. The test is performed bilaterally. If the test is negative, a lumbosacral lesion is suspected. The test is usually contraindicated in geriatrics.

Confirmation Procedures

Belt test, Goldthwait's sign, Smith-Petersen test

Reporting Statement

Gaenslen's test is positive on the left. This result indicates sacroiliac joint disease on the left.

~ **Clinical Pearl** ~

Sacroiliac joint involvement produces local pain over the joint, or pain that is referred to (1) the groin on the same side, (2) the posterior thigh on the same side, and (3) down the leg, which is less often. Pain is often increased by lying on the affected side.

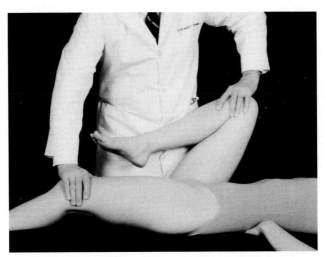

Fig. 9–11 The patient is supine with the affected side of the pelvis well to the side of the table. The unaffected thigh is flexed toward the abdomen. The examiner simultaneously exaggerates the thigh flexion on the unaffected side and the sacroiliac extension on the affected side. The test is positive if pain is felt in the affected sacroiliac joint as it is hyperextended.

～ Gapping Test ～
SACROILIAC STRETCH TEST

Comment

The normal movements that occur at the sacroiliac joints are determined by the direction of the articular surfaces, the muscles acting on the joint, and the symphysis pubis.

The movement is a rotation of the sacrum (or ilia) around the axis of the shortest and strongest part of the posterior interosseous sacroiliac ligament, which is situated in the angle between the posterosuperior and posteroinferior limbs of the auricular surfaces. When anterior rotation of the upper end of the sacrum occurs, the promontory of the sacrum will move in an anteroinferior direction, which narrows the anteroposterior diameter of the pelvic inlet. This rotation also increases the coronal width of the pelvic outlet and tightens the sacrotuberous and sacrospinous ligaments. During posterior rotation of the upper end of the sacrum, the reverse movements will occur. These movements produce a widening of the anteroposterior diameter of the pelvic inlet, a narrowing of the coronal width of the pelvic outlet, and a relaxation of the sacrotuberous and sacrospinous ligaments. The posterior sacroiliac ligaments will tighten and restrict this posterior rotation of the sacrum on the ilia.

In addition, because the auricular surfaces of the sacrum are inferiorly rather than superiorly closer to the median plane, anterior rotation of the sacrum will result in a slight widening of the symphysis pubis, while posterior rotation of the sacrum will result in compression of the symphysis pubis.

When a rotational force is applied to the hip bones in opposite directions—which occurs when extending one thigh while flexing the other, such as in stepping up to a stool—the extended thigh anchors the head of the femur on that side through the iliofemoral and ischiofemoral ligaments and the rectus femoris muscle. The flexed thigh, through the pull of the hamstring muscles, rotates the ilium in a posterior direction. In addition, the sacrum will move with the ilium on the flexed side because the pull of the hamstring muscle is transmitted to it via the sacrotuberous and sacrospinous ligaments. The result is that posterior rotation of the sacrum will occur at the sacroiliac joint on the extended side only.

Although these movements at the sacroiliac joints are small, especially in males, they are definite. The movements are increased when jumping from a height. They are also increased in females, especially toward the end of a pregnancy and up to three months after pregnancy because of the action of the hormone relaxin.

The finding that directs immediate attention to the sacroiliac joint as a possible cause of pain in the buttock and thigh, is that lumbar movements do not affect the gluteal symptom. With acute arthritis the lumbar movements do sometimes increase the pain a little because at the extreme of any lumbar motion, an added stress falls on the sacroiliac ligaments. If such an indirect strain on the joint hurts, much more severe pain is produced as soon as the sacroiliac joints are directly tested.

Procedure

The patient lies supine, and the examiner places both hands on the anterior superior spine of each ilium and presses laterally downward. Crossing the arms increases the lateral component of the strain on the ligaments. The pelvis must not be allowed to rock because the lumbar spine then moves. The examiner's hands can cause anterior iliac spine discomfort that is due to compression of the skin against the osseus structures. The expected finding is not local pain but rather aggravation of the gluteal symptoms. The response to the test is positive only if unilateral gluteal or posterior crural pain is elicited. The test is significant for anterior sacroiliac ligament sprain.

Confirmation Procedure

Yeoman's test

Reporting Statement

The gapping test is positive with pain elicited in the right gluteal area. This pain suggests sprain of the anterior sacroiliac ligaments on the right.

～ Clinical Pearl ～

Stretching the anterior ligaments in the manner described is the most delicate test for the sacroiliac joint. Patients recovering from a sacroiliac injury may say that all pain ceased some days before. Patients walk and bend painlessly; yet for a week to 10 days after subjective recovery, the straining of the joint that occurs in the gapping test still evokes discomfort. It is clear that this test applies more stress to sacroiliac ligaments than ordinary daily activities. If a patient has symptoms referable to the sacroiliac joint, this maneuver will elicit them.

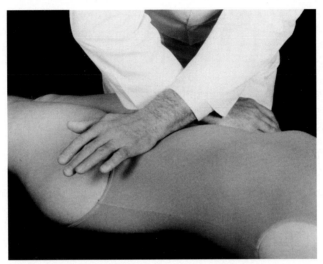

Fig. 9–12 The patient is supine on the examination table. The hips and knees are extended. With crossed arms the examiner places both hands on the opposite anterior superior iliac spines of each ilium. A downward and lateral pressure is applied to both ilia. Unilateral gluteal or posterior crural pain is a positive finding and indicates sprain of the anterior sacroiliac ligament.

Goldthwait's Sign

Comment

Because of their position at the juncture of the skeleton of the trunk and the pelvic girdle, sacroiliac articulations are of importance. In recent years, sacroiliac articulations have been the subject of extensive clinical study. It is largely the radiologists who have contributed to the knowledge of these articulations and who have described normal form and pathologic variations. The radiographic depiction of the sacroiliac synchondrosis is difficult because of its oblique and sinuous form. Severe fractures of the pelvis are sometimes associated with sacroiliac luxations and with marked displacement of the wings of the ilia. The sacroiliac joint may be the site of the infection, especially tuberculosis, with destruction of the articular surfaces and wandering abscess formation. Obliteration of these joints is an early finding in ankylosing spondylitis.

The most frequent morphologic change that is frequently associated with clinical symptoms is arthrosis deformans, which manifests itself by marginal osteophyte formation, particularly in the inferior portions of the synchondrosis and by subchondral osteosclerosis. These changes are responsible for a considerable degree of pain, especially with certain movements. These changes occur with advancing age in 90% of men and 77% of women. The healing of pelvic fractures that occurs with poor alignment of the sacroiliac articulations has a significant influence on the spine and the changes that are in these joints and are related to back pain.

Procedure

The patient is supine. The patient's affected leg is raised slowly, while one of the examiner's hands is under the lumbar portion of the patient's spine. If pain is brought on before the lumbar spine begins to move, a sacroiliac lesion is probably present. The lesion may be caused by arthritis or by a sprain of the ligaments that involve the sacroiliac joint. If pain does not come on until after the lumbar spine begins to move, the disorder is more likely to have its origin in the lumbosacral area or, less commonly, in the sacroiliac area. The test is repeated with the unaffected limb. A positive sign of a lumbosacral lesion is elicited if pain occurs at about the same height as it did with the affected limb. If the unaffected leg can be raised higher than the affected leg, it signifies sacroiliac involvement of the affected side.

Confirmation Procedures

Belt test, Gaenslen's test, Smith-Petersen test

Reporting Statement

Goldthwait's sign is present on the right and elicits pain in the sacroiliac joint prior to lumbosacral movement. This sign indicates sacroiliac joint sprain.

∽ Clinical Pearl ∽

This test is similar to the Lasègue test, straight-leg raising test and Smith-Petersen test. All have the use of the affected leg as a lever in common to stretch the suspect tissue, whether neural or ligamentous. The key to differentiation is the determination of the moment of L5-S1 separation, reflecting lumbosacral movement.

358 The Pelvis and Sacroiliac Joint

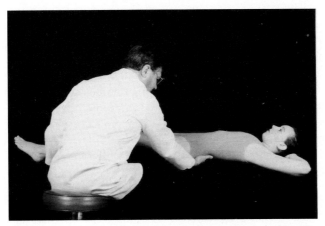

Fig. 9–13   The patient is supine on the examination table. The examiner places one hand under the lumbosacral portion of the patient's spine and palpates the L5 and S1 spinous processes. The examiner maintains contact with these two points.

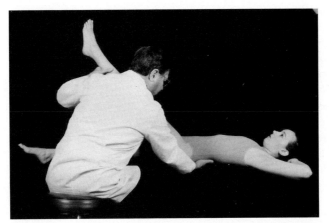

Fig. 9–14   The examiner elevates the affected leg as if performing a straight-leg raising maneuver. If pain is produced before the L5-S1 spinous processes separate, the lesion involves the sacroiliac joint. If the pain is produced as the L5-S1 spinous processes separate, it is more likely that a spinal lesion exists.

Comment

Tuberculous infection of the sacroiliac joint frequently is associated with tuberculosis of the spine at the lumbosacral area and the hip. This association suggests the ease with which tuberculosis spreads from the lumbosacral area to the sacroiliac joint by way of the psoas muscle. Destructive caseous lesions are the rule, and they often destroy the joint and form abscesses. The abscess may present dorsally over the joint or intrapelvically, erupting at the inguinal area. Rupture of the abscess results in a resistant sinus and secondary infection. Severe visceral lesions result in a serious condition. If the patient survives, spontaneous bony ankylosis of the sacroiliac joint occurs after 3 or 4 years. The disease may be bilateral.

The disease affects young adults and is rare in infancy and childhood. The onset of the disease is gradual and may follow trauma or pregnancy.

With this type of ankylosis there is pain over the sacroiliac joint. Most of the time, this pain is referred to the groin. Less commonly the pain is referred to the sciatic distribution. The pain is accentuated by direct pressure, such as during recumbency, and particularly when turning over in bed. Sitting on the buttock on the affected side is also painful. Sitting on the opposite buttock relieves the pain. Bending forward with the knee extended is painful, but bending forward while the knees are flexed is painless. Jarring that occurs during walking, coughing, or sneezing accentuates the discomfort.

The patient with this disease lists to the opposite side. With the lower extremities extended, forward bending is limited. When the knees and hips are flexed, the hamstrings are relaxed, tension is removed from the pelvis, and further forward bending is accomplished. Only the lower end of the joint is posteriorly superficial and displays tenderness and a boggy swelling. The swelling and tenderness may be more easily localized during rectal examination. Compressing the iliac crests together causes direct, painful pressure on the joint. Gaenslen's test for sacroiliac disease depends on twisting the ilium on the sacrum. The strain this move puts on the inflamed ligamentous structures around the sacroiliac joint produces the pain. The low-grade, inflammatory swelling of a cold abscess or sinus may be present.

Procedure

While the patient is in the prone position, the examiner stabilizes the pelvis on the nearest side by placing one hand firmly on the dorsum of the iliac bone. With the other hand around the patient's ankle, the opposite knee is flexed to a right angle. The knee is flexed to its maximum without elevating the thigh from the examination table. From this position the examiner slowly pushes the leg laterally, causing strong internal rotation of the femoral head. The test is performed bilaterally. The production of pelvic pain is a positive finding. The test is significant for a sacroiliac lesion. In the absence of hip involvement, stress is transmitted through the hip joints into the sacroiliac mechanism, producing pain.

Confirmation Procedures

Erichsen's sign, Laguerre's test

Reporting Statement

Hibb's test is positive on the right, suggesting sacroiliac disease.

∾ Clinical Pearl ∾

Tuberculosis is now rare in the developed countries but still a scourge elsewhere. Complications may be serious because of the formation of sinuses. These sinuses may become secondarily infected and may cause paraplegia (Pott's paraplegia) because of (1) pus and intracellular pressure, (2) mechanical injury to the nervous system (cord) caused by bony pressure, and (3) vascular embarrassment of the nervous system where it crosses the bony infection. Hibb's test is not specific for tuberculosis of the sacroiliac joint but is correlated with other systemic findings that may suggest the existence of this type of tuberculosis. At the least, Hibb's test reveals mechanical dysfunction of the sacroiliac joint.

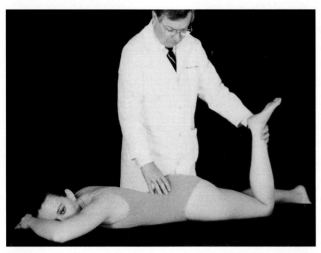

Fig. 9-15 The patient is prone on the examining table. The examiner stabilizes the unaffected side of the pelvis with one hand. With the other hand the examiner grasps the ankle of the affected leg and flexes the knee to 90 degrees.

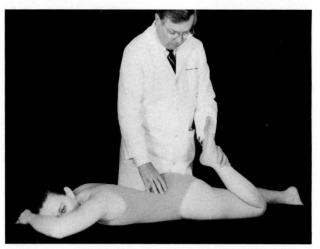

Fig. 9-16 The examiner flexes the patient's knee to its maximum without elevating the thigh from the examination table.

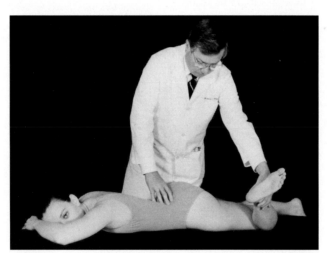

Fig. 9-17 The examiner slowly pushes the leg laterally, causing internal rotation of the femoral head. The production of pelvic pain is a positive finding. Even without a pathologic condition of the hip, the test is significant for a sacroiliac lesion.

∾ Iliac Compression Test ∾
COMPRESSION OF THE ILIAC CRESTS

Comment

Fracture of the wing of the ilium is not frequent. When such a fracture occurs, it is usually caused by a direct blow against the wing of the ilium. In most sports in which such an injury is likely, the iliac crest is padded to prevent the occurrence of this injury.

Fracture of the wing of the ilium is a painful injury not only at the time of the blow but also in the period immediately after the injury. This type of fracture is ordinarily recognized as a serious injury. Examination reveals extreme tenderness along the iliac crest and downward onto the wing of the ilium. The area of pain depends on the extent of the fracture. The patient will usually not permit deep enough palpation so that the examiner can actually feel a defect along the rim. Any attempt to use the involved muscles is extremely painful, and involuntary spasms of the abdominal or hip muscles may cause acute distress. It is necessary to have the patient completely relaxed before a definitive examination can be performed. If a lesion of this severity is suspected, an x-ray examination should be made. The fracture can be completely overlooked in the ordinary anteroposterior view of the pelvis. The fracture will be well delineated by an anteroposterior view of the ilium rather than of the pelvis.

Procedure

While the patient is in the side-lying position, the examiner's hands are placed over the upper part of the patient's iliac crest. The examiner then presses toward the floor. The movement causes forward pressure on the sacrum. An increased feeling of pressure in the sacroiliac joint indicates a possible sacroiliac lesion. The pressure may also indicate a sprain of the posterior sacroiliac ligaments. The test is significant for sacroiliac lesions, such as sprain, inflammation, subluxation, and fractures.

Confirmation Procedure

Diagnostic imaging

> ### Reporting Statement
>
> The iliac compression test is positive and pain is elicited at the left ilium, near the crest. This pain suggests fracture of the wing of the ilium.

∾ Clinical Pearl ∾

Fractures of the pelvis are serious in themselves and may result in long-term disability. However, even more important is that these fractures are frequently complicated by damage to the soft tissues, urethra, bladder, bowel, blood vessels, and nerves. These complications can be fatal. Genitourinary complications occur in about 20% of pelvic fractures and the overall mortality is 5%.

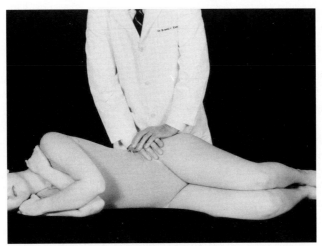

Fig. 9–18 The patient is in the side-lying position on an examination table with a firm surface. The examiner places both hands over the upper part of the superior iliac crest and exerts downward pressure. If the patient experiences an increased feeling of pressure in the sacroiliac joint, then the test indicates sacroiliac sprain, inflammation, subluxation, or fracture.

Comment

Septic arthritis is a disease process caused by the direct invasion of a joint space by infectious agents, usually bacteria. Joints become infected by direct penetration spread from contiguous structures or, more often, by hematogenous invasion through the blood stream. Septic arthritis occurs more often in large peripheral joints than in the lumbosacral spine. When a joint of the axial skeleton is involved, the sacroiliac joint is the one commonly affected.

Pyogenic sacroiliitis is an uncommon illness. The disease occurs most commonly in young adult men. The range of age is 20 to 66 years and the male to female ratio is 3:2.

Entry of the organisms into the sacroiliac joint is the initial factor that may result in joint infection. Most commonly infectious agents reach the sacroiliac joint by traveling through the blood stream. They lodge in the vascular synovial membrane that lines the lower portion of the sacroiliac joint. The infectious agents grow in the synovium and invade the joint space. The organisms also might lodge in the ilium, the most frequently infected flat bone in the body, and grow into the sacroiliac joint. The symmetric involvement of the ilium and sacrum in pyogenic sacroiliitis suggests that the joint is the initial area affected. Once an infection is established in the joint, rapid destruction may occur because of both the direct, toxic effects products or organisms have on joint structures and because of the host's inflammatory response to these products or organisms.

Any factor—such as intravenous drug abuse, skin infections, bone and urinary tract infections, endocarditis, pregnancy, and bowel disease—that promotes blood borne infection, or inhibits the normal defense mechanisms of the synovial joint, predispose the host to infection. Although the role of trauma in the pathogenesis of pyogenic sacroiliitis is unclear, buttock or hip injuries have been reported in patients before development of pyogenic sacroiliitis. Most patients however, deny a history of trauma, and its importance as a direct cause of the infection is in question. The histocompatibility typing associated with seronegative spondyloarthropathies, HLA-B27, is not associated with pyogenic sacroiliitis.

Another mechanism of joint infection is contamination by local spread from a contiguous suppurative focus. Extension of a pelvic infectious process may cause disruption of the joint capsule or of the periosteum of the ilium or sacrum. Infections spreading beneath the spinal ligaments may gain entry into the sacroiliac joints. Another mechanism of joint infection that is even more uncommon is direct seeding of organisms into the joint during diagnostic or surgical procedures.

Procedure

While the patient is in a supine position, the examiner fully flexes the patient's knee and hip and then adducts the hip. The sacroiliac joint is rocked by flexion and adduction of the patient's hip. The knee is moved toward the patient's opposite shoulder. Pain in the sacroiliac joint indicates a positive test. The test places a great amount of stress on the hip and sacroiliac joints. While performing the test, the examiner may palpate the sacroiliac joint to feel for a slight amount of movement that normally would be present. A positive test primarily indicates sacroiliac mechanical dysfunction. Correlated with other systemic findings, this result may suggest pyogenic sacroiliitis.

Confirmation Procedures

Anterior innominate test, Lewin-Gaenslen's test, Piedallu's sign, sacral apex test, sacroiliac resisted-abduction test

Reporting Statement

The knee-to-shoulder test is positive for the right sacroiliac joint. This result indicates an articular lesion. This afebrile finding implicates mechanical dysfunction.

The knee-to-shoulder test is positive for the right sacroiliac joint. This result, correlated with other systemic findings, implicates pyogenic sacroiliitis.

∽ Clinical Pearl ∽

With acute sacroiliac pyogenic infections, the onset is usually rapid and very painful. Swelling is tense and tenderness is widespread. The patient resists movement, and experiences pyrexia and general malaise. Pyogenic infections occurring in patients suffering from rheumatoid arthritis often have a much slower onset. Although the sacroiliac joint is swollen, other inflammatory changes are often suppressed, especially if the patient is receiving steroids. In the early stages, both modes of onset will mimic simple mechanical injury of the sacroiliac joint.

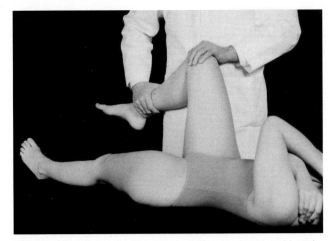

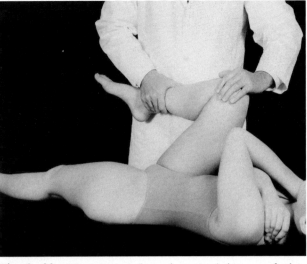

Fig. 9–19 The patient is supine on the examination table. The examiner flexes both the knee and hip of the affected leg to 90 degrees.

Fig. 9–20 The examiner flexes the patient's hip even further, toward the patient's abdomen.

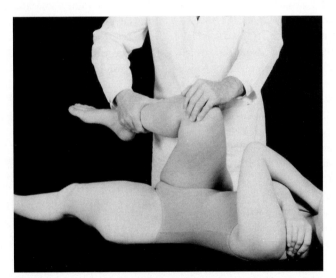

Fig. 9–21 The hip is adducted, approximating the knee of the affected leg to the contralateral shoulder. Pain in the sacroiliac joint indicates a positive test.

Comment

Osteitis condensans ilii is a disease characterized by mild back pain and unilateral or bilateral bony sclerosis of the lower ilium, with sparing of the sacral portion of the sacroiliac joints. The illness is not progressive and is not associated with functional disability. The major difficulty with osteitis condensans ilii is that it is frequently confused with ankylosing spondylitis.

The prevalence of osteitis condensans ilii has been estimated to be 1.6% in the Japanese and 3% in Scandinavians. The typical patient is a female 30 to 40 years old. The ratio of female to male is 9:1 or greater.

The pathogenesis of osteitis condensans ilii is unknown. Urinary tract infections, inflammatory diseases of the sacroiliac joint, and abnormal mechanical stresses have been suggested as possible etiologies in this illness. Urinary tract infection may reach the ilium via nutrient arteries, resulting in reactive sclerosis. The absence of a history of urinary tract infection in many individuals makes this mechanism unlikely. Osteitis condensans ilii may be a subset of ankylosing spondylitis. However, histocompatibility testing for HLA-B27 has not documented increased incidence of this antigen in osteitis patients. In addition, part of the confusion over differentiating osteitis condensans ilii and ankylosing spondylitis is the milder form of the latter illness in females.

A more likely cause of osteitis condensans ilii is mechanical stress across the sacroiliac joint in association with pregnancy and diastasis of the symphysis pubis. A normal physiologic zone of hyperostosis on the anterior iliac margin of the sacroiliac joint may become exaggerated in response to abnormal stresses. Abnormal stresses are placed on the sacroiliac joints during pregnancy. However, these stresses alone would not explain the occasional male with osteitis or female who develops osteitis without having been pregnant. Therefore it must be said that the mechanical stresses that cause osteitis condensans ilii are commonly, but not exclusively, associated with pregnancy. Diastasis of the symphysis pubis may explain this clinical occurrence. Diastasis of the pubis occurs frequently during pregnancy and is secondary to the release of relaxin, a product of the corpus pregnancy, which allows greater laxity of the supporting structures (ligaments) of the pelvis. Patients may actually notice movement or a popping sensation in the sacroiliac joints and pubis. Diastasis is not exclusively related to pregnancy because it may occur secondary to trauma. Individuals, both male and female, with diastasis related to trauma may be at risk of developing osteitis condensans ilii.

Procedure

The patient lies in a supine position. The examiner then flexes, abducts, and laterally rotates the patient's hip. The examiner then applies an overpressure at the end of the range of motion. The examiner must stabilize the pelvis on the opposite side by holding the opposite ASIS down. Pain in the sacroiliac joint on the affected side constitutes a positive test. This test should be performed with caution for patients with pathologic hip conditions because hip pain may ensue.

Confirmation Procedures

Erichsen's sign, Hibb's test, diagnostic imaging

Reporting Statement

Laguerre's test is positive for the right sacroiliac joint and suggests a pathologic condition that is of an intraarticular origin.

~ **Clinical Pearl** ~

With osteitis condensans ilii there is a disturbance of the normal architecture of the ilium, in which increased condensations of bone occur in the auricular portion of the ilium, without a corresponding change in the sacroiliac joint or the sacrum. Osteitis condensans ilii must be differentiated from ankylosing spondylitis, which also causes condensations around the sacroiliac joint. Laguerre's test reveals a mechanical problem of the sacroiliac joint. Involvement of the joint in osteitis condensans ilii can only be confirmed by diagnostic imaging.

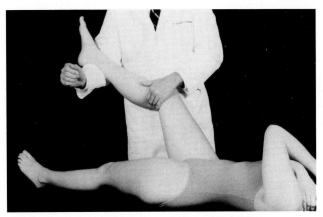

Fig. 9–22 The patient is supine. The examiner flexes and abducts the patient's hip on the affected side. The patient's foot rests on the examiner's forearm.

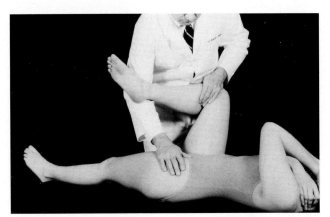

Fig. 9–23 The examiner laterally rotates the hip, applying an overpressure at the end of the range of motion. The contralateral pelvis is stabilized by holding the anterior superior iliac spine down. Pain in the sacroiliac joint on the affected side constitutes a positive test.

Comment

The sacroiliac joint is subject to several different processes that may damage it. Sprain is common, and sacroiliac joint subluxation can occur. Sprain may occur when heavy loads are placed upon the joints, during a fall, or with blows to the sacroiliac joint. The pain that occurs will be felt unilaterally over the sacroiliac joint and can radiate into the ipsilateral hip or buttock. The pain will be made worse by movement of the joint or by axial loading of the joint. During palpation, the joint is extremely tender, particularly near an area just inferomedial to the posterior superior iliac spine. When examining the patient for global motions, extending the joint may produce some pain, but flexion is typically not painful. Lateral flexion of the pelvis may be painful but is not universally so, particularly if the motion is very smoothly performed. Straight-leg raising tests produce pain at approximately 70 degrees of flexion. There are no muscular changes noted, and reflex testing will be normal.

Pain from sacroiliac joint lesions, other than sprain, will typically be dull in nature and perceived in the region of the buttock. The pain may radiate into the area of the anterior groin, the posterior thigh, the knee, or even the lower abdomen, causing possible misdiagnosis as an intraabdominal lesion. A neurologic symptom is rare, so paresthesia is not often experienced. Patients suffering from mechanical lesions of the sacroiliac joint experience the pain unilaterally. The pain is exacerbated by motions that produce stress on the joint. Disorders of the sacroiliac joint can be classified into the following groups: (1) inflammatory lesions, (2) infectious lesions, (3) mechanical lesions, (4) degenerative lesions, and (5) osteitis condensans ilii.

Procedure

Lewin-Gaenslen's test is a modification of Gaenslen's test, in which the patient lies on the unaffected side and pulls the knee of that side to the chest. The patient holds the affected thigh in extension for the examiner. The examiner, positioned behind the patient, then provides pressure by hyperextending the affected thigh. Pain produced in the sacroiliac joint is a positive finding. The test is significant for sacroiliac lesions.

Confirmation Procedures

Anterior innominate test, knee-to-shoulder test, Piedallu's sign, sacral apex test, sacroiliac resisted-abduction test

Reporting Statement

Lewin-Gaenslen's test is positive on the right and indicates an articular pathologic condition of the sacroiliac joint.

∼ Clinical Pearl ∼

Because of the strength of the sacroiliac ligaments, sprain of these structures is uncommon. Bending movements—such as lifting and hyperextension, which produce a torsion sprain upon the joint—are more likely to cause sprain of the thinner capsular ligaments in the small lumbosacral joints.

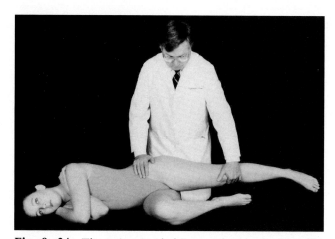

Fig. 9–24 The patient is side-lying on the examination table, on the unaffected side. The knee and hip of the unaffected leg are flexed. The examiner abducts the affected leg slightly, supporting its weight with one hand. The examiner's other hand fixes the pelvis to the table with firm downward pressure.

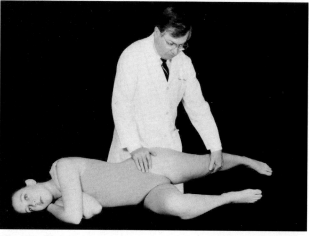

Fig. 9–25 The affected leg is extended by the examiner. Pain elicited during this maneuver constitutes a positive sign and indicates a sacroiliac lesion.

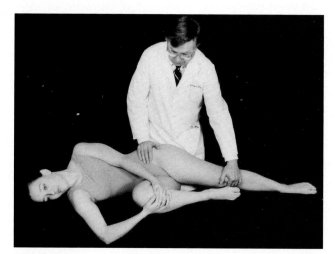

Fig. 9–26 In a slight variation of this test, the patient maximally flexes the thigh of the unaffected leg onto the abdomen and holds it in place.

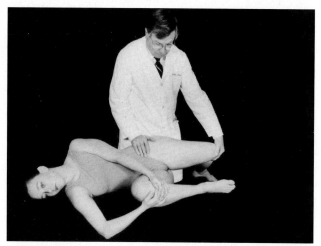

Fig. 9–27 The examiner extends the affected leg, allowing flexion of the knee. With the unaffected thigh in fixed flexion, very little extension motion is required to elicit a pain response in the affected leg.

Comment

There are many inflammatory disorders that affect the sacroiliac joint. Most of these disorders fall under the general heading of the seronegative arthropathies, such as ankylosing spondylitis, Reiter's syndrome, and psoriatic arthritis. When an inflammatory disorder exists, a combination of radiographic and laboratory tests can be used to confirm the presence of a particular disease. Each disease has it own characteristics, such as a predisposition for ankylosing spondylitis in the sacroiliac joint that migrates superiorly in the spine.

Infections within the sacroiliac joint are caused most frequently by staphylococcus bacteria, as well as tuberculous or brucellar infection. X-ray can once again be used to show typical changes and bone scans will be useful in demonstrating the hot spot appearance of such an infection. Aspiration biopsy is needed to culture the organism.

Mechanical lesions of the sacroiliac joint are common and consist of both hypo- and hypermobility lesions. Causes of hypomobility lesions include rotational stress on the joint, pregnancy, trauma, and unequal leg length. Hypermobility lesions are only due to an unstable symphysis pubis or to pregnancy, which also affects the symphysis pubis via the release of the hormone relaxin.

Degenerative changes may occur within the sacroiliac joint, as well as in any other joint in the body. The changes that occur in the joint are similar to those in other joints. There is pitting of the bone accompanied by subchondral sclerosis and osteophytic changes. This condition has a tendency to occur with aging. This is in concert with greater amounts of stress placed upon the joint, such as increasing weight or damage from fracture or biomechanical abnormality.

Osteitis condensans ilii is a condition in which bone condenses along the ilium near the sacroiliac joint. The cause of this condition is not known, but it may be associated with increased stress, ankylosing spondylitis, urinary tract infection, and circulatory problems. Osteitis condensans ilii can lead to lower back pain. During diagnostic imaging, there is a characteristic triangular area of sclerosis located near the medial ilium.

Sacroiliac subluxation may produce irritative microtrauma to the articular structures, induction of spinal curvatures, induction of spinal or pelvic subluxation and fixation, and biomechanical abnormalities in stance and locomotion. Evaluation of the sacroiliac joint for the presence of such subluxation or fixation will need to combine both static and dynamic palpation as well as a plumb line analysis. There may be tenderness during palpation of the posterior superior iliac spine when there is innominate rotation. A full, range-of-motion palpation procedure is needed to evaluate the joint for motion abnormalities or fixation. Both the static and organic procedures need to be performed to evaluate the joint for subluxation or fixation.

Procedure

The patient is seated on a hard, flat surface. This position keeps muscles, such as the hamstrings, from affecting the pelvic-flexion symmetry. The seated position also increases the stability of the ilia. In effect, sitting provides a test of the sacrum on the ilia. The examiner finds the posterior superior iliac spines and compares their height. If one PSIS, usually the painful one, is lower than the other, the patient is directed to forward flex while remaining seated. If the lower PSIS becomes the higher one during forward flexion, the test is positive, and it is that side that is affected. Because the affected joint does not move properly and is hypomobile, it goes from a low to a high position. The presence of this sign indicates an abnormality in the torsion movement at the sacroiliac joint.

Confirmation Procedures

Anterior innominate test, knee-to-shoulder test, Lewin-Gaenslen's test, sacral apex test, sacroiliac resisted-abduction test

Reporting Statement

Piedallu's sign is present for the right sacroiliac joint and indicates an abnormality in the torsion movement of the joint.

∾ Clinical Pearl ∾

In the sacroiliac joint fixation complex, an irregular prominence of one articular surface becomes wedged upon another prominence of the opposing articular surface. When reduction is successful, the pain is relieved immediately.

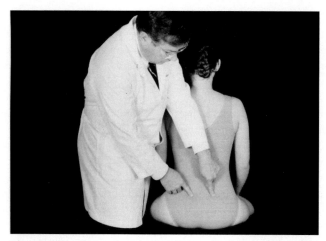

Fig. 9–28 The patient is seated on a hard, flat surface. The examiner notes pelvic symmetry and compares the height of the iliac crests.

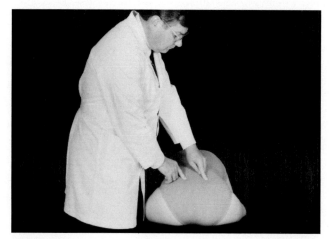

Fig. 9–29 If the posterior superior iliac spine on the affected side is lower than the other, the patient flexes forward while remaining seated. If the lower posterior superior iliac spine now becomes higher, the test is positive for an abnormality of torsion motion of the sacroiliac joint.

Comment

The forces for sacroiliac joint motion are gravity, ground reaction force, and muscle power. Sacroiliac joint motion is initiated by the muscles of the vertebral column, thighs, and respiratory system. The vertebral column muscles initiate sacroiliac joint motion of the sacrum, relative to the ilium, by changing posture (lying down, sitting, and standing) and by changing the shape of the spinal column (flexion, extension, lateral flexion, and rotation). The movement is due to change in the center of gravity, with the apex of the lordotic curve moving up or down, which causes the sacrum to nutate and the ilium to flare. As a result, the articular surfaces move anterosuperiorly to posteroinferiorly and superomedially to inferolaterally. The two posterior superior iliac spines will approximate and separate. During lateral flexion, both iliac and sacral auricular surfaces move together but gapping at different times in the anterior or posterior part of the joint as well as the upper or lower margins.

The thigh muscles initiate sacroiliac joint motion of the ilium, relative to the sacrum, again by altering posture and causing motion of the thigh rather than the spine. Here, motions will include thigh flexion, extension, supination, pronation, abduction, and adduction. The two thighs can act together or independently. Abduction and adduction create sacroiliac joint gapping but no shearing of cartilage.

Respiration aids sacroiliac joint motion during inspiration and expiration. During inspiration, the erector spinae muscles contract and the rectus abdominis relaxes by decreasing abdominal pressure. The pelvic diaphragm also relaxes and decreases abdominal pressure. When the erector group pulls the posterior part of the pelvic ring up and the rectus abdominis is relaxed, the pelvic ring will be tilted anteriorly. This tilt causes the sacral promontory to move backward and superiorly. During expiration, the erector group relaxes, the rectus abdominis contracts, and the pelvic diaphragm contracts. Action of the rectus abdominis pulls the symphysis pubis up and tilts the pelvic ring posteriorly. Abdominal pressure is increased, which causes the sacral promontory to move anteriorly and inferiorly.

Procedure

The patient lies in a prone position on a firm surface while the examiner places the base of both hands at the apex of the patient's sacrum. Pressure is then applied to the apex of the sacrum, causing a shear of the sacrum on the ilium. The test may indicate a sacroiliac joint problem if pain is produced over the joint. The test causes a rotational shift of the sacroiliac.

Confirmation Procedures

Anterior innominate test, knee-to-shoulder test, Lewin-Gaenslen's test, Piedallu's sign, sacroiliac resisted-abduction test

---

Reporting Statement

The sacral apex test is positive and indicates an abnormal rotational shifting of the right sacroiliac joint.

~ **Clinical Pearl** ~

Sciatic neuritis is a term used to describe pain or other discomfort that is experienced anywhere along the distribution of the sciatic nerve and is due to a primary disease of the nerve or, more commonly, a mechanical disorder affecting the nerve. A sacroiliac subluxation-sprain may be the true cause of sciatic neuritis. The piriformis muscle is most often affected, and it may involve the L5-S1 and S2 distribution.

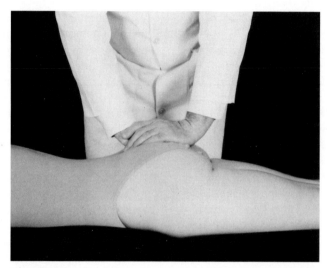

Fig. 9–30 The patient is prone on a firm examination table. The examiner places both hands at the apex of the patient's sacrum and applies pressure to the apex, causing a shear stress of the sacrum on the ilium. Pain produced in a sacroiliac joint is a positive test.

Sacroiliac Resisted-Abduction Test

HIP-ABDUCTION STRESS TEST

Comment

The sacroiliac joint has well-developed cartilage surfaces, a synovial membrane, strong anterior and posterior ligaments, and a large internal sacroiliac ligament. After the fifth decade of life, fibrosis takes place between the cartilage surfaces. By the sixth or seventh decade, the joint has usually undergone fibrous ankylosis. Bony ankylosis is a rare phenomenon late in life. The joint surfaces can rotate 3 to 5 degrees in the younger, symptom-free patient. The joint has two functions, which are to provide elasticity to the pelvic ring and to serve as a buffer between the lumbosacral and hip joints.

The sacroiliac syndrome causes pain over one sacroiliac joint in the region of the posterior superior iliac spine. This pain may be accompanied by referred pain in the leg.

The mechanism of injury is not well understood. Until late in middle age, a small amount of movement (3 to 5 degrees) is usually present in the sacroiliac joint. After that age, movement is reduced by articular cartilage degeneration, fibrosis, and rarely ankylosis. It is possible that minor dysfunction in the sacroiliac joint leads to pain, but it is more reasonable to suppose that pain results from sustained contraction of the muscle overlying the joint. This hypertonicity may accompany dysfunction in the sacroiliac joint or in the L4-L5 or L5-S1 posterior lumbar joints.

A typical symptom is pain that varies in its degree of severity and is over the back of the sacroiliac joint. Another typical symptom is referred pain in the groin, over the greater trochanter; down the back of the thigh to the knee; and occasionally, down the lateral or posterior calf to the ankle, foot, and toes.

The signs include tenderness when pressure is applied over the posterior superior iliac spine, in the region of the sacroiliac joint, or in the buttock. Movement of the joint is usually reduced. Normally the joint moves by rotating in the sagittal plane. Restricted movement can be detected in two ways.

The first way to detect restricted movement is to have the patient stand with one hand resting on the examining table for support. To examine the left sacroiliac joint, the examiner places the thumb of the right hand over the spinous process of L5 and the thumb of the left hand over the left posterior superior iliac spine. The patient then flexes both the left hip and the left knee and lifts the knee toward the chest. As this move is performed, the examiner can detect a small but definite amount of movement. Rotation in the joint causes the iliac spine to move downward in relation to the spinous process of L5. When the sacroiliac joint is fixed in position, this movement of the iliac spine, relative to the spinous process, is reduced or absent.

Confirmation can be obtained by the second test. To examine the left sacroiliac joint, the examiner places the right thumb over the apex of the patient's sacrum and the left thumb over the ischial tuberosity. In a normal joint, flexing the left knee and hip and bringing the knee toward the chest causes the ischial tuberosity to move laterally, away from the apex of the sacrum. When the joint is fixed in position, the lateral movement does not take place. The sacroiliac joint on the right is examined, using the same method.

During forward flexion the strain falls first on the iliolumbar ligament. Next, the strain is transmitted to the interspinous ligaments from L5 upward and then to the lumbodorsal fascia, particularly to the sacral triangle. During extension the impingement signs prevail over the tension effects: the articulation comes first, then the interspinous ligaments. The ligamentum flava escapes impingement. During axial rotation, the iliolumbar ligament becomes strained first, then the intertransverse. During lateral flexion the sequence is quadratus, ligamentum flava, and the interspinous ligament on the convex side.

The legs transmit their effect through the pelvis. Single leg raising causes no pelvic movement, though it causes contraction of the contralateral gluteus maximus. Double leg raising tilts the pelvis backwards; the ischial tuberosities serve as fulcrums. Forcible hyperextension of the hip puts strain on the sacroiliac ligamentous structures and is an important sign of sacroiliac strain. Abduction and outward rotation of the hip joint is transmitted to the pelvis and rotates the ilium against the sacrum. This rotation is also a practical sign for sacroiliac strain.

Through the sacroiliac joints, the weight of the body above the sacrum is transmitted to the bony pelvis and lower extremities. The upper portion of the sacrum is wider than the lower portion. The sacrum is wedged between the ilia, and its upper end extends farther forward than its lower end.

Each sacroiliac joint is formed by the internal or medial surface of the ilium and the lateral aspect of the first, second, and third sacral vertebrae. The sacroiliac joints have an articular capsule and a synovial membrane. The joint cavity is a narrow, irregular slit, and the articular surfaces of the sacrum and the ilium are covered with a layer of cartilage. The lower portion of the joint is oblique in relation to the frontal plane of the body, and, at the level of these joints, the ilia are posteriorly wrapped around the lateral portion of the sacrum. The tuberosities of the ilia extend medially beyond the sacroiliac joints and cover the upper portions of the joints, at the points where the joints are most superficial. A series of strong but short intraarticular fibers (the interosseous sacroiliac ligament) connect the tuberosities of the sacrum and ilium, filling the narrow space between these bones in the posterior portion of the joint. The sacroiliac joints are stabilized by unusually strong, dense extracapsular ligaments that resist the tendency of the upper end of the sacrum to rotate anteriorly and the lower end of the sacrum to rotate posteriorly during weight bearing. There is very little motion occurring in these joints. Whatever motion does occur, disappears with increasing age and is usually gone by middle age.

Procedure

The patient lies on the unaffected side with the affected leg extended and slightly abducted. The unaffected limb can be flexed at the hip and knee to provide stability. The examiner then exerts downward pressure on the abducted leg against the patient's resistance. The test is repeated on the opposite side. If the test elicits pelvic pain near the posterior superior iliac spine, it is positive. The test is specific for a sacroiliac sprain or subluxation.

Confirmation Procedures

Anterior innominate test, knee-to-shoulder test, Lewin-Gaenslen's test, Piedallu's sign, sacral apex test

---

Reporting Statement

Sacroiliac resisted-abduction test is positive on the right and indicates generalized abductor muscular weakness. The pain elicited implicates the sacroiliac joint and indicates sprain or subluxation of the joint.

∾ Clinical Pearl ∾

Slight, unilateral hip-abductor weakness is found in association with lateral pelvic tilt. The abductors are weak on the slightly elevated side of the pelvis. The beginning weakness in the abductors, as seen in nonparalytic individuals, is usually associated with handedness and is a strain weakness from postural or occupational causes.

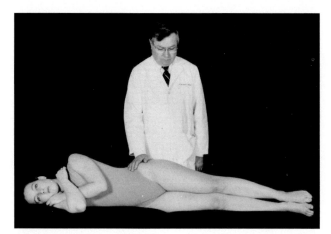

Fig. 9–31 The patient is in a side-lying position on the unaffected side.

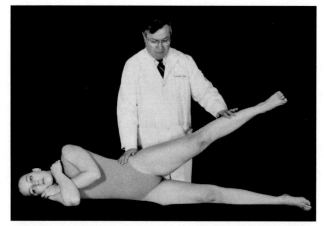

Fig. 9–32 The patient actively abducts the affected leg. At the end of the range of movement the examiner applies downward pressure on the affected limb. The patient tries to resist this pressure. When positive, the test elicits pain at the posterior superior iliac spine. The test is specific for sacroiliac sprain or subluxation.

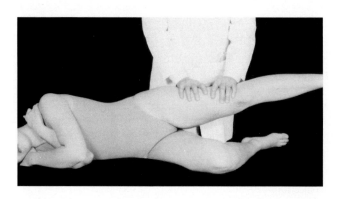

Fig. 9–33, left. In a slight modification that is only for more stability of the pelvis, the patient may flex the knee of the unaffected leg.

Comment

Sacroiliac joint injuries may take four forms, (1) a dislocation, where the articular surfaces are completely displaced from each other, (2) a subluxation, where the articular surfaces remain in contact although they are displaced, (3) a sprain, in which there is a tear of the capsular ligament without a disturbance in its relationship to the opposing surfaces, and (4) a fracture-dislocation, where a fracture of part of one of the bones has taken place in order for the articular surfaces to be completely displaced from each other.

For complete separation of the articular surfaces in a normal sacroiliac joint to be possible, the capsule of the joint must be completely torn through. This is, therefore, an injury that resulted from considerable violence applied to the joint. The soft-tissue damage may cause some residual stiffness because of scarring. At certain sites, where the cavity is shallow, residual capsular laxity may leave an unstable joint. There also may be an unhealed rent that leads to recurrent dislocation. Pathologic dislocations may occur where there is some inherent ligamentous laxity or abnormal muscle pull, such as in certain neurologic disorders leading to paralytic dislocations. Pathologic dislocations also may occur where the joint lining has been destroyed by an infective process.

Partial displacement of the articular surfaces of the sacroiliac joint, when the bones remain in contact with each other, is a subluxation. In these cases, residual laxity usually persists.

Tears of the capsular lining of the sacroiliac joint may be of a trivial nature, or they may be severe, involving a complete disruption of one of the posterior ligaments. In the latter case, momentary subluxation will have taken place, and unless the ligamentous rent heals, recurrent sprains from minor violence occurs.

The fracture of the bony margin of the sacroiliac joint, as it is dislocated, is most frequently seen in the more severe rotational injuries.

Procedure

The Smith-Petersen test is often confused with and thought to be synonymous with the Goldthwait's sign or Lasègue test. The Smith-Petersen test is also performed with the patient in the supine posture. Straight-leg raising is performed slowly, while one hand is placed under the lower part of the patient's spine. As the hamstrings tighten, leverage is progressively applied to the sacroiliac joint and then to the lumbosacral articulation. If pain is brought on before the lumbar spine begins to move, Smith-Petersen considers that a sacroiliac condition is present. If, however, pain does not come on until after the lumbar spine begins to move, either sacroiliac or lumbosacral involvement may be present. Straight-leg raising of both sides should be accomplished. If, on the unaffected side, the leg can be raised much higher, sacroiliac involvement is likely. If discomfort is elicited when both legs are brought to the same level, lumbosacral involvement is likely.

Confirmation Procedures

Belt test, Gaenslen's test, Goldthwait's test

Reporting Statement

Smith-Petersen test is positive on the right and strongly indicates sacroiliac joint involvement on that side.

Smith-Petersen test is positive bilaterally and indicates lumbosacral involvement.

∽ Clinical Pearl ∽

An acute sacroiliac flexion sprain is caused by lifting heavy objects. Often, however, the patient with chronic sacral pain has also sustained an ancient fall or flexion sprain. In cases of partial tearing of the sacroiliac ligaments, where poor healing has taken place, a painful fibrous area persists, and this results in a chronic, weak area of the joint. This area becomes symptomatic when placed under tension and stress.

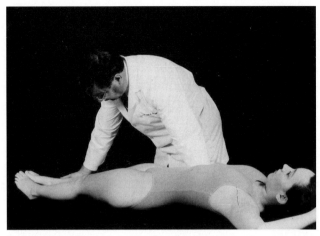

Fig. 9-34 The patient is supine on the examination table. The examiner stands on the side of the affected leg. The examiner places one hand under the patient's lumbar spine and palpates the L5-S1 spinous processes.

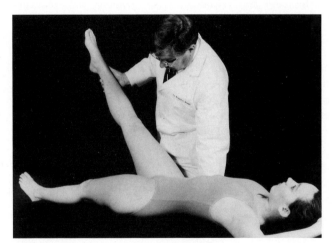

Fig. 9-35 While maintaining contact with the lumbosacral bony landmarks, the examiner performs a straight-leg raising maneuver on the affected leg. If pain occurs before the L5-S1 spinous processes separate, a sacroiliac lesion is present. If pain occurs as the L5-S1 spinous processes separate, either a sacroiliac or lumbosacral lesion may be present. The test is performed bilaterally.

Comment

Injuries to the bony pelvis are of two types: (1) isolated fractures of the pubic rami or ilium, or (2) double fractures of the pelvic ring. The latter may occur in three forms. With the first type the anterior portion of the ring may be broken if all four pubic rami are broken, and the loose portion of the ring will get driven posteriorly. With the second type, one side of the pubis may be fractured anteriorly and posteriorly and may roll laterally. With the last type, one side of the pelvic ring may be fractured and not only may it roll laterally but also it may be superiorly displaced.

As with all bony injuries of the trunk, the possibility of visceral damage must be constantly borne in the examiner's mind. With pelvic injuries this possibility is particularly applicable because the rectum, bladder, and urethra are contained within the pelvic cavity. As the membranous urethra passes through the pelvic diaphragm, this structure is especially vulnerable. A blow hard enough to disrupt the pubic bones is also very capable of rupturing a distended bladder.

Isolated pelvic fractures follow direct blows and occur, therefore, rather more readily in the more osteoporotic bones of the elderly. Fractures of the ilium alone, although less common than fractures of the pubic rami, usually result from greater trauma and therefore cause more constitutional upset to the patient. Fractures of the pubic rami on one side are of little significance unless they extend into the hip joint.

Detachment of the whole anterior segment of the pubis follows a severe blow on the front of the pelvis. This injury usually results from road accidents or sometimes from falls from a height when the patient lands prone and strikes this region on some hard object.

With lateral disruption of the pelvic ring, the pelvic ring is broken both posterior and anterior to the hip. The natural tendency for the lower limb to roll laterally will open the pelvis anteriorly. The plane of cleavage in the anterior will be either through both pubic rami on the affected side or through the pubic symphysis (diastasis of the symphysis pubis). Posteriorly, the break may be through the ilium, at the sacroiliac joint, or through the ala of the sacrum itself.

The most severe fracture is a combined lateral and superior displacement. With this form of pelvic fracture, the displaced fragment, which is attached to the lower limbs, not only has rolled laterally, but also is displaced superiorly.

Procedure

While the patient is supine, the examiner places both hands on the patient's anterior superior iliac spines and iliac crests and pushes down at a 45-degree angle. This movement will test the posterior sacroiliac ligaments. Pain indicates a positive test.

Confirmation Procedures

Gapping test, Yeoman's test

Reporting Statement

The squish test is positive on the right. This result indicates damage to the posterior sacroiliac ligaments.

∼ Clinical Pearl ∼

In the elderly, fractures of the pubic rami and ischial rami are often caused by a trivial fall. The fractures usually occur in pairs. Fracture of one ramus alone is unusual. A positive squish test in an elderly patient indicates a possible fracture of a ramus and a posterior sacroiliac sprain. The fracture can be confirmed with diagnostic imaging.

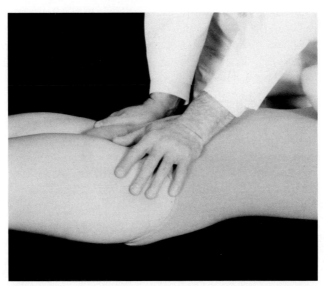

Fig. 9—36   The patient is supine on the examination table. The examiner places both hands on the patient's anterior superior iliac spines and iliac crests. The examiner pushes inferior and caudal at a 45 degree angle. Pain indicates a positive test and indicates sprain of the posterior sacroiliac ligaments.

Comment

When certain lumbosacral spinal mesodermal structures—such as ligaments, periosteum, joint capsule, and the annulus—are subjected to abnormal stimuli—such as excessive stretching—a deep, ill-defined, and dull aching is noted. This aching may be referred into areas of the lumbosacral spine, sacroiliac joint, and the buttocks as well as the legs. The referral pattern is to the area designated as the sclerotome, which has the same embryonic origin as the mesodermal tissues stimulated. Although this peripheral pathway can explain the referred pain pattern, the significant individual variations that are encountered necessitate the consideration of central neural pathways. Referred pain distribution depends not only on segmental innervation but also on the severity of pain and the extent to which an individual is cognizant of the stimulated components of the axial skeleton.

Pain of this type can often present concurrently with radicular pain that results from nerve root tension. The deeper, penetrating pain is usually attributed to distribution along the myotome and sclerotomes, and the sharper and more-localized superficial pain is conveyed via the dermatomes. The two types of pain may easily be confused. Moreover, sympathetic dystrophic signs and symptoms caused by nerve root encroachment can further confuse the presentation because the causalgia may exist with or without the more classic complaints associated with radiculopathy. Thus all lower-extremity pain is not a result of nerve root compression.

Procedure

The patient is lying prone. With one hand the examiner applies firm pressure over the suspected sacroiliac joint, fixing the pelvis to the table. With the other hand the examiner flexes the patient's leg on the affected side and hyperextends the thigh by lifting the knee off the examining table. If pain is increased in the sacroiliac area, this increase in pain indicates a sacroiliac lesion. This pain is due to the strain placed on the anterior sacroiliac ligaments. In a normal patient pain will not be felt during this maneuver.

Confirmation Procedures

Gapping test, Squish test

Reporting Statement

Yeoman's test is positive for the right sacroiliac joint. This result indicates injury of the anterior sacroiliac ligaments.

∼ Clinical Pearl ∼

Ruptured sacroiliac ligaments do not heal soundly, even if they are accurately repaired, because the scar tissue, which forms at the site of the repair, stretches and is never as tough as the original. Surgical repair is often attempted after severe rupture of these ligaments, but conservative management may be equally effective.

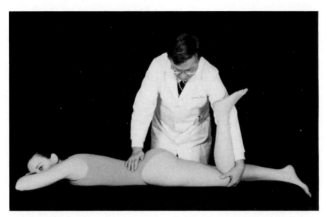

Fig. 9–37 The patient is prone on the examination table. With one hand the examiner stabilizes the affected sacroiliac joint. The examiner flexes the knee of the affected leg to 90 degrees.

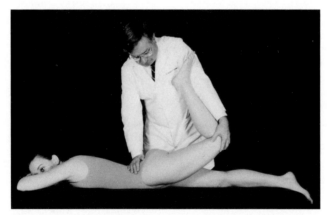

Fig. 9–38 The examiner hyperextends the thigh of the affected leg by lifting it off the examination table. Pressure is maintained over the affected sacroiliac joint. Increased sacroiliac pain constitutes a positive test and indicates a sacroiliac joint lesion.

Bibliography

American Medical Association: *Guides to the evaluation of permanent impairment,* ed 3, Chicago, 1990, The Association.

Apley AG, Solomon L: *Concise system of orthopaedics and fractures,* London, 1988, Butterworth-Heinemann.

Aston JN: *A short textbook of orthopaedics and traumatology,* Philadelphia, 1967, JB Lippincott.

Beal MC: The sacroiliac problem, review of anatomy, mechanics and diagnosis, *J Am Osteopath Assoc,* 82(June): 667, 1982.

Berens DL: Roentgen features of ankylosing spondylitis, *Clin Orthop,* 74:20, 1971.

Berghs H, Remans J, Dieskens L, Kieboom S, Polderman J: Diagnostic value of sacroiliac joint scintigraphy with 99m technetium pyrophosphate in sacroiliitis, *Ann Rheum Dis,* 37:190, 1978.

Borenstein DG, Wiesel SW: *Low back pain medical diagnosis and comprehensive management,* Philadelphia, 1989, WB Saunders.

Bowen V, Cassidy JD: Macroscopic and microscopic anatomy of the sacroiliac joint from embryonic life until the eighth decade, *Spine,* 6:620, 1981.

Brand C, Warren R, Luxton M, Barraclough D: Cryptococcal sacroiliitis: Case report, *Ann Rheum Dis,* 44:126, 1985.

Carrera GF, Foley WD, Kozin F, Ryan L, Lawson TL: CT of sacroiliitis, *AJR Am J Roentgenol,* 136:41, 1981.

Cipriano JJ: *Photographic manual of regional orthopaedic and neurological tests,* ed 2, Baltimore, Williams and Wilkins, 1991.

Colachis SC: Movement of sacroiliac joint in adult male, *Arch Phys Med Rehabil,* 44(September): 490, 1963.

Cox JM: *Low back pain, mechanism, diagnosis and treatment,* ed 5, Baltimore, 1990, Williams and Wilkins.

Coy JT, Wolf CR, Brower TD, Winter WG Jr: Phygenic arthritis of the sacro-iliac joint: Long-term follow-up, *J Bone Joint Surg,* 58A:845, 1976.

Cyriax J: *Textbook of orthopaedic medicine, vol. 1, diagnosis of soft tissue lesions,* London, 1982, Bailliere Tindall.

D'Ambrosia RD: *Musculoskeletal disorders regional examination and differential diagnosis,* Philadelphia, 1977, JB Lippincott.

Dandy DJ: *Essential orthopaedics and trauma,* Edinburgh, 1989, Churchill Livingstone.

deBlecourt JJ, Poleman A, deBlecourt-Meindersma T: Hereditary factors in rheumatoid arthritis and ankylosing spondylitis, *Ann Rheum Dis,* 20:215, 1961.

DeBosset P, Gordon DA, Smythe HA, Urowitz MB, Koehler BE, Singal DP: Comparison of osteitis condensans ilii and ankylosing spondylitis in female patients: Clinical, radiological and HLA typing characteristics, *J Chron Dis,* 31:171, 1978.

Delbarre F, Rondier J, Delrieu F, Evrard J, Cuyla J, Menkes CJ, Armor B: Pyogenic infection of the sacroiliac joint, *J Bone Joint Surg,* 57A:819, 1975.

Dihlmann W: Diagnostic radiology of the sacroiliac joints, New York, 1980, George Thieme Verlag.

Dilsen N et al: A comparative roentgenologic study of rheumatoid arthritis and rheumatoid (ankylosing) spondylitis, *Arthritis Rheum,* 5:341, 1962.

Doherty M, Doherty J: *Clinical examination in rheumatology,* London, 1992, Wolfe Publishing.

Dulhunty JA: Sacroiliac subluxation, facts, fallacies and illusions, *J Aust Chiro Assoc,* 15(3):91-99, 1985.

Dunn DJ, Bryan Dm, Nugent JT, Robinson RA: Pyogenic infections of the sacroiliac joint, *Clin Orthop,* 118:113, 1976.

Elliott FA, Schutta HS: The differential diagnosis of sciatica, *Orthop Clin North Am,* 2:477, 1971.

Epstein MC: Cause of low back problem, *Dig Chiro Econ,* (January/February):52-54, 1983.

Farfan HF: *Mechanical disorders of the low back,* Philadelphia, 1973, Lea & Febiger.

Finneson BE: Low back pain, ed 2, Philadelphia, 1980, JB Lippincott.

Gifford DB, Patzakis M, Ivler D, Swezey RL: Septic arthritis due to pseudomonas in heroin addicts, *J Bone Joint Surg,* 57A:631, 1975.

Goldberg, J, Kovarsky J: Tuberculous sacroiliitis, *South Med J,* 76:1175, 1983.

Goldstein MJ, Nasr K, Singer HC, Anderson JG: Osteomyelitis complicating regional enteritis, *Gut,* 10:264, 1969.

Gordon G, Kabins SA: Pyogenic sacroiliitis, *Am J Med,* 69:50, 1980.

Gorse GJ, Pais MJ, Kusske JA, Cesario TC: Tuberculous spondylitis: A report of six cases and a review of the literature, *Medicine (Baltimore),* 62:178, 1978.

Greenman PE: Innominate shear dysfunction in sacroiliac syndrome, *Jmm,* 2:114, 1986.

Hendrix RW, Lin PJP, Kane WJ: Simplified aspiration or injection techniques for the sacroiliac joint, *J Bone Joint Surg,* 64A:1249, 1982.

Iczkovitz JM, Leek JC, Robbins DL: Pyogenic sacroiliitis, *J Rheumatol,* 8:157, 1981.

Jenkins DH, Young MH: The operative treatment of sacroiliac subluxation and disruption of the symphysis pubis, *Injury,* 10:139, 1978.

Kapandji LA: *The physiology of the joints, vol 3: The trunk and vertebral column,* New York, 1974, Churchill Livingstone.

Katz WA: Rheumatic diseases diagnosis and management, Philadelphia, 1977, JB Lippincott.

Kellgren JH: The anatomical source of back pain, *Rheum Rehab,* 16:3, 1977.

Kendall HO, Kendall FP, Wadsworth GE: Muscles testing and function, ed 2, Baltimore, 1971, Williams and Wilkins.

Kirkaldy-Willis WH: Managing low back pain, New York, 1983, Churchill Livingstone.

Lewkonia RM, Kinsella TD: Phygenic sacroiliitis: Diagnosis and significance, *J Rheumatol,* 8:153, 1981.

Lisbona R, Rosenthall L: Observation on the sequential use of 99mTc-phosphate complex and 67Gd imaging in osteomyelitis and septic arthritis, *Radiology,* 123:123, 1977.

Longoria RK, Carpenter JL: Anaerobic phygenic sacroiliitis, *South Med J,* 76:649, 1983.

Magee DJ: *Orthopedic physical assessment,* Philadelphia, 1987, WB Saunders.

Maigne R: *Orthopaedic medicine: A new approach to vertebral manipulation,* Springfield, 1972, Charles C. Thomas.

Maitland GD: *Vertebral manipulation,* ed 5, London, 1986, Butterworth.

Mazion JM: *Illustrated manual of neurological reflexes/signs/tests, part I, orthopedic signs/tests/maneuvers for office procedure, part II,* Orlando, 1980, Daniels Publishing.

McRae R: *Clinical orthopaedic examination,* ed 3, Edinburgh, 1990, Churchill Livingstone.

Medical Economics Books: *Patient care flow chart manual,* ed 3, Oradell, NJ, 1982, Medical Economics Books.

Mitchell FL: *Structural pelvic function,* Mosby, 2:178, 1965.

Mooney V, Robertson J: The facet syndrome, *Clin Orthop,* 115:149, 1976.

Murphy ME: Primary pyogenic infection of sacroiliac joint, *NY State J Med,* 77:1309, 1977.

Norman GF: Sacroiliac disease and its relationship to lower abdominal pain, *Am J Surg,* 116:54-56, 1968.

Numaguci Y: Osteitis condensans ilii, including its resolution, *Radiology,* 98:1, 1971.

O'Donoghue DH: *Treatment of injuries to athletes,* ed 3, Philadelphia, 1976, WB Saunders.

Omer GE, Spinner M: *Management of peripheral nerve problems,* Philadelphia, 1980, WB Saunders.

Polley HF, Hunder GG: *Rheumatologic interviewing and physical examination of the joints.* ed 2, Philadelphia, 1978, WB Saunders.

Resnick D, Dwosh I, Goergen TG, Shapiro R, Utsinger PD, Wiesner K, Bryan B: Clinical and radiographic abnormalities in ankylosing spondylitis, a comparison of men and women, *Radiology,* 119:293, 1976.

Rothman RH, Simeone FA eds: *The spine,* vol 1, 2, Philadelphia, 1975, WB Saunders.

Schafer RC: *Clinical biomechanics,* ed 2, Baltimore, 1987, Williams and Wilkins.

Schlosstein L et al: High association of an HL-A Antigen W 27 with ankylosing spondylitis and rheumatoid arthritis, *Ann Rheum Dis,* 20:47, 1961.

Schmorl G, Junghanns H: *The human spine in health and disease,* Am ed 2, (Translated by EF Bessmann), New York, 1971, Grune and Stratton.

Singal DP, deBosset P, Gordon DA, Smyth HA, Urowitz MB, Koehler BE: HLA antigens in osteitis condensans ilii and ankylosing spondylitis, *J Rheumatol* 4 (Suppl 3):105, 1977.

Smith-Petersen MN: Painful affections of lower back, in Christopher F: Textbook of surgery, ed 5, Philadelphia, 1949, WB Saunders.

Strange FGS: The prognosis in sacro-iliac tuberculosis, *Br J Surg,* 50:561, 1963.

Szlachter BN, Quagliarello J, Jewelewicz R, Osathanondh R, Spellacy WN, Weiss G: Relaxin in normal and pathologenic pregnancies, *Obstet Gynecol,* 59:167, 1982.

Taylor RW, Sonson RD: Separation of the pubic symphysis, an underrecognized peripartum complication, *J Reprod Med,* 31:203, 1986.

Thurston SE: *The little black book of neurology,* Chicago, 1987, Mosby.

Turek SL: *Orthopaedics principles and their application,* ed 3, Philadelphia, 1977, JB Lippincott.

Veys EM, Govaerts A, Coigne E, Mielants H, Verbruggen A: HLA and infective sacroiliitis, *Lancet,* 2:349, 1974.

Wallace R, Cohen AS: Tuberculous arthritis: A report of two cases with review of biopsy and synovial fluid findings, *Am J Med,* 61:277, 1976.

Wiesel SW, Bernini P, Rothman RH: The aging lumbar spine, Philadelphia, 1982, WB Saunders.

Withrington RH, Sturge RA, Mitchell N: Osteitis condensans ilii or sacro-iliitis?, *Scand J Rheumatol,* 14:163, 1985.

Wood J: *Motion of sacroiliac joint,* Palmer College Research Forum, Davenport, Ia (Spring):1-16, 1985.

~ 10 ~

The Hip Joint

*T*he hip joint is the largest and most stable joint in the body. If the hip joint is injured or if it exhibits a pathologic condition, the presence of a lesion is immediately perceptible during walking. Because pain from the hip can be referred to the sacroiliac joint or the lumbar spine, it is imperative, unless there is direct trauma to the hip, that these joints be examined with the hip.

The hip joint is a multiaxial ball and socket joint that has maximum stability because of its deep insertion into the head of the femur into the acetabulum. The hip joint has a strong capsule and very strong muscles that control its actions. The acetabulum is formed by the fusion of the ilium, ischium, and pubis and is deepened by a labrum. The acetabulum, which opens outward, forward, and downward, is half of a sphere, and the femoral head is two thirds of a sphere.

The hip joint has three different degrees of freedom. The resting position of the hip is 30 degrees of flexion, 30 degrees of abduction, and slight external rotation. The capsular pattern of the hip is flexion, abduction, and internal rotation. These three movements will always be affected the most in a capsular pattern, but the order may be altered. For example, internal rotation may be most limited, followed by flexion and abduction. The close packed position of the joint is maximum extension, internal rotation, and abduction.

Under low loads, the joint surfaces are incongruous. Under heavy loads, the joint surfaces become congruous, providing maximum surface contact. The maximum contact brings the load per unit area down to a tolerable level. An example of the forces involved in the hip are (1) standing while supporting one third of the body weight, (2) standing on one limb while supporting 2.4 to 2.6 times the body weight, and (3) walking while supporting 1.3 to 5.8 times the body weight.

Index of Tests

Actual leg length test

Allis' sign

Anvil test

Apparent leg-length test

Chiene's test

Gauvain's sign

Guilland's sign

Hip telescoping test

Jansen's test

Ludloff's sign

Ober's test

Patrick's test

Phelp's test

Thomas test

Trendelenburg's test

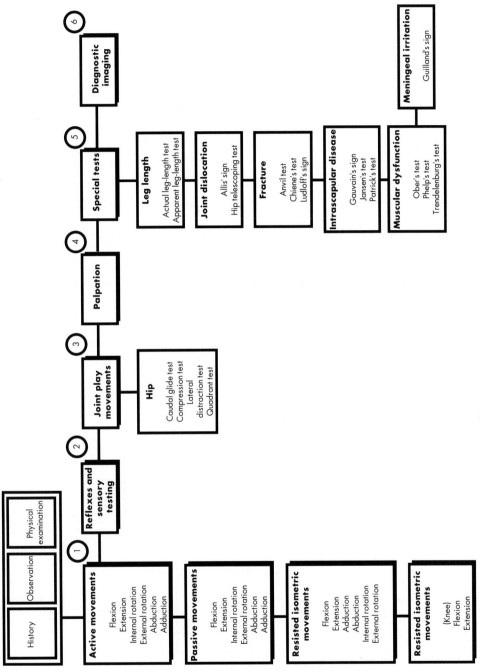

Fig. 10—1 Hip joint assessment.

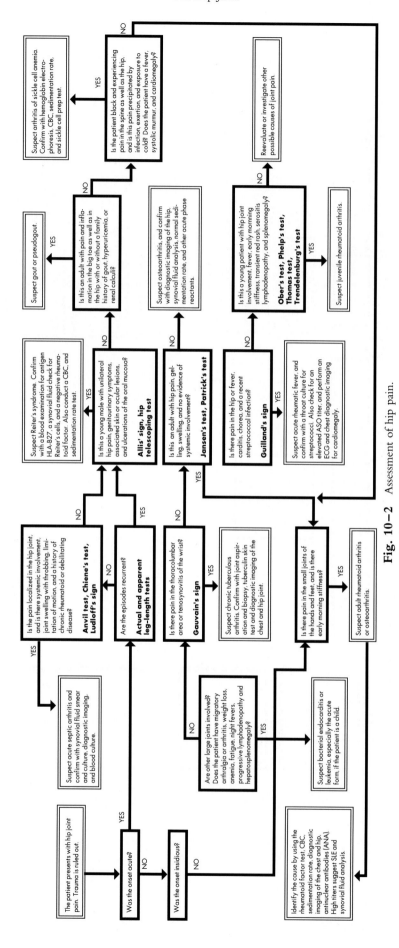

Fig. 10–2 Assessment of hip pain.

RANGE OF MOTION

The hip has a wide range of motion that permits flexion, extension, adduction, abduction, rotation, and circumduction. The angulation between the neck and the shaft of the femur partially converts the angular movements of flexion, extension, adduction, and abduction, into rotary movements of the femoral head within the acetabulum. When the hip is flexed and abducted, it loses much of the stability that is observed in the extended position. This loss of stability is because only a part of the femoral head is covered by the acetabulum and the remaining portion is covered only by the articular capsule.

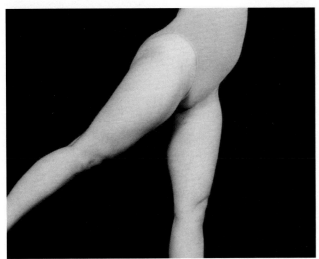

Fig. 10–3 Extension of the hip is defined as the upward (or backward) motion of the hip from the zero starting position. Motion beyond the neutral position (0 degrees) is sometimes alternatively called hyperextension. Extension of the hip is likely to reflect some motion of the back, but this is infrequent. Extension normally may measure 10 to 20 degrees less when the patient is prone or supine than when the patient is standing. The difference is attributed to a greater extensor torque, which is created by the weight of the torso, centered slightly posterior to the hip joint in a normal standing position.

In the usual method of clinical examination for extension of the hip, the patient is prone. The examiner applies downward pressure to the sacrum with a flattened hand. The examiner's other hand, which is placed midway against the anterior aspect of the patient's thigh, is used to lift the thigh on the side that is being examined.

With the available methods of eliminating exaggerated lumbar lordosis and accomplishing fixation of the pelvis, 15 degrees of extension or hyperextension of the hip may be obtained. With less adequate fixation or with abnormal laxity of the ligaments of the hip (a rarity), the thigh may be hyperextended about 30 to 40 degrees. Retained extension range of motion (standing or prone) of 20 degrees or less is an impairment of the hip in the activities of daily living.

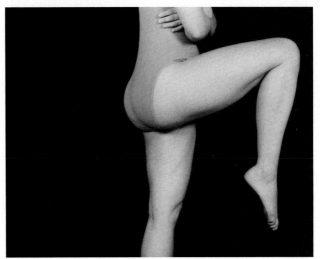

Fig. 10–4 The greatest degree of flexion of the hip while in the standing position is possible when the knee is also flexed. The thigh can be flexed to 120 degrees from the neutral or extended position (0 degrees), if the knee has first been flexed to 90 degrees. Sometimes, the hip can be flexed until the anterior surface of the thigh presses against the anterior abdominal wall.

If the knee cannot be flexed, flexion of the hip can be tested by raising the extended leg off the surface of the examination table. If the knee remains extended, tension of the hamstring muscles will limit flexion of the hip. The angle between the thigh and the long axis of the body, when the hip is normal, may not be more than a right angle (90 degrees).

However, some individuals with apparently normal hips are only able to flex the hip to form an angle of about 75 degrees, when the leg is extended. In other individuals, the range of motion is much greater than 90 degrees. Retained flexion range of motion of 90 degrees or less is an impairment of hip function in the activities of daily living.

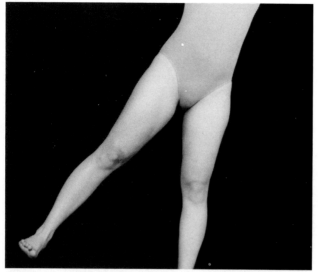

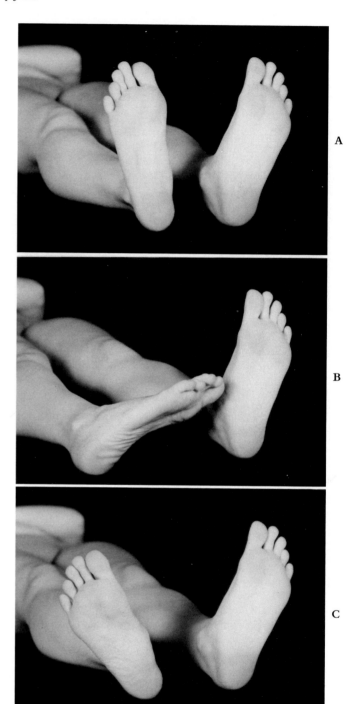

Fig. 10-5   Abduction and adduction are measured while both thighs and legs are in the extended position and are parallel to each other. The patient can be standing or supine. Measurement is made from the angle formed between an imaginary midline that is extended from the long axis of the body and the long axis of the leg. The amount of abduction permitted increases with flexion and decreases with extension of the hip. Normally, when the leg and thigh are extended, the hip abducts to approximately 40 to 45 degrees, from the neutral position, before the pubofemoral and medial portions of the iliofemoral ligaments restrict this abduction. Retained abduction range of motion of 30 degrees or less is an impairment of the hip in the activities of daily living.

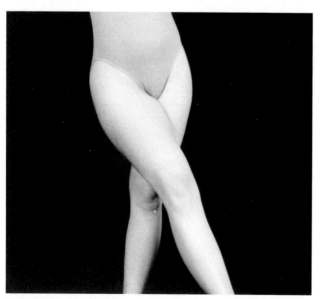

Fig. 10-6   Adduction with the leg straight out is limited by the legs and thighs, which come into contact with each other. When it is possible to adduct the hip with enough flexion to permit crossing one leg over the other and then reversing the procedure, the degree of adduction of the hip of the extremity that is on top can be measured. Adduction is usually possible to approximate 20 to 30 degrees from the neutral (starting) position.

Fig. 10-7   External and internal rotation of the hip can be tested with the patient's hip and knee fully extended while the patient is supine (**A**), by rolling the thigh, leg, and foot inward (**B**) and outward (**C**). The hip normally rotates inward approximately 40 degrees and outward approximately 45 degrees, but the range of motion varies among normal individuals and both sides should be compared. External rotation is limited by the lateral band of the iliofemoral ligament. Internal rotation is limited by the ischiocapsular ligament. Rotation of the hip increases with flexion and decreases with extension of the hip. Limitation of internal rotation of the hip is the earliest and most reliable sign of disease of the hip.

Retained internal rotation of 30 degrees or less or retained external rotation range of motion of 40 degrees or less is an impairment of the hip in the activities of daily living.

MUSCLE TESTING

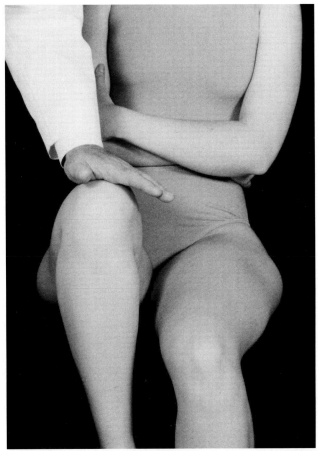

Fig. 10–8 The iliopsoas is the primary flexor of the hip, and it is innervated by the femoral nerve, which is composed of the L1, L2, and L3 nerve roots. To test the strength of the iliopsoas, the patient is examined while seated on the examining table. The examiner asks the patient to flex the hip against manual resistance, which the examiner provides. Accessory muscles involved are the rectus femoris, sartorius, tensor fasciae latae, pectineus, adductor brevis, and adductor longus muscles and the oblique fibers of the adductor magnus muscle. Flexion of the hip also may be tested while the patient is lying supine with the knee extended. Tension of the hamstring muscles, when they are stretched, may limit flexion and interfere with interpretation of the test.

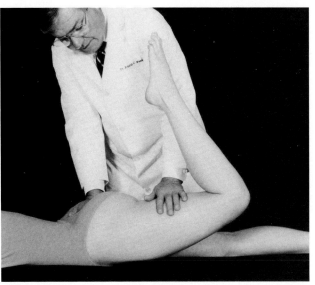

Fig. 10–9 Prime movers in extension of the hip are the gluteus maximus (inferior gluteal nerve, L5, S1, and S2), semitendinosus (tibial branch of sciatic nerve, L4, L5, S1, and S2), and semimembranosus (tibial branch of sciatic nerve, L5, S1, and S2) muscles, and the long head of the biceps femoris (tibial branch of the sciatic nerve, S1, S2, and S3) muscle. To measure the strength of the gluteus maximus, the patient is placed prone on the examining table and is directed to extend the hip against the examiner's hand, which is placed on the thigh and pelvis.

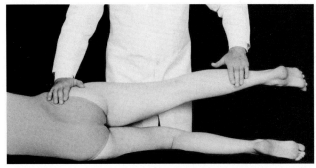

Fig. 10–10 The gluteus medius muscle (superior gluteal nerve, L4, L5, and S1) is the primer mover in abduction of the hip. The gluteus minimus, tensor fasciae latae, and upper fibers of the gluteus maximus muscles are accessory to this motion. The strength of these can be estimated by observing the patient's gait and using Trendelenburg's test. An additional test can be performed by placing the patient in a side-lying position on the examination table and having the patient abduct the hip against resistance provided by the examiner.

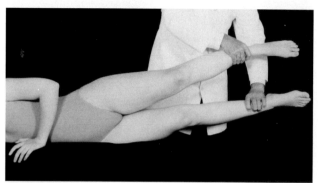

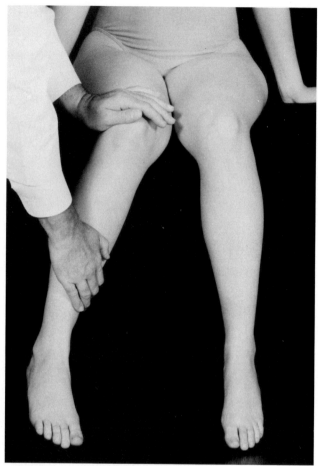

Fig. 10–11 Prime movers in adduction of the hip are the adductor magnus (obturator and sciatic nerves, L3, L4, L5, and S1), adductor brevis (obturator nerve, L3, and L4), adductor longus (obturator nerve, L3, and L4), pectineus (femoral nerve, L2, L3, and L4 and occasionally obturator nerve, L3, and L4) and gracilis (obturator nerve, L3, and L4) muscles. Adduction is tested while the patient is lying on one side with the legs extended. The upper leg, which is supported by one of the examiner's hands, is held in approximately 25 degrees of abduction. The patient then adducts the lower leg off the table, toward the elevated leg, without rotating the leg or tipping the pelvis. The examiner's free hand provides graded resistance proximal to the knee joint.

Fig. 10–12 Prime movers in external rotation of the hip are the obturator externus (obturator nerve, L3, and L4), obturator internus (sacral plexus, L4, L5, and S1) piriformis (sacral plexus, S1, and S2) gemellus superior (sacral plexus, L5, S1, and S2) gemellus inferior (sacral plexus, L4, L5, and S1) and the gluteus maximus (inferior gluteal nerve, L5, S1, and S2) muscles. The sartorius muscle is accessory to this motion. Lateral rotation of the hip is tested while the patient sits with the legs hanging over the edge of the table. The examiner places one hand over the lateral aspect of the thigh, just above the knee, and applies counterpressure to the thigh to prevent abduction and flexion of the hip. The patient grasp the edge of the table to help stabilize the pelvis. The patient then rotates the hip and thigh laterally and the lower leg rotates medially while the examiner's other hand applies graded resistance above the ankle against the motion being tested.

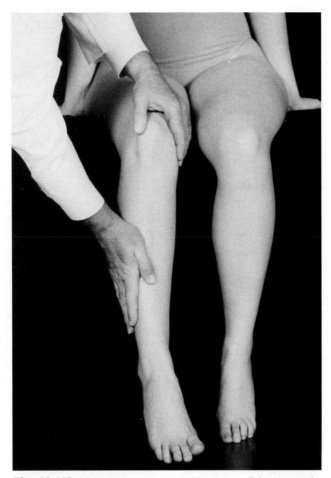

Fig. 10–13 Prime movers in internal rotation of the hip are the gluteus minimus (superior gluteal nerve, L4, L5, and S1) and the tensor fasciae latae (superior gluteal nerve, L4, L5, and S1) muscles. Anterior fibers of the gluteus medius, semimembranosus, and semitendinosus muscles are accessory to this motion. Medial rotation of the hip is tested while the patient sits with the legs over the edge of a table, as if testing lateral rotation of the hip. The examiner uses one hand to apply counterpressure above the knee and over the medial aspect of the thigh to prevent adduction of the hip. The patient holds the edge of the table to stabilize the pelvis. The patient then rotates the thigh medially and rotates the lower leg laterally while the examiner's other hand provides graded resistance above the ankle joint.

Comment

Methods of measuring the lower limbs are often confusing. Accuracy in measurement is of more than academic significance. Accurate measurement is of practical importance when corrective operations or adjustments to the shoes are contemplated. Limb length can be measured clinically within an error of 1 cm. If greater accuracy is needed, radiographic measurement (scanography) is recommended.

First, it is necessary to measure the real, or true, length of each limb. Second, it is necessary to determine whether there is any apparent, or false, discrepancy in the length of the limbs due to fixed pelvic tilt. It is always necessary to measure the true leg length. It is necessary to measure apparent discrepancy only when there is a correctable pelvic tilt.

The anterior superior iliac spine (ASIS) is significantly lateral to the axis of hip movement. This positioning does not matter if the angle between the limb and the pelvis is the same on each side. The measurements will be fallacious if the angle between limb and pelvis is not the same for each side. Abduction of a hip brings the medial malleolus nearer to the corresponding anterior superior iliac spine. Adduction of the hip carries the medial malleolus away from the (ASIS). Thus if measurements are made while the patient lies with one hip adducted and the other abducted (a common posture in cases of hip disease), inaccurate readings will be obtained. The length will be exaggerated on the adducted side and diminished on the abducted side.

To obtain an accurate comparison of true length by surface measurement, the two limbs must be placed in comparable positions relative to the pelvis. If one limb is adducted and cannot be brought out to the neutral position, the other limb must be adducted through a corresponding angle, by crossing it over the first limb before the measurements are taken. Similarly, if one hip is in fixed abduction, the other hip must be abducted to the same angle before the measurements of true length are made.

In fixing the tape measure to the anterior superior iliac spine, a flat metal end is essential. The metal end is placed immediately distal to the (ASIS), and this end is pushed up against the spine. The thumb is then pressed firmly backwards against the bone and the tape end. This procedure provides rigid fixation of the tape measure against the bone.

When taking the reading at the medial malleolus, the tip of the index finger should be placed immediately distal to the medial malleolus and should be pushed up against it. The thumbnail is brought down against the tip of the index finger so the tape measure is pinched between them. The point of measurement is indicated by the thumbnail.

If measurements reveal real shortening of a limb, it is necessary to determine whether the shortening is above the trochanteric level (suggesting an affection in or near the hip), or below the trochanteric level (suggesting an affection of the limb bones).

Tests for shortening that occurs above the trochanteric level are (1) the measurement of Bryant's triangle, (2) the construction of Nélaton's line, and (3) construction of Shoemaker's line.

In principle, Bryant's triangle is nothing more than a method of comparing the distance between the greater trochanter and the wing of the ilium on the two sides. While the patient is lying supine, a perpendicular is dropped from the anterior superior spine of the ilium (ASIS) toward the examining table. A second line is projected upwards from the tip of the greater trochanter to meet the first line at a right angle. The second line is the important line of the triangle because it is measured and compared bilaterally. The third side of the triangle is unimportant. This third line joins the anterior superior iliac spine to the tip of the greater trochanter. Measurement of Bryant's triangle allows for comparison of the distance between the pelvis and the trochanter on each side. Relative shortening on one side indicates that the femur is displaced upward as a result of a lesion in or near the hip. If there is a possibility that both sides are abnormal, measurement of Bryant's triangle is not helpful.

Nélaton's line is measured while the patient is lying on the unaffected side. A tape measure or string is stretched on the affected side from the tuberosity of the ischium to the anterior superior spine of the ilium. Normally, the greater trochanter lies on or below that tape measure line. If the trochanter lies above the line, the femur has been displaced upward.

Shoemaker's line is a similar test. The test involves projection of two lines, one on each side of the body, from the greater trochanter through and beyond the anterior superior iliac spine. Normally the two lines meet in the midline above the umbilicus. If one femur is displaced upward, because of shortening above the greater trochanter, the lines will meet away from the midline on the opposite side. If both femora are displaced, the lines will meet at or near the midline but below the umbilicus.

True shortening is sometimes caused by an abnormality—such as a congenital defect of development, impaired epiphyseal growth, or previous fracture with overlapping of the fragments—that occurs below the trochanteric level. To investigate this possibility, measurements of the femur (tip of the greater trochanter to the line of the knee joint) and of the tibia (line of the knee joint to the medial malleolus) on each side should be obtained.

Procedure

The patient is lying supine with the feet together, the knees and hips straight, the anterior superior iliac spines and the iliac crests exposed. The examiner, by way of palpation, marks the apex of the anterior iliac spines and the crests of the ilia. The examiner then measures the distance between these features and the medial malleolus. The distance is recorded and compared with the opposite side. These distances represent the actual leg length. Actual leg length discrepancies are caused by an abnormality above or below the trochanter level.

Confirmation Procedures

Apparent leg-length measurements

Reporting Statement

Leg-length measurements reveal a true leg-length discrepancy on the right. This discrepancy is corroborated by Bryant's triangle as a discrepancy that results from a lesion in or near the hip joint.

∽ Clinical Pearl ∽

Causes of true shortening above the trochanter include (1) coxa vara, resulting from neck fractures, slipped epiphysis, Perthes disease, congenital coxa vara; (2) loss of articular cartilage from infection or arthritis; and (3) dislocation of the hip. It is rare that lengthening of the other limb gives relative, true shortening. This relative, true shortening may be due to (1) stimulation of bone growth from increased vascularity, which may occur after long bone fracture in children or bone tumor, and (2) coxa valga, which follows polio.

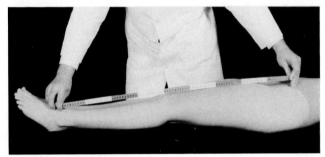

Fig. 10–14 The patient is lying supine with the feet together. The knees and hips are straight. With a tape measure the examiner measures the length of the affected leg from the apex of the anterior superior iliac spine to the medial malleolus. The distance is recorded and compared with the opposite leg. Actual leg-length shortening is caused by an abnormality above or below the trochanteric level.

∾ Allis' Sign ∾
SALEAZZI'S SIGN

Comment

Congenital dislocation of the hip is a spontaneous dislocation of the hip that occurs either before, during, or shortly after birth. It is clear that several factors are causative agents. Some of the factors are genetic and some environmental. One such factor, acting alone, may not always be sufficient by itself to bring about dislocation, and it may be that a combination of factors is often at work.

Generalized ligamentous laxity is found in some patients, and it may also be present in a parent or relatives. This laxity leads to a lack of stability at the hip, so dislocation may occur easily in certain positions of the joint.

It is possible that, in females, a ligament-relaxing hormone (relaxin) may be secreted by the fetal uterus in response to estrogen and progesterone that reaches the fetal circulation. This relaxin may cause instability as does genetically determined joint laxity. It is also possible that laxity of the hip ligaments from this cause might help to explain the greater incidence of dislocation in females.

Defective development of the acetabulum and the femoral head can be inherited. The defect appears always to be bilateral and is probably as common in males as in females. Defective development of the acetabulum predisposes a fetus to hip dislocation, which may indeed occur before birth. If dislocation does not occur, the defect may show itself in adult life in the form of an unduly shallow acetabulum that has a tendency to subluxate. Later, osteoarthritis (acetabular dysplasia) may occur.

The incidence of congenital hip dislocation is slightly higher when an infant is delivered by a breech rather than normal delivery. It is possible that the act of extending the hips during delivery may precipitate dislocation, when there is already a predisposition to it from ligamentous laxity or acetabular dysplasia.

There may be two distinct types of congenital dislocation of the hip. The first type of dislocation is caused by ligamentous laxity, whether genetically determined or hormonal. With this type of dislocation, the dislocation occurs almost accidentally when some precipitating movement, such as extension of the hips during delivery, occurs. This dislocation is the type that is often unilateral and readily correctable. The second type of dislocation is due to genetically determined dysplasia of the acetabulum, which is always bilateral and often much more difficult to treat.

Procedure

The patient is lying supine with the knees flexed and the soles of the feet flat on the table the great toes and malleoli being approximated bilaterally. The examiner observes the heights of the knees from a viewpoint at the foot of table. If one knee is lower than the other, ipsilateral hip dislocation or severe coxa disorder is indicated. Tibial length discrepancies are also discerned in this position. From side-viewing the position the examiner can assess femoral length discrepancies.

Confirmation Procedures

Hip telescoping test, diagnostic imaging

Reporting Statement

Allis' sign is present in the right leg, and demonstrates a femoral portion deficiency. The presence of this sign suggests congenital dislocation of the hip joint.

Allis' sign is present in the right leg, and demonstrates a tibial portion deficiency. The presence of this sign suggests bone dysplasia of the lower leg.

∾ Clinical Pearl ∾

Congenital dislocation of the hip (CDH) is a condition in which one or both hips are dislocated at birth or are dislocated in the first few weeks of life. There is a familial tendency and a well-established geographic distribution for the disorder. The disorder may occur with other congenital defects.

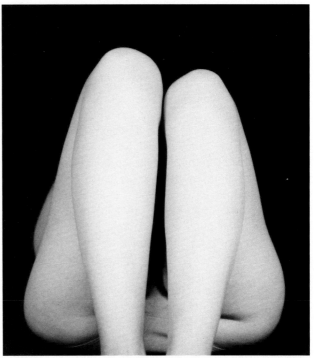

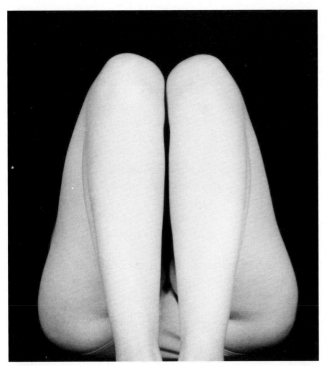

Fig. 10–15 The patient is lying supine. The knees are flexed, and the feet are flat on the examination table. The great toes and malleoli are approximated bilaterally.

Fig. 10–16 From the foot of the table, the examiner observes the height of the knees. If one is lower than the other, it indicates a femoral deficiency that is due to a pathologic condition of the ipsilateral coxa (dislocation). This may also indicate a tibial length discrepancy.

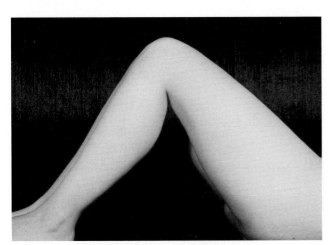

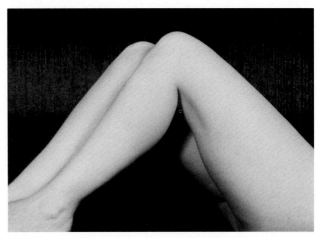

Fig. 10–17 From the side of the table, the examiner observes the position of the patient's knees. Again, the great toes and malleoli are approximated bilaterally.

Fig. 10–18 If one knee is ahead of the other, it indicates femoral length discrepancy (dysplasia) or ipsilateral coxa pathology (dislocation).

Comment

All fracture-dislocations of the hip have a history of severe trauma in common. The type of trauma and the mechanism of injury are extremely important in identifying the fracture-dislocations. Physical examination and simple observation of the attitude of the limp will aid in differentiating the type of fracture-dislocation even before diagnostic imaging. Laboratory data are usually of no help unless there are extremely low hemoglobin and hematocrit counts. When these counts are low, the possibility of pelvic fracture must be a paramount consideration, because enormous quantities of blood can be lost in the retroperitoneal area from pelvic fractures.

Fractures of the head of the femur usually occur in association with a dislocation of the head of the femur but have been known to occur without a dislocation. There is nothing unique about the presentation of these fractures that aids in their differentiation. The examiner must rely on diagnostic imaging for help identifying the type fracture. The examiner should look for fractures of the superior aspect of the head of the femur with anterior dislocation and fractures of the inferior aspect with posterior dislocations.

Fractures of the neck of the femur may be displaced or undisplaced. The undisplaced fractures are due to stress, which usually occurs in young athletic individuals; impaction, which usually occurs in instances of minor trauma and associated osteoporosis; or postirradiation of the pelvis, which occurs after treatments for cervical cancer. The patient presents with mild to moderate pain in the groin and no rotational deformity or length discrepancy of the extremity. Often the patient is able to walk but has an antalgic gait. Routine anteroposterior diagnostic imaging of the hip will often be normal. Oblique x-rays and tomograms are indicated.

On the other hand, displaced fractures of the neck of the femur have a usual mode of presentation. These fractures occur in osteoporotic individuals, usually older females, and are associated with a minor fall or severe trauma, although the latter is rare. These patients experience severe pain throughout the hip, and the leg is held in external rotation and mild abduction. Some shortening occurs. X-rays are diagnostic and make fractures readily apparent with the displacement and disruption of Shenton's line.

In older people, the average age being 70 years, intertrochanteric fractures occur more frequently than do neck fractures. These neck fractures are more common in females, in a ratio of 8:1 over males. Neck fractures usually occur in a major fall or an associated automobile injury, with both direct and indirect forces acting on the hip. The indirect forces are the iliopsoas, with its attachment on the lesser trochanter, and the abductors, with their attachment on the greater trochanter. These indirect forces explain why separate fragments often occur within this type of injury. There will be marked external rotation of the extremity, especially in the comminuted fracture, with the foot often resting on its lateral surface. This rotation occurs because of the attachment of the iliopsoas, which, because of the fracture, can now rotate the shaft of the femur externally. The leg shortening varies with the degree of comminution.

Patients with subtrochanteric fractures are usually younger than those with neck or intertrochanteric fractures. More force is needed to produce a subtrochanteric fracture than a intertrochanteric fracture. The physical findings are the same and the differentiation can only be made by diagnostic imaging.

Procedure

While the patient is lying supine, the inferior calcaneus is struck with the examiner's fist. Localized pain in the thigh indicates a femoral fracture or a severe pathologic condition of the joint. Localized pain in the leg indicates a tibial or fibular fracture. Pain localized to the calcaneus indicates calcaneal fracture.

Confirmation Procedures

Chiene's test, Ludloff's sign, diagnostic imaging

Reporting Statement

Anvil test is positive on the right side and elicits a sharp pain in the hip joint. This result suggests fracture of the femoral neck or head.

~ Clinical Pearl ~

Two questions must be answered in the assessment of a hip fracture. Is there a fracture? Is the fracture displaced? Usually the break becomes obvious when viewed with diagnostic imaging, but an impacted fracture can be missed. The assessment is important because impacted or undisplaced fractures have a good prognosis. Displaced fractures have a high rate of nonunion and avascular necrosis.

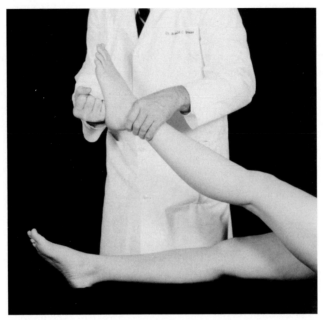

Fig. 10–19 The patient is lying supine. The examiner elevates the affected leg while keeping the knee extended. The calcaneus is struck with the examiner's fist. Localized pain in the thigh indicates a femoral fracture or a severe pathologic condition involving the joint. Localized pain in the leg indicates a tibial or fibular fracture. Pain localized to the calcaneus indicates calcaneal fracture. Markedly reactive patients may be tested with the affected leg resting completely on the examination table.

Comment

Apparent, or false, discrepancy in limb length is due entirely to sideways tilting of the pelvis. The usual cause is an adduction deformity in one hip, which gives an appearance of shortening on that side, or an abduction deformity, which gives an appearance of lengthening. An exception is a fixed pelvic obliquity that is caused by severe lumbar scoliosis.

To measure apparent discrepancy the limbs must be placed parallel to one another and in line with the trunk. Measurement is made from any fixed point in the midline of the trunk (for example the xiphisternum) to each medial malleolus. True length must be evaluated when apparent discrepancy is determined.

Procedure

Measurement is made bilaterally from the umbilicus or xiphisternum to the apex of the medial malleolus. This measurement is an index of the functional length of the lower extremities. An abduction contracture deformity causes apparent lengthening of the limb and an adduction contracture deformity causes an apparent shortening. Because the pelvis is tilted sideways to make the legs parallel, the heel of the shorter side cannot be placed on the ground when the knees are straight. The difference between the lower limbs is caused only by pelvic obliquity and measuring for a structural short leg is highly inaccurate when done in this manner.

Confirmation Procedures

Actual leg-length measurements

Reporting Statement

Measurements of leg length reveal an apparent discrepancy. This discrepancy is corroborated by accurate and equal measurements for true leg length. This result suggests a leg-length discrepancy due to pelvic obliquity.

∽ Clinical Pearl ∽

Pelvic tilting accompanied by a heel discrepancy indicates apparent shortening of the limb. This apparent shortening may be accompanied by some true shortening. The discrepancy at the heels provides a measure of its degree.

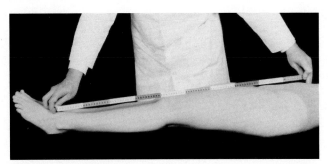

Fig. 10–20 The patient is lying supine with the legs extended on the examination table. With a tape measure the examiner measures the length of the affected leg from the medial malleolus to the umbilicus. The distance is recorded and compared with the measurement obtained for the opposite leg. The difference in the length of the legs is probably due to pelvic obliquity.

Comment

Fracture about the hip is unusual in the adolescent and young adult because the bone is exceptionally resilient. In young patients the hip is much more likely to dislocate than it is to break.

If a fracture does occur, it is a major injury and should be treated as a medical emergency. The patient with a broken hip is completely disabled at once. The patient has severe pain in the hip and resists any attempt to manipulate the limb. The extremity is usually held with the thigh internally rotated and adducted while the knee rests above and against its fellow on the opposite side. The trochanter appears prominent. Any attempt to move the thigh from this position of flexion adduction and internal rotation causes pain. Diagnosis is confirmed by diagnostic imaging, and the images should be carefully studied to be sure there is not an accompanying fracture in the femoral shaft or acetabulum. The posterior acetabular margin, vulnerable in the adult, is seldom broken in the adolescent or young adult.

Nonunion of femoral neck fractures occurs in approximately 15% of the cases. The reasons for nonunion are (1) meager blood supply and (2) inaccurate approximation and rigid fixation of the fragments.

The outstanding manifestations of nonunion of fracture of the neck of the femur are (1) pain in the hip when bearing weight, (2) shortening and external rotation of the limb, and (3) grating in the hip during motion. Additional complicating factors that may be present include avascular necrosis of the femoral head, which appears on diagnostic images as density changes and collapse of the head, and osteoarthritis that may restrict the mobility of the head of the acetabulum.

Procedure

Determine if a fracture of the neck of the femur has occurred by using a tape measure. The patient is supine with the legs extended on the examination table. Using a tape measure, the examiner measures the circumference of the thigh, passing the tape over the level of the greater trochanter. The distance is recorded and compared to that of the opposite leg. An increased diameter indicates that the trochanter has rolled laterally. This increased measurement correlates with fracture of the neck of the femur.

Confirmation Procedures

Anvil test, Ludloff's sign, diagnostic imaging

Reporting Statement

Chiene's test is positive for the right hip. This result suggests a fracture of the neck of the femur.

~ **Clinical Pearl** ~

A fracture of the neck of the femur occurs mainly among elderly females whose bones are osteoporotic. The patient may fall but more often the patient catches a foot on something and ends up twisting the hip. The femoral neck is broken by rotational force. In most cases the fracture is markedly displaced and completely unstable. In some cases the fragments are impacted and the patient may even walk about, albeit with some pain.

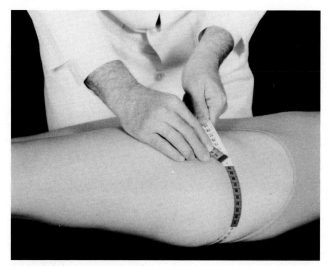

Fig. 10−21   The patient is lying supine with the legs extended on the examination table. Using a tape measure, the examiner measures the circumference of the thigh by passing the tape over the level of the greater trochanter. The distance is recorded and compared with the measurement obtained for the opposite leg. An increased diameter indicates that the trochanter has rolled laterally. This result correlates with fracture of the neck of the femur.

Comment

Tuberculosis of the hip joint may appear at any age, but it occurs most commonly in children. An intermittent limp is the first, constant sign. At first, tuberculosis of the hip may come on after exercise, but later it is present after rest, such as in the early morning. Initially pain may be only a slight discomfort that occurs in the groin or the knee and thigh (referred pain). Startling pain at night occurs at a later stage and is due to relaxation of the protective muscle contraction. At an even later stage, the patient may suffer from stiffness of the joint.

In the early stages of the disease, when it is limited to the synovium or bone, the position of the joint is that of slight flexion, abduction, and lateral rotation (greatest fluid capacity). At a later stage, when arthritis supervenes, the leg becomes flexed, adducted, and internally rotated. At an early stage, muscle wasting is not a very pronounced sign, but soon afterward it becomes obvious. In a longstanding case, atrophy of the quadriceps and glutei becomes very pronounced. At a later stage swelling that is due to the formation of an abscess may be present. This abscess commonly points anteriorly. Apparent lengthening may be present in the active stage because of fixed abduction. Apparent shortening occurs later and is due to fixed adduction.

True shortening may occur as a result of (1) bone destruction that occurs in the acetabulum, which tends to enlarge upward and is called a *wandering acetabulum*; (2) damage that occurs to the upper femoral epiphysis and that may cause retardation of growth, and, if the hip is also treated with prolonged immobilization, may result in premature fusion of the lower epiphysis; and (3) pathologic dislocation that may occasionally occur and add to the shortening.

In the early stage, deep tenderness can often be elicited in the groin. At a later stage, if an abscess is present, a soft swelling may be palpable. Atrophy of the muscles occurs later, and the trochanter may be raised on the affected side.

At first, only the extremes of movement are limited and painful. Thomas test becomes positive at an early stage and reveals concealed flexion contracture. Limitation of extension is also a valuable sign. Later, when arthritis supervenes, movements are restricted by muscular spasm, and attempted movement becomes very painful.

General malaise and pallor accompany tuberculous arthritis, and slight evening pyrexia is not uncommon. In the healing stage the general condition improves, and the joint is no longer painful.

Procedure

The patient is lying supine with the affected thigh extended. The examiner carefully rotates the thigh. The sign is positive if contraction of the abdominal muscles is noted on the same side that is being maneuvered. The sign is significant for reflex muscle spasm, which is commonly elicited in tuberculosis of the coxa. The test may be performed with the patient in a side-lying position.

Confirmation Procedure

Jansen's test, Patrick's test, diagnostic imaging

Reporting Statement

Gauvain's sign is present in the right hip. The presence of this sign suggests tuberculous arthritis of the joint.

❦ Clinical Pearl ❦

Tuberculosis of the hip is now rare in the United States. A child infected with this disease walks with a limp and often complains of pain in the groin or knee. Night pain is another feature. In early cases complete resolution may be hoped for by antituberculous therapy, bed rest, and traction. In the advanced case, joint débridement is carried out with efforts to obtain a bony fusion of the joint.

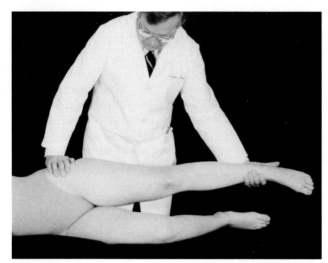

Fig. 10–22 The patient is in a side-lying position on the unaffected hip. The affected leg is extended, and the examiner slightly abducts the affected leg.

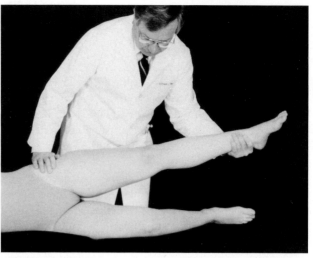

Fig. 10–23 The examiner cautiously externally rotates the leg (internally rotates the femoral head).

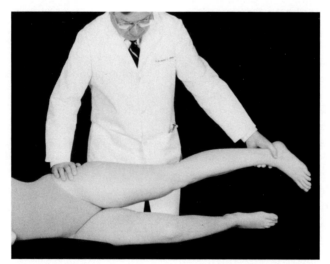

Fig. 10–24 Next the examiner internally rotates the leg (externally rotating the femoral head). If abdominal muscular contraction occurs on the same side, it is a positive sign. The sign indicates reflex muscle spasm due to tuberculosis of the hip. This condition is usually not common after adolescence.

Comment

The signs and symptoms of meningitis may develop explosively de novo or may appear in the waning stages of an infection that is localized elsewhere. Headache, backache, nausea, and vomiting are common symptoms, and nuchal rigidity occurs in more than 80% of the cases. Kernig/Brudzinski sign is often present. Only in the neonate and very young infant is meningitis often unattended by evidence of increased pressure and meningeal irritation. At this stage, even fever may be absent. Photophobia may be a prominent, early symptom and is related in some way to the meningeal inflammation.

Disturbances in mental status occur in nearly all cases of acute bacterial meningitis. Irritability, confusion, delirium, and stupor are common. Coma occurs in about 10% of the cases and indicates a poor prognosis. Focal or generalized seizures occur in about a fourth of all patients with meningitis. Seizures are encountered much more frequently in infants, who have a greater susceptibility to them. Signs of cerebral dysfunction, other than altered consciousness and seizures, are infrequent in cases of acute bacterial meningitis. The signs of cerebral dysfunction appear most often when treatment has been delayed. These signs include a disturbed conjugate gaze, dysphagia, paresis of extremities, and visual field defects. Striking and persistent signs are usually due to infarction of tissue as a result of cortical venous thrombosis. The latter complication commonly develops during the second week of disease when signs of infection and meningeal irritation are subsiding. Bilateral neurologic signs and convulsions occurring first on one side then on the other always suggest an associated thrombosis of the superior saggital sinus. Prominent and slowly progressive focal signs appearing early in the meningitis should indicate an associated focus of sepsis such as subdural endocarditis with cerebral embolism.

Between 5% to 20% of the patients with bacterial meningitis will develop cranial nerve palsies during the acute stage of the disease. Impaired ocular movement, deafness, and labyrinthine dysfunction are most frequently seen, but blindness and facial paralysis also occur. Most cranial nerve palsies are probably attributable to the meningeal exudate, but the eighth nerve complex may be damaged by bacteria or their toxins, which act directly on the inner ear. Although the cerebrospinal fluid pressure is usually elevated in patients with bacterial meningitis, papilledema is rare and is more characteristic of a brain abscess, subdural empyema, or venous sinus thrombosis. The infrequent occurrence of papilledema in uncomplicated meningitis is probably explained by the short duration of the increased pressure.

Procedure

While the patient is in a supine position, there is a brisk flexion of the hip and the knee when the quadriceps muscle on the opposite limb is irritated, such as by a firm pinch. The sign is present in cases of meningeal irritation.

Confirmation Procedures

Kernig/Brudzinski sign, clinical laboratory assessment, neurologic assessment

> **Reporting Statement**
>
> Guilland's sign is present on the right. The presence of this sign suggests meningeal irritation.

∾ Clinical Pearl ∾

Acute meningitis (associated with a cortical encephalitis and, often, with ventriculitis) is an emergency and should be suspected in any patient with the acute onset of nonlocalizing CNS signs. Fever, nuchal rigidity, headache, altered mental status, vomiting, and photophobia are typically present. The absence of fever is not uncommon. Meningeal signs are not usually present in infants younger than 6 months of age. Acute signs may also be less apparent in the elderly, alcoholic, immunocompromised, or comatose patients.

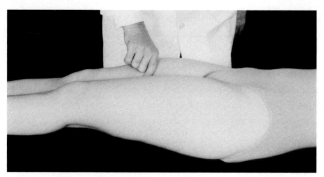

Fig. 10–25 The patient is lying supine with the legs extended on the examination table. The examiner firmly irritates (pinches) one of the quadriceps muscles.

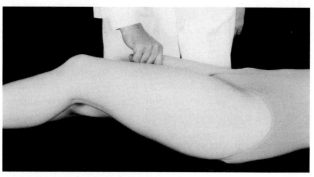

Fig. 10–26 If the sign is present, brisk flexion of the opposite hip and knee occurs. The sign is only present in meningeal irritation.

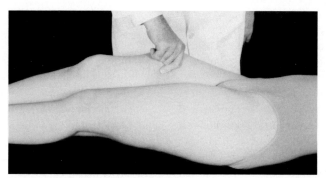

Fig. 10–27 The sign is not exclusive to brisk flexion of the contralateral hip and knee. Ipsilateral flexion, as a function of spasmophilia due to meningeal irritation, can occasionally be observed.

Comment

Congenital dislocation of the hip occurs as the result of underlying dysplasia of the joint. There are several theories as to the etiology of this type of dislocation, but the precise cause is still unknown. The disorder exhibits familial and racial tendencies and is often seen in Mediterranean and Scandinavian countries.

There are two general degrees of the pathologic condition: complete dislocation and subluxation. Subluxation is the more common type and if the condition goes untreated, it may develop into complete dislocation.

As a consequence of a defective acetabulum, the roof of the acetabulum slopes vertically instead of lying in its normal horizontal position. The acetabulum is shallow and the glenoid labrum (limbus) may be folded into the cavity. The femoral head is dislocated upward and laterally out of the acetabulum. There is usually marked forward torsion of the axis of the femoral neck (anteversion). Adaptive changes take place in the capsule and muscles, and the acetabulum is filled with fatty tissue.

Dislocation is much more common in females than in males, and it is often bilateral. In the infant the obvious clinical findings in unilateral cases are the asymmetrical skin folds on the medial aspect of the thigh, the exaggerated vertical angle of the inguinal crease, and the shortening of the affected extremity. The lengths of the patient's femurs are compared while the hips and knees are flexed at 90 degrees. Shortening is readily apparent from the lower level of the knee on the involved side. Abduction of the flexed thigh, which is normally possible up to approximately 90 degrees, is sharply limited. While the thigh is flexed to 90 degrees, a telescopic movement may be apparent by a gentle push-pull technique. During palpation the absence of the femoral head in Scarpa's triangle and its abnormal posterior position are noted. A click may be felt as the femoral head passes in and out of the acetabulum, when the flexed hip is abducted or adducted.

After walking starts, an abnormality of gait is noted. If the condition is unilateral, the child walks with an abduction lurch and if the condition is bilateral the child walks with a typical duck-waddling gait.

Congenital subluxation of the hip presents with the clinical findings of asymmetrical of skin folds and limited abduction of the flexed hip. The diagnosis of congenital subluxation is established by diagnostic imaging. The acetabular roof shows an obliquity and the underdeveloped capital epiphysis, which lies slightly lateral and superior, although in the acetabulum.

Procedure

The telescoping sign is evident in patients who have a dislocated hip. While the patient is lying in the supine position, the examiner flexes the patient's knee and hip to 90 degrees. The femur is pushed down into the examining table. The femur and leg are then lifted from the examining table. With a normal hip, little movement occurs during this action. However, with a dislocated hip there will be a lot of relative movement. This excessive movement is called *telescoping of the hip*.

Confirmation Procedures

Allis' sign, diagnostic imaging.

Reporting Statement

The telescoping test is positive in the right hip. This result suggests congenital dislocation of the articulation.

~ **Clinical Pearl** ~

Where treatment in childhood for congenital dislocation of the hip has been unsuccessful, or even where the condition has not been diagnosed, a patient may seek help during the third and fourth decades of life. Symptoms may arise from the hips or the spine. In the hips, secondary arthritic changes occur in the false joint that may form between the dislocated femoral head and the ilium. In the spine, osteoarthritic changes are the result of long-standing scoliosis. The telescoping test may remain positive for as long as the cause of the dislocation goes untreated.

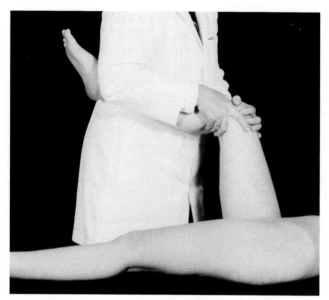

Fig. 10-28 The patient is lying supine. The examiner flexes the affected hip to 90 degrees and the knee to 90 degrees. The femur is pushed toward the examining table and then pulled up from the table. If the test is positive, a distinct pistoning of the hip is noted. The positive finding indicates dislocation of the hip. Although this test is usually used with neonates, the effect of the test may be observed throughout adult life in individuals with untreated or undiagnosed congenital hip dislocations.

Comment

Osteoarthritis involves a few joints, so symptoms and signs are localized in nature. Early on in the disease, osteoarthritis is associated with few or no symptoms. Pain is usually the earliest symptom, and it comes on with use, particularly after prolonged inactivity of the joint, and is relieved by rest. The pain is usually a low-grade ache that is often difficult for the patient to localize well. As the disease progresses in severity, pain occurs even during rest. Cold, damp weather exacerbates the pain. In some patients, pain may be aggravated by heat. The pain that is experienced by patients with osteoarthritis is of multiple origins. The pain may result from periosteal elevation associated with cartilage and bone proliferation, from pressure on exposed bone, from microfractures of bone, or from trauma to the synovium. Synovitis occurs in advanced cases of the disease and may cause pain as a result of inflammation. Spasm of muscles or pressure on nerves in the region of the joint may also be a major source of pain.

Stiffness is another common complaint, and it is usually more severe when a patient awakens in the morning or after inactivity during the day. Frequently, pain and stiffness are worse just before changes in the weather. Although stiffness is an important symptom in other forms of connective tissue disease, the stiffness, or fibrositis, associated with osteoarthritis is short lived and usually lasts less than 15 minutes. Limited joint motion eventually develops, as a result of abnormalities in the joint surface, muscle spasm, contracture of soft tissues and the interfering effect of spurs and loose bodies.

During physical examination, the joints may show slight tenderness, and pain occurs as the joint is moved. Palpation of the joint will often reveal crepitus, a sensation of grating as the joint is moved. Joint enlargement is seen, primarily due to proliferative reactions in cartilage and bone. Later, both deformity and subluxation become more apparent.

Osteoarthritis of the hip usually occurs in older persons, but it may begin at an earlier age. Osteoarthritis is progressive in nature, and bilateral involvement is not uncommon. Pain is often associated with a limp early on in the disease. Hip pain is felt at the side or the front of the joint or along the inner aspect of the thigh. Errors in diagnosis often arise because pain that originates in the hip may be referred to other regions and may present elsewhere. Hip pain may present as pain in the buttocks or sciatic region. Frequently, pain is referred along the obturator nerve, down the front of the thigh and knee. In some patients most or all the pain of the hip disease is felt in the knee. The pain in this area may be so severe that its hip origin is overlooked. Conversely, pain in the region of the hip may originate elsewhere, such as in the lumbosacral spine. Varying degrees of limited hip motion can be noted during examination when osteoarthritis is present. For example, the leg is held in external rotation with the hip flexed and adducted. Functional shortening may occur. Walking is awkward, and the patient finds difficulty sitting, rising from a seated position, and ascending stairs. Sexual intercourse becomes a stressful activity.

Procedure

In osteoarthritis deformans of the hip, the patient is asked to cross the legs, with a point just above the ankle resting on the opposite knee. If significant disease exists, this test and motion are impossible.

Confirmation Procedure

Gauvain's sign, Patrick's test, diagnostic imaging

Reporting Statement

Jansen's test is positive for the right hip. This result suggests osteoarthritis of the joint.

∽ Clinical Pearl ∽

Primary osteoarthritis of the hip occurs in middle-aged and elderly patients and is often associated with obesity and overuse. However, often no obvious cause can be found. The symptoms of secondary osteoarthritis of the hip are identical to those of primary osteoarthritis. The condition occurs most frequently as a sequel to congenital hip dislocation.

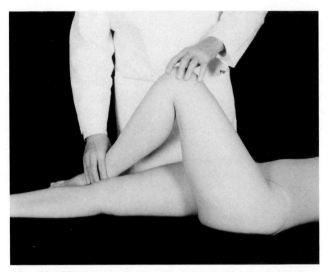

Fig. 10–29 The patient is lying supine. The examiner flexes and externally rotates the affected hip, crossing the patient's ankle over the contralateral knee.

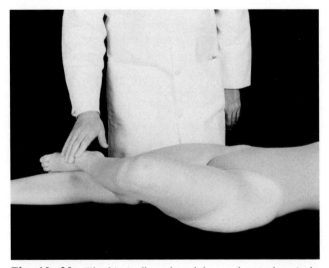

Fig. 10–30 The hip is allowed to abduct and extend passively. The distance between the lateral surface of the thigh and the examination table is noted. The distance is compared with the distance obtained on the opposite side. The test is positive when the motion is impossible to complete. A positive test indicates osteoarthritis of the hip joint.

Comment

Occasionally the tip of the greater trochanter is cracked as a result of a direct blow. Other than protecting the limb by avoiding weight bearing for a few weeks until the reaction to the trauma has settled down, no specific treatment is required for such a trochanteric crack.

The lesser trochanter may be avulsed by the pull of the psoas muscle. By itself this avulsion is of no importance, but sometimes this avulsion occurs because the bone at this level is weakened through pathologic change or a secondary neoplastic deposit. The examiner must bear this possibility in mind and should perform a biopsy if necessary.

There are many varieties of malignant tumor. The picture of any of them may vary depending on the age of the patient, the site, and duration of the lesion. A picture common for one tumor at one stage may be similar to that of a different tumor at a different stage. The examiner does not encounter enough examples of a rare tumor to make generalizations.

Two points are imperative for the examiner to remember. There is a constant need to be aware of the possibility that a malignant lesion may be present. There is also a need to simplify the problem. These needs can be accomplished, but even so, the examiner should maintain the attitude that the diagnosis, though highly probable, does not become established until the tissue is actually examined.

Although it is said that any metastatic tumor may appear in bone, for many tumors this is true only when they have existed long enough and are in the terminal stage. Tumors of this type should have been recognized much earlier. Several of the tumors are so rare that the whole group represents less than 2% of the cases involving the structural tissues.

These considerations serve to reduce the list of malignant lesions for practical purposes to approximately 13 varieties, and two of these, metastatic carcinomas of the breast and prostate, are differentiated by the sex of the patient.

The following is list of the 13 common lesions.
1. Neuroblastoma
2. Ewing's sarcoma
3. Lymphoma
4. Primary osteogenic sarcoma or chondroma
5. Secondary osteogenic sarcoma or chondroma
6. Metastatic carcinoma of the thyroid
7. Metastatic carcinoma of the breast in females
8. Metastatic carcinoma of the prostate in males
9. Metastatic carcinoma of the bronchus
10. Metastatic carcinoma of the kidneys
11. Hypernephroma
12. Myeloma
13. Neurogenic carcinoma

These few lesions can be separated into conveniently small groups when the usual age of onset of the particular disease is considered.

Procedure

In traumatic separation of the epiphysis of the lesser trochanter, swelling and ecchymosis are present at the base of Scarpa's triangle and the patient cannot raise the thigh when in the seated position.

Confirmation Procedure

Anvil test, Chiene's test, diagnostic imaging

Reporting Statement

Ludloff's sign is present on the right side. The presence of this sign suggests a traumatic separation of the lesser trochanter.

∼ Clinical Pearl ∼

As with femoral neck fractures, this fracture is common in elderly, osteoporotic females. However, in sharp contrast to the intracapsular neck fractures, the extracapsular trochanteric fractures unite very easily and seldom cause avascular necrosis.

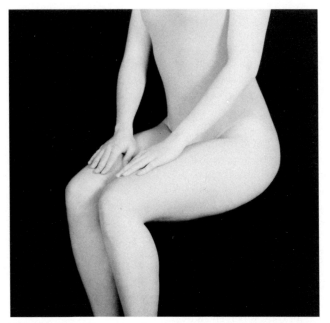

Fig. 10–31 The patient is seated on the edge of the examination table. The feet may touch the floor.

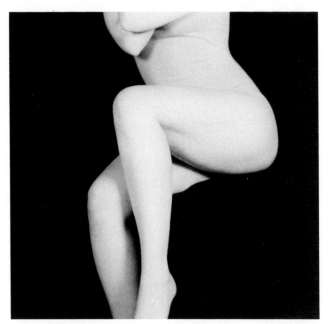

Fig. 10–32 While remaining seated, the patient tries to raise the affected thigh from the table surface. The sign is present when this move cannot be accomplished. When accompanied by swelling and ecchymosis in Scarpa's triangle, this sign indicates fracture of the lesser trochanter.

Comment

The iliotibial band is a thickened portion of the tensor fascia latae along its lateral aspect. The tensor fascia latae arises from the coccyx, the sacrum, the iliac crest, Poupart's ligament, and the pubic ramus. Between two layers the band encloses the gluteus maximus and the tensor fasciae femoris, giving attachment to the latter muscle and most of the former. The fibers of the fasciae converge to form the iliotibial band along the lateral side of the thigh. The iliotibial band is continuous medially with the lateral intermuscular septum, which attaches to the linea aspera. Distally the band gives origin to the short head of the biceps. At the level of the knee joint the band spreads out and attaches to the lateral tibial condyle and the head of the fibula. The iliotibial band lies in a plane anterior to the hip joint and posterior to the knee.

Involvement of the attached muscles is responsible for increased tension, under which the band is placed during the acute and convalescent stages. The taut band is perceived by deep palpation while adducting and extending the thigh. Spasm in the gluteus maximus is demonstrated by resistance to passive flexing of the hip while the knee is fully extended. Spasm in the short head of the biceps is demonstrated by flexing the hip, which relaxes the iliopsoas band, and finding resistance to extension of the knee. The patient assumes the most comfortable position in which the thigh is flexed, abducted, and externally rotated at the hip while the knee is flexed. This position relaxes the tension of the band. If tension is not overcome by stretching during the acute stage, band contracture becomes progressive and permanent deformity ensues.

Procedure

The patient is side lying on the unaffected hip and thigh. The examiner places one hand on the pelvis to steady it and grasps the patient's ankle lightly with the other hand, holding the knee flexed at a right angle. The thigh is abducted and extended in the coronal plane of the body. In the presence of iliotibial band contracture, the leg will remain abducted; the degree of abduction depends on the amount of contracture present. The sign is present both in the conscious and anesthetized patient. Ober calls attention to the frequency of a negative roentgenogram in the presence of clinical signs and symptoms of irritation of the sacroiliac or lumbosacral joints. He refers to the importance of the iliotibial band as a factor to consider in the occurrence of lumbosacral spinal disorders with or without associated sciatica.

Confirmation Procedures

Phelp's test, Thomas test, Trendelenburg's test

Reporting Statement

Ober's test is positive on the right. This result indicates an iliotibial band contracture.

∾ Clinical Pearl ∾

Transient synovitis of the hip is the most common cause of an irritable hip and can produce a limp and a positive Ober's test. There is sometimes a history of preceding minor trauma, which in some cases is at least coincidental. Radiographs of the hip sometimes give confirmatory evidence of synovitis, but no other pathologic condition is demonstrable.

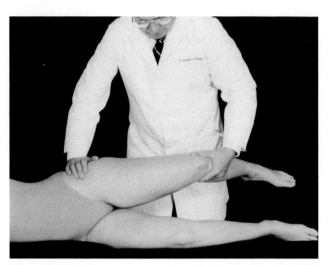

Fig. 10–33 The patient is in a side-lying position on the unaffected hip. The affected leg is extended. The examiner slightly abducts the affected leg.

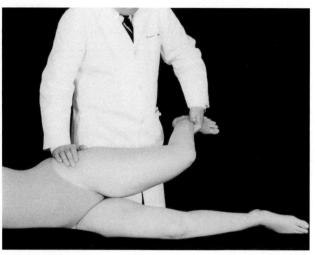

Fig. 10–34 The examiner stabilizes the pelvis with one hand and grasps the ankle of the affected leg with the other hand. The examiner flexes the knee to 90 degrees. The thigh is abducted and extended. The test is positive if the leg remains abducted. A positive test indicates iliotibial band contracture.

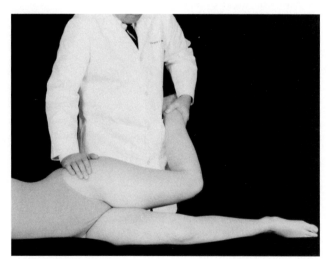

Fig. 10–35 The same procedure used on a normal hip demonstrates the normal adduction movement of the leg.

Patrick's Test

FABERE (FLEXION, ABDUCTION, EXTERNAL, ROTATION, EXTENSION) SIGN

Comment

Degenerative arthritis that is confined to the hip joint is a common affliction that occurs in the middle and later years of adult life. The cause of degenerative arthritis is not completely understood, but obesity, trauma, congenital hip dysplasia, avascular necrosis of the femoral head, and slipped capital femoral epiphysis are all factors in its onset.

Pathologically, the articular cartilage becomes progressively thinned and worn away. New bone proliferation around the femoral head and acetabulum occurs, and the synovium becomes chronically thickened and congested.

The clinical course is gradual and both hips may be affected. The onset of symptoms may be precipitated by a minor injury. Pain after activity and stiffness after rest are characteristic. The stiffness frequently subsides with activity and the pain frequently subsides with rest. The pain is often referred to the knee joint region. With the passage of time, the pain increases, sometimes even occurring during rest. Crepitus and grating in the hip may develop, and a painful limp is common.

Examination reveals tenderness over the anterior and posterior hip joint and restriction of motion, especially internal rotation and abduction. Pain is usually present at the extremes of motion, and a flexion contracture frequently develops. This contracture can be measured by Thomas test.

Procedure

Patrick's test is of particular value for use in geriatric cases because it indicates hip joint disease. The patient lies supine, and the examiner grasps the ankle and the flexed knee. The thigh is flexed, abducted, externally rotated, and extended. The first letters of these words form the acronym FABERE. Pain in the hip during the maneuver, particularly on abduction and external rotation, is a positive sign of a coxa pathologic condition.

Confirmation Procedures

Gauvain's sign, Jansen's test, diagnostic imaging

Reporting Statement

Patrick's test is positive on the right and indicates a coxa pathologic condition.

∾ Clinical Pearl ∾

An intracapsular fracture, which can cause a positive Patrick's test, can cut off the blood supply to the femoral head completely, which can lead to aseptic necrosis, nonunion, or both. Because the fracture line is inside the capsule, blood is contained within it. This trapped blood raises the intracapsular pressure, damaging the femoral head still further, and prevents visible bruising because the blood cannot reach the subcutaneous tissues.

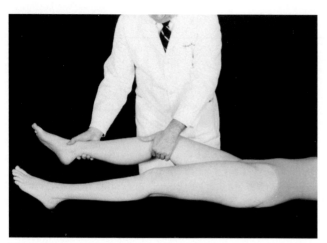

Fig. 10–36 The patient is lying supine on the examination table. The examiner grasps the affected leg.

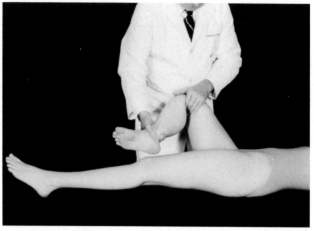

Fig. 10–37 The examiner flexes the hip, abducts the thigh, crosses the ankle over the contralateral knee, and externally rotates the hip.

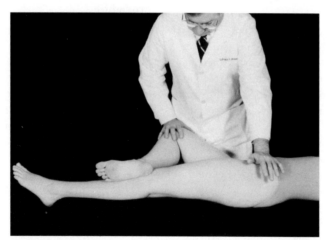

Fig. 10–38 The examiner then extends the hip by applying downward pressure on the knee. The contralateral side of the pelvis is fixed to the table and not allowed to rock upward. Pain during abduction and external rotation is a positive finding and indicates a coxa pathologic condition.

Comment

The majority of patients seeking help because of a hip-joint problem may do so because of pain, stiffness, limp, or deformity.

Pain of a hip-joint origin may be localized to the groin and from there may radiate down the medial or anterior aspect of the thigh. The pain also may arise in the region of the greater trochanter and radiate laterally along the course of the tensor fasciae latae, toward the knee. Hip-joint pain may present posteriorly in the region of the ischial tuberosity and must be carefully differentiated from the complaint of sciatica. Frequently the pain is referred to the lower back or knee and can be reproduced or accentuated by movements of the hip joint.

Subjective stiffness of the hip joint may be noted by the patient following periods of immobility, such as after prolonged sitting or upon arising from bed in the morning. In more advanced degenerative states affecting the hip joint, objective stiffness may be noted by the examiner. In degenerative arthritis of the hip joint, for example, the patient will lose hip-joint motion sequentially, with the ability to rotate the hip being lost first, followed by abduction and adduction loss, and finally hip flexion. For this reason, many patients with degenerative arthritis of the hip describe difficulty in putting a shoe or stocking on the affected leg because this action usually requires the ability to rotate the hip joint externally.

A limp is a pathologic asymmetrical gait, and several mechanisms, singly or in combination, may be operating on the hip joint to produce it. Shortening of the lower extremity and marked stiffness of the hip joint may be sufficient to alter gait pattern. The limp may be protective because of weight-bearing pain. This type of abnormal gait, called an antalgic gait, is characterized by a very short stance phase. However, the gait most characteristic of hip-joint disease is called a gluteal lurch, and it relates directly to a structural or functional weakness of the gluteus medius on the affected side. Any abnormality of the pelvic-femoral lever arm may weaken the gluteus medius muscle. If this weakening occurs, the muscle can no longer support the pelvis and trunk on the lower extremity, and the patient's trunk lurches to the affected side during weight bearing.

Visible deformity of the lower extremity is frequently associated with injuries or disease affecting the hip joint. A patient with a fracture of the hip joint usually presents with the lower extremity held in marked external rotation. A patient who has sustained a traumatic dislocation of the hip joint usually presents with the lower extremity held in internal rotation. Degenerative arthritis of the hip joint is frequently associated with flexion-adduction-external rotation contractures. Flexion and adduction contractures about the hip, external rotation position of the lower extremity, shortening of the leg, and a limp are characteristic deformities that may be produced by hip joint disorders.

Procedure

The patient is lying prone, the knees are extended, and the thighs are maximally abducted. Pain and resistance should be used as criterion for maximum abduction. The patient's knees are flexed bilaterally to a right angle. The examiner notes if the maneuver allows more hip abduction. The test is positive if knee flexion increases or knee extension decreases hip abduction. The test indicates contracture of the gracilis muscle.

Confirmation Procedure

Ober's test, Thomas test, Trendelenburg's test

Reporting Statement

Phelp's test is positive on the right. This result suggests contracture of the gracilis muscle, which is associated with a pathologic condition of the hip joint.

～ Clinical Pearl ～

Two, nonspecific gait abnormalities commonly result from hip disease. The antalgic gait usually indicates a painful hip. The patient shortens the stance phase on the affected hip, leaning over the affected side, to avoid painful contraction of the hip abductors. The Trendelenburg gait, or abductor limp, indicates weakness of the abductors on the affected side. During the stance phase, on the affected side, the contralateral pelvis dips down and the body leans to the unaffected side. If the condition is bilateral, this produces a waddling gait.

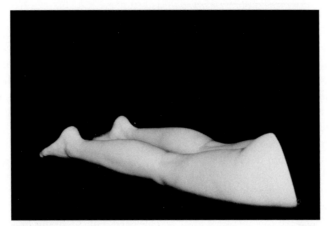

Fig. 10–39 The patient is lying prone with the knees extended. The thighs are maximally abducted as far as the patient can tolerate.

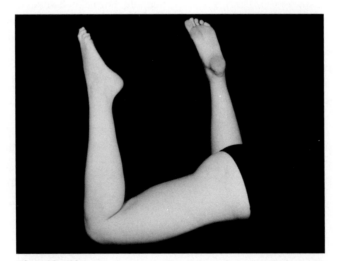

Fig. 10–40 The knees are flexed actively or passively to 90 degrees. If flexion of the knees allows more hip abduction, the test is positive. A positive test indicates gracilis muscle contracture.

Comment

Osteochondritis deformans juvenilis, or coxa plana, is largely limited by age and sex. The disease was described separately in the United States, Germany, and France by Legg (1910), Perthes (1910) and Calvé (1910). It is seen almost exclusively in children 3 to 12 years old, but the disease has been reported in children as young as 2 and in others as old as 18. More boys are affected than girls by a ratio of 4:1. The disease is usually unilateral, and a familial history of the disease is present in 20% of the cases.

The most widely accepted cause for the disease is interruption of the blood supply to the head of the femur. This interrupted blood supply is thought to be produced by excessive fluid pressure of a synovial effusion in the hip joint. The head of the femur is at risk between the ages of 3 and 10 because, of the three blood supplies to the femoral head, only the lateral epiphyseal vessels are functional during this period. The blood supply to different segments of the head of the femur varies. For instance, the blood supply to the posterior segment is more generous than the supply to the anterior segment. The posterior portion of the head of the femur is often spared from this disease.

Subchondral fractures occur early in the disease, and these may be the initiating factor in a sequence of events that results in Legg-Calvé-Perthes disease.

Abnormal blood clotting processes, caused by substances that create a state of hypercoagulability, are thought to result in formation of platelet aggregations and fibrin thrombi that could block the limited vascular supply to the head of the femur.

This process has a relationship with previous transient synovitis or other inflammatory processes because of the presence of thickened blood vessels and capsules.

During physical examination, pain can range from mild to severe and will be felt in the groin, thigh, and very often the knee. This pain is associated with a limp or slightly abnormal gait. The gait is an antalgic one, in which the patient tries to protect the hip by rapidly shifting body weight off the foot of the involved side.

With a flexion contracture (positive Thomas test) motion—particularly abduction, internal rotation, extension, and flexion—at the hip is limited. A patient may experience muscle spasm of the adductor and psoas muscle and muscle wasting of the thigh and buttock. The anterior and posterior aspects of the hip joint may also be tender.

The erythrocyte sedimentation rate (ESR) might be elevated, but the results of other laboratory investigations are normal.

Procedure

The patient lies supine, and the thigh is flexed with the knee bent upon the abdomen. The patient's lumbar spine should normally flatten, or flex. If the spine maintains a lordosis, the test is positive and indicates hip flexion contracture, as from a shortened iliopsoas muscle.

Confirmation Procedures

Ober's test, Phelp's test, Trendelenburg's test

Reporting Statement

Thomas test is positive on the right and indicates a flexion contracture involving the iliopsoas musculature.

∾ Clinical Pearl ∾

Restricted hip flexion may be compensated by an increase in lumbar lordosis. This increase masks the fixed flexion deformity. Fixed flexion, external rotation, and abduction accumulate sequentially as the hip disease progresses.

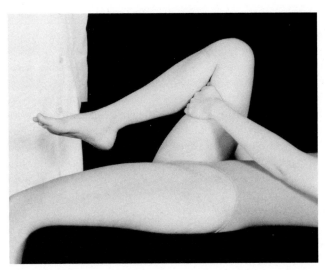

Fig. 10—41 The patient is lying supine on the examination table. The thigh of the unaffected leg is actively flexed toward the abdomen. The patient holds the leg in this position with both hands. The examiner observes the posture of the lower back and the affected leg. The lumbar spine should flatten and the opposite leg should remain flat on the table.

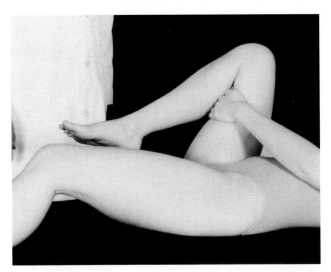

Fig. 10—42 If the lumbar spine maintains a lordosis and the affected leg flexes, and if the patient is unable to lay the leg flat on the table, the test is positive. A positive test indicates a shortened iliopsoas muscle.

Comment

Trendelenburg's test tests stability of the hip and particularly of the ability of the hip abductors (gluteus medius and gluteus minimus) to stabilize the pelvis on the femur.

Normally, when one leg is raised from the ground, the pelvis tilts upward on that side because of the action of the hip abductors of the supporting limb. This automatic mechanism allows the lifted leg to clear the ground while walking. If the abductors are inefficient, they are unable to sustain the pelvis against the body weight. The result is that the pelvis tilts downward instead of rising on the side of the lifted leg.

There are three fundamental causes for a positive Trendelenburg's test. (1) Paralysis of the abductor muscles, which can occur with poliomyelitis. (2) Marked approximation of the insertion of the muscles to their origin by upward displacement of the greater trochanter causing the muscles to be slack. This slackening may occur in severe coxa vara or congenital dislocation of the hip. (3) Absence of a stable fulcrum causes a positive test. This result occurs in the ununited fracture of the femoral neck. Sometimes two of these factors will operate together. For instance, in a case of upward dislocation of the hip there is an unstable fulcrum as well as approximation of the origin of the abductor muscles to their insertion.

Procedure

The patient with a suspected hip involvement stands on one foot, on the side of involvement and raises the other foot and leg for thigh flexion and knee flexion. If the hip and its muscles are normal, the iliac crest will be low on the standing side and high on the side of the elevated leg. If there is hip-joint involvement and muscle weakness, the iliac crest will be high on the standing side and low on the side of the elevated leg. The test is commonly positive in a developing Legg-Calvé-Perthes disease, poliomyelitis, muscular dystrophy, coxa vara, Otto's pelvis, epiphyseal separation, coxa ankylosis, dislocation, fracture, or subluxation.

Confirmation Procedure

Ober's test, Phelp's test, Thomas test

Reporting Statement

Trendelenburg's test is positive on the right. This result suggests insufficiency of the hip abductor system.

∼ Clinical Pearl ∼

The Trendelenburg's test is positive as a result of (1) gluteal paralysis or weakness (from polio), (2) gluteal inhibition (from pain arising in the hip joint), (3) from gluteal insufficiency from coxa vara, or (4) congenital dislocation of the hip (CDH). Nevertheless, false positives have been recorded in approximately 10% of the patients with hip pain.

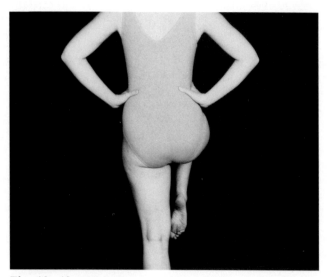

Fig. 10–43   The patient is standing and is instructed to raise the foot of the unaffected leg off the floor. If normal, the iliac crest may be low on the standing side and high on the side of the elevated leg.

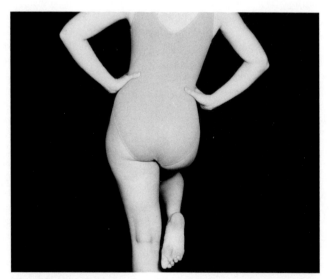

Fig. 10–44   If the test is positive, the iliac crest will be high on the standing side and low on the side of the elevated leg. A positive test indicates a coxa pathologic condition.

Bibliography

Adams JA: Transient synovitis of the hip joint in children, *J Bone Joint Surg,* 45B:471, 1963.

Adams JC: *Standard orthopaedic operations,* Edinburgh, 1985, Churchill Livingstone.

Adams JC, Hamblen DL: *Outline of orthopaedics,* Edinburgh, 1990, Churchill Livingstone.

Adams RD: *Diseases of muscle,* ed 3, London, 1975, Henry Kimpton.

Alexander CJ: The etiology of femoral epiphyseal slipping, *J Bone Joint Surg,* 48B:299, 1966.

American Academy of Orthopaedic Surgeons: *Atlas of limb prosthetics,* St. Louis, 1981, Mosby.

American Academy of Orthopaedic Surgeons: *Instructional course lectures,* vol 36, Chicago, 1987, AAOS.

American Academy of Orthopaedic Surgeons: *Instructional course lectures,* vol 37, Chicago, 1988, AAOS.

American Medical Association: *Guides to the evaluation of permanent impairment,* ed 3, Chicago, 1990, The Association.

American Orthopaedic Association: *Manual of orthopaedic surgery,* Chicago, 1972, The Association.

Apley AG, Solomon L: *Concise system of orthopaedics and fractures,* London, 1988, Butterworth-Heinemann.

Aston JN: *A Short textbook of orthopaedics and traumatology,* Philadelphia, 1967, JB Lippincott.

Barlow TG: Congenital dislocation of the hip, *Hospital Medicine,* 2:571, 1968.

Barnes R: Fracture of the neck of the femur, *J Bone Joint Surg,* 49B:607, 1967.

Beeson PB, McDermott W: *Textbook of medicine,* ed 13, Philadelphia, 1971, WB Saunders.

Bennett JT, MacEwen GD: Congenital dislocation of the hip: Recent advances and current problems, *Clin Orthop,* 247:15, 1989.

Benson MKD, Evans DCJ: The pelvis osteotomy of chiari, *J Bone Joint Surg,* 58B:164, 1976.

Berkeley ME, Dickson JE, Cain TE, Donovan MM: Surgical therapy for congenital dislocation of the hip in patients who are twelve to thirty-six months old, *J Bone Joint Surg,* 66A:412, 1984.

Birch R: The place of microsurgery in orthopaedics. In *Recent advances in orthopaedics,* ed 5, Edinburgh, 1987, Churchill Livingstone.

Blockey NJ: Derotation osteotomy in the management of congenital dislocation of the hip, *J Bone Joint Surg,* 66B:485, 1984.

Bombelli R: *Osteoarthritis of the hip: Pathogenesis and consequent therapy,* New York, 1976, Springer-Verlag.

Bowen JR, Foster BK, Hartzell C: Legg-Calvé-Perthes disease, *Clin Orthop,* 185:97, 1984.

Bradley GW et al: Resurfacing arthroplasty: Femoral head viability, *Clin Orthop,* 220:137, 1987.

Brashear HR, Raney RB: *Shands' handbook of orthopaedic surgery,* St. Louis, 1978, Mosby.

Burnett W: *Clinical science for surgeons,* London, 1981, Butterworth.

Burwell RG, Harrison HM, editors: Perthes disease (symposium), *Clin Orthop,* 209:2, 1986.

Butler WT, Alling DW, Spickard A, Utz JP: Diagnostic and prognostic value of clinical and laboratory findings in cryptococcal meningitis, *New Eng J Med,* 270:59, 1964.

Caffey J: The early roentgenographic changes in essential coxa plana, their significance in pathogenesis, *Am J Roentgenol,* 103:620, 1968.

Camp WA: Sarcoidosis of the central nervous system: A case with postmortem studies, Chicago, *Arch Neurol,* 7:432, 1962.

Campbell WC: *Operative orthopaedics,* ed 7, London, 1981, Henry Kimpton.

Campion GV, Dixon A: *Rheumatology,* Oxford, 1989, Blackwell.

Carter CO, Wilkinson JA: Genetic and environmental factors in the etiology of congenital dislocation of the hip, *Clin Orthop,* 33:119, 1964.

Catterall A: The natural history of Perthes disease (symposium), *J Bone Joint Surg,* 53B:37, 1971.

Catterall A: *Recent advances in orthopaedics,* ed 5, Edinburgh, 1987, Churchill Livingstone.

Charnley J: Total hip replacement by low-friction arthroplasty, *Clin Orthop,* 72:7, 1970.

Cipriano JJ: *Photographic manual of regional orthopaedic and neurological tests,* ed 2, Baltimore, 1991, Williams and Wilkins.

Clarke NMP, Clegg J, Al-Chalabi AN: Ultrasound screening of hips at risk for congenital dislocation, *J Bone Joint Surg,* 71B:9, 1989.

Copperman DR, Stulberg SD: Ambulatory containment treatment in Perthes disease, *Clin Orthop,* 203:289, 1986.

Cruess RL, Rennie W: *Adult orthopaedics,* New York, 1987, Churchill Livingstone.

Currey HLF: *Essentials of rheumatology,* ed 2, Edinburgh, 1988, Churchill Livingstone.

Cyriax JH: *Textbook of orthopaedic medicine,* ed 8, London, 1983, Bailliere, Tindall.

D'Ambrosia RD: *Musculoskeletal disorders regional examination and differential diagnosis,* Philadelphia, 1977, JB Lippincott.

Dandy DJ: *Essential orthopaedics and trauma,* Edinburgh, 1989, Churchill Livingstone.

DeRosa GP, Feller N: Treatment of congenital dislocation of the hip, management before walking age, *Clin Orthop,* 225:77, 1987.

Dixon AS et al: A double-blind controlled trial of Rumalon in the treatment of painful osteoarthrosis of the hip, *Ann Rheum Dis,* 29:193, 1970.

Dobbs HS: Survivorship of total hip replacements, *J Bone Joint Surg,* 62B:168, 1980.

Dodge PR, Swartz MN: Bacterial meningitis: Special neurologic problems, postmeningitic complications and clinicopathologic correlations, *New Eng J Med,* 272:954, 1965.

Doherty M, Doherty J: *Clinical examination in rheumatology,* London, 1992, Wolfe Publishing.

Duthie RB, Bentley G, editor: *Mercer's orthopaedic surgery,* ed 8, London, 1983, Edward Arnold.

Eastcott HHG: *Arterial surgery,* ed 2, London, 1973, Pitman.

Eftekhar NS editor: Low friction arthroplasty, *Clin Orthop,* 211:2, 1986.

Eyre-Brook A: Septic arthritis of the hip and osteomyelitis of upper end of the femur in infants, *J Bone Joint Surg,* 42B:11, 1960.

Eyre-Brook AL, Jones DA, Harris FC: Pemberton's acetabuloplasty for congenital dislocation of subluxation of the hip, *J Bone Joint Surg,* 60B:18, 1978.

Ferguson AB Jr.: The pathology of degenerative arthritis of the hip and the use of osteotomy in its treatment, *Clin Orthop,* 77: 118, 1971.

Fisk JW, Balgent ML: Clinical and radiological assessment of leg length, *N Z Med J,* 81:477, 1975.

Gage JR, Winter RB: Avascular necrosis of the capital femoral epiphysis as a complication of closed reduction of congenital dislocation of the hip, *J Bone Joint Surg,* 54A:373, 1972.

Galasko CSB, editor: *Neuromuscular problems in orthopaedics,* Oxford, 1987, Blackwell.

Galasko CSB, Nobel J editor: *Current trends in orthopaedic surgery,* Manchester, 1988, Manchester University Press.

Galpin RD et al: One-stage treatment of congenital dislocation of the hip in older children, *J Bone Joint Surg,* 71A:734, 1989.

Gartland JJ: *Fundamentals of orthopaedics,* ed 2, Philadelphia, 1974, WB Saunders.

Gartland JJ: Orthopaedic Clinical Research, *J Bone Joint Surg,* 70A:1357, 1988.

Gillis L: *Diagnostic in orthopaedics,* London, 1969, Butterworths.

Graham S et al: The Chiari osteotomy, *Clin Orthop,* 208:249, 1986.

Grauer JD et al: Resection arthroplasty of the hip, *J Bone Joint Surg,* 71A:669, 1989.

Gruebel-Lee DM: *Disorders of the hip,* Philadelphia, 1983, JB Lippincott.

Hadlow V: Neonatal screening for congenital dislocation of hip, *J Bone Joint Surg,* 70B:740, 1988.

Hall AJ: Perthes Disease: Progression in aetiological research, In *Recent advances in orthopaedics* ed 5, (edited by Catteral), Edinburgh, 1987, Churchill Livingstone.

Hansson G: Congenital dislocation of the hip joint: Problems in diagnosis and treatment, *Curr Orthop,* 2:104, 1988.

Hardinge K: The etiology of transient synovitis of the hip in childhood, *J Bone Joint Surg,* 52B:100, 1970.

Harris CM, Baum J: Involvement of the hip in juvenile rheumatoid arthritis, *J Bone Joint Surg,* 70A:821, 1988.

Harris WH: Etiology of osteoarthritis of the hip, *Clin Orthop,* 213:20, 1986.

Heikkila E, Ryoppy S, Louchimo I: The Management of Primary Acetabular Dysplasia, *J Bone Joint Surg,* 67B:25, 1985.

Heinmann WG, Freiberger RH: Avascular necrosis of the femoral and humeral heads after high-dosage corticosteroid therapy, *New Eng J Med,* 263:627, 1960.

Henderson RS: Osteotomy for unreduced congenital dislocation of the hip in adults, *J Bone Joint Surg,* 52B:468, 1970.

Hirsch C, Frankel VH: Analysis of forces producing fractures of the proximal end of the femur, *J Bone Joint Surg,* 42B:633, 1960.

Hughes S, Benson MKD, Colton CL: *The principles and practice of musculo-skeletal surgery,* Edinburgh, 1987, Churchill Livingstone.

Jones DA: Irritable hip and campylobacter infection, *J Bone Joint Surg,* 71B:227, 1989.

Jones JP Jr, Engelman EP: Osseous avascular necrosis associated with systemic abnormalities, *Arthritis Rheum,* 5:728, 1966.

Katz WA: *Rheumatic diseases diagnosis and management,* Philadelphia, 1977, JB Lippincott.

Kendall HO, Kendall FP, Wadsworth GE: *Muscles testing and function,* ed 2, Baltimore, 1971, Williams and Wilkins.

Keret D, Harrison MHM, Clarke NMP et al: Coxa plana: The fate of the physis, *J Bone Joint Surg,* 66A:870, 1984.

Lawrence JS: Generalized osteoarthrosis in a popular sample, *Am J Epidemiol,* 90:381, 1969.

Lloyd-Roberts GG: Suppurative arthritis in infancy, *J Bone Joint Surg,* 42B:706, 1960.

Lorber J: Long-term follow-up of 100 children who recovered from tuberculous meningitis, *Pediatrics,* 28:778, 1961.

Love BRT, Stevens PM, William PF: A long-term review of shelf arthroplasty, *J Bone Joint Surg,* 62B:321, 1980.

Lynch AF: Tuberculosis of the greater trochanter, *J Bone Joint Surg,* 64B:185, 1982.

MacAusland WR Jr., Mayo RA: *Orthopedics: A concise guide to clinical practices,* Boston, 1965, Little, Brown.

MacEwen GD: Treatment of congenital dislocation of the hip in older children, *Clin Orthop,* 225:86, 1987.

Magee DJ: *Orthopedic physical assessment,* Philadelphia, 1987, WB Saunders.

Maxted MJ, Jackson RK: Innominate osteotomy in Perthes' disease, *J Bone Joint Surg,* 67B:399, 1985.

Mazion JM: *Illustrated manual of neurological reflexes/signs/tests, Part I, orthopedic signs/tests/maneuvers for office procedure, Part II,* Orlando, 1980, Daniels Publishing.

McAndrew MP, Weinstein SL: A long-term follow-up of Legg-Calvé-Perthes disease, *J Bone Joint Surg,* 66A:860, 1984.

McRae R: *Clinical orthopaedic examination,* ed 3, Edinburgh, 1990, Churchill Livingstone.

McKee GK: Development of total prosthetic replacement of the hip, *Clin Orthop,* 72:85, 1970.

McKibbin B: Anatomical factors in the stability of the hip joint in the newborn, *J Bone Joint Surg,* 52B:148, 1970.

McKibbin B, editor: *Recent advances in orthopaedics,* ed 4, Edinburgh, 1983, Churchill Livingstone.

Medical Economics Books: *Patient care flow chart manual,* ed 3, Oradell, NJ, 1982, Medical Economics Books.

Menelaus MB: Lessons learned in the management of Legg-Calvé-Perthes disease, *Clin Orthop,* 209:41, 1986.

Mercier LR, Pettid FJ: *Practical orthopedics,* Chicago, 1980, Mosby.

Meyer HM Jr., Johnson RT, Crawford IP, Dascomb HE, Rogers NG: Central nervous system syndromes of "viral" etiology—a study of 713 cases, *Amer J Med,* 29:334, 1960.

Moll JMH: *Manual of rheumatology,* Edinburgh, 1987, Churchill Livingstone.

Moore FH: Examination of infant's hips: Can it do harm?, *J Bone Joint Surg,* 71B:4, 1989.

Muirhead-Allwood W, Catterall A: The treatment of Perthes disease, *J Bone Joint Surg,* 64B:282, 1982.

Noble HB, Hajek MR, Porter M: Diagnosis and treatment of iliotibial band tightness in runners, *Sports Med,* 10:67, 1982.

Nobel J, Galasko CSB: *Recent developments in orthopaedic surgery,* Manchester, 1987, Manchester University Press.

Nunn D: The ring uncemented plastic-on-metal total hip replacement, *J Bone Joint Surg,* 70B:40, 1988.

Ober FB: The role of the iliotibial and fascia lata as a factor in the causation of low-back disabilities and sciatic, *J Bone Joint Surg,* 18:105, 1936.

O'Donoghue DH: *Treatment of injuries to athletes,* ed 3, Philadelphia, 1976, WB Saunders.

Omer GE, Spinner M: *Management of peripheral nerve problems,* Philadelphia, 1980, WB Saunders.

Owen R, Goodfellow J, Bullough P, editors: *Scientific foundations of orthopaedics and traumatology,* London, 1980, Heinemann.

Paterson D, Salvage JP: The nuclide bone scan in the diagnosis of Perthes disease, *Clin Orthop,* 209:23, 1986.

Patterson RJ, Bickel WH, Dahlin DC: Idiopathic avascular necrosis of the head of the femur: A study of fifty-two cases, *J Bone Joint Surg,* 42A:267, 1964.

Polley HF, Hunder GG: *Rheumatologic interviewing and physical examination of the joints,* Philadelphia, 1978, WB Saunders.

Post M: *Physical examination of the musculoskeletal system,* Chicago, 1987, Mosby.

Radin EL: The physiology and degeneration of joints, *Arthritis Rheum,* 2:245, 1972.

Ranawat CS: Surgery for rheumatoid arthritis: The hip, *Curr Orthop,* 3, 146, 1989.

Rang M, editor: *The growth plate and its disorders,* Edinburgh, 1969, Livingstone.

Ratliff AHC: Perthes disease: A study of thirty-four hips observed for thirty years, *J Bone Joint Surg,* 49B:102, 1967.

Renne JW: The iliotibial band friction syndrome, *J Bone Joint Surg,* 57A:1110, 1975.

Renshaw TS: *Pediatric orthopaedics,* Philadelphia, 1987, Saunders.

Ring PA: Complete replacement arthroplasty of the hip by the ring prosthesis, *J Bone Joint Surg,* 50B, 720, 1968.

Roach HI, Shearer JR, Archer C: The choice of an experimental model: A guide for research workers, *J Bone Joint Surg,* 71B:549, 1989.

Russotti GM, Conventry MB, Stauffer RN: Cemented total hip arthroplasty with contemporary techniques, *Clin Orthop,* 235:141, 1988.

Scott JT, editor: *Copeman's textbook of the rheumatic diseases,* ed 6, Edinburgh, 1986, Churchill Livingstone.

Sherlock DA, Gibson PH, Benson MKD: Congenital subluxation of the hip, *J Bone Joint Surg,* 67B:390, 1985.

Smith ET, Pevey JK, Shindler TO: The erector spinae transplant—a misnomer, *Clin Orthop,* 20:144, 1963.

Smith WS, Ponseti IV, Ryder CT, Salter RB: Congenital dislocation of the hip in the older child (symposium) (instructional Course Lectures, American Academy of Orthopaedic Surgeons), *J Bone Joint Surg,* 48A:1390, 1966.

Solomon L: Patterns of osteoarthritis of the hip, *J Bone Joint Surg,* 58B:176, 1976.

Somerville EW: A long-term follow-up of congenital dislocation of the hip, *J Bone Joint Surg,* 60B:25, 1978.

Staheli LT: Medial femoral torsion, *Orthop Clin North Am,* 11:39, 1980.

Stewart JDM, Hallett JP: *Traction and orthopaedic appliances,* Edinburgh, 1983, Churchill Livingstone.

Susuke S et al: Diagnosis by ultrasound of congenital dislocation of the hip joint, *Clin Orthop,* 217:171, 1987.

Swartout R, Compere EL: Ischiogluteal bursitis: The pain in the arse, *JAMA,* 227:551, 1974.

Swartz MN, Dodge PR: Bacterial meningitis: General clinical features, special problems and unusual meningeal reactions mimicking bacterial meningitis, *New Engl J Med,* 272:725, 1965.

Tachdjian MO: *Pediatric orthopedics,* Philadelphia, 1972, WB Saunders.

Tergesen T, Berdland T, Berg V: Ultrasound for hip assessment in the newborn, *J Bone Joint Surg,* 71B:767, 1989.

Thurston SE: *The little black book of neurology,* Chicago, 1987, Mosby.

Tronzo RG, editor: *Surgery of the hip joint,* Philadelphia, 1973, Lea & Febiger.

Turek SL: Orthopaedics principles and their application, ed 3, Philadelphia, 1977, JB Lippincott.

Wainwright D: The shelf operation for hip dysplasia in adolescence, *J Bone Joint Surg,* 58B:159, 1976.

Weisl H: Intertrochanteric osteotomy for osteoarthritis, *J Bone Joint Surg,* 62B:37, 1980.

Weiss W, Flippen HJ: The changing incidence and prognosis of tuberculous meningitis, *Amer J Med Sci,* 250:46, 1965.

Williams PF, editor: *Orthopaedic management in childhood,* Oxford, 1982, Blackwell.

Woerman AL: Binder-Macleod SA: Leg-length discrepancy assessment: Accuracy and precision in five clinical methods of evaluation, *J Orthop Sports Phys Ther,* 5:230, 1984.

Wynne-Davis R: Acetabular dysplasia and familial joint laxity: Two etiological factors in congenital dislocation of the hip, *J Bone Joint Surg,* 52B:704, 1970.

CHAPTER

~ *11* ~

The Knee

The knee joint is particularly susceptible to traumatic injury. The joint is at the ends of two long lever arms: the tibia and the femur. The knee joint depends on the ligaments and muscles that surround it rather than its bony configuration, for its strength and stability.

Knee stability depends on four ligaments—the tibial collateral, fibular collateral, and the anterior and posterior cruciates—and on the surrounding musculature. Little stability is furnished by the rounded contour of the femoral condyles and the flat tibial plateaus which are deepened by the semilunar cartilages. The quadriceps muscle and its tendinous expansions are great contributors to the stability and function of the knee. The earliest clinical indication of internal knee derangement is atrophy of the quadriceps.

The knee is not a hinge joint. The tibia navigates a helical course on the condyles of the femur. Most traumatic arthritis of the knee, in middle-aged and elderly people, is due to minor derangements of the soft tissues, especially the menisci.

The knee joint represents a real challenge for treatment. The knee lacks the stability of the hip, which has its ball and socket, or the ankle, which has its mortise and tendon. Both the hip and ankle have structures that give some degree of bony stability. In the knee joint the socket of the top of the tibia is so minimal that the lateral tibial plateau may be flat or even convex. The little bit of buffering provided by the menisci gives minimal increase in stability because the menisci are unstable themselves. For stability the knee must depend largely upon the soft tissues, the ligaments, capsule, and muscles. It is extremely important to make an accurate diagnosis about the exact nature of the patient's knee injury.

It is vital that a definitive diagnosis be made early so treatment can be started early. Examination must determine what part of the knee is injured and how bad the injury is. The parts that may be injured include: (1) ligaments, (2) muscle tendon, (3) capsule, (4) meniscus, (5) cartilage, (6) bone, (7) bursae, and (8) any combination of these.

Index of Tests

Abduction stress test
Adduction stress test
Apley's compression test
Apprehension test for the patella
Bounce home test
Childress duck waddle test
Clarke's sign
Drawer test
Dreyer's sign
Fouchet's sign
Lachman test
Lateral pivot shift maneuver
Losee test
McMurray sign
Noble compression test
Patella ballottement test
Payr's sign
Q-angle test
Slocum's test
Steinmann's sign
Thigh circumference test
Wilson's sign

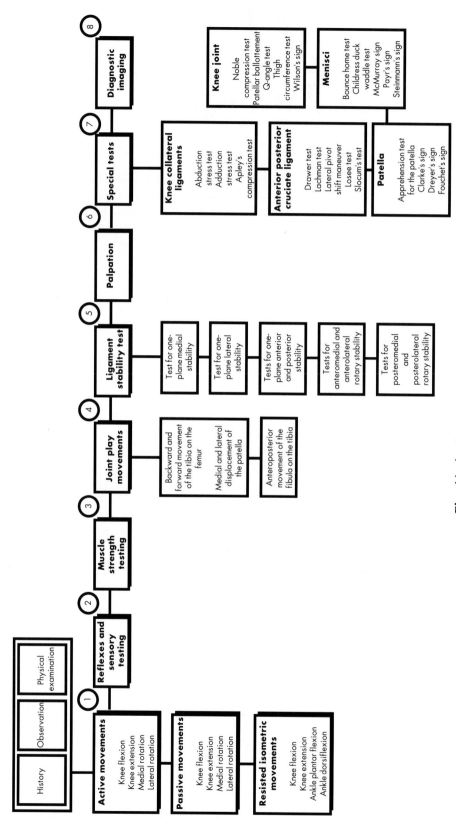

Fig. 11–1 Knee joint assessment.

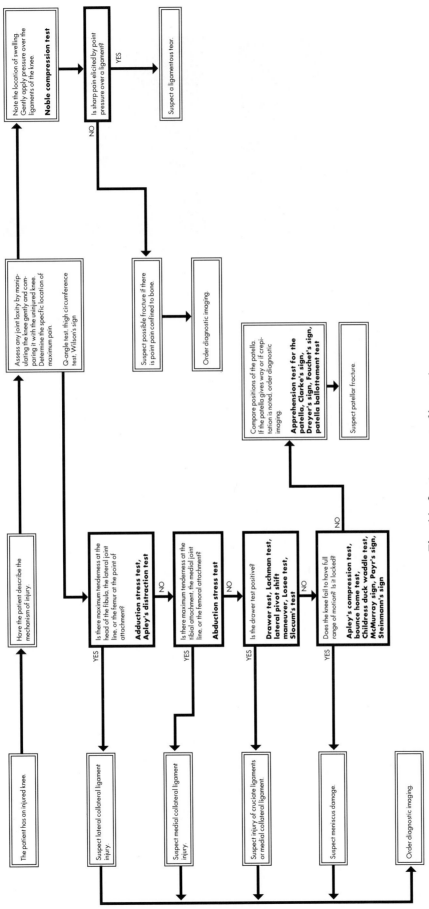

Fig. 11-2 Assessment of knee pain.

RANGE OF MOTION

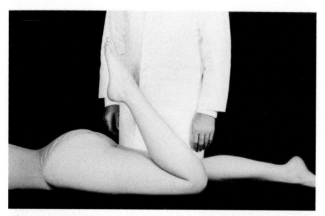

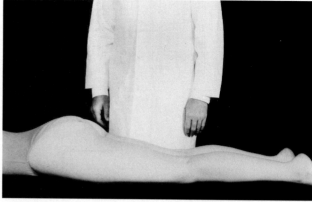

Fig. 11−3 The normal angle of knee flexion ranges from 130 to 150 degrees. A simple and useful but less-precise method for comparing the flexion of both knees can be used. This method involves comparing the distance between the heel and buttock when both knees are maximally flexed. Less than 140 degrees of retained active flexion range of motion is an impairment of the knee joint in the activities of daily living.

Flexion contractures (limitation of extension) of the knee often complicate chronic involvement of the joint. Varying degrees of subluxation or dislocation of the knee are most often the result of posterior displacement of the tibia on the femur or occasionally from destruction of one condyle and the supporting plate of the tibia. When, as a result of such destruction, the tibia is dislocated laterally or medially, abnormal lateral or medial mobility is present, although the range of flexion and extension of the knee is limited.

A catch or jerky motion sometimes can be felt or seen during passive flexion and extension of the knee when the joint space harbors loose bodies. When the motion is repeated, the catch occurs at the same position in the arc of movement. The knee may lock or become suddenly fixed in partial extension while flexion from the point of limitation may remain unrestricted. A catching or jerky motion also may result from the absence of both menisci, whether from surgical removal or from disintegration that is secondary to articular inflammatory diseases, such as rheumatoid arthritis.

Fig. 11−4 The knee should normally extend to a straight line (0 degrees), and occasionally can be hyperextended up to 15 degrees. The degree of extension is determined by measuring the angle formed between the thigh and the leg. A flexion angle that is 10 degrees or greater in the fully extended knee is an impairment of the knee in the activities of daily living.

MUSCLE TESTING

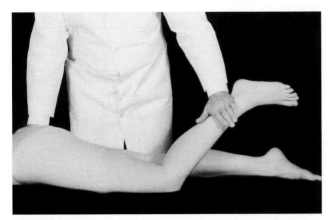

Fig. 11–5 The prime movers involved in flexion of the knee are the biceps femoris (sciatic nerve, tibial branch, S1, S2, and S3 to the long head; peroneal branch, L4, L5, S1, and S2 to the short head), semitendinosus (sciatic nerve, tibial branch, L4, L5, S1, S2, and S3), and the semimembranosus (sciatic nerve, tibial branch, L4, L5, S1, S2, and S3) muscles. Accessory muscles to this motion are the popliteus, sartorius, gracilis, and gastrocnemius muscles. Flexion of the knee is tested while the patient is lying in a prone position with the knees extended. The examiner places one hand over the lateral aspect of the pelvis to immobilize it and applies graded resistance just proximal to the ankle with the other hand. The patient flexes the knee through its range of motion. If knee flexion is tested with the ankle rotated laterally, the biceps femoris is tested more directly because it is placed in better alignment. If knee flexion is tested with the ankle rotated medially, the semimembranosus and semitendinosus muscles are tested more directly during flexion. To prevent substitution by the gastrocnemius muscle, plantar flexion of the foot should not be allowed during knee flexion.

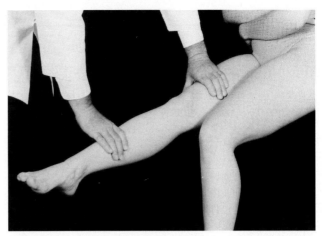

Fig. 11–6 The prime mover involved in extension of the knee is the quadriceps femoris (rectus femoris, vastus intermedius, vastus medialis, and vastus lateralis) muscle (innervated by the femoral nerve, L2, L3, and L4). Extension of the knee is tested while the patient sits with the legs hanging over the edge of a table. The examiner stabilizes the thigh by placing one hand over the pelvis or the proximal part of the thigh. The examiner should not exert pressure over the origin of the rectus femoris or induce pain. While the examiner provides stabilization, the patient then extends the knee through its range of motion. The examiner's free hand applies graded resistance proximal to the leg or ankle. As an alternative, the examiner can observe quadriceps femoris weakness if the patient is not able to rise from a low chair (height less than 65 cm) or from a squatting to a standing position without using the hands or other supports.

Abduction Stress Test

Comment

The medial ligament is the main strut of the capsular tissues of the knee. The deep portion of the ligament is a thickened part of the capsule itself and is adherent to the medial meniscus. The superficial part forms a strong, broad, and triangular strap. Originating from a point just distal to the adductor tubercle, the ligament keeps free of the meniscus and the joint margins and has an extensive insertion into the medial surface of the tibia, at least 1.5 inches below the joint level. The posterior border of the ligament has continuity with the strong posterior capsule of the knee joint. Anteriorly, there are fibrous connections with the quadriceps expansion and the patellar ligament. The whole medial capsule, which is accompanied by its ligament, is adequately designed to take strong control of the tibia in all movements of the knee, both by structure and by the intimate connections that the capsule forms with the anterior and posterior muscles of the thigh.

A ligament is a fibrous structure designed to prevent abnormal motion of a joint. Any ligamentous injury that is caused by an abnormal motion may be defined as a sprain. A sprain can vary from a complete dislocation of the joint, accompanied by total loss of ligament integrity, to a slight tearing of a few isolated fibers with no loss of function. A sprain should include avulsion of the ligament from the bone, with or without a small fragment (sprain-fracture); partial avulsion of the ligament from the bone; or tearing—either transversely, obliquely, or longitudinally—of the ligament within its substance. In the last instance the ligament will be elongated although it will still be intact. The function of the ligament depends not only on its strength but also on its length. A ligament that is elongated does not carry out its function of preventing abnormal motion of the joint. The severity of the injury is of more significance than the exact location or type of tear.

Procedure

While the patient is lying supine and the knee is in complete extension, the examiner, who is on the ipsilateral side, places one palm against the lateral aspect of the patient's knee, at the joint line. While the other hand is gripping the ankle, the examiner laterally draws the leg to open the medial side of the joint. If the patient is indifferent to this action, the examiner repeats it while the knee is in approximately 30 degrees of flexion, a position of lesser stability. This maneuver makes the medial joint vulnerable to torsion stress. The production or increase of pain, especially below, above, or at the joint line, is evidence of medial collateral ligament injury.

Confirmation Procedures

Adduction stress test, Apley's compression/distraction test

Reporting Statement

Abduction stress test is positive on the right. This result indicates medial collateral ligament injury.

∞ Clinical Pearl ∞

The knee is an unusual joint because it contains ligaments deep within the joint. There are also medial and lateral collateral menisci that can be damaged. Finally, the normal motions of the knee are very complex, including two planes of rotation. It is very common to see multiple and complex injuries.

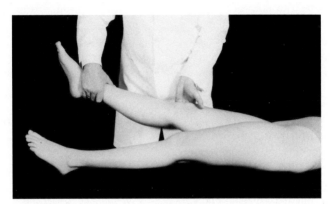

Fig. 11-7 The patient is lying supine, and the knee is in complete extension. The examiner, who is on the ipsilateral side, places one palm against the lateral aspect of the patient's knee, at the joint line. With the other hand gripping the ankle, the examiner draws the leg laterally, to open the medial side of the knee joint. The production or increase of pain—especially below, above, or at the joint line—is evidence of medial collateral ligament injury.

Adduction Stress Test

VARUS STRESS TEST

Comment

The lateral ligament extends, in two layers, from the lateral condyle of the femur to the head of the fibula, where the ligament inserts on the biceps tendon. The tendon of the popliteus and frequently a bursa separates the ligament from the knee joint and the lateral meniscus. The only connection the ligament has with the fibrous capsule is at the posterior border of the lateral ligament, which is continuous with the fascia covering the popliteus and therefore is continuous with that muscle's attachments to the posterior horn of the lateral meniscus. The lateral ligament plays its part in stability of the leg on the thigh through the superior tibiofibular joint. The lateral ligament is independent of rotary movements of the tibia. Where the ligament attaches to the lateral meniscus, rotation is prevented and flexion of the knee is restricted. The lateral capsule is thinner and weaker than the one on the medial side.

Ligament instability may be defined as abnormal rotational or translational motion of the tibial plateaus in relation to the femoral condyles. This rotational or translational motion occurs around one or more axes or in one or more planes of motion and results in a functional deficit. The key to evaluating ligament instability is the term *functional deficit*. Although two patients may have identical degrees of ligamentous instability, the functional deficit in each is not the same because the demands each patient places on the knees are different. A moderate amount of instability in an individual who wants to take part in vigorous physical activity may create a serious handicap, but a more sedentary patient may find that the same degree of instability is not a serious problem.

Stability of the knee is provided by static and dynamic elements that work together as an integrated mechanism. Static support is a function of the ligaments, capsule, menisci, and bony contour of the joint. Dynamic support is the function of the surrounding muscles. Attempting to assign a specific function to each ligament has led to confusion in evaluating ligamentous instability. The examiner must bear in mind that the static stabilizers are an integral part of a mechanism that must provide support to an inherently unstable joint that is subject to a variety of forces. It is rare for an injury to affect only one element in this complex system. Usually an injury influences more than one other structure either directly or indirectly. The knee joint is not merely a hinge joint that allows flexion and extension. The joint also has the element of rotation and even some valgus and varus motion.

Even with normal ligaments, knee stability is a rather tenuous situation, because the knee does not have the dynamic support of the various thigh and calf muscles, which protect the static elements. The static structures define the limits of motion, and the musculotendinous structures control the motion through voluntary and kinesthetic mechanisms. These structures create appropriate motion and simultaneously serve as energy-absorbing mechanisms for extrinsic and intrinsic forces that might otherwise injure the static structures.

Procedure

While the patient is lying supine and the knee is in complete extension, the examiner, who is on the ipsilateral side, places one palm against the medial aspect of the patient's knee, at the joint line. While the examiner's other hand grips the ankle, the examiner draws the leg medially to open the lateral side of the joint. If the patient is indifferent to this procedure, the examiner repeats it with the knee in approximately 30 degrees of flexion. An initiation or increase of pain above, below, or at the joint line is evidence of lateral collateral ligament injury.

Confirmation Procedures

Abduction stress test, Apley's compression/distraction test

Reporting Statement

Adduction stress test is positive for the right knee. This result indicates lateral collateral ligament injury.

Clinical Pearl

There is little congruency between the articular surfaces of the tibia and the femur. As a result, there is a well-developed system of ligaments for stability, and an arrangement of intraarticular menisci that reduce the contact loading between the femur and tibia.

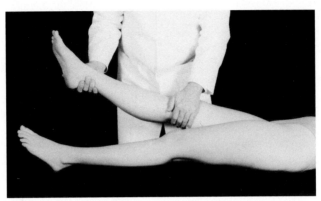

Fig. 11–8 The patient is lying supine and the knee is in complete extension. The examiner, who is standing on the ipsilateral side, places one palm against the medial aspect of the patient's knee, at the joint line. With the other hand gripping the ankle, the examiner draws the leg medially, to open the lateral side of the knee joint. The production or increase of pain that is above, below, or at the joint line is evidence of lateral collateral ligament injury.

Apley's Compression Test

APLEY'S DISTRACTION TEST
APLEY'S GRINDING TEST

Comment

When bearing weight, the tibia rotates laterally as the knee joint extends, and it rotates medially as the knee flexes. If this synchrony is forcibly prevented, such as by the weight of the patient's falling body, the rotator mechanism of the knee is injured. Certain cartilage tears are caused by this disruption of the rotator mechanism of the knee. In a geriatric patient the transverse fracture of the fibrotic medial meniscus, which takes place at the junction of the anterior two thirds and the posterior one third, may be due to pressure and grinding between the femur and the tibia. All other tears can be explained by the violent stretching that must occur if medial rotation of the tibia is prevented when the knee is flexed, or if lateral rotation is prevented when the knee is extended. Similar forces are brought into play when weight is taken on while squatting or kneeling. For example, a sudden twisting may occur without extension or further flexion, or the tibia may twist laterally while the body lurches backward and increases flexion of the knee.

At first the meniscus straightens. To allow it to do so, a transverse or oblique split forms in the shorter or free edge. This minor split is the most frequent finding and is usually deeper in the lateral meniscus than in the medial meniscus, because of the longer curve of the latter. If no more damage occurs, the knee might be symptomless after recovery from the acute injury, but the split itself would not heal. However, occasionally the split extends obliquely to form a mobile tag, which causes an irritating, recurring, and painful catch in the knee.

The split usually occurs at the apex of the curve or in the anterior portion of the meniscus. This location is to be expected because the straightening under tension would take place first in the more mobile portion. The posterior segments are more firmly fixed to the capsule.

Should the range of unaccommodated movement be greater, it is achieved either by pulling the cartilage away from its attachments to the anterior cruciate and from its capsular moorings at the back or by splitting the cartilage longitudinally to allow the free border to bowstring across the joint.

Procedure

The test involves four steps, and if any or all of them elicit knee pain or clicking, then the test is positive. (1) The patient is lying prone with the lower limbs straight and the ankles hanging over the table edge. The examiner grasps the foot of the involved lower extremity, strongly rotates the leg internally, and flexes the knee past 90 degrees. (2) This maneuver is repeated with the leg strongly rotated in external rotation. (3) The examiner anchors the patient's thigh to the examination table by placing a knee in the patient's popliteal space. A small pillow or towel should be used for cushioning. The examiner strongly distracts the patient's knee joint by lifting the foot. This move is followed by rapid rotating, both internally and externally, of the leg. (4) This procedure is repeated with strong downward pressure on the patient's foot. An intermediate maneuver may be performed. The examiner flexes the patient's knee to 90 degrees and rapidly rotates the foot and leg, both internally and externally, without anchorage to rule out a rotational strain or collateral ligament tear. The test is significant for meniscus tear.

Confirmation Procedures

Abduction stress test, adduction stress test, bounce home test, Childress duck waddle test, McMurray sign, Payr's sign, Steinmann's sign

---

Reporting Statement

Apley's compression test is positive on the right and indicates injury to the medial meniscus.

Apley's knee compression testing is positive on the right and indicates injury to the lateral meniscus.

Apley's distraction test is positive on the right and indicates injury to the lateral collateral ligaments.

Apley's distraction test is positive on the right and indicates injury to the medial collateral ligaments.

∾ Clinical Pearl ∾

The phrase *internal derangement of the knee* is a common provisional diagnosis for any patient with mechanical symptoms of the knee. The initials of this phrase, IDK, also stand for "I don't know," and the temptation to use these initials, instead of making a complete diagnosis, must be avoided.

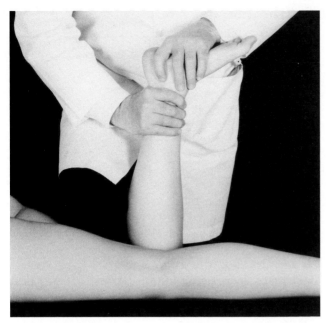

Fig. 11–9 The patient is lying prone with the leg extended and the ankles hanging over the table edge. The examiner grasps the foot and strongly and internally rotates the leg and then flexes the knee to 90 degrees.

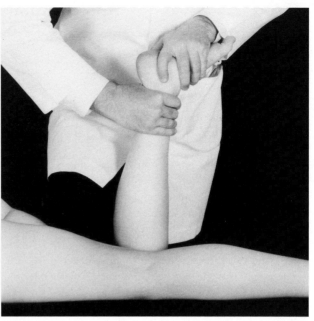

Fig. 11–10 The examiner repeats the maneuver described in Fig. 11–9 while the leg is strongly rotated externally and strong downward pressure is applied to the patient's foot. The production of pain is significant for meniscus tear.

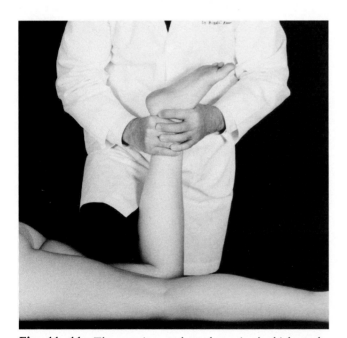

Fig. 11–11 The examiner anchors the patient's thigh to the table by placing a knee in the patient's popliteal space. The maneuver can be cushioned by a small pillow or towel. The examiner strongly distracts the patient's knee joint by lifting the foot.

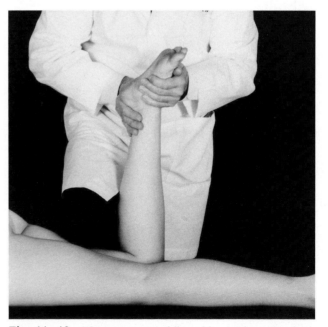

Fig. 11–12 This maneuver is followed by rapid rotation, both internally and externally, of the leg. Pain elicited is significant for collateral ligament tear.

Comment

Recurrent dislocation, or subluxation, of the patella that occurs to the lateral side while the knee is flexed is commonly encountered in adolescents. This type of dislocation is often bilateral, and it occurs in females more often than in males.

The first dislocation is initiated by trauma. A mild hypoplasia of the anterior surface of the lateral femoral condyle and genu valgum are predisposing factors. This type of trauma usually occurs while the patient is engaged in an active sport. The patient falls and strikes the medial aspect of the patella, forcing it laterally over the condyle. Pain is severe, and the patient is unable to straighten the leg. The displacement may be reduced immediately, either by the patient or a companion or spontaneously.

After this type of fall some patients have no further difficulty. In other cases, dislocation becomes more and more frequent, and the patient complains that the knee is unstable and gives way. Occasionally a patient is able to describe the maneuver by which the dislocation can be reduced. This maneuver involves straightening the knee and forcing the lateral border of the patella in a medial direction. Following reduction, the knee is usually painful for 2 or 3 days. There may also be mild effusion. With recurrent episodes, degenerative changes develop on the undersurface of the patella and on the femoral condyle.

When the patient is examined after recurrent episodes of dislocation, tenderness occurs along the medial aspect of the patella and suggests a partial tear of the insertion of the vastus medialis. Effusion of the knee and slight quadriceps atrophy also occurs. The range of knee motion is normal.

Procedure

The apprehension test for the patella is a test for vulnerability to recurrent dislocation of the patella. For the test the patient is either supine or seated with the quadriceps muscles relaxed. The knee is flexed to 30 degrees. The examiner carefully and slowly pushes the patella laterally. If the patella feels as if it is about to dislocate, the patient will contract the quadriceps muscles and bring the patella back into line. This action indicates a positive test. The patient will also exhibit a look of apprehension.

Confirmation Procedures

Clarke's sign, Dreyer's sign, Fouchet's sign

Reporting Statement

The apprehension test for the patella is positive on the right. This result indicates a vulnerability to recurrent dislocation of the patella.

~ Clinical Pearl ~

The examiner should observe for genu recurvatum and the position of the patella in relation to the femoral condyles. A high patella (patella alta) is a predisposing factor to recurrent lateral dislocation of the patella. The recurrent dislocation of the patella is also most common in females with the genu valgum deformity.

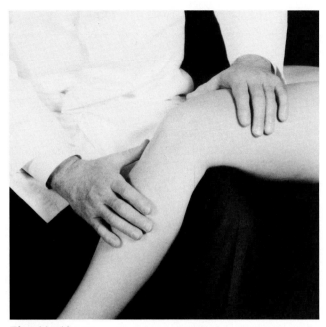

Fig. 11–13 The patient is seated, with the quadriceps muscles relaxed and the knee flexed to approximately 30 degrees over the examiner's leg.

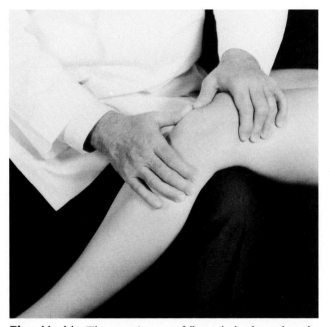

Fig. 11–14 The examiner carefully and slowly pushes the patella laterally. If the patella feels as if it is about to dislocate, the patient will contract the quadriceps muscle, to bring the patella back into line. This action indicates a positive test. A positive test indicates a vulnerability or predisposition for recurrent dislocation of the patella.

Comment

The congenital discoid meniscus most frequently involves the lateral meniscus and it often presents symptoms in childhood. With this defect the meniscus is not in the usual semilunar form but rather more *D* shaped, with its central edge extending toward the tibial spines. The meniscus may produce a very pronounced clicking from the lateral compartment, a block to the extension of the joint, and other derangement signs.

The most common cause of meniscal tears in young adults is a sporting injury, such as when a twisting strain is applied to the flexed, weight-bearing leg. In this case the entrapped meniscus often splits longitudinally, and its free edge may displace inward, toward the center of the joint. This is called a *bucket-handle tear.* This type of tear prevents full extension (locking), and if an attempt is made to straighten the knee, a painful, elastic resistance (a springy block to full extension) is felt. The injury of the medial meniscus, which involves prolonged loss of full extension, may lead to stretching and eventual rupture of the anterior cruciate ligament. Lateral meniscus tears are often associated with cysts that restrict the mobility of the meniscus. Major meniscus tears are treated by excision of the meniscus, but with bucket-handle tears the removal of only the central portion may decrease the risk of late, secondary osteoarthritis. In some lesions involving the periphery of the meniscus, repair by direct suture is sometimes attempted.

Loss of elasticity in the menisci, through degenerative changes associated with the aging process, may cause horizontal cleavage tears within the substance of the meniscus. These tears may not be associated with any remembered incident. Sharply localized tenderness in the joint line is a common feature.

Ganglion-like cysts occur in both menisci. However, these cysts are much more common in the lateral meniscus. There is often a history of a blow on the side of the knee, over the meniscus. The cysts are tender, and because they restrict mobility of the menisci, the cysts render them more susceptible to tears. Medial meniscus cysts must be carefully differentiated from ganglion cysts that arise from the pes anserinus (the insertion of the sartorius, gracilis, and semitendinosus).

Procedure

The patient lies supine, and the heel of the patient's foot is cupped in the examiner's hand. The patient's knee, which is at first completely flexed, is allowed to extend. If the extension is not complete or if it has a rubbery, end feel (springy block), then something is blocking the extension. The most likely cause of a block is a torn meniscus.

Confirmation Procedures

Childress duck waddle test, McMurray sign, Payr's sign, Steinmann's sign

---

Reporting Statement

The bounce home test is positive for the right knee and indicates a torn meniscus.

∾ **Clinical Pearl** ∾

Meniscus lesions are the most common internal derangement. Although the menisci are damaged by trauma, the incident is often so trivial that the patient cannot remember any injury at all. Because of this, patients with meniscal injuries are rarely seen in emergency rooms.

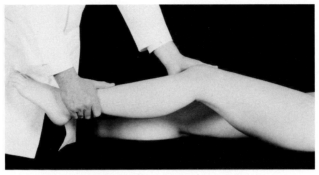

Fig. 11–15 The patient is lying supine, and the heel of the patient's foot is cupped in the examiner's hand, or the examiner may grasp the patient's leg at the ankle. The patient's knee is flexed.

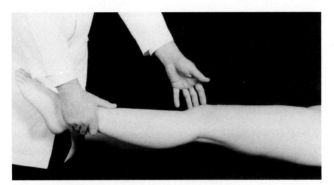

Fig. 11–16 The knee is allowed to extend. If the extension is not complete or if it has a rubbery end feel (springy block), there is something blocking the extension. This result is a positive finding, and indicates a torn meniscus.

Comment

The term internal derangement is used to group together a variety of knee joint conditions, usually of traumatic origin, in which the internal structure of the joint is affected to such an extent that its function and mechanics are compromised.

A rotary force applied to the knee joint may trap a meniscus between the femur and the tibia, and produce the familiar torn-cartilage lesion. A meniscus cannot be torn while the knee is in extension. To produce a tear, the knee joint must be first rotated in the flexed position to trap the meniscus and then extended to produce the tearing force on the tissue. This combination of motions is frequently encountered on the football field or basketball court.

Tears of the medial meniscus are encountered about nine times more frequently than tears of the lateral meniscus. This difference in frequency is believed to be because the medial meniscus is attached to the deep layer of the medial collateral ligament, and because the mechanisms that cause the tearing are more frequently applied to the medial aspect of the joint.

A tear of the medial meniscus is associated with pain that is referred to the medial side of the joint and is accompanied by synovial effusion. The pain caused by the torn meniscus is frequently aggravated by forced rotation of the foot and leg. Pain or a clicking may be produced by testing for the McMurray sign. Locking of the joint may or may not be present, depending upon the location of the tear.

Two types of tears occur most frequently. The first type is punch-press effect of the femoral condyle on the trapped meniscus, which may cause a splitting of the meniscus, along its longitudinal axis, producing the so-called *bucket-handle tear.* In this instance, the inner portion of the torn cartilage may displace into the joint and cause locking. The joint may be unlocked by manipulation, but the healing of the tear does not occur because the meniscus cannot totally regenerate.

The second type of tear occurs under certain circumstances, when the meniscus may be torn along its transverse axis. This type of tear usually does not cause locking of the joint. The pain is produced by momentary impingement of the irregular meniscus between the femur and the tibia during motions of the joint. Lesions of the lateral meniscus include tears, cystic degeneration, and discoid meniscus.

Tears similar to those seen in the medial meniscus may involve the lateral meniscus, but these tears are less common.

On the other hand, cystic degeneration is a much more common event in the lateral meniscus than in the medial meniscus. In this condition, multiple cysts containing gelatinous material appear within the peripheral border of the meniscus. Repeated trauma causes the appearance of these cysts. Once developed, cartilage cysts may cause pain and often can be seen and palpated along the lateral border of the knee joint.

A discoid meniscus is a congenitally abnormal lateral meniscus, in which the structure assumes a thickened and rounded shape. Because of its thickness, the meniscus does not glide smoothly between the femur and the tibia. Rather the meniscus must force its way through. As a result, a loud clicking noise is heard when the knee flexes or extends, but locking does not occur.

Procedure

The patient stands with the feet somewhat apart and the legs in maximal internal rotation. A full squat is attempted. During this maneuver, the patient's heels may come up from the floor, with weight bearing passing to the balls of the feet. The maneuver is repeated, with the lower limbs in maximal external rotation. A positive test consists of pain, inability to fully flex the knee, or a clicking sound on either posterior side of the joint. The test is significant in internal rotation for a medial meniscus tear or during external rotation for a lateral meniscus tear.

Confirmation Procedures

Bounce home test, McMurray sign, Payr's sign, Steinmann's sign

---

Reporting Statement

Childress duck waddle test is positive for the right knee in external rotation. This result indicates a lateral meniscus tear.

Childress duck waddle test is positive for the right knee in internal rotation. This result indicates a medial meniscus tear.

∾ Clinical Pearl ∾

The menisci are important parts of the load-bearing mechanism of the knee because they absorb the downward thrust of the convex femoral condyles. The menisci are so effective that if they are removed, the force that is taken by the articular cartilage during peak loading increases about five times. Therefore a meniscectomy exposes the articular cartilage to much greater forces than normal. Evidence of degenerative osteoarthritis is seen in 75% of patients 10 years after a total meniscectomy.

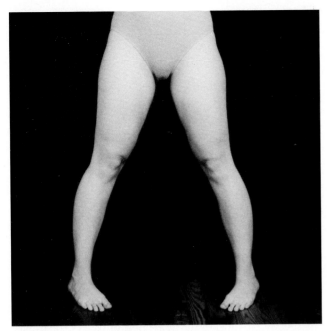

Fig. 11–17 The patient stands with the feet apart and the legs in maximum internal rotation.

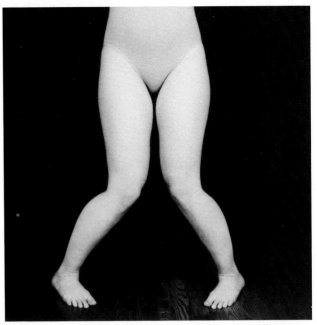

Fig. 11–18 The patient attempts a full squat. During this maneuver the patient's heels may come up from the floor and weight may be shifted to the balls of the feet.

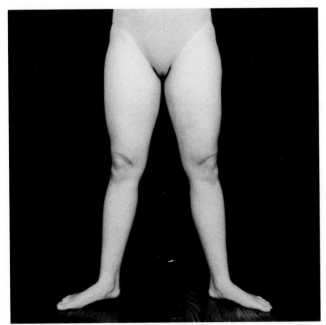

Fig. 11–19 The maneuver is repeated with the lower limbs in maximum external rotation.

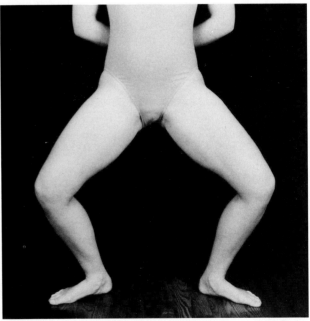

Fig. 11–20 A full squat is attempted again. A positive test consists of pain, inability to fully flex the knee, or a clicking sound on either posterior side of the joint. With internal rotation the test is significant for a medial meniscus tear. During external rotation the test is significant for a lateral meniscus tear.

Comment

The term patellar malacia has been used as a catchall to include the many processes that involve the undersurface of the patella. True malacia is a softening or breaking down of a part of the tissue. When chronic synovitis of the knee causes the patellar cartilage to break down and the bed to eburnate so that denuded bone is exposed the condition is called *malacia*. This is the same condition that occurs in a young individual who has fragmentation of the patellar cartilage with no signs of arthritis. Patellar malacia falls into three groups.

Group I is trauma related. There may be a chondral fracture or infraction that is caused either by acute trauma or by repeated, lesser traumata to the patella. Infraction of the patellar cartilage causes irritation of the patellar groove on the femur, and gradual changes supervene with fissuring, absorption, and fragmentation of the cartilage.

Group II is associated with a disturbance of the rhythm of the patellar function. These disturbances are commonly called *tracking disorders*. This is the type of malacia that accompanies intrinsic injury to the knee. Any condition that causes a disturbance in the rhythm of the knee action frequently results in involvement of the undersurface of the patella. The knee is checked abruptly, motion is reversed, and the patella is driven against the femur. There is a relationship between the locking of the knee and the degree of malacia present. These two factors are much more important for indicating the amount of malacia present than is the age of the patient. The exact mechanism of the breakdown of the patella has never been wholly explained. This condition also probably occurs as the result of various other causes including direct trauma, synovitis of the joint, and general chondrolytic changes. The particular pathologic changes described usually accompany other intrinsic conditions of the knee.

Group II is primary malacia of the patella, usually a bilateral condition, without any demonstrable etiologic factor. These cases are puzzling. The examiner cannot rule out the effect of repeated trauma, since the young patients are usually very physically active. These patients should be expected to traumatize the patella repeatedly. However, the simultaneous involvement of both knees, with relative lack of involvement of other chondral surfaces equally susceptible to trauma, prompts the examiner to seek a cause other than a simple contusion.

Careful evaluation of the anatomic development of the knee may give a definite indication of the cause of the idiopathic malacia. Patella alta is very prone to alter the mechanism of the gliding surface of the patella on the trochlear groove and to contribute to the malacia. Lateral subluxation of the patella, as the knee comes into complete extension, may cause malacia of the patella without actually giving any evidence of gross displacement.

Procedure

This test assesses the presence of chondromalacia patellae. The examiner presses down with the web of the hand at a site slightly proximal to the upper pole or base of the patella. The patient lies relaxed with the knee extended while the examiner exerts this pressure. The patient is instructed to contract the quadriceps muscles while the examiner pushes down. If the patient can complete and maintain the contraction without pain, the test is negative. If the test causes retropatellar pain and the patient cannot hold the contraction, the test is considered positive. A positive test can result in any patient if sufficient pressure is applied to the patella as the patient contracts the quadriceps. The amount of pressure applied must be controlled. The way to do this is to repeat the procedure several times, increasing the pressure each time and comparing results with those obtained on the unaffected side. For testing different parts of the patella, the knee should be tested in 30, 60, and 90 degrees of flexion as well as in full extension.

Confirmation Procedures

Apprehension test for the patella, Dreyer's sign, Fouchet's sign

---

Reporting Statement

Clarke's sign is present at the right knee. The presence of this sign indicates patellar chondromalacia.

～ Clinical Pearl ～

In examining the patella the examiner should note any tenderness over the anterior surface and whether a bipartite ridge is present. Upper and lower pole tenderness occurs in Sinding-Larsen-Johannson disease and jumper's knee (an extensor apparatus traction injury).

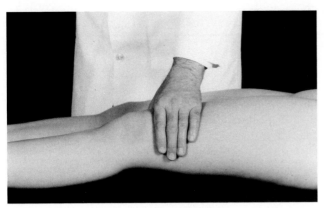

Fig. 11–21 The patient is lying supine with the affected knee extended. The examiner presses down with the web of the hand at a site that is slightly proximal to the upper pole or base of the patella.

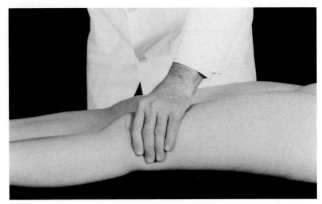

Fig. 11–22 The examiner pushes the patella into an inferior position, which stretches the quadriceps muscle and tendon.

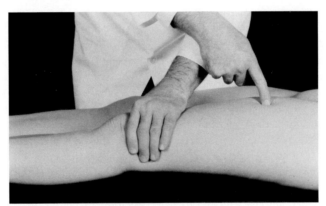

Fig. 11–23 The patient is instructed to contract the quadriceps muscle, as the examiner restricts the movement of the patella by continuing to push down. If this maneuver causes retropatellar pain and the patient cannot hold the contraction, the test is positive. A positive test is significant for chondromalacia patellae.

Comment

Damage to the anterior cruciate ligament occurs most frequently as a sequel to tears of the medial meniscus. Many longitudinal meniscus tears produce a block to extension of the joint. Attempts to obtain full extension lead to attrition rupture of the ligament. Anterior cruciate ligament tears also may accompany severe collateral ligament injuries.

Isolated rupture of the anterior cruciate ligament are uncommon and are not usually treated surgically, unless they are accompanied by avulsion of the bone at the anterior tibial attachment. When the tear accompanies a meniscus lesion, the meniscus is preserved, if possible, to reduce the risks of tibial subluxation and secondary osteoarthritic changes. Nevertheless, the damage may be such that excision cannot be avoided. When an acute tear is associated with damage to the collateral ligaments, a combined repair or reconstruction is usually attempted. Problems from tibial subluxation are common, particularly when anterior cruciate tears are accompanied by damage to the medial or lateral structures. When anterior tibial subluxation is the main source of symptoms, surgical reconstruction may be indicated if simple measures, such as quadriceps strengthening, are not successful.

Posterior cruciate ligament tears are produced when the tibia is forcibly pushed backwards while the knee is flexed (for example, in a car accident, in which the upper part of the leg strikes the dashboard). Surgical repair is always advised if the injury is seen at the acute stage. The persisting instability and osteoarthritis are the usual sequelae in the untreated case.

In this group of conditions, which are characterized by rotary instability in the knee, the tibia may sublux forward or backwards on either the medial or lateral side when the knee is stressed. This subluxation may cause pain and a feeling of instability in the joint. There are four main forms of this condition. (1) The medial tibial condyle subluxes anteriorly (anteromedial instability). In the more severe cases the anterior cruciate and the medial structures (medial ligament and meniscus) are torn. (2) The lateral tibial condyle subluxes anteriorly (anterolateral rotary instability). In the most severe cases the anterior cruciate ligament and lateral structures are torn, and there may be an associated lesion of the anterior horn of the lateral meniscus. (3) The lateral tibial condyle subluxes posteriorly (posterolateral rotary instability). This subluxation may follow rupture of the lateral structures and the posterior cruciate ligaments and is recognized by the presence of instability of the knee on applying varus stress. This subluxation is associated with an abnormal, posterior drawer test. (4) Combinations of these lesions may be found, especially where there is major ligamentous disruption of the knee.

Procedure

The drawer test is a test for one-plane anterior and one-plane posterior instability. The patient's knee is flexed to 90 degrees and the hip to 45 degrees. In this position, the anterior cruciate ligament is almost parallel with the tibial plateau. The patient's foot is held on the table by the examiner, who sits on the patient's forefoot. The examiner's hands are placed around the tibia to ensure that the hamstring muscles are relaxed. The tibia is then drawn forward on the femur. The normal amount of movement that should be present is approximately 6 mm. This part of the test is an assessment for one-plane anterior instability. If the test is positive, which occurs when the tibia moves forward more than 6 mm on the femur, the following structures may have been injured to some degree: (1) the anterior cruciate ligament, especially the anteromedial bundle, (2) the posterolateral capsule, (3) the posteromedial capsule, (4) the medial collateral ligament, especially the deep fibers, (5) the iliotibial band, (6) the posterior oblique ligament, and (7) the arcuate-popliteus complex.

The examiner must ensure that the posterior cruciate ligament is not torn or injured. If this ligament has been torn, it will allow the tibia to drop back on the femur. When the examiner pulls the tibia forward, a large amount of movement will occur, giving a false-positive sign.

Following the anterior movement of the tibia on the femur, the posterior movement of the tibia on the femur should be completed. In this part of the test the tibia is pushed back on the femur. This phase is a test for one-plane posterior instability. If the test is positive, the following structures may have been injured to some degree: (1) the posterior cruciate ligament, (2) the arcuate-popliteus complex, (3) the posterior oblique ligament, and (4) the anterior cruciate ligament.

If the anterior or posterior cruciate ligaments are torn (third-degree sprain), some rotary instability will be evident when the appropriate ligamentous tests are done.

Confirmation Procedures

Lachman test, Lateral pivot shift maneuver, Losee test, Slocum's test

---

Reporting Statement

The drawer test is positive for the right knee, and anterior instability is greater than 6 mm. This result indicates insufficiency of the anterior cruciate ligament.

The drawer test is positive for the right knee, and a posterior instability is greater than 6 mm. This result indicates insufficiency of the posterior cruciate ligament.

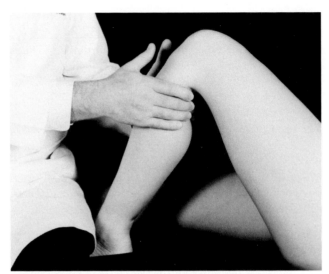

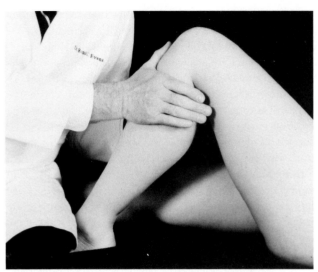

Fig. 11–24 The patient is lying supine, the knee is flexed to 90 degrees, and the hip is flexed to 45 degrees. The patient's foot is held on the table by the examiner, who is sitting on the patient's forefoot. The examiner's hands are placed around the tibia to ensure that the hamstring muscles are relaxed. The tibia is then drawn forward on the femur. The normal amount of movement that should be present is approximately 6 mm.

If the test is positive, that is, the tibia moves forward more than 6 mm on the femur, the following structures may have been injured to some degree: (1) the anterior cruciate ligament, especially the antero-medial bundle, (2) the posterolateral capsule, (3) the posteromedial capsule, (4) the medial collateral ligament, especially the deep fibers, (5) the iliotibial band, (6) the posterior oblique ligament, and (7) the arcuate-popliteus complex.

Fig. 11–25 Following the anterior movement of the tibia on the femur, the posterior movement of the tibia on the femur should be assessed. In this part of the test the tibia is pushed posterior on the femur. If the test is positive, which is demonstrated by a large amount of posterior movement, the following structures may have been injured to some degree: (1) the posterior cruciate ligament, (2) the arcuate-popliteus complex, (3) the posterior oblique ligament, and (4) the anterior cruciate ligament.

Comment

Fracture of the patella is not as common as chondral fractures of the patella. Fractures of either the superior or inferior pole or along the medial or lateral margins are usually actually either strain fractures or sprain fractures. The examiner should suspect chondral fracture to accompany stellate fracture of the patella without displacement.

Fracture of the patella by direct contusion is not infrequent. The fracture usually involves the lateral portion of the patella because the bone is thinner in this area. A fracture of the patella differs from the avulsion type, in which the fragment is torn away by the tension on the fragment. The avulsion fracture is usually on the medial side and occurs as the patella is forced laterally. A patella fracture also differs from the explosive type of fracture that is caused by a forceful blow against the patella while the quadriceps are in violent contraction. This situation may occur when the knee hits the dashboard in a car accident. The contusion fracture is due to a sharp blow in a localized area. This same force may cause chondral damage.

The bipartite or tripartite patella should not be confused with acute injury. The partite patella is usually bilateral and symmetrical and is asymptomatic. Careful examination will demonstrate that the symptoms are not in the area of the anomaly. It is possible for the quadriceps lateralis to avulse or partially avulse the separate piece, in which the condition will be symptomatic.

Procedure

While lying supine with the knee extended, the patient is unable to raise the leg. When the examiner applies compression to the thigh, by using the hands to give anchorage to the quadriceps, the patient is able to lift the leg. When this force is removed, the patient is again unable to raise the leg. The test is significant for a fracture of the patella.

Confirmation Procedures

Apprehension test, Clarke's sign, Fouchet's sign, diagnostic imaging

---

Reporting Statement

Dreyer's sign is positive for the right knee. The presence of this sign indicates a fracture of the patella.

~ **Clinical Pearl** ~

The quadriceps muscle gains insertion into the tibia through the medium of the patella, which is enclosed within the quadriceps expansion, and the patellar tendon. Complete rupture may occur as a disruption through the patella. This area is the usual site of rupture for a common variety of fractured patella. The injury occurs mainly in adults of middle age.

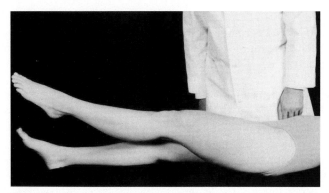

Fig. 11-26   The patient is lying supine with the knee extended. The patient attempts to raise the leg. In the presence of patellar fracture, this raising motion is painful and difficult to accomplish.

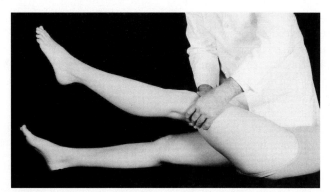

Fig. 11-27   The examiner applies forceful, circumferential grasp to the thigh with the hands, which give anchorage to the quadriceps. The patient attempts to lift the leg. The sign is present when the patient can lift the leg with minimal distress. When this force is removed, the inability to raise the leg recurs. The presence of the sign is significant for a fracture of the patella.

Comment

The patella is a pulley, and its excursion is controlled by the direction of action of the quadriceps group of muscles and the position of the tibial tubercle, which carries the patellar ligament.

The articular surface of the patella is divided into a large lateral and a small medial area. These areas are separated by a vertical, rounded ridge. During full extension, the shape of the patella fits into the trochlear surface of the femur. The ridge then lies in the hollow, or trough, of the trochlear surface. When the knee is flexed, the patella is carried downward and backward on the under aspect of the femur, where the trochlear surface is prolonged onto the inner condyle. During flexion, the patella tilts away from the lateral condyle so only the inner part of its articular surface rests against the medial condyle.

So long as the tibial tubercle rotates smoothly, the patella travels its short course smoothly and under even tension. However, any derangement of the joint that prevents lateral rotation of the tibia during extension of the knee would affect the normal tension because contraction of the quadriceps would force the inner border of the patella against the medial condyle of the femur. This forced meeting explains the patellar symptoms and signs produced by certain cartilage injuries. Some of these symptoms and signs include retropatellar pain experienced during climbing and descension of stairs, tenderness of the medial border of the patella, and the pattern of cartilage erosion that develops only on the medial surfaces of the patella and the femur. This pattern differs from that produced by retropatellar arthritis, which complicates recurring dislocation, when the lateral surface of the patellar cartilage undergoes fibrillation. Later the medial surface is damaged from repeated drag over the lateral condyle of the femur during reduction. This repeated dragging results in erosion of the articular cartilage. By this time both sides of the patella are tender.

Procedure

While the patient is lying supine and the knee is in full extension, the examiner uses the flat of a hand to compress the patella against the femur. If this produces point tenderness and pain at the patellar margin, the sign is present. If pain is not produced by this maneuver, the examiner then rubs the patella transversely, against the femur. Audible or palpable grating and pain confirm the presence of the sign. When the patella has peripheral tenderness upon medial or lateral displacement, this is known as Perkins' sign. Perkins' sign is significant for patellar tracking disorder, peripatellar syndrome, or patellofemoral dysfunction.

Confirmation Procedures

Apprehension test for the patella, Clarke's sign, Dreyer's sign, diagnostic imaging

---

Reporting Statement

Fouchet's sign is present in the right knee. The presence of this sign indicates a patellar tracking disorder, peripatellar syndrome, or patellofemoral dysfunction.

∾ Clinical Pearl ∾

Placing a palm of the hand over the patella and the thumb and index finger along the joint line as the joint is flexed and extended will distinguish the source of the crepitus from damaged articular surfaces.

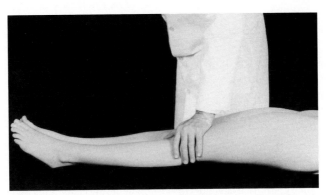

Fig. 11−28 The patient is lying supine, and the affected knee is in full extension. With the flat of a hand the examiner compresses the patella against the femur. If this produces point tenderness and pain at the patellar margin, the sign is present. If no pain is produced, the patella is then rubbed transversely, against the femur. Audible or palpable grating and pain confirm the presence of the sign. The sign is significant for patellar tracking disorders, peripatellar syndrome, or patellofemoral dysfunction.

Comment

Ligamentous injuries to the knee are among the most serious of all knee disorders. Because of the importance of the ligaments in stabilizing the joint, early diagnosis of the injury is mandatory. Any delay in diagnosis and treatment may lead to a chronically unstable knee, which predisposes the knee to early traumatic arthritis.

The mechanism is usually one of forceful stress against the knee while the extremity is bearing weight. A valgus stress against the knee may sprain or tear the medial collateral ligament, and a varus stress will injure the lateral collateral ligament. Tears of the cruciate ligaments, menisci, and capsule also may occur with the collateral ligament injury.

The history of a ligamentous injury is often difficult to reconstruct, but it will provide clues to the type of force applied to the knee. After the injury, the extremity's ability to bear weight is often lost. Swelling from an acute ligament or capsular tear is usually immediate and is due to hemorrhage. A pop or tearing sensation may be heard or felt. Incomplete tears or sprains are often more painful than complete ligamentous ruptures.

Patients with chronically unstable knees that are due to old injuries often complain of the knee going out or giving way and of not being able to depend on the extremity. These symptoms are always most noticeable during vigorous activities. A chronic effusion is often present.

With an acute injury the examination is of utmost importance. Any swelling or discoloration is noted. The lesion can frequently be localized by palpation alone. The palpation should begin away from the suspected area to promote patient cooperation. A point of maximum tenderness is often present along the course of the collateral ligament or capsule.

The knee should always be tested for stability while the patient is in a relaxed, supine position. If the examination cannot be adequately performed because of pain or hamstring spasm, it may have to be repeated while the patient is under local or general anesthesia. The injured knee is always compared to the opposite, uninvolved knee.

Procedure

The Lachman test is a good indicator of injury to the anterior cruciate ligament, especially the posterolateral band. It is a test for one-plane, anterior instability. The patient lies in a supine position with the involved leg beside the examiner. The examiner holds the patient's knee between full extension and 30 degrees of flexion. The patient's femur is stabilized with one of the examiner's hands while the proximal aspect of the tibia is moved forward with the other hand. A positive sign is indicated by a mushy, or soft, end feel when the tibia is moved forward on the femur and the infrapatellar tendon slope disappears. A positive sign indicates that several structures may have been injured to some degree. These structures include: (1) the anterior cruciate ligament, especially the posterolateral bundle, (2) the posterior oblique ligament, and (3) the arcuate-popliteus complex.

Confirmation Procedures

Drawer test, lateral pivot shift maneuver, Losee test, Slocum's test

---

Reporting Statement

Lachman test is positive for the right knee. This result indicates injury to the anterior cruciate ligament.

∼ Clinical Pearl ∼

When both medial and lateral or both anterior and posterior, as well as the medial and lateral compartments are torn, combined complex instability exists. Transitory dislocation, or at least subluxation of the knee, is a preliminary symptom. In many instances the peroneal nerve has been injured.

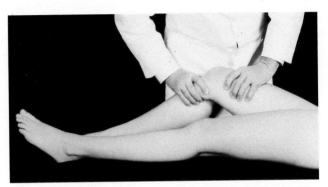

Fig. 11—29 The patient is lying supine with the involved leg beside the examiner. The examiner holds the patient's knee between full extension and 30 degrees of flexion. The patient's femur is stabilized with one of the examiner's hands, while the proximal aspect of the tibia is moved forward with the examiner's other hand. A positive sign is indicated by a mushy or soft end feel when the tibia is moved forward on the femur, and the infrapatellar tendon slope disappears. A positive sign indicates that the following structures may have been injured to some degree: (1) the anterior cruciate ligament, especially the posterolateral bundle, (2) the posterior oblique ligament, and (3) the arcuate-popliteus complex.

Lateral Pivot Shift Maneuver

TEST OF McINTOSH

Comment

Lateral instabilities of the knee may involve both varus and rotational instabilities. The rotation instabilities are anterolateral rotary instability, which involves a lateral tibial plateau that displaces anteriorly and posterolateral instability, which involves a lateral tibial plateau that displaces posteriorly. The most frequently encountered lateral instability is the anterolateral rotary instability. A lateral rotary instability is called the lateral pivot shift, which should not be confused as something other than anterolateral rotary instability. Clinically this instability is characterized by a sensation that the knee "gives way" as the patient decelerates suddenly and pivots on the involved extremity.

Anterolateral instability is created by incompetency of the anterior cruciate ligament, the midlateral capsule, some degree of laxity of the arcuate ligament, and occasionally laxity of the iliotibial tract. If the iliotibial tract has been stretched or injured, then the McIntosh-type testing for anterolateral rotary instability will not be positive in eliciting the classic jumping sensation. With most anterolateral instabilities the iliotibial tract is intact and the instability can be more graphically demonstrated with some form of the McIntosh test.

Procedure

The lateral pivot shift maneuver is the primary test used to assess anterolateral rotary instability of the knee. During this test, the tibia moves away from the femur on the lateral side and moves anteriorly in relation to the femur.

Normally the knee's center of rotation changes constantly through its range of motion because of the shape of the condyles, the ligamentous restraint, and muscular tension. The path of movement of the tibia on the femur is described as a combination of rolling and sliding. Rolling predominates when the instant center shifts distally from the contact area. The McIntosh test (lateral pivot shift maneuver) is a duplication of the anterior subluxation-reduction phenomenon that occurs during the normal gait cycle, when the anterior cruciate ligament is torn. The test illustrates a dynamic sub-

luxation. This shift occurs between 20 and 40 degrees of flexion (0 degrees occurs when the knee is in the extended position). It is this phenomenon that gives the patient the clinical description of feeling that the knee gives way.

The patient lies supine with the hip flexed to 20 degrees and relaxed in slight medial rotation 20 degrees. The examiner holds the patient's foot with one hand while the other hand flexes the knee slightly (5 degrees). This flexing is done by placing the heel of the hand behind the fibula, over the lateral head of the gastrocnemius muscle, and with the tibia medially rotated, which causes the tibia to sublux anteriorly. As the knee approaches extension, the secondary restraints (hamstrings, lateral femoral condyle, and lateral meniscus) are less sufficient than in flexion. The examiner then applies a valgus stress to the knee while maintaining a medial rotation torque on the tibia at the ankle. If the leg is then flexed 30 to 40 degrees, the tibia will reduce, or jog backward, and the patient will say that is what the "giving way" feels like. This response constitutes a positive test. The reduction is due to the change in position of the iliotibial band moving from an extensor function to a flexor function, thus pulling the tibia back to its normal position. If the test is positive, the following structures have been injured to some degree: (1) the anterior cruciate ligament, (2) the posterolateral capsule, (3) the arcuate-popliteus complex, (4) the lateral collateral ligament, and (5) iliotibial band.

Confirmation Procedures

Drawer test, Losee test, Slocum's test

Reporting Statement

The lateral pivot shift maneuver is positive for the right knee. This result indicates injury to the anterior cruciate ligament.

～ Clinical Pearl ～

Normally the knee's center of rotation changes constantly through its range of motion as a result of the shape of the femoral condyles, the ligamentous restraint, and the muscle pull. A positive pivot shift test usually suggests damage to the anterior cruciate, the posterior capsule, or the lateral collateral ligament.

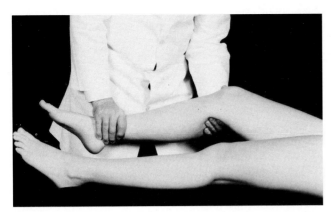

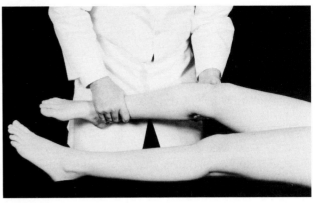

Fig. 11–30   The patient is lying supine with the hip flexed to 20 degrees and relaxed in slight medial rotation of 20 degrees. The examiner holds the patient's foot with one hand, while the other hand flexes the knee slightly (5 degrees). This flexing is done by placing the heel of the hand behind the fibula, over the lateral head of the gastrocnemius muscle, with the tibia medially rotated, which causes the tibia to sublux anteriorly.

Fig. 11–31   The examiner then applies a valgus stress to the knee, while maintaining a medial rotation torque in the tibia and at the ankle.

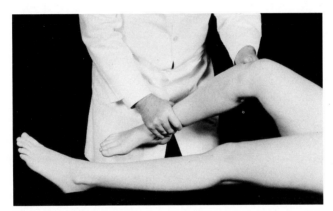

Fig. 11–32   If the leg is then flexed 30 to 40 degrees, the tibia will reduce or jog backward, and the patient will say that is what it feels like when the knee gives way. This indicates a positive test. If the test is positive, the following structures have been injured to some degree: (1) the anterior cruciate ligament, (2) the posterolateral capsule, (3) the arcuate-popliteus complex, (4) the lateral collateral ligament, and (5) the iliotibial band.

Comment

The most serious injuries to the knee involve instability. Forceful overrotation of the flexed knee while the leg is fixed may disrupt many parts of the knee.

Simple instability denotes that only one compartment of the knee is involved. The medial complex structures, such as the medial collateral ligament, can be torn without involving the posterior capsule and can produce a valgus deformity or one-plane laxity. This laxity can result from a blow to the side of the leg or from a fall from a height. Immediate pain, a feeling of weakness, and valgus laxity are the cardinal signs. The medial collateral ligament usually tears at its upper pole. Motion may not be particularly affected for the first 12 hours, but motion is later impeded by hemarthrosis. Clinically, medial laxity of the joint is what determines the diagnosis.

Lateral instability of the simple type involves primarily varus rather than rotational laxity. However, pure lateral instability is unusual. When present, the lateral ligament and usually the iliotibial band and the popliteal tendon are torn. In both instances the patient feels a pop, and the knee becomes quite wobbly. Pain during flexion is localized to the upper end of the fibula and over the joint line. The lateral side of the knee is slightly lax in flexion.

Acute anterolateral instability occurs when the leg is hit from the posterior side, while the foot is planted, with the tibia internally rotated and the strain placed on the lateral side. A part of the lateral quadruple complex, the anterior cruciate, and the lateral meniscus are torn. Internal-external rotation is increased, but an intact posterior cruciate ligament prevents backward tibia displacement. An anterior drawer test and lateral laxity are present.

Procedure

The patient lies in a supine position. The examiner holds the patient's ankle and foot so the leg is laterally rotated. The patient's knee is flexed to 30 degrees, and the examiner ensures that the hamstring muscles are relaxed. The lateral rotation ensures that the subluxation of the knee is reduced at the beginning of the test. While the examiner's other hand is positioned so the thumb is hooked behind the fibular head, a valgus force is applied to the knee. The patient's knee is extended and forward pressure is applied behind the fibular head with the thumb. The valgus stress compresses the structures in the lateral compartment and makes the anterior subluxation more noticeable if it is present. The foot and ankle are allowed to drift into medial rotation. If the foot and ankle are not allowed to rotate medially, the anterior subluxation of the lateral tibial plateau may be prevented. If the test is positive, then just before full extension of the knee, there will be a "clunk" forward and the patient will recognize the movement as the instability that was previously experienced. This clunk means that the tibia has subluxed anteriorly and indicates injury to the same structures listed with the lateral pivot shift maneuver. The Losee test assesses anterolateral rotary instability.

Confirmation Procedures

Drawer test, lateral pivot shift maneuver, Slocum's test

Reporting Statement

The Losee test is positive for the right knee. This result indicates anterolateral rotary instability of the knee.

∾ Clinical Pearl ∾

If rotary instability is present, then as full extension is reached, a dramatic clunk will occur as the lateral tibial condyle subluxes forward. The patient should relate this to the sensations experienced during activity.

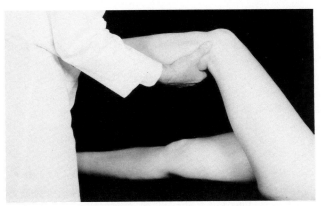

Fig. 11–33 The patient is lying supine and the knee is extended and relaxed. The examiner holds the patient's ankle and foot so the leg is laterally rotated. The knee is then flexed to 30 degrees.

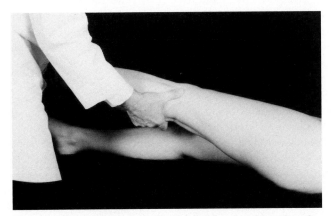

Fig. 11–34 With the examiner's other hand positioned so that the thumb is hooked behind the fibular head, a valgus force is applied to the knee. The examiner extends the patient's knee and applies forward pressure behind the fibular head with the thumb. At the same time the foot and ankle are allowed to drift into medial rotation. If a "clunk" is heard or felt just before full extension of the knee, the test is positive. This clunk means that the tibia has subluxed anteriorly. The Losee test assesses anterolateral rotary instability.

Comment

Injuries of the menisci are common in males younger than 45. A tear is usually caused by a twisting force while the knee is semiflexed or flexed. This tear is usually the result of an athletic injury, but it is also common among males who work in a squatting position, such as coal miners and flooring installers. The medial meniscus is torn much more often than the lateral.

There are three types of tears. All of these tears begin as longitudinal splits. If this split extends throughout the length of the meniscus, it becomes a bucket-handle tear, in which the fragments remain attached at both ends. This tear is the most common type. The bucket handle, the central fragment, is displaced towards the middle of the joint, so the condyle of the femur rolls upon the tibia, through the rent in the meniscus. Because of the femoral condyleo's shape, it requires the most space when the knee is straight. The main effect of a displaced bucket-handle fragment is that it limits full extension (locking).

If the initial longitudinal tear emerges at the concave border of the meniscus, a pedunculated tag is formed. With a posterior horn tear, the fragment remains attached at the posterior horn. With an anterior horn tear, the fragment remains attached to the anterior horn. A transverse tear through the meniscus is nearly always an artifact.

The menisci are almost avascular. Consequently, when the menisci are torn, there is not an effusion of blood into the joint. However, there is an effusion of synovial fluid, which is secreted in response to the injury. Major tears of the menisci do not heal spontaneously, probably because the torn surfaces are separated by fluid.

The patient is usually 18 to 45 years old. This history is characteristic, especially with bucket-handle tears. In consequence of a twisting injury, the patient falls and has pain at the anteromedial aspect of the joint. The patient is either unable to continue the activity or does so with difficulty. The patient is unable to straighten the knee fully. The next day the patient notices swelling of the whole knee. The knee is rested, and during the next 14 days the swelling decreases. The knee straightens, and the patient resumes activities. Within weeks or months the knee suddenly gives way again during a twisting movement. Pain and swelling occurs as before. Similar incidents occur repeatedly.

Locking means inability to extend the knee fully and is not a true jamming of the joint because there is free range of flexion. Locking is a common feature of a torn medial meniscus, but the limitation of extension is often so slight that it is not noticed by the patient. Persistent locking can occur only in bucket-handle tears. Tag tears cause momentary catching, but not locking in the true sense.

The meniscal tears described are uncommon in patients older than 50, which is when the menisci begin to show degenerative changes. A degenerative meniscus suffers a different type of lesion. The medial meniscus, in particular-,may split horizontally, at a point that is often near the middle of its convexity. Such a split is usually of small dimensions. Because there is no separation of the fragments, natural healing can occur.

Clinically, there is troublesome and persistent pain at the medial aspect of the knee at the joint level. The pain may be noticed after a minor injury, but it often comes on spontaneously, without any preceding incident. In the early stages there is usually a small effusion of fluid into the joint.

Procedure

The patient is lying supine, and the thigh and leg are flexed until the heel approaches the buttock. One of the examiner's hands is on the knee, and the other is on the heel. The examiner internally rotates then slowly extends the leg. Then examiner externally rotates and slowly extends the leg. McMurray sign is present if, at some point in the arc, a painful click or snap is heard. This sign is significant in meniscal injury. The point in the arc where the snap is heard locates the site of injury of the meniscus. If noted with internal rotation, the lateral meniscus will be involved. The higher the leg is raised when the snap is heard, the more posterior the lesion is in the meniscus. If noted with external rotation, the medial meniscus will be involved. The higher the leg is raised when the snap is heard, the more posterior the lesion is.

Confirmation Procedures

Bounce home test, Childress duck waddle test, Payr's sign, Steinmann's sign

---

Reporting Statement

McMurray sign is present in the right knee. The presence of this sign indicates injury to the medial meniscus.

McMurray sign is present in the right knee. The presence of this sign indicates injury to the lateral meniscus.

~ **Clinical Pearl** ~

Observe for tenderness in the joint line and test for a springy block to full extension of the knee. These two signs, in association with evidence of quadriceps atrophy, are the most consistent and reliable signs of a torn meniscus.

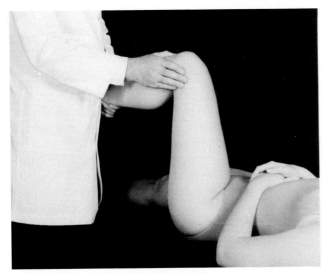

Fig. 11—35   The patient is lying supine. The examiner flexes the thigh and leg to 90 degrees, respectively.

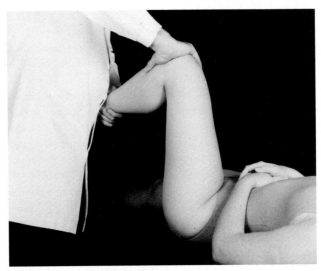

Fig. 11—36   The examiner places one hand on the knee, the other hand grasps the patient's heel.

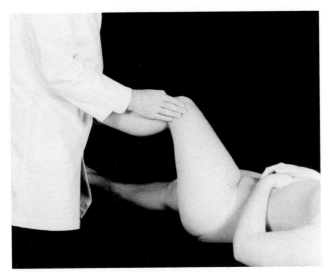

Fig. 11—37   The examiner internally rotates the lower leg, then slowly extends the knee, applying valgus pressure to the joint. Then the examiner externally rotates the leg, then slowly extends the leg. The test is positive if, at some point in the arc, a painful click or snap is heard. This test is significant for a meniscal injury. If the click is noted with internal rotation, the lateral meniscus is involved. If the click is noted with external rotation, the medial meniscus is involved. The higher the leg is raised when the snap is heard, the more posterior the lesion is.

Comment

The biceps femoris and the iliotibial band are both active in stabilizing the fully extended knee. Contraction of these muscles is a preliminary to strong action by the extensors of the knee. In the initial stages of contraction, until the quadriceps group of muscles has shortened sufficiently to exert full power, the position and stability of the knee must be controlled by the action of the biceps and the iliotibial band. The biceps tendon is inserted into the head of the fibula with the fibular collateral ligament, but the iliotibial band finds insertion into the tibia through the lateral capsule and into the fibula through the lateral ligament. The biceps muscle is also a flexor of the knee, and both the biceps and iliotibial band play a part in external rotation of the tibia. With paralytic contracture of the knee, the iliotibial band may indeed be the main contributor to the flexion-external rotation deformity.

However, the most important function of the biceps femoris and iliotibial band is probably to stabilize the fibular component of the leg during weight bearing. Through their attachments, the biceps and iliotibial band exert control on the superior tibiofibular joint. When the knee is fully extended, rotation of the tibia on the femur is not possible. Also the weight-bearing knee cannot indulge in any change of its exact ratio of flexion-extension to rotation. The flexion and extension movements of the ankle and inversion and eversion of the foot do not take place in isolation in the ankle and the subtaloid and midtarsal joints. The foot and ankle movements require a component of rotation in the leg. This necessary movement must take place in the inferior and superior tibiofibular joints, a factor more easily appreciated when it is realized that the increasing width of the articular surface of the talus needs posterior changing accommodation in the ankle mortise. Indeed, one might generalize by saying that most actions of the weight-bearing leg are accomplished by adaptatory movements of all the joints of the leg, from the hip downward. The coordination of the joints, whether stationary or in motion, is a fundamental part of bodily posture and movement.

Procedure

The Noble compression test is a test for iliotibial band friction syndrome. The patient lies in a supine position, and the examiner flexes the patient's hip and then the knee to 90 degrees. The examiner uses the thumb to apply pressure to the lateral femoral condyle, or within 1 to 2 cm of this condyle. While the pressure is maintained, the patient's knee is passively extended. At about 30 degrees of flexion (0 degrees being straight), the patient will complain of severe pain over the lateral femoral condyle. The patient will state that it is the same pain that occurs during activity.

Confirmation Procedures

Patella ballottement test, Q-angle test, thigh circumference test, Wilson's sign

---

Reporting Statement

The Noble compression test is positive for the right knee. This result indicates iliotibial band friction syndrome.

~ **Clinical Pearl** ~

This syndrome produces a line of tenderness that extends from the anterolateral tibia, across the joint line, and up the side of the thigh. Tenderness is usually maximal over the lateral femoral condyle, and a painful arc occurs at about 30 degrees of flexion.

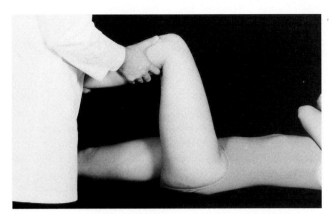

Fig. 11–38 The patient is lying in a supine position. The examiner flexes the patient's knee to 90 degrees and then flexes the hip.

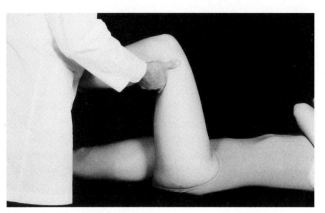

Fig. 11–39 With the thumb the examiner applies pressure to the lateral femoral condyle, or 1 to 2 cm proximal to it.

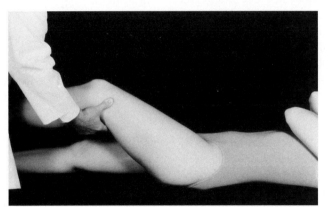

Fig. 11–40 While maintaining pressure, the examiner extends the patient's knee. At about 30 degrees of flexion (0 degrees being straight) the patient will complain of severe pain over the lateral femoral condyle. This pain is a positive finding and indicates iliotibial band friction syndrome.

Comment

The swollen knee is the result of conditions that create an inflammatory response of the synovial membrane. The basic inflammatory process in each condition is similar and, if left to proceed unhindered, the process results in secondary degenerative changes of the joint. The differential diagnosis of these conditions is difficult at the onset, but with sufficient information the diagnosis usually becomes apparent.

Undoubtedly trauma is the most common cause of effusion within the knee joint. Effusion is caused by intrinsic factors such as internal derangements that damage the synovial membrane, creating bleeding within the joint, or from extrinsic factors, such as a direct blow to the knee or a twisting injury. In most instances of trauma, the history is sufficient to make a diagnosis of a traumatic effusion or hemarthrosis. However, such a history may not be apparent in the infant or young child, who is unable to communicate. It also is not apparent in the adult, in whom the effusion is secondary to microtrauma. The microtrauma may be secondary to some activity related to the patient's occupation, such as one requiring the repeated use of the knee to perform a certain maneuver, or repeated minor blows to the knee, which may not be of any significance to the patient.

Idiopathic effusion has its beginnings as a traumatic synovitis, which creates synovial effusion that leads to rest and immobility with resultant quadriceps atrophy. The loss of muscle protection makes the knee more susceptible to the minor trauma of everyday usage. Reinjury creates repeated synovial effusions and sets up a vicious cycle that promotes chronic synovitis. A patient in this condition presents with a painful, swollen knee that is held in a semiflexed position—the position of maximum comfort. The suprapatellar pouch may be distended and quite tense. The patella is ballottable, and the knee may be somewhat warm, but it does not give the appearance of a septic joint. Motion is resisted because attempts at flexion or extension create more tension which causes pain within the joint.

Differentiation of traumatic hemarthrosis from traumatic synovitis can be a diagnostic problem. Swelling from a traumatic hemarthrosis begins within a few minutes after the injury, while a traumatic synovial effusion begins several hours after the injury and progresses more slowly. The aspiration of blood from the joint confirms a traumatic hemarthrosis, and fat globules that float in the blood indicate an interarticular fracture as well. A traumatic synovial reaction may have synovial fluid that appears normal but, in some instances, is tinged with blood. The joint is somewhat warmer to the touch than usual but does not have the warmth or redness of the skin that is found with acute septic arthritis.

Procedure

While the patient's knee is extended or flexed to the point of discomfort, the examiner applies a slight tap or pressure over the patella. When doing so, a floating of the patella should be felt. This test can detect a large amount of swelling in the knee.

Confirmation Procedures

Fouchet's test, Q-angle test, thigh circumference test, Wilson's sign

> ### Reporting Statement
>
> Patellar ballottement confirms the existence of intraarticular swelling in the right knee.

~ Clinical Pearl ~

If popliteal swelling is found, it is possible to confirm communication with the joint, by massaging its contents back into the main synovial cavity, while the knee is in flexion. The examiner maintains pressure on the popliteal fossa, extends the knee, then removes the pressure. The swelling will not reappear until the patient flexes the knee several times, confirming a valve-like communication between the main cavity and the "cyst."

The Knee

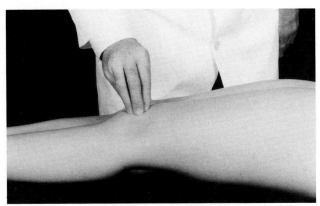

Fig. 11–41   The patient is lying supine with the knee extended or flexed to comfort. The examiner applies pressure over the patella. A floating sensation of the patella is a positive finding and indicates a large amount of swelling in the knee.

Comment

The medial meniscus is C-shaped. Its anterior attachment is on top of the tibia near the midline and in front of the tibial spines. The posterior attachment is on top of the tibia, behind the tibial spines. In each case the attachment is near the periphery of the tibia so the two ends are widely separated from each other. The meniscus is attached by the coronary ligament (which has its origins around the top of the tibia) to the medial collateral ligament and then to the tibia. This attachment is firm, and while it does allow a little movement, extensive motion is not permitted in the normal medial meniscus.

In sprain of the medial collateral ligament the tibia and femur separate on the medial side, and stress is applied in the area of the attachment of the meniscus to the medial collateral ligament. The cartilage may be forced to accompany either the femur or the tibia, depending on the location of the ligament injury. Because the structure of the meniscus does not allow much flexion stress, it will tear transversely or, more commonly, split around its periphery. If the tear is actually in the attachment to the ligament, it may heal. If the tear is within the substance of the meniscus, it will not. Meniscus injury accompanies repeated sprains of the knee more frequently than it does the initial, single sprain. With an acute injury, there is no way to determine if the meniscus is torn, unless the knee is locked. If the knee is locked, and the ligaments are stable, the episode is the first. If the meniscus has been detached at its periphery, this attachment may heal. This possibility is much more likely if the meniscus has slipped into the knee, locked, and then immediately unlocked.

Procedure

While the patient is in the Turkish seated position, with the feet and ankles crossed, the examiner applies downward pressure on the knee joint. Pain is elicited on the medial side of the joint when the sign is present. The test is significant when a lesion of the posterior horn of the medial meniscus is present.

Confirmation Procedures

Bounce home test, Childress duck waddle test, McMurray sign, Steinmann's sign

---

Reporting Statement

Payr's sign is present in the right knee. This sign indicates injury to the posterior horn of the medial meniscus.

∼ **Clinical Pearl** ∼

Meniscal cysts lie in the joint line, feel firm during palpation, and are tender to deep pressure. Cysts of the menisci may be associated with tears. Lateral meniscus cysts are by far the most common. Cystic swellings on the medial side are sometimes due to ganglions that arise from the pes anserinus (insertion of the sartorius, gracilis, and semitendinosus).

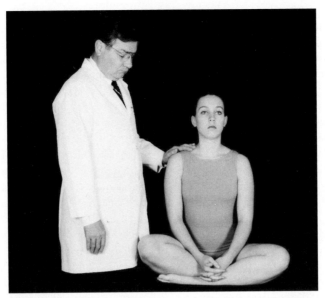

Fig. 11—42 The patient is lying in the Turkish seated position, with the feet and ankles crossed.

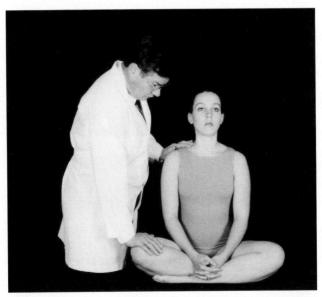

Fig. 11—43 The examiner applies downward pressure on the affected knee joint. Pain is elicited on the medial side of the joint when the sign is present. The sign is present when there is a lesion of the posterior horn of the medial meniscus.

∾ Q-Angle Test ∾

Comment

The true, congenital dislocation of the patella implies actual and constant dislocation of the patella. This dislocation is usually lateral to the femoral condyle. This condition, if fully developed, will interdict athletic participation. Of much greater importance is the dislocation that occurs infrequently and under certain circumstances. This type of dislocation is due to repeated episodes of acute dislocation in a normal knee. There is no true congenital dislocation, but there are certain physical characteristics that predispose a patient to subluxation or luxation. One predisposing anatomic condition is an abnormally acute angle between the axis of the patellar tendon and the axis of the quadriceps mechanism, the Q-angle.

If the patellar tendon tends to angulate sharply and laterally to reach its tibial attachment, then this angulation, combined with a quadriceps mechanism that tends to angulate medially at the knee, results in an increased angle between the patellar tendon and the long axis of the quadriceps tendon. As the quadriceps muscle is contracted, there is a tendency for this angle to straighten, by slipping the patella laterally. This action may be inhibited anteriorly by the prominence of the lateral femoral condyle. The general tendency is for the patella to slide laterally with each forceful extension of the knee. The female, with a widened pelvis and internally angulated femora, is much more prone to patellar subluxation or dislocation than the male. A similar situation arises in patients with tibial torsion or genu valgum. A dislocated patella in a patient with genu varum is uncommon, because in such a patient the axis of the patellar tendon and the quadriceps muscle is parallel. However, in some genu varum patients, this bow is part of the internal torsion of the femur, so the femoral condyles are rotated toward the midline. Such a patient often has an associated external rotation of the tibia, to compensate and straighten the long axis of the leg. In this instance the Q-angle may be markedly more acute as the patellar tendon moves from the internally rotated patella, down to the externally rotated patellar tubercle.

Procedure

The Q-angle is defined as the angle between the quadriceps muscle (primarily the rectus femoris) and the patellar tendon. The angle is obtained first by ensuring that the lower limbs are at a right angle to the line that joins each anterior superior iliac spine (ASIS). A line is then drawn from the ASIS to the midpoint of the patella and from the tibial tubercle to the midpoint of the patella. The angle formed by the intersection of these two lines is the Q-angle. The foot and hip should be placed in a neutral position. Different foot and hip positions alter the Q-angle. Normally theQ-angle (quadriceps angle or patellofemoral angle) is 13 to 18 degrees. When the knee is straight, the normal angle for males is 13 degrees and for females it is 18 degrees. Any angle less than 13 degrees may be associated with patellofemoral dysfunction or patella alta. Any angle greater than 18 degrees is often associated with patellofemoral dysfunction, subluxing patella, increased femoral anteversion, genu valgum, or increased lateral tibial torsion. During the test the quadriceps should be relaxed. If measured in the seated position, the Q-angle should be 0 degrees.

Confirmation Procedures

Noble compression test, patella ballottement test, thigh circumference test, Wilson's sign

---

Reporting Statement

The Q-angle of the right knee is less than 13 degrees and suggests patellofemoral dysfunction or patella alta.

The Q-angle of the right knee is greater than 18 degrees and suggests patellofemoral dysfunction, subluxing patella, or increased tibial torsion.

∾ Clinical Pearl ∾

In children an increased Q-angle presents as genu valgum. The examiner must note whether the genu valgum is unilateral or, as is usual, bilateral. The severity of the deformity is recorded by measuring the intermalleolar gap. The examiner grasps the child's ankles and rotates the legs until the patellae are vertical. The legs are brought together to touch lightly at the knees. A measurement is made between the malleoli. Serial measurements, often every 6 months, are used to check progress. Note that with growth, a static measurement is an angular improvement.

The Knee

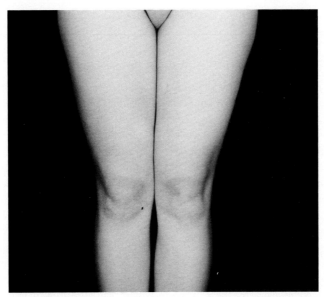

Fig. 11—44 A line is drawn from the ASIS to the midpoint of the patella and from the tibial tubercle to the midpoint of the patella. The angle formed by the intersection of these two lines is the Q-angle. Normally, the Q-angle (quadriceps angle or patellofemoral angle) is 13 to 18 degrees (13 degrees for males and 18 degrees for females), when the knee is straight. Any angle less than 13 degrees may be associated with patellofemoral dysfunction or patella alta.

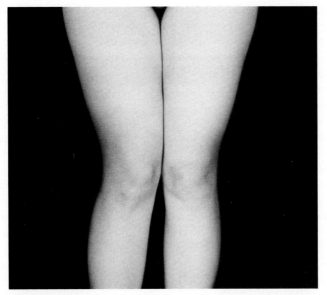

Fig. 11—45 Any angle greater than 18 degrees is often associated with patellofemoral dysfunction, subluxing patella, increased femoral anteversion, genu valgum, or increased lateral tibial torsion.

Comment

The cruciate ligaments are valuable stabilizers of the knee, which not only assist in knee flexion and extension but also limit rotation as well as extension and flexion. The anterior cruciate ligament varies in length. The ligament is taut when the knee is in full extension and when the knee is externally rotated at the femorotibial joint. The ligament remains taut until 5 to 20 degrees of flexion, at which point it relaxes. The ligament is most relaxed at 40 to 50 degrees of flexion and becomes taut again when the knee flexes to 70 to 90 degrees.

Rotation (internal) increases the tension of the anterior cruciate ligament even when the knee is flexed to 40 or 50 degrees. External rotation increases the tautness of the ligament as does abduction of the knee. Anterior shear of the tibia upon the femur is permitted to 5 mm of distance but then is checked. Excessive external rotation can tear the anterior cruciate ligament, especially if there is added abduction. Hyperextension and anterior shear may tear this ligament. With the knee flexed to 90 degrees and externally rotated the first limiting soft tissue that tears is the medial capsular ligament. With further rotation and abduction the next tissue to tear is the tibial medial collateral ligament then the anterior cruciate ligament. Isolated tears of the anterior cruciate ligament, when they do happen, probably occur from a posterior force, which causes shear stress but also may occur from internal rotation.

The anterior cruciate ligament can be torn as an isolated injury that is the result of an acute deceleration from a sharp stop-and-cut movement. As the forward motion of the patient is abruptly halted, the quadriceps muscle decelerates the leg and simultaneously pulls the tibia forward upon the femur. This shearing disrupts the anterior cruciate ligament. With the abrupt stop, the patient frequently makes a rapid rotation, or cut, to form the direction of movement. This rotation places anterior shear and rotatory stress on the knee. The rotational stress depends on the direction of the cut. After a jump, the knee absorbs the impact by being slightly flexed. Thus, shear also occurs at this point because of deceleration. The patient who makes the stop and cuts or jumps feels a pop as the knee gives way. Swelling occurs within 3 or 4 hours.

Procedure

Slocum's test assesses both anterior and rotary instabilities. While the patient is supine, the involved knee is flexed to 80 or 90 degrees and the hip is flexed to 45 degrees. The foot is placed in 30-degree internal rotation. The foot is held in position, and the tibia is drawn forward. If the test is positive, movement will occur primarily on the lateral side of the knee. This movement would be excessive when compared to the unaffected side and indicates anterolateral rotary instability. Excessive movement indicates that the following structures may have been injured to some degree: (1) the anterior cruciate ligament, (2) the posterolateral capsule, (3) the arcuate-popliteus complex, (4) the lateral collateral ligament, (5) the posterior cruciate ligament, and (6) the iliotibial band (tensor fascia lata).

If the examiner finds anterolateral instability during the first position of Slocum's test, then the second part of the test, which assesses anteromedial rotary instability, is of less importance.

While the foot is placed in 15 degrees of external rotation, the tibia is drawn forward by the examiner. If the test is positive, the movement will occur primarily on the medial side of the knee. This movement, which would be excessive when compared to the unaffected side, indicates anteromedial rotary instability. With anteromedial rotary instability the following structures may have been injured to some degree: (1) the medial collateral ligament, especially the superficial fibers, although the deep fibers also may be affected, (2) the posterior oblique ligament, (3) the posteromedial capsule, and (4) the anterior cruciate ligament.

For Slocum's test the examiner must medially and laterally rotate the foot to the degrees indicated. If the examiner rotates the tibia as far as it will go, the test will be negative because this action tightens all the remaining structures. If a stress radiograph is taken during the test, minimal or no movement indicates a negative test, 1 mm or less indicates a grade-1 injury, 1 to 2 mm indicates a grade-2 injury, and more than 2 mm indicates a grade-3 injury.

The test also may be performed while the patient is seated with the knees flexed over the edge of the examination table. The examiner applies an anterior or posterior force to the knee while holding the foot medially or laterally rotated. If this procedure is used, the examiner must remember that the anterior force is testing for anterior rotary instability, while the posterior force is testing for posterior rotary instability. The examiner should note whether the movement is excessive on the medial or lateral side of the knee as compared with the knee. Excessive movement indicates a positive test.

Confirmation Procedures

Drawer test, lateral pivot shift maneuver, Losee test, Lachman test

---

Reporting Statement

Slocum's test is positive on the right. This result indicates anterolateral rotary instability of the knee.

Slocum's test is positive on the right. This result indicates anteromedial instability of the right knee.

∾ Clinical Pearl ∾

This maneuver tightens the lateral capsule, giving enough stability to eliminate the anterior drawer sign. If the anterior drawer sign is still positive while the patient is in this position (most anterior movement occurring on the lateral side), it is likely that the lateral capsule (or lateral collateral ligament) is also damaged.

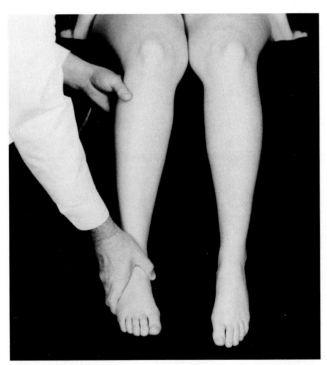

Fig. 11–46 The patient is seated with the knees flexed and hanging over the edge of the examination table.

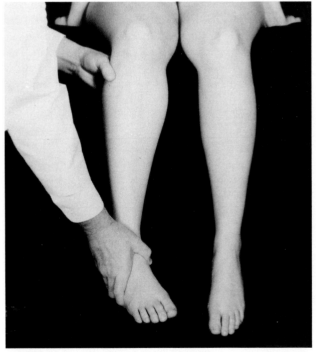

Fig. 11–47 The examiner applies an anterior or posterior force to the tibia (by pulling the tibia forward), while holding the foot medially or laterally rotated. If this procedure is used, the examiner must remember that the anterior tibial force is testing for anterior rotary instability, and the posterior tibial force is testing for posterior rotary instability. The examiner should note whether the movement is excessive on the medial or lateral side of the knee compared to the normal knee. Excessive movement is a positive test, which indicates cruciate ligament instability.

～ Steinmann's Sign ～
STEINMANN'S TENDERNESS DISPLACEMENT TEST

Comment

During normal movements of the knee the anterior mobile portion of the medial semilunar cartilage slides slightly backwards, into the interior of the joint, as flexion occurs. If the joint is simultaneously abducted, the medial side of the joint is opened, and the mobility of the cartilage is increased further. Turning of the trunk toward the opposite side produces a movement of external rotation on the fixed tibia in relation to the femur. The medial meniscus is forced toward the back of the joint and the medial collateral ligament becomes taut.

The ligament initially steadies the posterior part of the cartilage. If the ligament can withstand the strain, the anterior mobile part of the meniscus is injured and either of the following may occur: (1) the anterior part of the ligament may be detached where it joins with the fixed posterior portion, or (2) the ligament may sustain any variety of transverse or oblique tears.

A fragment may slip into the interior of the joint. When the knee is extended and an attempt is made to screw the condyle home, the fragment is impacted between the condyles, and the joint locks. When the medial rotator strain is more severe, the collateral ligament is stretched to such an extent that the attachment between it and the meniscus is destroyed. With even more severe strain the ligament may become avulsed from its tibial attachment and from the cartilage. In either of the two cases the whole cartilage slips into the interior of the joint. When the knee is extended, the free border is trapped between the condyles, and a longitudinal split occurs in the substance of the meniscus to form the bucket-handle tear.

Detachment or longitudinal tears of the posterior horn are caused by forceful lateral rotation of the femur on the fixed tibia, when the rotation is combined with flexion.

Although the lateral semilunar cartilage is much less frequently injured than the medial cartilage, tears and displacements do occur. The mechanism is the opposite of that which damages the medial cartilage.

For tears of the cartilage to occur the following three factors have to be present: (1) the knee must be bearing weight, (2) the knee must be flexed, and (3) there must be a rotation strain.

Procedure

Steinmann's sign is indicated by point tenderness and pain on the joint line. The pain appears to move anteriorly when the knee is extended, and it moves posteriorly when the knee is flexed. This pain indicates a meniscus tear. Medial pain is elicited by lateral rotation, and lateral pain is elicited by medial rotation.

Confirmation Procedures

Bounce home test, Childress duck waddle test, McMurray sign, Payr's sign

---

Reporting Statement

Steinmann's sign is present in the right knee. The presence of this sign indicates a medial meniscus tear.

Steinmann's sign is present in the right knee. The presence of this sign indicates a lateral meniscus tear.

～ Clinical Pearl ～

Patient's use "locking" to describe episodes of severe pain in the knee, or even collapsing of the knee. It is curious that the word is not applied in this way to any other joints. "Locking" denotes mechanical jamming of the knee joint and nothing more.

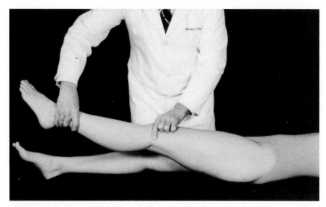

Fig. 11–48 The patient is lying supine with the knee extended. With one hand the examiner grasps the leg at the ankle and palpates for tenderness at the knee joint with the other hand.

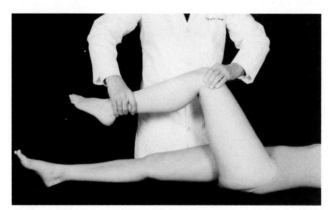

Fig. 11–49 If the pain is found during initial palpation while the knee is extended, and if the pain moves posteriorly as the knee is flexed, the sign is present. The sign indicates a meniscal tear.

Comment

The quadriceps and, to a lesser extent, the hamstrings rapidly atrophy after injury to the cartilage and the ligaments of the knee. This reaction varies in degree and is due to disturbance of the neurotrophic relationships between the joint and its controlling musculature. Muscle bulk, tone, and control are diminished rapidly and in some instances severely. This diminishment is not due to muscle inactivity alone, although this factor does aggravate both atrophy and weakness. Conscientious muscle exercise cannot prevent but does minimize muscle atrophy. Although effusion remains, atrophy is generalized, but the tendency is for the medial vasti to show greater atrophy in sympathy with a medial meniscus injury. Lateral ruptures are associated with atrophy of the lateral vastus.

Although muscle weakness is present, effusion persists and is increased with any activity beyond the power and the endurance of the residual muscle bulk. In turn the effusion affects the trophic reflexes and further atrophy occurs.

Displacement of a meniscus remains and, despite arduous exercise, muscle bulk and tone cannot recover significantly. If the cartilage is reduced or removed so that the knee recovers full movement, then exercise will increase both power and bulk of the muscle.

Procedure

The examiner selects an area of the thigh where muscle bulk or swelling is greatest and measures the circumference of the leg. It is important to record how far above the patella the examiner is measuring. The examiner also must note if muscle bulk or swelling is being measured. There is no correlation between muscle bulk and strength.

Confirmation Procedures

Noble compression test, patella ballottement test, Q-angle test, Wilson's sign

---

Reporting Statement

The thigh circumference test indicates increased muscle bulk dimension on the right when compared with the left.

The thigh circumference test indicates decreased muscle bulk dimension on the right when compared to the left.

∾ Clinical Pearl ∾

Although all the quadriceps atrophy uniformly, atrophy of the bulky vastus medialis (particularly in a fit young male) may be the most conspicuous. Quadriceps atrophy is a difficult sign to detect, particularly in the middle-aged, the elderly, and females. Some asymmetry of muscle bulk is common.

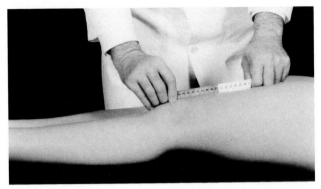

Fig. 11–50 The examiner selects an area of the thigh where muscle bulk or swelling is greatest. It is important to record how far above the patella the examiner is measuring. The examiner also must note whether muscle bulk or swelling is being measured.

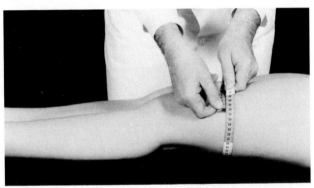

Fig. 11–51 At that point the circumference of the muscle is measured and recorded. This is compared with the uninvolved leg. There is no correlation between muscle bulk and strength.

Comment

Loose bodies, or joint mice, are most commonly osteo-cartilaginous fragments of traumatic origin from tangential osteochondral fractures. However, joint mice can also originate from pathologic processes, such as osteochondritis dissecans. Other types of loose bodies may consist of chondral fragments (pieces of articular cartilage), remnants of menisci, foreign bodies, fibrous tissues, and interarticular tumors. Some loose bodies may obtain a synovial attachment, but it is more common for them to remain loose in the joint. A tangential osteochondral fragment, with its normal bone, is more likely to become attached to the synovium than is a fragment from osteochondritis dissecans, with its necrotic bone fragment. Fragments of articular cartilage can enlarge as they are nourished by the synovial fluid. Small, loose bodies are more likely to cause symptoms than larger ones, because the former may be more easily impinged between the articular surfaces.

The most likely origins for a loose body, in a male, are (1) osteochondritis dissecans at the lateral border of the medial femoral condyle, (2) a marginal fracture that is from the lateral margin of the lateral femoral condyle and is secondary to direct trauma or patellar dislocation, and (3) medial tangential osteochondral fracture of the patella from dislocation. This order is reversed in the female patient.

Osteochondritis dissecans is an ischemic condition that involves the subchondral bone and is probably either the result of or in association with repeated trauma to the area. The involved area of ischemic bone demarcates and may eventually separate with the overlying articular cartilage. This separation leaves behind a defect, a fragment that becomes a loose body within the joint. The knee is the most commonly involved joint, and the incidence is higher in males than in females. The most common sites are (1) the lateral border of the medial femoral condyle, (2) the inferior, central area of the lateral femoral condyle, and (3) the inferior, central region of the medial femoral condyle. Osteochondritis dissecans occurs at the classic site and is due to repeated trauma to the area from contact with a prominent medial tibial spine. The central lesions in the femoral condyles are usually associated with a meniscal lesion that traumatizes the area. Often there is a family history of osteochondritis dissecans, and it is not unusual for both knees to be involved.

Classically the problem occurs in a teenage male, who complains of pain and a giving way of the knee. There may be effusion and transient episodes of locking as opposed to the more persistent locking that is seen with a torn meniscus. Before the fragment separates there is nothing diagnostic about the complaints, but after the fragment separates, episodes of transient locking are frequent, and the patient may be aware of something loose in the knee.

Procedure

Wilson's sign tests for osteochondritis dissecans. The patient sits with the knee flexed and the leg hanging over the edge of the examining table. The knee is then actively extended while the tibia is medially rotated. At about 30 degrees of flexion (0 degrees being a straight leg), the pain in the knee increases, and the patient stops the rotated movement. The tibia rotates laterally, and the pain disappears. This finding indicates a positive test. The positive test indicates osteochondritis dissecans of the femur. The test is positive only if the lesion is at the classic site for osteochondritis dissecans of the knee: the medial femoral condyle, near the intercondylar notch.

Confirmation Procedures

Noble compression test, patella ballottement test, Q-angle test, thigh circumference test

---

Reporting Statement

Wilson's sign is present in the right knee. The presence of this sign indicates osteochondritis dissecans of the knee.

～ **Clinical Pearl** ～

Patients with loose bodies give a classic account of a loose fragment in the knee and will usually be able to describe its size and shape. Loose bodies are sometimes called *joint mice,* which is an appropriate description because these loose bodies can be recognized instantly, but they disappear and may be impossible to find again. Loose bodies should not be called foreign bodies. Foreign bodies, including bullets and bits of gravel, come from outside the body and are rare in joints.

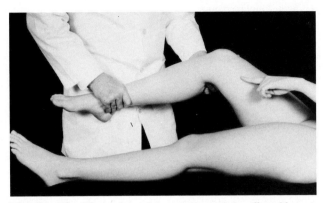

Fig. 11–52   The patient is lying supine, and the affected knee is flexed to 90 degrees by the examiner. The knee is extended with the tibia medially rotated. At or about 30 degrees of flexion (0 degrees being a straight leg), the pain in the knee increases, and the patient attempts to stop the movement.

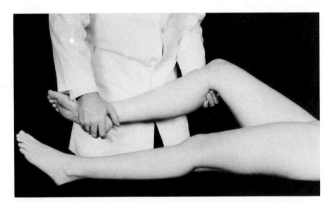

Fig. 11–53   The tibia is rotated laterally, and the pain disappears. This disappearance of pain indicates that the sign is present, which indicates osteochondritis dissecans of the femur.

Bibliography

Aegerter E, Kirkpatrick JA: *Orthopaedic diseases,* ed. 3, Philadelphia, 1968, WB Saunders.

American Medical Association: *Guides to the evaluation of permanent impairment,* ed. 3, Chicago, 1990, The Association.

Apley AG, Solomon L: *Concise system of orthopaedics and fractures,* London, 1988, Butterworth-Heinemann.

Baker CL, Norwood LA, Hughston JC: Acute combined posterior and posterolateral instability of the knee, *Am J Sports Med,* 12:204, 1984.

Barnett CH, Davies DV, MacConaill MA: *Synovial joints: Their structure and mechanics,* New York, 1961, Longmans Green.

Butler DL, Noyes FR, Grood ES: Ligamentous restraints to anterior-posterior drawer in the human knee, *J Bone Joint Surg,* 622A:259, 1980.

Cailliet R: *Knee pain and disability,* ed. 2, Philadelphia, 1983, FA Davis.

Childress HM: Popliteal cysts associated with undiagnosed posterior lesions of the medial meniscus, *J Bone Joint Surg,* 52A:1487, 1970.

Cipriano JJ: *Photographic manual of regional orthopaedic and neurological tests,* ed. 2, Baltimore, 1991, Williams and Wilkins.

Clark K, Williams P, Willis W, McGavran W: Injection injury to the sciatic nerve, *Clin Neurosurg,* 17:111, 1970.

Clawson DK, Seddon HJ: The late consequences of sciatic nerve injury, *J Bone Joint Surg,* 42B:213, 1960.

Crosby EB, Insall J: Recurrent dislocation of the patella, *J Bone Joint Surg,* 58A:9, 1976.

D'Ambrosia RD: *Musculoskeletal disorders regional examination and differential diagnosis,* Philadelphia, 1977, JB Lippincott.

Dandy DJ: *Essential orthopaedics and trauma,* Edinburgh, 1989, Churchill Livingstone.

Dandy DJ, Jackson RW: The impact of arthroscopy on the management of disorders of the knee, *J Bone Joint Surg,* 57B: 346, 1975.

Detenbeck LC: Function of the cruciate ligaments in knee stability, *Am J Sports Med,* 2:217, 1974.

Dinham, JM: Popliteal cysts in children, *J Bone Joint Surg,* 57B:69, 1975.

Doherty M, Doherty J: *Clinical examination in rheumatology,* London, 1992, Wolfe Publishing.

Fetto JF, Marshall JL: Injury to the anterior cruciate ligament producing the pivot shift sign: An experimental study on cadaver specimens, *J Bone Joint Surg,* 61A:710, 1979.

Ficat RP, Hungerford DS: *Disorders of the patello-femoral joint,* Baltimore, 1977, Williams and Wilkins.

Furman W, Marshall JL, Girgis FG: The anterior cruciate ligaments: A functional analysis based on postmortem studies, *J Bone Joint Surg,* 58A:179, 1976.

Galway HR, MacIntosh DL: The lateral pivot shift: symptoms and sign of anterior cruciate ligament insufficiency, *Clin Orthop,* 147:45, 1980.

Gartland JJ: *Fundamentals of orthopedics,* ed. 2, Philadelphia, 1974, WB Saunders.

Gillis L: *Diagnosis in orthopaedics,* London, 1969, Butterworths.

Girgis FG, Marshall JL, Al Monajem ARS: The cruciate ligaments of the knee joint: Anatomical, functional and experimental analysis, *Clin Orthop,* 106:216, 1975.

Goodfellow J, Hungerford DS, Woods C: Patello-femoral joint mechanics and pathology: Chondromalacia patella, *J Bone Joint Surg,* 58B:291, 1976.

Goodfellow J, Hunderford DS, Zindel M: Patello-femoral joint mechanics and pathology: Functional anatomy of the patello-femoral joint, *J Bone Joint Surg,* 58B:287, 1976.

Helfet A: *Disorders of the knee,* Philadelphia, 1974, JB Lippincott.

Helfet AJ: Diagnosis and management of internal derangement of the knee joint. In *American Academy of Orthopaedic Surgeons Instructional Course Lectures,* vol 19, St. Louis, 1970, Mosby.

Helfet AJ: *Disorder of the knee,* Philadelphia, 1974, JB Lippincott.

Hughston JC et al: The classification of knee ligament instabilities: I. The medial compartment and cruciate ligaments, *J Bone Joint Surg,* 58A:159, 1976.

Hughston JC et al: The classification of knee ligament instabilities: II. The lateral compartment, *J Bone Joint Surg,* 58A:173, 1976.

Hughston JC, Walsh WM, Puddu G: *Patellar subluxation and dislocation,* Philadelphia, 1984, WB Saunders.

Hughston JC, Norwood LA: The posterolateral drawer and external rotational recurvatum test for posterolateral rotary instability of the knee, *Clin Orthop,* 147:82, 1980.

Insall J, Falvo KA, Wise DW: Chondromalacia patella, *J Bone Surg,* 58A:1, 1976.

Jakob RP, Hassler H, Staeubli HU: Observations on rotary instability of the lateral compartment of the knee, *Acta Orthop Scand Suppl,* 191 (52):1, 1981.

Jonsson T, Althoff B, Peterson L, Renstrom P: Clinical diagnosis of ruptures of the anterior cruciate ligament: A comparative study of the Lachman test and the anterior drawer sign, *Am J Sports Med,* 10:100, 1982.

Katz WA: *Rheumatic diseases diagnosis and management,* Philadelphia, 1977, JB Lippincott.

Kendall HO, Kendall FP, Wadsworth GE: *Muscles testing and function,* ed. 2, Baltimore, 1971, Williams and Wilkins.

Kennedy JC: *The injured adolescent knee,* Baltimore, 1979, Williams and Wilkins.

Laurin CA et al: The abnormal lateral patellofemoral angle: A diagnostic roentgenographic sign of recurrent patellar subluxation, *J Bone Joint Surg,* 60A:55, 1978.

Lipscomb PR Jr., Lipscomb PR Sr., Bryan RS: Osteochondritis dissecans of the knee with loose fragments, *J Bone Joint Surg,* 60A:235, 1978.

Losee RE, Ennis TRJ, Southwick WO: Anterior subluxation of the lateral tibial plateau: A diagnostic test and operative review, *J Bone Joint Surg,* 60A:1015, 1978.

MacAusland WR, Mayo RA: *Orthopedics: A concise guide to clinical practices,* Boston, 1965, Little, Brown.

Magee DJ: *Orthopedic physical assessment,* Philadelphia, 1987, WB Saunders.

Maquet PGJ: *Biomechanics of the knee: With application of the pathogenesis and the surgical treatment of osteoarthritis,* New York, 1976, Springer-Verlag.

Martin AF: The pathomechanics of the knee joint, *J Bone Joint Surg,* 42A:13, 1960.

Mazion JM: *Illustrated manual of neurological reflexes/signs/tests, part I, orthopedic signs/tests/maneuvers for office procedure, part II,* Orlando, 1980, Daniels Publishing.

McMurray TP: *The robert joint birthday volume,* London, 1928, Humphrey Milford.

McMurray TP: The semilunar cartilages, *Br J Surg,* 29:407, 1942.

McRae R: *Clinical orthopaedic examination,* ed. 3, Edinburgh, 1990, Churchill Livingston.

Medical Economics Books: *Patient care flow chart manual,* ed. 3, Oradell, NJ, 1982, Medical Economics Books.

Mercier LR: *Practical orthopedics,* Chicago, 1982, Mosby.

Muller W: *The knee: Form, function and ligament reconstruction,* New York, 1983, Springer-Verlag.

Nicholas JA: The five-one reconstruction for anteromedial instability of the knee, *J Bone Joint Surg,* 55A:899, 1973.

Noble HB, Hajek MR, Porter M: Diagnosis and treatment of iliotibial band tightness in runners, *Sports Med,* 10:67, 1984.

Noyes FR, Butler DL, Grood ES et al: Clinical paradoxes of anterior cruciate instability and a new test to detect its instability, *Orthop Trans,* 2:36, 1978.

O'Donoghue DH: *Treatment of injuries to athletes,* ed. 3, Philadelphia, 1976, WB Saunders.

Omer GE, Spinner M: *Management of peripheral nerve problems,* Philadelphia, 1980, WB Saunders.

Polley HF, Hunder GG: *Rheumatologic interviewing and physical examination of the joints,* ed. 2, Philadelphia, 1978, WB Saunders.

Renne JW: The iliotibial band friction syndrome, *J Bone Joint Surg,* 57A:1110, 1975.

Ricklin P, Ruttiman A, Del Buono MA: *Meniscus lesions: Practical problems of clinical diagnosis, arthrography and therapy,* New York, 1971, Grune and Stratton.

Slocum DB, Larson RL: Rotary instability of the knee, *J Bone Joint Surg,* 50A:211, 1968.

Slocum DB, James SL, Larson RL, Singer KM: A clinical test for anterolateral rotary instability of the knee, *Clin Orthop,* 118:63, 1976.

Smillie IS: *Diseases of the knee joint,* New York, 1974, Longman.

Smillie IS: *Injuries of the knee joint,* Edinburgh, 1970, E and S Livingstone.

Tamea CD, Henning CD: Pathomechanics of the pivot shift maneuver, *Am J Sports Med,* 9:31, 1981.

Thurston SE: *The little black book of neurology,* Chicago, 1987, Mosby.

Turek SL: *Orthopaedics principles and their application,* ed. 3, Philadelphia, 1977, JB Lippincott.

Waldron VD: A test for chondromalacia patella, *Orthop Rev,* 12:103, 1983.

CHAPTER

∾ *12* ∾

Lower Leg, Ankle, and Foot

*I*t is estimated that 80% of the population of modern times has foot problems that can often be corrected by proper assessment and treatment. Lesions of the ankle and foot can alter the mechanics of gait and, as a result, place stress on other lower-limb joints. This, in turn, leads to a pathologic condition in these joints.

The foot and ankle combine flexibility with stability because of the many bones that are present and because of their shape. The lower leg, ankle, and foot have two main functions. These functions are propulsion and balance. For propulsion the joints act as a flexible lever. For support the joints act like a rigid structure that holds up the entire body. The functions of the foot include acting as a base support that is sufficient to provide the necessary stability for upright posture with minimal muscle effort. The leg, ankle, and foot provide a mechanism for rotation of the tibia and fibula during the stance phase of gait. The leg, ankle, and foot provide flexibility to adapt to uneven terrain. The leg, ankle, and foot provide flexibility for absorption of shock by becoming a rigid structure in the pronated position, and they act as a lever during stride push off.

Although the joints of the lower leg, ankle, and foot are often discussed as separate joints, they act as a functional group and not in isolation. The movement occurring at each joint is minimal. However, taken together, there is normally a sufficient range of motion in all the joints to allow normal mobility while providing stability.

The leg, ankle, and foot are subject to static deformities more than any other skeletal unit. The weight-transmitting and propulsive functions of these structures are restricted daily by nonyielding foot coverings. Anatomic variations in the shape and stability of joint surfaces may predispose, resist, or modify the deforming force of common footwear.

Modern civilization disregards the physiology of the ankle and foot. Fashion and eye appeal rather than function determine shoe design, especially in the fore part of the shoe, where most disabilities and deformities of the foot occur.

The restrictive force of poorly fitting shoes produces little deformity on the tarsus because the tarsus is made up of short heavy bones. Normal movement in the tarsal joints is limited because the articular surfaces of the tarsal joints are flat. However, the phalanges and metatarsals are long thin bones with a normally wide range of joint motion. Restrictive force on these bones produces most of the static deformities of the forefoot. These static deformities include first metatarsophalangeal joint deformities, hammertoe, tailor's bunion, overlapping toes, and many other conditions that are deviations from the normal.

The human foot is uniquely specialized. The metatarsals and toes enable the body to stand erect. The versatility of the forefoot permits the human to retain an upright stance and allows for grace during walking, dancing, and athletics.

A well-developed and strong foot withstands surprising abuse. Morbid changes take place only when maltreatment becomes excessive. An underdeveloped and frail foot, ankle, and lower-leg mechanism may fail under ordinary stress and strain.

Index of Tests

Anterior drawer sign of the ankle
Buerger's test
Calf circumference test
Claudication test
Duchenne's sign
Foot tourniquet test
Helbings' sign
Hoffa's test
Homans' sign
Keen's sign
Morton's test
Moszkowicz test
Moses' test
Perthes' test
Strunsky's sign
Thompson's test
Tinel's foot sign

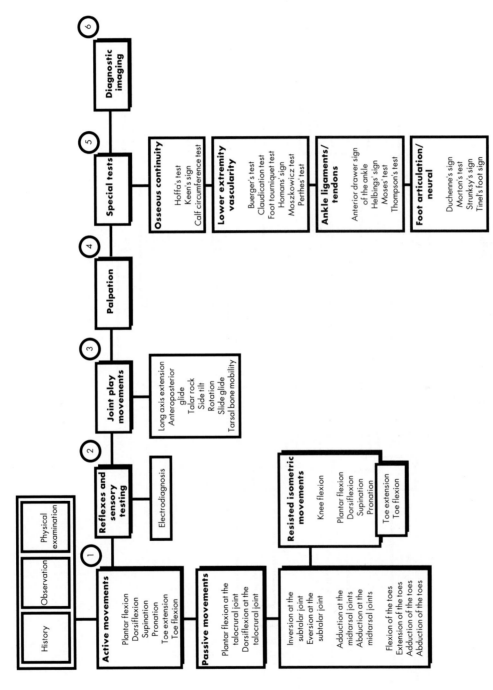

Fig. 12–1 Lower leg, ankle, and foot assessment.

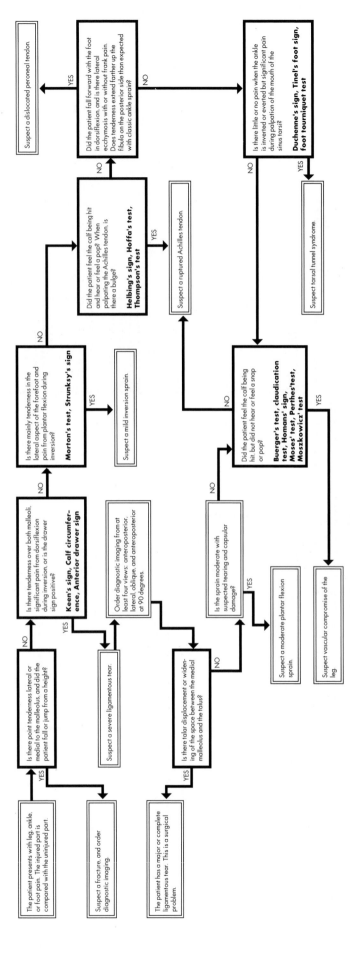

Fig. 12-2 Assessment of lower leg, ankle, and foot pain.

RANGE OF MOTION

For the sake of simplicity, motions are tested along three different axes. Dorsiflexion and plantar flexion are movements at the ankle joint that occur around a transverse axis that passes through the body of the talus. Because the normal foot toes out approximately 16 degrees, this motion occurs at an angle of 16 degrees to the transverse axis of the body. Inversion and eversion are movements of rotation of the foot along its long axis. These movements are assigned to the subtalar joint, which forms an axis of approximately 42 degrees with the ground. Abduction and adduction of the forefoot, occurring along a vertical axis, are movements of the midtarsal joints. These movements cannot occur independently of the movements of eversion and inversion. Moreover, inversion usually occurs with plantar flexion and eversion with dorsiflexion of the ankle. Further confusion is added by the improper use of the terms pronation and supination as substitutes for eversion and inversion. The terms pronation and supination refer to a weight-bearing foot. The complex movements of eversion and inversion indicate changes in the form of the whole foot when it is not bearing weight.

Forefoot adduction and abduction occur mainly at the midtarsal joints and are tested passively. The examiner moves the forefoot laterally and medially in relation to the calcaneus. Compare the range of motion to the opposite foot. This test is important in children with congenital forefoot deformities. Exact measurements are not possible, and it is sufficient to record whether the movement appears normal, abnormally free, or restricted. The direction in which the movement is restricted should also be recorded. The other tarsal joints allow little more than gliding motion, which is an important attribute of the foot in conforming to uneven surfaces. This gliding motion cannot be accurately recorded, but a note is made about suppleness or stiffness of the forefoot.

The other joints that allow significant motion in the forefoot are the metatarsophalangeal and interphalangeal joints. Of particular importance are the joints of the great toe. The patient's foot is placed in the neutral position, which is 45 degrees of flexion at the knee and 90 degrees of flexion of the foot to the leg. Record the dorsiflexion of the first metatarsophalangeal joint. Normal dorsiflexion of the great toe is approximately 50 degrees. Plantar flexion of the metatarsophalangeal and interphalangeal joints of the great toe is approximately 30 degrees. Retained dorsiflexion of the great toe that is 40 degrees or less is an impairment of the foot in the activities of daily living. Retained plantar flexion of the great toe that is 20 degrees or less is an impairment of the foot in the activities of daily living.

Movements of the lesser toes can be similarly measured. Clinically, it is adequate to note if there are fixed contractures or if the joints are supple. Restriction of joint motion can be the result of soft-tissue contractures, bony abutment, or intraarticular adhesions. Motion may be restricted because of pain that results from inflammation or injuries.

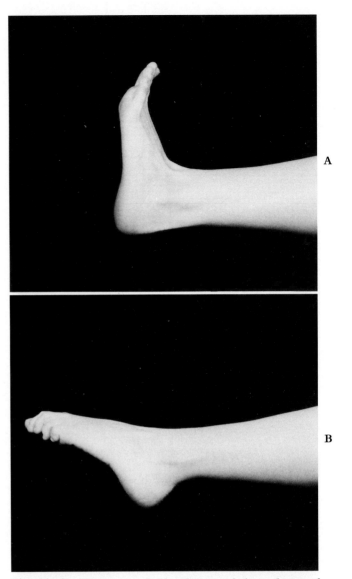

Fig. 12–3 When testing the dorsiflexion and plantar flexion of the ankle joint, neutral position for the ankle is when the lateral border of the foot is at 90 degrees in relation to the leg and the knee is in full extension. A normal ankle allows 20 degrees of dorsiflexion (**A**) and 40 degrees of plantar flexion from this position (**B**). Retained dorsiflexion of 10 degrees or less and retained plantar flexion range of motion of 30 degrees or less are impairments of the ankle for the activities of daily living. The measurements of dorsiflexion and plantar flexion can be repeated while the knee is held in 45 degrees of flexion. If the arc of motion is different from the previous finding, it indicates the presence of Achilles tendon tightness. For all practical purposes, movements of the ankle jointare considered limited to dorsiflexion and plantar flexion. In some individuals with hypermobility of the ankle joint, medial tilt of the talus can occur within the ankle mortise. This tilt is the result of a congenital laxity of the lateral collateral ligaments and predisposes the patient to recurrent ankle sprains.

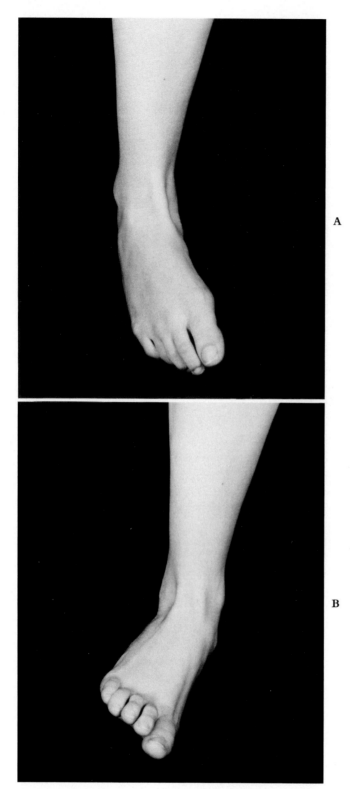

A

B

Fig. 12–4 Inversion and eversion of the foot occur mainly at the subtalar joint and are tested while the patient is lying supine. The ankle is first dorsiflexed to a neutral position. The patient rocks the foot into inversion (**A**) and eversion (**B**). A normal joint allows 20 degrees of eversion and about 30 degrees of inversion. Retained inversion range of motion that is 20 degrees or less and retained eversion range of motion that is 10 degrees or less are impairments of the foot-ankle mechanism in the activities of daily living.

MUSCLE TESTING

The motions in the ankle joint are plantar flexion and dorsiflexion. The muscles in the posterior compartment, which are innervated by the tibial nerve, are primarily responsible for plantar flexion motion. The major muscles for plantar flexion are the gastrocnemius and soleus, and they are supplemented by the tibialis posterior, peroneus longus, flexor digitorum longus, and hallucis longus. The power of the gastrocnemius-soleus group is weakened when the knee is in flexion because the gastrocnemius is a two-joint muscle.

However, while the knee is in flexion, the passive range of ankle dorsiflexion increases slightly. The muscles of the anterior compartment, innervated by the deep peroneal nerve, are primarily responsible for dorsiflexion motion. Dorsiflexion is performed by the tibialis anterior and the extensor digitorum longus. When these two muscles act together, their individual actions of inversion and eversion are neutralized. The extensor hallucis longus and peroneus tertius also aid in dorsiflexion.

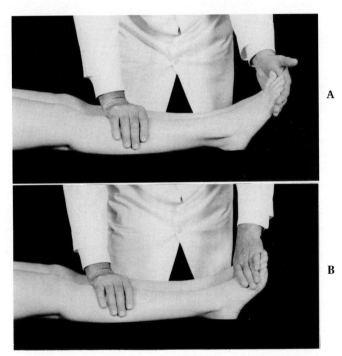

Fig. 12–5 The soleus and gastrocnemius should be evaluated separately. The soleus is evaluated by applying a dorsiflexion force to the foot while the patient plantar flexes the foot (**A**). The maneuver is performed with the knee in extension to evaluate the muscle power of the gastrocnemius. The tibialis anterior is tested by exerting a counterforce to the dorsiflexion and inversion movement of the foot and ankle (**B**).

A

B

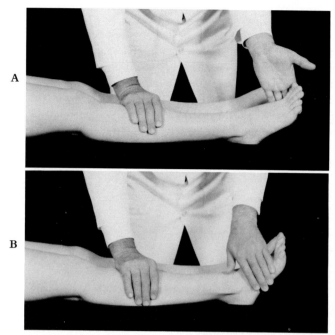

A

B

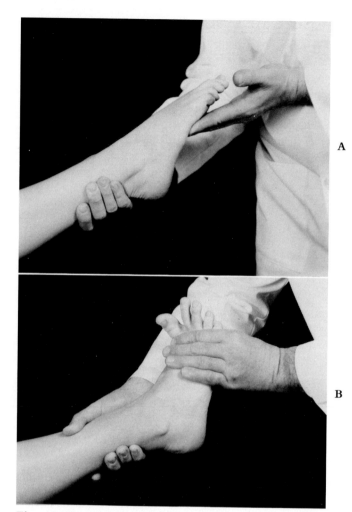

Fig. 12–6 The prime motions at the intertarsal joints are inversion and eversion, and these motions occur primarily at the subtalar joint. Inversion is achieved principally by the tibialis posterior and the tibialis anterior, but is supplemented by the long toe flexors and gastrosoleus. Eversion is achieved primarily by the peroneus brevis and peroneus longus, which are innervated by the superficial peroneal nerve and is supplemented by the extensor digitorum longus and peroneus tertius. The tibialis posterior is evaluated by exerting a counterforce to the foot while the patient inverts and plantar flexes the foot (**A**). The peroneus longus is tested by exerting a counterforce to a foot that is held in plantar flexion while the patient actively everts it (**B**). The peroneus brevis is evaluated the same way, but the foot is held in the neutral position.

Fig. 12–7 The main motions at the metatarsophalangeal and interphalangeal joints are extension and flexion. Flexion of the metatarsophalangeal joint is achieved primarily by the lumbricales, interossei, and flexor hallucis brevis, which are augmented by the flexor hallucis longus and the flexor digitorum longus and brevis (**A**). Extension of these joints is achieved primarily by the extensor digitorum longus and the extensor hallucis longus, which are supplemented by the extensor digitorum brevis and the extensor hallucis brevis (**B**). The interphalangeal joints are hinge joints that allow flexion and extension but more flexion than extension. Flexion is achieved by the flexor digitorum longus at the distal interphalangeal joint and is supplemented by the flexor digitorum brevis at the proximal interphalangeal joints.

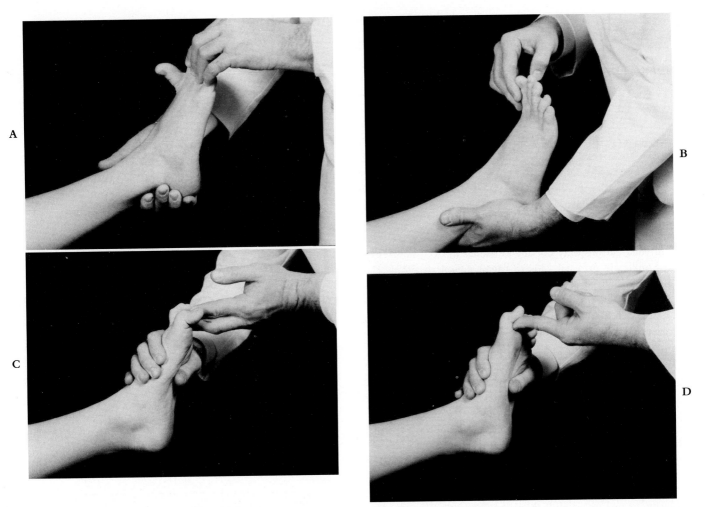

Fig. 12–8 The muscle power of the long toe extensors is tested by exerting a counterforce to the toes while the patient extends the metatarsophalangeal joints (**A**), (**B**). The long toe flexors are tested by exerting a counterforce to the tip of the toes while the patient flexes the interphalangeal joints (**C**), (**D**).

Comment

With injuries to the ankle there is such a close association between sprain dislocation and fracture that it is unwise to place them in separate categories. This is particularly true because the same forces may well cause a combination of injuries. Resultant pathologic conditions may be determined more by the strength and duration of the forces that cause the injury than by the exact type of stress. The injury is usually caused by stresses that may result in either a sprain, a dislocation, a fracture, or all three.

Because the ankle is functionally a hinge joint that normally permits only dorsal and plantar flexion, injuries to the ankle are primarily due to lateral stresses that force the ankle through an arc of motion that it does not normally possess. Less frequently injuries are due to hyperflexion or hyperextension. The injuries that are due to lateral stresses may readily be divided into two categories, inversion injuries and eversion injuries.

Inversion injuries to the ankle are usually not due to pure inversion. The force consists of inversion, internal rotation, and plantar flexion of the foot in relation to the leg, so the foot is inverted and the ankle and foot are thrown laterally. In this injury mechanism the push is against the medial malleolus, and the pull is away from the lateral malleolus. As the foot inverts in relation to the leg, strain is put upon the lateral collateral ligament, the ligament primarily constructed to resist this motion. As a result of this overinversion, the ligament will tear slightly, partially, or completely according to the severity of the force. If the inverting force continues as the lateral ligament gives way, the ankle opens on the lateral side and the talus is forcibly thrust against the medial malleolus. The medial malleolus acts as a fulcrum, and its tip impinges against the central portion of the medial face of the talus. The talus rotates over the malleolus rather than pushes off it. In such a case the injury will probably be confined to the lateral side, and there will be complete laceration of the lateral collateral ligaments. It is unusual for this type of force to break off the lateral malleolus. In the geriatric patient in whom the bone is osteoporotic, the lateral malleolus may break before the ligament tears.

Procedure

The patient may be seated or supine. The examiner places one hand around the anterior aspect of the lower tibia, just above the ankle, while gripping the calcaneus in the palm of the other hand. While the tibia is pushed posteriorly, the calcaneus and talus are drawn anteriorly. Normally there is no movement from this action. The sign is present when the talus slides anteriorly under the ankle mortise. The test indicates anterior talofibular ligament instability, which is usually secondary to rupture.

Confirmation Procedures

Keen's sign, calf circumference test, diagnostic imaging

Reporting Statement

Anterior drawer sign of the ankle is positive for the right ankle. The presence of this sign implicates the anterior talofibular ligament and may represent a sprain.

∼ Clinical Pearl ∼

The drawer sign is a sensitive indicator of the amount of ligamentous damage in the ankle. Often, ankles with drawer sign present will require casting or rigid immobilization, at the least, in acute-stage management. Instability may sometimes follow tears of the anterior talofibular portion of the lateral ligament. This instability may be confirmed by radiographs after local anesthesia. Support the heel on a sandbag and press firmly downward on the tibia for 30 seconds before exposure. A gap that is between the talus and the tibia and is greater than 6 mm is regarded as a pathologic condition.

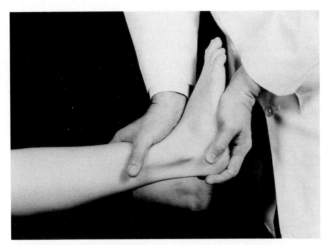

Fig. 12–9 The patient may be seated or supine. The examiner places one hand around the lower tibia, slightly above the ankle mortise. The calcaneus and talus are gripped in the palm of the other hand. The tibia is pushed posteriorly, while the calcaneus and talus are drawn anteriorly. The sign is present if any movement of the talus is detected in the ankle mortise. The presence of this sign represents a talofibular ligament instability.

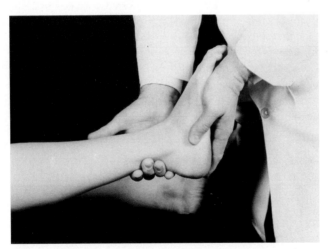

Fig. 12–10 In a reversal of this maneuver, the tibia is drawn anteriorly as the calcaneus and talus are pushed posteriorly. In this maneuver a positive sign is indicated by a greater degree of mortise definition in the anterior. This may indicate insufficiency of the posterior talofibular portion of the lateral ligament.

Comment

Knowledge of the smaller, peripheral, vascular bed structures is important to the understanding of diseases that cause peripheral vascular compromise. After leaving the mainstream artery the efferent circulatory system branches into smaller and smaller muscularly walled precapillaries and arterioles. Arterioles can lead directly to venules through arteriovenous anastomoses (thin-walled arterioles that contain contractile smooth muscle for control of shunting). However, more frequently arterioles channel into precapillaries and then capillaries connect to the venules and larger venous system. Fine tuning of the systemic blood pressure can be controlled by the small, muscularly walled vessels as well as by shunting blood through collateral channels around the capillary bed. The pressures in capillaries of skeletal muscle range between 20 and 30 mm Hg. Therefore external pressures that exceed this value may occlude these capillaries, which deliver oxygen and remove carbon dioxide during the normal blood flow. It is at this microvascular level that increased interstitial fluid pressure first affects compartmental contents and leads to a progressive pathologic condition.

Similar to the varying types of muscles, different patterns of blood supply within the muscles exist. Muscles in general have isolated vascular support systems with limited internal and external anastomoses, and therefore anatomic relationships may be inconsistent. In some muscles, abundant communications between arteriolar systems exist (longitudinal anastomotic chains, such as the soleus and peroneus longus). In other muscles, several mainstream arteries send arterial branches into the muscle, so damage to a single vessel, such as the anterior tibialis and the flexor hallucis longus, may not be critical. However, some muscles, such as the extensor hallucis longus, have a single blood supply with few anastomoses. These latter systems are extremely susceptible to any circulatory compromise by virtue of their single vascular stem. Tendons have a substantial and constant blood supply that may form an anastomosis with the muscular system. The vascularity of muscles may be isolated from the surrounding tissue and therefore susceptible to arterial injury.

In general every major artery in a limb has one or two veins traveling with it. Any stasis or engorgement in this system may retard blood flow. This retardation causes increased pressure in the small arteriolar capillary system and leads to an alteration of the Starling equilibrium. This could then cause fluid extrusion from the capillary walls, and add to or create increased pressure in a closed compartment.

Because the venous walls are thinner and less muscular than comparable arterial channels, the venous walls are more compressible and therefore more susceptible to changes surrounding muscle and interstitial fluid pressure. The extremities have two venous flow networks, the superficial and the deep. Deep veins are apparently more efficient in maintaining blood flow. Through the forces of external muscular pumping and the system of intimal valves and communicating branches, the blood is shunted to and transported through the deep vessels.

Procedure

While the patient is lying supine, the examiner elevates the leg and extends the knee to a point of comfortable tolerance, approximately 45 degrees, for no less than 3 minutes. The examiner lowers the limb, and the patient sits up with both legs dangling side by side over the examining table. The test measures arterial blood supply to the lower limbs. The blood supply is deficient if the dorsum of the foot blanches and the prominent veins collapse when the leg is initially raised. The test is also positive if, when the leg is lowered, it takes 1 to 2 minutes for a ruddy (reddish) cyanosis to spread over the affected part and for the veins to fill and become prominent.

Confirmation Procedures

Claudication test, foot tourniquet test, Homans' sign, Moszkowicz test, Moses' test, Perthes' test, vascular assessment

Reporting Statement

Buerger's test is positive for the right leg. This result suggests vascular compromise of the right lower extremity.

∽ Clinical Pearl ∽

It is not uncommon in lower extremity vascular disorders for sciatic-like pain to be produced. This test allows for quick determination of neurogenic versus vascular pain. The test demonstrates loss of vascular integrity, but as circulation diminishes, the primary complaint is produced.

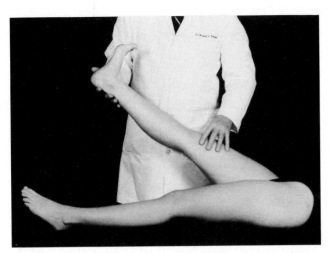

Fig. 12–11 The patient is lying supine. The examiner elevates the patient's leg to 45 degrees while the knee is fully extended. The patient actively dorsiflexes the foot.

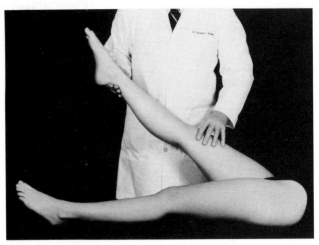

Fig. 12–12 After dorsiflexing the foot, as in Fig. 12–11, the patient plantar flexes the foot for at least 3 minutes. This maneuver diminishes the amount of blood in the distal vessels.

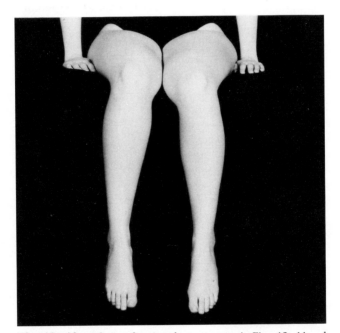

Fig. 12–13 After performing the maneuvers in Figs. 12–11 and 12–12, the patient sits at the edge of the examining table and dangles the legs. The test is positive for circulatory deficiency if the foot is blanched and the veins are collapsed. Also, the test is considered positive if it takes more than 2 minutes for the circulation to return to the dangling leg.

~ Calf Circumference Test ~

Comment

In the anterior compartment of the leg the anterior tibial, the extensor hallucis, and the extensor digitorum longus muscles arise from the sides of the tibia, fibula, and interosseous membrane. These muscles completely fill the anterior compartment. This compartment is tightly roofed by the anterior fascia of the leg. With the anterior tibial syndrome there is a rapid swelling of the muscle within its compartment. This swelling may come on following active exercise alone. In theory this is because muscles that have not been previously conditioned are overused, so they respond with swelling and edema. The swelling also may come on following a direct injury in which there is excessive swelling and hemorrhage into the space. The condition also can be caused by localized infection within the space. In fact, anything that causes intractable swelling may cause this syndrome.

At the onset of anterior tibial syndrome, there is severe pain over the involved area and a loss of function. Contraction of the muscles contained in the space rapidly becomes impossible and foot drop can ensue. Even passive stretching of the muscles quickly becomes painful. However, this condition is not ordinarily preceded by the symptoms of tenosynovitis. The skin over the area becomes red, glossy, warm, and markedly tender. There is a feeling of woody tension over the point of real hardness of the fascia over the space. There may occasionally be involvement of the peroneal nerve with sensory loss. The loss of muscle function is usually not due to nerve involvement but to pathologic change within the muscle itself. The muscles develop ischemic necrosis, which is often called Volkmann's ischemia of the leg. Volkmann's ischemia is characterized by swelling, edema, extravasation of red blood cells, destruction of blood cells, and replacement of muscle tissue by a fibrous scar. The result is a firm, inelastic, and noncontractile muscle group. This condition can be extremely disabling and defies reconstructive treatment.

Procedure

While the patient is lying supine, the circumference of the bellies of the gastrocnemius and soleus muscles are measured. The measurement is compared with the calf circumference of the opposite leg. Because the dominance of a leg is not established except in highly specialized sports or occupations, the measurements should be equal. A diminished calf circumference may represent simple loss of muscle tone, but it also may represent atrophy of muscle fibers. An increased calf circumference, corroborated with other pathologic findings, may indicate a fulminating compartment syndrome.

Confirmation Procedures

Keen's sign, anterior drawer sign of the ankle, vascular assessment, diagnostic imaging

---

Reporting Statement

Calf circumference measurements reveal a diminished size, when compared with the uninvolved leg. This size difference suggests loss of muscular tone or atrophy.

Calf circumference measurements reveal an increased size relative to the uninvolved leg. This difference suggests an increase in muscular bulk, muscular compartment pressures, or hypertrophy.

~ Clinical Pearl ~

In knee injuries the first sign of internal joint derangement is loss of tone in the quadriceps. Internal derangement of the ankle joint produces the same phenomenon in its controlling musculature. The gastrocnemius-soleus mechanism weakens and loses tone to a degree sufficient enough to be quantified with a tape measure. This measuring can help differentiate the degree of ankle involvement.

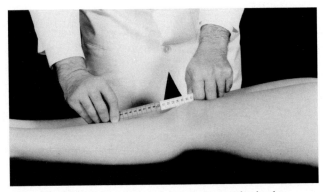

Fig. 12–14 The patient is lying supine with the knees extended. The examiner establishes a point in the leg 6 inches below the midline of the patella.

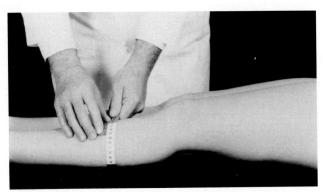

Fig. 12–15 The circumference of the leg is measured at the point selected in Fig. 12–14. The examiner should be cautious when drawing the tape measure tight. The tape should be snug, but no skin depressions should be observed. The measurement is recorded and compared with the circumference of the same point in opposite leg.

Comment

Muscle is dependent on its peripheral and central nervous system for control and on its vascular supply for survival. Total interruption of the vascular supply to a region will result in necrosis of the nerves and muscles. A clinical example of this is the anterior tibial compartment syndrome. In the early stages there is a loss of voluntary control. With electrodiagnostic procedure, movement of the electrode needle reveals normal or slightly reduced insertional activity. When the condition has been present for a longer period, even this insertional activity will disappear. After this point it is probable that decompressive procedures will not prevent necrosis of the nerves and muscles.

The most common cause of small vessel diseases are arteriosclerosis and the collagen vascular diseases. Microembolization will produce histologic changes in muscles that are comparable to those seen in myopathic diseases. An acute obstruction of small vessels is an example of such a change. The clinical conditions are chronic and usually progressive. The collagen vascular diseases may have periods of acute exacerbation. During these periods the diseases are rapidly progressive. In this case the EMG findings would be myopathic in nature and would resemble polymyositis. The nerve conduction studies would show normal or slightly slowed velocities, and the M-wave would probably be reduced slightly. With slowly progressive arteriosclerosis, EMG studies are rarely performed. The changes would be very slow and would represent loss of individual muscle fibers from the motor units as well as loss of small nerve fibers. The EMG findings would demonstrate myopathic and neuropathic, large-amplitude and small-amplitude motor units of brief duration. Fibrillation potentials would be a rare finding.

Procedure

The patient walks at a rate of 120 steps per minute, for 60 seconds. This goal can be accomplished by having the patient walk on a treadmill. The time that elapses between the start of the test and the occurrence of leg cramping, is the claudication time. The site of the cramping and often the color change (pallor) in the tissues identifies the level of the lesion. The test indicates peripheral vascular disease of chronic arterial occlusion.

Confirmation Procedures

Buerger's test, foot tourniquet test, Homans' sign, Moszkowicz test, Moses' sign, Perthes' test, vascular assessment

---

Reporting Statement

The claudication test is positive on the right. This result suggests chronic arterial occlusive disease.

∼ Clinical Pearl ∼

The claudication test may be an assumed finding in patients who complain of leg cramps during distance walking. The pain of neurogenic origin is differentiated from pain of arterial origin when the patient relates sitting with almost immediate cramp relief.

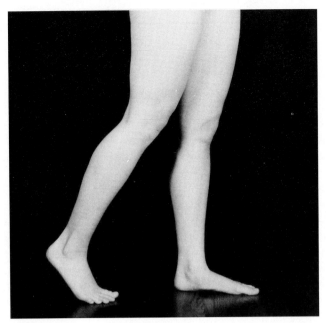

Fig. 12–16   The patient begins marching in place. The pace should be about 120 steps per minute and should be continued for 60 seconds. This maneuver also may be accomplished by using a treadmill.

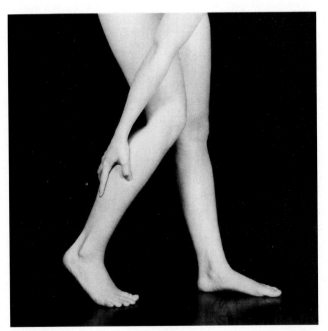

Fig. 12–17   The time elapsing between the start of the test and the onset of the leg cramping is the claudication time. The normal leg should not cramp. When positive, the test indicates chronic arterial occlusion.

Comment

Compression or distortion of the superficial peroneal nerve may occur where the nerve exits the muscular layer of the leg and pierces the crural fascia at the level between the middle and distal third of the leg.

At the entrance into the peroneal tunnel, near the head of the fibula, the common peroneal nerve divides into two terminal branches, the deep and the superficial peroneal nerve. This terminal branch point may vary as well as the course of the superficial peroneal nerve. The superficial branch continues distally between the fibula and the peroneus longus muscle, which lies on the intermuscular septum of the anterior compartment. The nerve also lies proximally between the peroneus longus and the extensor digitorum longus muscles and distally between the peroneus longus and brevis muscles. At the level between the middle and distal third of the leg, the nerve pierces the crural fascia and continues subcutaneously as the cutaneous dorsalis medialis and the cutaneous dorsalis intermedius nerves. Before piercing the fascia, the superficial peroneal nerve supplies the peroneus longus and brevis muscles. The cutaneous branches of the superficial nerves supply the skin of the anterolateral side of the leg; the dorsum of the foot; the dorsum of the first, second, and third toes; and the medial side of the fourth toe. The sural nerve, via the cutaneous dorsalis lateralis nerve, supplies the lateral sides of the fourth and fifth toes.

Trauma represents the most commonly proposed etiology of this rarely diagnosed syndrome of the superficial peroneal nerve. Surgical trauma, lipomas, muscular hernias, tight boots, repetitive compression of the foot in sports, and dynamic compression of the narrow fascial tunnel have been offered as possible etiologies. Trauma in this area may lead to local inflammation, reactive swelling, and eventual compression of the fascial tunnel.

Dynamic compression, based on the functional anatomy of the leg, places the nerve at risk. The superficial peroneal nerve is fixed. Therefore forced inversion and extension of the foot further stretches the nerve over the fascial border. While typically 1 cm in length, surgical evidence shows that the tunnel may actually extend up 3 to 11 cm in length.

Repetitive activities may cause scarring of the nerve or fascial borders, which narrows the tunnel even further.

Described as mononeuralgia, pain caused by compression or damage to the superficial peroneal nerve appears on the dorsum of the foot and is occasionally accompanied by dysesthesia or complete anesthesia in the nerve's dermatome. There are three additional tests for evaluating patients for the syndrome: (1) resisted dorsiflexion and eversion with pressure applied over the tunnel, (2) passive plantar flexion and inversion, (3) stretching of the nerve, as in the second test, with percussion over the tunnel. A positive result for these provocative tests is the production of pain or paresthesia over the nerve's dermatome. Electromyographic studies of the peroneal and anterior tibial muscles and conduction velocities help in identifying the syndrome.

Procedure

The examiner pushes up the head of the first metatarsal with the thumb, and the patient plantar flexes the foot. The sign is present when the medial border of the foot dorsiflexes, with the lateral border plantar flexing. The head of the first metatarsal offers no resistance to the pushing thumb. The plantar crease runs laterally from the medial side of the big toe to the heel, and the arch disappears. This result is caused by paralysis of the peroneus longus, which is due to a lesion of the superficial peroneal nerve or a lesion at or above the L4, L5, and S1 roots.

Confirmation Procedures

Tinel's foot sign, electrodiagnosis

Reporting Statement

Duchenne's sign is positive in the right foot. The presence of this sign suggests a lesion of the superficial peroneal nerve.

∼ Clinical Pearl ∼

Before diagnosing pes planus that is due to structural problems, the examiner should attempt to elicit Duchenne's sign. The presence of this sign indicates a pes planus phenomenon that is due to neural lesions at a much higher level than the arch itself.

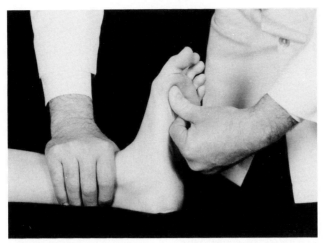

Fig. 12–18 The patient is lying supine, and the leg is extended. The examiner grasps the lower tibia with one hand, slightly above the ankle mortise. With the thumb of the other hand, the examiner applies pressure to the head of the first metatarsal.

A

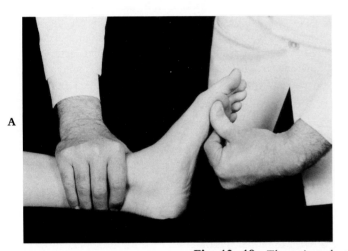

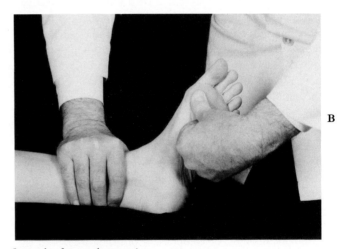

B

Fig. 12–19 The patient plantar flexes the foot as the examiner maintains pressure on the first metatarsal (**A**). The sign is present when the medial border of the foot dorsiflexes, the lateral border of the foot plantar flexes, and the arch of the foot disappears (**B**). The presence of this sign indicates paralysis of the peroneus longus muscle that is due to a lesion of the superficial peroneal nerve.

~ Foot Tourniquet Test ~

Comment

Significant diminution of blood flow to individual toes or to an entire foot results in pale nail beds, slow capillary recovery after skin compression, diminished bleeding after skin puncture, lowering of the skin temperature, and pain of varying intensity. Symptoms and signs of pain, pulselessness, pallor, paresthesia, and paralysis indicate arterial insufficiency or inadequate capillary perfusion. The coexistence of pallor with cyanosis and rubor (mottling) is consistent with vaso-constriction and later vasodilation.

The spectrum of causes for diminished blood flow is apparent by observing the alterations that occur in the healthy extremity, which is affected temporarily by decreased blood flow, as a result of environmental alterations, such as cooling of the feet, contact of a toe with ice, or sympathetic nervous stimulation from anxiety or fear. In each instance the occurrence of pallor and a significant drop in skin temperature will cause pain that is moderately severe and is described as a deep, aching sensation. As the ischemic state persists, pain becomes more intense.

The phrase *Raynaud's disease* is used to describe the occurrence of vasospasm within an underlying primary disease. If vasospasm is associated with a known connective-tissue disease, then a Raynaud's phenomenon is implied. Recognition of Raynaud's syndrome and the patient's response to this condition is important in explaining pain and cold tolerance associated with a known pathologic condition. When the symptoms of pain occur in a toe, the foot, or the entire lower extremity, the existence of adequate blood flow in the large and small vessels must be determined.

In patients known to have a nerve compression lesion, such as superficial peroneal nerve compression at the fascial tunnel, diminished blood flow will cause abnormal sensory changes to occur earlier than would happen in the normal patient. Motor weakness occurs more quickly when partial or complete ischemia occurs.

Various conditions—such as atherosclerotic stenosis, thromboembolism, or compression of major arteries in the lower abdomen—cause pain, claudication, paresthesia, and intermittent episodes of pallor. The lesions may be partial or complete, and the clinical symptoms may vary according to the degree of ischemia.

Acute occlusion of an artery is associated with unrelenting pain and pallor, followed by rubor and cyanosis. Cold toler-ance is diminished, and intrinsic muscle weakness occurs.

Obliteration of the artery is due to trauma and the occurrence of an anterior compartment compression of the lower leg muscles, vessels, and nerve. This compression causes pallor of the foot, diminished pulse volume, and severe pain. The effect of diminished arterial inflow and lessened venous outflow during pain has been well calibrated by analyzing the effects of traumatic lesions at various levels of the extremity. Decompression of a tight compartment that is anterior to the leg will diminish pain almost immediately. Elimination of nerve compression syndromes at the ankle will provide measurable relief of pain.

Causalgia is considered a mixed nerve lesion with accompanying or secondary vascular insufficiency. The residual pain may require direct treatment of the peripheral nerve.

Sympathetic dystrophy is one condition that may occur, although a specific nerve injury cannot be demonstrated. However, there is a vasospastic element that occurs second-ary to a major or minor insult of the extremity or an adjacent organ.

Procedure

Application of a pneumatic tourniquet, with pressure elevated to 20 mm Hg above the patient's resting diastolic blood pressure to a normal extremity will obliterate arterial inflow and venous outflow, slow motor nerve conduction, decrease sensory conduction, and cause pain in the foot and at the site of tourniquet compression. Anoxia and nerve com-pression occur simultaneously, and muscle weakness is evident within 3 to 5 minutes. Digital paresthesia occur and sensation diminishes gradually to anesthesia in about 30 minutes. These painful sensations are a combination of muscle and nerve ischemia as well as nerve compression.

Confirmation Procedures

Buerger's test, claudication test, Homans' sign, Moszkow-icz test, Moses' test, Perthes' test, vascular assessment

---

Reporting Statement

The tourniquet test is positive for the right leg and ankle. This result indicates arterial insufficiency.

∿ Clinical Pearl ∿

Tenderness at the front of the leg is characteristic in (1) Osgood–Schlatter disease, (2) Brodie's abscess, or osteitis, (3) anterior tibial compartment syndrome, (4) stress fracture, and (5) shin splints. Tenderness at the back of the leg is characteristically situated (1) in the plantaris tendon in partial and complete ruptures, (2) over varicosities in superficial thrombophlebitis, and (3) over the tendocalcaneus in partial tears and complete ruptures.

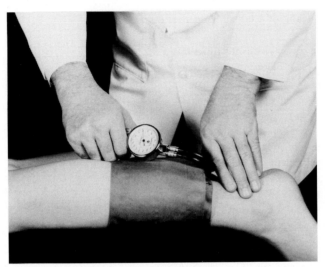

Fig. 12–20   The patient is lying prone on the examining table, and the leg is extended. The foot dangles over the end of the examining table. The calf musculature should be as relaxed as possible. A blood pressure cuff is applied to the leg, near the ankle, above the area of complaint. The cuff is inflated to 20 mm above the patient's resting diastolic blood pressure. Pressure may need to be increased to reach blanching of the distal extremity. Foot pain, paresthesia, and muscle weakness appearing in less than 5 minutes indicate arterial insufficiency.

Comment

Pes planus is attributed to deficiencies in the structure of the talus and calcaneus. Conversely, strong and well-shaped feet are attributed to the result of tarsal bones so shaped and so integrated into one another that they cannot shift when weight is imposed on them. In symptomatic pes planus that does not involve osseous anomalies, the condition is often related to weak posterior tibial muscle function. This weakness permits an abnormal excursion of the talonavicular joint.

Rupture of the tendon of the posterior tibialis muscle is an etiologic factor in pes planus. These ruptures have occurred in middle-aged individuals who have had one or more injections of a corticosteroid into the sheath of the tendon. Such an injection is used to relieve local discomfort or to alleviate an obvious synovitis. Rupture of the tendon occurs with prompt development of a markedly pronated foot. When the patient attempts to rise on the toes, the patient has difficulty doing so on the involved side because the heel fails to invert and the longitudinal arch fails to rise during this maneuver. Rupture of the posterior tibial tendon should be suspected in any case in which unilateral pes planus suddenly appears.

The symptomatic weak foot may be flat or may have a high longitudinal arch, especially when at rest. The flat foot usually has a degree of abduction of the forefoot and eversion of the ankle. The Achilles tendon may be shortened and pulled at an angle instead of following a plumb line. The long, narrow, flaccid foot with a normal arch is likely to become symptomatic.

Procedure

Medial curving of the Achilles tendon, when viewed posteriorly, indicates foot pronation.

Confirmation Procedures

Hoffa's test, Thompson's test

Reporting Statement

Helbings' sign is present for the right foot. The presence of this sign suggests pes planus.

∿ Clinical Pearl ∿

The arches of the foot do not become fully formed until a child has been walking for some years. The young child's foot is normally flat. If the arches fail to establish, then an awkward gait and rapid, uneven wear and distortion of the shoes may occur but it is rare for pain or other symptoms to develop. Persistent flatfoot may be associated with knock-knees, torsional deformities of the tibia and valgus deformities of the heel.

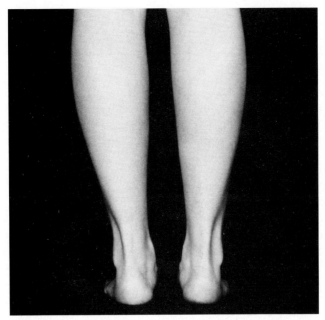

Fig. 12–21 The patient is standing, with the feet resting on a smooth, flat surface. From the posterior, the examiner observes the positions of the Achilles tendons. Normally, there should be no curving of the tendons as the patient bears weight.

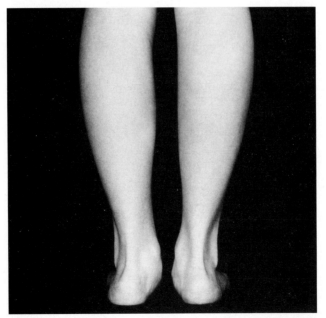

Fig. 12–22 The sign is present when a medial curving of the Achilles tendon is observed (as on the left). The sign indicates a pes planus condition.

~ Hoffa's Test ~

HOFFA'S SIGN

Comment

The posterior portion of the foot is rarely fractured, if sprain-fractures are excluded. The ordinary fracture of the calcaneus is by direct compression as in a fall from a height or from driving the foot into a hard surface. Fortunately, neither of these causes is common. Certain fractures do occur in special situations. Abnormal, forceful motion may cause avulsion or snubbing fractures of the talus. Also the sustentaculum tali may be broken by forceful eversion of the foot. It is extremely important to restore the contour of the calcaneus and particularly the integrity of the talocalcaneal joint. Adduction or abduction of the foot may cause a snubbing or avulsion fracture of the superior portion of the calcaneus at the calcaneocuboid joint.

Fracture of the calcaneus is the most common tarsal bone injury. A fracture involving the body of the calcaneus is the most common calcaneal fracture, and it often extends into the subtalar joint, with the posterior portion of the body displaced upward. This type of fracture is caused by a direct vertical force onto the calcaneus that usually occurs after a fall from a height. The spine should always be carefully examined because a compression fracture of the spine in the dorsolumbar area is frequently associated with calcaneal fractures.

The other types of calcaneal fractures, such as an avulsion fracture of the Achilles tendon insertion and fracture of the sustentaculum tali or anterior process, are seen less frequently.

Anteroposterior and lateral diagnostic imaging of the foot are necessary to evaluate the involvement of the subtalar joint. Fracture of the sustentaculum tali is demonstrable only in the axial views.

Procedure

While the patient is lying prone, the ankles hang well over the edge of the examining table, in a symmetrical position. Hoffa's test is positive if the examiner, using movement and palpation, finds the Achilles tendon on the injured side less taut than on the contralateral side. There may also be increased dorsiflexion of the foot in the relaxed position on the affected side. A loose fragment may be observed and felt behind either malleolus. The test is significant for fracture of the calcaneus.

Confirmation Procedures

Helbings' sign, Thompson's test, diagnostic imaging

Reporting Statement

Hoffa's test is positive for the right foot. This result implicates fracture of the calcaneus.

~ Clinical Pearl ~

In geriatric patients the Achilles tendon insufficiency that is due to attrition also produces a positive Hoffa's test. In this instance the calcaneus remains intact.

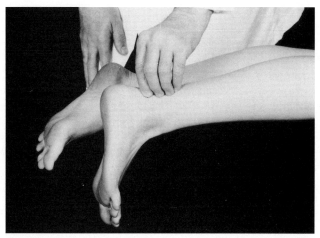

Fig. 12–23 The patient is prone on the examining table. The knees are extended and the ankles hang well over the end of the table. The sign is present when the affected foot rests in a more dorsiflexed position than the opposite foot (as noted on the right). The test is positive when the examiner determines by palpation the loss of Achilles tendon integrity. The sign implicates calcaneal fracture.

Comment

Intermittent claudication is the term applied to a condition that denotes an insufficient blood supply to the muscles of the lower extremities when they are called into activity during locomotion. Intermittent claudication occurs in atheroma, with or without thrombosis, and in embolism, Buerger's disease, and rarely, syphilitic endarteritis. The condition is aggravated by anemia.

The patient complains of pain that occurs in one or both legs and in the calf muscles and comes on after walking a certain distance. The pain disappears during rest. The pain becomes so intolerable that the patient is obliged to stand or sit still until it passes. As time goes on, the distance that the patient can walk in comfort becomes progressively shorter. Examination of the affected limb reveals nothing obvious. The legs are well nourished and normal in sensation and reflexes. The arteries at the ankle will be pulseless and the popliteal pulsation behind the knee joint may not be felt. The femoral artery can usually be felt to pulsate in a normal manner.

After walking, the foot may appear unduly pale. With rest, normal color returns and spreads gradually over the surface of the foot. The ankle jerk may be diminished or absent as a result of ischemia of the posterior tibial nerve. In later cases, paresthesia and objective sensory loss occur in the toes and foot. Intermittent claudication is not uncommon and its diagnosis is not difficult. The importance of recognizing the condition is paramount because of the tendency for the condition to develop into gangrene.

Procedure

While the patient is lying in the supine position, the examiner dorsiflexes the patient's foot and squeezes the calf. Deep-seated pain in the posterior leg or calf indicates thrombophlebitis.

Confirmation Procedures

Buerger's test, claudication test, foot tourniquet test, Moszkowicz test, Moses' sign, Perthes' test, vascular assessment

---

Reporting Statement

Homans' sign is present in the right leg. The presence of this sign suggests thrombophlebitis.

∽ Clinical Pearl ∽

The use of Homans' sign does not aid differentiation between a muscular lesion and a thrombophlebitis. The differentiation occurs when the test is concluded. When the pain remits quickly, thrombophlebitis is suspected. When the pain persists or lags on as an ache, calf strain is suspected.

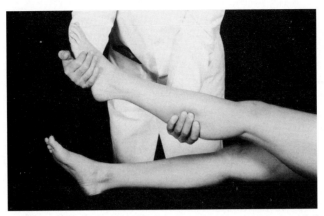

Fig. 12–24   The patient is lying supine with the knees extended and the legs resting on the examining table. The examiner elevates the affected leg to 45 degrees, and the calf is squeezed firmly.

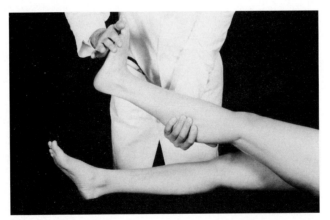

Fig. 12–25   As the calf pressure is maintained, the examiner dorsiflexes the foot. Deep calf or leg pain during this maneuver indicates thrombophlebitis.

Comment

Fracture of the tibia is infrequent, but fracture of the fibula is common. In any fracture of the fibula, associated injury of the ankle must be investigated. Whenever there is a complete fracture of the fibula, above the level of the tibiofibular syndesmosis, complete rupture of the inferior tibiofibular ligaments must be investigated. The possibility of rupture is the most serious and most important consideration in the fracture of the fibula. The actual fracture of the fibula is usually inconsequential, except that it does require a certain period of healing. If the fracture is accompanied by a rupture of the tibiofibular ligaments and results in instability or separation of the ankle mortise, then a serious and permanent disability results.

Fractures of the fibula result from direct blows that usually occur in the lower one third of the fibula. These blows may be caused by contact with a shoe or other hard object. With fracture of the fibula there is immediate pain but not severe disability. Upon examination local tenderness will be present at the site of the injury. There may or may not be local crepitus. There is usually prompt swelling with localized hematoma formation. The individual can usually walk quite well. In fact the patient may be able to complete a walking task because with a fracture of the fibula by direct blow the integrity of the ankle is not involved and disability is due to contraction of the muscle attachments on the fibular shaft. Diagnosis is confirmed by diagnostic imaging, which should always be made in a case of localized tenderness over any bone.

Of all bones the fibula is particularly prone to stress fracture and is second only to the metatarsals in this respect. This condition arises early in athletic or new job training and first appears as an ache, with some soreness and distress during function. The ache is usually localized near the neck of the fibula. There is no history of injury.

Procedure

If a fracture of the distal fibula exists (as in Pott's fracture), there is an increased diameter around the malleoli area of the affected ankle.

Confirmation Procedures

Calf circumference test, anterior drawer sign of the ankle, diagnostic imaging

---

Reporting Statement

Keen's sign is present in the right ankle. This sign indicates a distal fibular fracture.

∽ Clinical Pearl ∽

Keen's sign is an early indicator of ankle fracture. When present, the sign mandates diagnostic imaging of the joint.

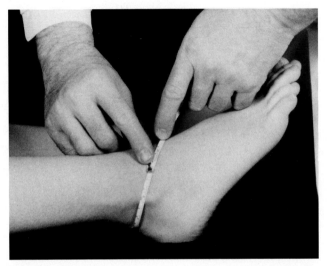

Fig. 12–26 The patient is lying supine on the examination table. The foot and ankle are in a resting position. A tape measure is placed around the ankle, passing over both malleoli. The diameter of the ankle is recorded and compared to the opposite ankle. An increased diameter, correlated with other pathologic findings, indicates a fracture of the distal fibula.

Comment

Morton's neuroma is a common disorder in the adult. A fibroneuromatous reaction between the third and fourth metatarsal heads, over the deep transverse metatarsal ligaments, affects the lateral terminal branch of the median plantar nerve. The impinging effect on the nerve is accentuated during weight bearing, particularly during the push-off phase of walking or when the metatarsal heads are compressed. Localized tenderness between the third and fourth metatarsal heads on the plantar surface also occurs. Hypesthesia over the lateral and medial side of the third and fourth toes, respectively, may be present. Morton's neuroma can occur in the web spaces that involve the corresponding terminal branch of either the medial or lateral plantar nerve, but this is not a frequent occurrence.

The term *metatarsalgia* denotes pain in the metatarsals and is a very common condition in adults. This pain is caused by various foot deformities or arthritis of the metatarsophalangeal joints. This latter type of pain is most commonly due to rheumatoid arthritis. The term metatarsalgia is used to refer to a pain syndrome and is not disease nomenclature per se. The disease may occur as an isolated condition or in association with hallux valgus or rigidus. The patient complains of pain in the metatarsal heads or toes when standing during the push-off phase of gait. On examination, there is localized tenderness directly under the plantar surface of the metatarsal head. The most common sites for the pain are the second and third metatarsal heads. Excessive pressure over the metatarsal heads is a primary cause of the pain. This pain is aggravated by ill-fitting shoes that squeeze the toes into a narrow toe-box and is differentiated from Morton's neuroma by having its most severe tenderness directly under the metatarsal heads with no associated hypesthesia of the involved toes.

Procedure

Transverse pressure across the heads of the metatarsals causes sharp pain in the forefoot. This pressure indicates metatarsalgia or neuroma.

Confirmation Procedures

Strunsky's sign, diagnostic imaging

Reporting Statement

Morton's test is positive for the right foot and indicates a neuroma at the third and fourth interspace.

Morton's test is positive for the right foot and indicates a metatarsalgia at the first through third metatarsal heads.

∾ Clinical Pearl ∾

Anterior metatarsalgia is particularly common in the middle-aged female and is also often associated with some splaying of the forefoot. Symptoms may be triggered by periods of excessive standing or by an increase in weight, and there is often concurrent flattening of the medial longitudinal arch. Weakness of the intrinsic muscles is usually present, so there is a tendency for clawing of the toes.

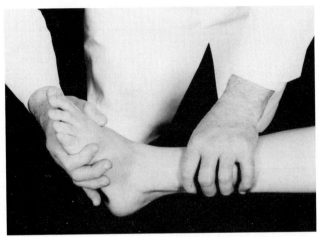

Fig. 12—27 The patient is lying supine on the examination table. The examiner grasps the affected forefoot with one hand and applies transverse pressure to the metatarsal heads. Sharp pain in the foot indicates a positive test and suggests metatarsalgia or neuroma.

Comment

Arteriovenous fistulas are abnormal communications, single or multiple, between arteries and veins, by which arterial blood enters the veins directly without traversing a capillary network.

Acquired arteriovenous fistulas, usually single and saccular, may develop after a bullet or stab wound involving an artery and a contiguous vein. Fistulas of the iliac vessels may occur following surgery for intervertebral disc disease. Congenital fistulas, which are present from birth, are usually multiple, and they result from defects in the differentiation of the common embryologic tissue into artery and vein. There is no special sex incidence, and any part of the body may be involved.

Arterial blood, following the path of least resistance, flows directly into the vein and bypasses the corresponding capillary bed. The arterial blood pressure is transmitted to the venous side of the fistula. The distal vein pressure is increased, but the proximal vein pressure may actually be negative. The elevated venous pressure leads to the development of varicose veins and venous stasis changes in the leg. Increased blood flow makes the tissues near the fistula abnormally warm, and diminished flow distal to the fistula may produce peripheral coldness and trophic changes. Large fistulas impose a burden on the heart. The cardiac output must be increased above normal by an amount proportional to the size of the fistula to maintain the general circulation. Total blood volume may be increased. The low peripheral resistance of the involved area decreases diastolic and increases systolic and pulse pressure systemically. Large fistulas may lead to cardiac decompensation.

In the region of the fistula the intima and the media of the involved veins become thickened and newly developed elastic fibers appear. The arteries show a thinning of their walls with a loss of elastic tissue and muscular fibers in the media.

Patients complain of ache, pain, edema, varicosities, or hypertrophied legs. Occasionally cardiac symptoms—such as palpitations, substernal pain, and dyspnea on exertion—are present. Examination reveals tortuous, dilated superficial veins in the leg. The venous pulsation can be felt unless the fistula is small and deeply placed. With congenital fistulas the skin temperature is usually elevated locally but decreased distal to the fistulas, although in acquired lesions, the temperature of the toes may be greater than in the opposite normal foot. Bruits or thrills are common over acquired fistulas. The bruit lasts throughout systole and diastole and has a coarse machinery-like quality. The tissues near the fistula may be tender, edematous, and either red or slightly cyanotic. The circumference of the leg is increased by edema or true hypertrophy, but bony structures are hypertrophied only if the fistula was present before epiphyseal closure. Temporary compression of the artery that supplies the large fistula diminishes the heart rate (Branham's sign) and may be a helpful diagnostic sign.

Procedure

The patient's lower extremity is elevated and an elastic bandage is wrapped firmly around the limb. The elevated position is maintained for 5 minutes, and then the extremity is placed in a horizontal position, and the examiner quickly removes the applied bandage. If the circulation is normal, a hyperemic blush occurs and rapidly flows into the area as the bandage is removed. The test is positive when the blush is absent or lags slowly behind the unbandaged area. The test demonstrates inadequacy of the collateral circulation as in an arteriovenous fistula.

Confirmation Procedures

Buerger's test, claudication test, foot tourniquet test, Homans' sign, Moses' test, Perthes' test, vascular assessment

Reporting Statement

Moszkowicz test is positive for the right leg. This result suggests an arteriovenous fistula at the level of the iliac artery.

∼ Clinical Pearl ∼

Thrombosis in the superficial veins of the calf and with local inflammatory changes is a common cause of recurrent calf pain and the presence of tenderness and other inflammatory signs along the course of the calf vein make diagnosis easy. Thrombosis in the deep veins is often silent and its importance in the postoperative situation is well known.

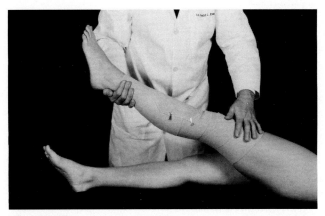

Fig. 12–28 The patient is lying supine on the examination table. The patient's legs are extended at the knees. The affected leg is elevated or flexed at the hip. While maintaining the leg in an elevated position, the examiner wraps the leg firmly with a 6-inch wide elastic bandage and maintains the elevation of the leg for 5 minutes.

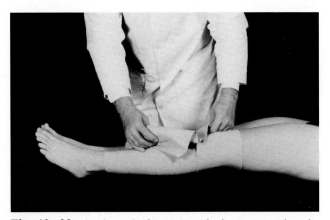

Fig. 12–29 At the end of 5 minutes the leg is returned to the horizontal position, and the bandage is quickly removed. The test is positive if the area of the leg previously wrapped has no hyperemic blush. The lack of hyperemic blush indicates arteriovenous fistula formation.

Comment

Arteriosclerosis obliterans is caused by arteriosclerotic narrowing or obstruction of large and small arteries that supply the extremities. Symptoms and signs are produced by ischemia.

Arteriosclerosis obliterans is the leading cause of obstructive arterial disease of the lower extremities after the age of 30. The superficial femoral artery is affected by stenosis or obstruction in approximately 90% of the patients. The aortoiliac and popliteal arteries are the next most common sites. The greatest incidence of superficial femoral and more distal arterial disease occurs in the seventh decade, but aortoiliac disease has its peak a decade earlier. The disease is more common in males than in females, especially before menopause. Patients with diabetes mellitus develop arteriosclerosis obliterans more frequently and at an earlier age than nondiabetics.

The most common symptom of arteriosclerosis obliterans is intermittent claudication (intermittent limping). The patient experiences cramping pain, tightness, numbness, or severe fatigue in the muscle group being exercised. The amount of exercise producing the pain is constant in each patient. The pain is relieved promptly by rest. In a few patients pain may disappear after further walking because of an unconscious slowing of the gait. Intermittent claudication is most frequent in the calf muscles because femoral artery disease is so common. However, the calf is the most common site of claudication because these muscles do the most work during walking. Lower back, buttock, thigh, and foot claudication also may occur. The site of the symptom localizes the obstruction proximally.

Rest pain is the other important symptom of obstructive arterial disease. Rest pain is a grave sign that indicates that the blood supply is not sufficient even for the small nutritional requirements of the skin. Rest pain may be localized to one or more toes, but often has a stocking distribution. The latter distribution means that ischemic neuritis is not usually the cause of rest pain. Rest pain is worse at night and is relieved somewhat by dependency and by cooling.

Other symptoms of arteriosclerosis obliterans include coldness, numbness, paresthesia, and color changes in the involved extremity.

Procedure

Moses' test is performed by grasping the patient's calf, which creates pain if phlebitis or vascular occlusion is present.

Confirmation Procedures

Buerger's test, claudication test, foot tourniquet test, Homans' sign, Moszkowicz test, Perthes' test, vascular assessment

Reporting Statement

Moses' test is positive for the right leg. This result indicates arteriosclerosis obliterans.

∼ Clinical Pearl ∼

Pain in the calf is common for patients suffering from prolapsed intervertebral discs. Claudication pain is a feature of vascular insufficiency and spinal stenosis. Lesions of the foot and ankle that lead to protective muscle spasm, during standing and walking, frequently cause marked calf and leg pain.

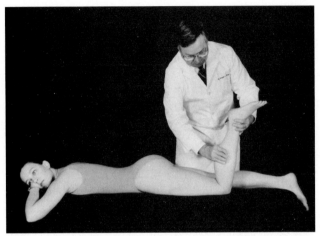

Fig. 12–30 The patient is lying prone on the examining table. The examiner flexes the patient's knee to 90 degrees. The examiner grasps and squeezes the calf of the affected leg. The sign is present if pain is elicited. The pain suggests phlebitis.

Comment

Varicose veins are distended, tortuous veins with incompetent valves. The *postphlebitic syndrome* denotes the chronically swollen lower extremity with trophic changes secondary to chronic venous stasis. Despite the name, a history of thrombophlebitis is often not obtainable.

Varicose veins are caused either by congenitally defective valves or by a condition that deforms valves or obstructs venous outflow over a long period. Varicosities that result from congenital defects are most common and may develop early in life. Because increased forearm vein distensibility has been demonstrated in patients with leg varicosities, a generalized abnormality of the veins has been suggested as the predisposing factor. Thrombophlebitis leads to deformation or destruction of venous valves and venous obstruction, and it is the second most frequent etiologic factor of venous problems. Pregnancy, ascites, abdominal tumor, excessive weight and height, or prolonged weight bearing may lead to increased venous pressure in the legs, distention of the veins, and finally incompetency of the valves.

Varicose veins is rather common. The condition appears in approximately 40% of all females, but the incidence is less in males. The saphenous veins in the lower extremity are most frequently the veins affected.

The dilated, tortuous, sacculated varices are easily visible. Some patients with extensive superficial varicosities have no other symptoms or signs, but some patients experience aching or easy fatigability of the calf muscles, and edema after weight bearing. The edema usually disappears with bed rest overnight. When the communicating or deep veins are incompetent, symptoms and signs are more common. Chronic venous insufficiency is manifested by edema, which may later become fibrosed to produce brawny induration. Extravasation of blood locally may cause a brownish pigmentation. An itchy eczematoid rash may appear in the area. Finally the skin may ulcerate, which produces an indolent, painless lesion that is usually above the medial malleolus, near a palpable, incompetent communicating vein. This picture of chronic swelling and stasis dermatitis is called the *postphlebitic syndrome*. Arterial pulses are normal. When the deep venous system is blocked, pain similar to intermittent claudication may rarely occur.

Procedure

While the patient is standing, an elastic tourniquet is applied around the upper thigh to compress only the long saphenous vein. The patient then exercises the limb briskly, by walking, kicking, or twisting, for up to 60 seconds. The examiner then notes the prominence of the varicosities. Normally the muscular action of the exercise should empty the blood from the superficial system (long saphenous) through the communicating veins into the deep system. If superficial varicosities disappear, the valves of the communicating and deep veins are competent. If superficial varicosities remain the same, then both the superficial and communicating valves are incompetent. If the varicosities become distended and more prominent and pain develops, the deep veins are obstructed and the valves of the communicating veins are incompetent.

Confirmation Procedures

Buerger's test, claudication test, foot tourniquet test, Homans' sign, Moszkowicz test, Moses' test, vascular assessment

---

Reporting Statement

Perthes' test is positive for the right leg. This result indicates varicosities that are due to incompetency of the valves of the saphenous vein.

~ **Clinical Pearl** ~

Vascular damage may lead to gangrene of the foot and ankle. The circulation must always be observed if it is likely that the vessels have been traumatized seriously by stretching or contusion, and the findings must be recorded. Neurologic damage often accompanies vascular injury.

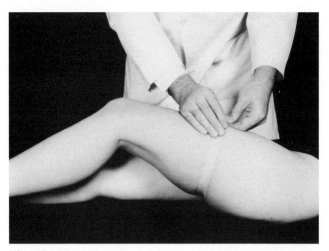

Fig. 12−31 The patient is lying supine on the examining table. A tourniquet is applied at the upper thigh of the affected leg. The tourniquet is only tight enough to compress the long saphenous vein.

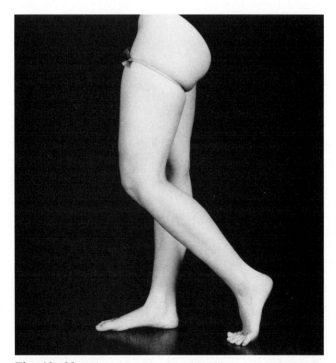

Fig. 12−32 The patient stands and briskly exercises the leg for up to 60 seconds. Prominent varicosities that do not disappear with exercise suggest that the valves of the communicating and deep veins are incompetent.

Comment

The metatarsals are arranged in an arch both in an anteroposterior and in a transverse direction. The transverse arch, in which the central three bones lie at a higher level than the peripheral bones, is pronounced proximally at the tarsometatarsal junctions and becomes shallower toward its distal extremity. The term metatarsal arch refers to the shallow concavity over the plantar aspect of the metatarsal heads. The central three heads are elevated by the transverse metatarsal ligaments and the transverse head of the adductor hallucis muscle. The mechanism is ineffective during weight bearing, but it transfers pressure toward the medial and lateral tarsal heads when the arch is obliterated. During the take-off movement of a step, the intrinsic muscles flex the toes and help elevate the central metatarsal heads off the ground, thus relieving them of pressure. Paralysis of these muscles results in clawed toes, dropped metatarsal heads, and the inevitable plantar calluses.

Stretching of the transverse metatarsal ligaments is a major cause of pain in the forefoot. This pain is due to congenital laxity, which typically results in flatfoot, in which the heel is everted, the longitudinal arch depressed, the metatarsals and the toes widely spread (splayfoot), and the forefoot supinated in relation to the hindfoot. An acquired stretching occurs as a result of obesity, prolonged standing, degenerative changes of aging, and following acute illness. The three central metatarsal heads drop and are prominent in the sole when palpated through the thinned subcutaneous fat.

Weakness of the intrinsics deprives the toes of strong flexor power, and the metatarsal heads drop. With poliomyelitis, paralysis of the foot dorsiflexors results in equinus that throws the weight forward on the foot. In addition, the common cavus deformity, which follows this disease, causes a downward tilting of the metatarsals and added pressure is brought to bear distally.

Any form of arthritis can affect the metatarsophalangeal joints. In young and middle-aged patients, rheumatoid arthritis is suspected. Severe degenerative arthritis favors the first metatarsophalangeal articulation. Degenerative changes in a single joint, other than the first, suggest an antecedent osteochondrosis.

An acute exacerbation of gout characteristically develops around the first metatarsophalangeal joint. Pain is severe and continuous and is aggravated by weight bearing and movement of the large toe.

Prolonged walking will cause a sprain of the transverse metatarsal ligament. Pain occurs throughout the distal metatarsal area during weight bearing and is intensified by spreading the toes passively.

Any deformity of the foot that changes the axis of the metatarsal to a more vertical direction throws forward the pressure of weight bearing.

Procedure

Sudden passive flexing of the toes is painless in a normal foot, but if inflammation exists, pain is experienced in the anterior arch of the foot.

Confirmation Procedures

Morton's test, diagnostic imaging

Reporting Statement

Strunsky's sign is present in the right foot. The presence of this sign indicates metatarsalgia.

◇ Clinical Pearl ◇

Pain in the forefoot, which is called metatarsalgia, can be due to many etiologies. A prominent metatarsal head is a common cause of pain and can follow any operation on the forefoot, including Keller's operation, or dislocation of the second toe.

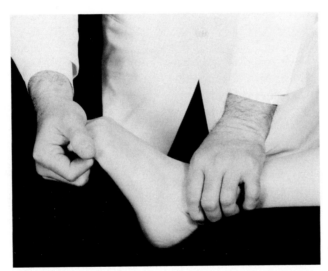

Fig. 12–33.   The patient is lying supine, and the affected leg is extended on the examining table. The examiner grasps the toes of the affected foot. The examiner causes a sudden, passive flexion of the toes. The sign is present if the maneuver causes pain. The presence of this sign indicates inflammation of the anterior arch of the foot (metatarsalgia).

Comment

The calf muscle may be partially or completely ruptured at any place, from its origin on the posterior part of the femoral condyles and back of the tibia to its attachment to the calcaneus. The tear may be in the muscle belly, but it occurs more frequently in the musculotendinous junction between the gastrocnemius and the conjoined tendon with the soleus. The muscle unit may rupture through the tendon or at the attachment to the heel, sometimes avulsing a fragment of bone. As with a muscle rupture anywhere, determination of the location and extent of injury is extremely important. The location is usually determined when the injury is examined early because the tenderness will be quite localized. After several hours, swelling, edema, and inflammation become diffuse and the exact location may be in doubt. Both active and passive stretching will cause pain. If there is complete severance of the whole muscle-tendon unit from the head of the gastrocnemius or the entire gastrocnemius from the conjoined tendon or rupture of the tendon, then loss of function will be noted so the muscle will bunch up during contraction rather than flatten down, as it normally does. If the rupture is in the distal tendon or musculotendinous junction, a palpable defect often can be felt. The condition is quite disabling even with a minor degree of tearing, and it interdicts running or any activity that causes the patient to be on the toes. This loss of function may be due to actual loss of continuity of the tendon, but it more frequently is due to muscle spasm and pain.

Procedure

The patient is prone with the feet hanging over the edge of the examining table. The examiner flexes the knee of the affected leg to 90 degrees and squeezes the calf muscles just below the widest level of the posterior portion of the leg. Normally this maneuver causes a reflex plantar flexion motion of the foot. The test is positive when the foot does not respond. The test indicates a complete rupture of the Achilles tendon.

Confirmation Procedures

Helbings' sign, Hoffa's test, diagnostic imaging

Reporting Statement

Thompson's test is positive for the right ankle. This result indicates loss of integrity of the Achilles tendon.

∾ Clinical Pearl ∾

The Achilles tendon can be torn by the same movements, such as a forward lunge on the sports field or a squash court, that tear the medial head of the gastrocnemius. The patient will feel as though someone has kicked the Achilles tendon. There are legendary stories, in which the victim of such a tear turns around and punches the person behind, in retribution.

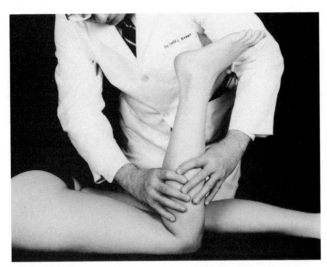

Fig. 12-34 The patient is lying prone on the examination table. The knee of the affected leg is flexed to 90 degrees by the examiner. The examiner grasps the patient's calf with both hands. The patient's musculature is relaxed.

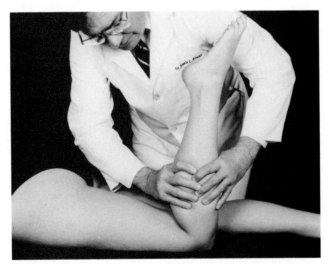

Fig. 12-35 The examiner squeezes the calf musculature at a point just distal to the widest level of the posterior portion of the leg. The test is positive if the foot does not plantar flex with this maneuver. A positive test indicates a rupture of the Achilles tendon.

Comment

Accompanied by their corresponding arteries and veins, the tibial nerve's two terminal branches, the medial and the lateral plantar nerves, pass around the medial malleolus through a fibroosseous tunnel, which is the tarsal tunnel.

Although the etiologies of tarsal tunnel syndrome may be diverse, nerve compression or irritation is a common feature of them all. Mechanical pressure from changes in the tissue relationships within the tunnel remains the common denominator of the proposed etiologies. Therefore trauma and congenital or acquired anomalies predispose these individuals to a higher risk of nerve compression because their tarsal tunnels are abnormally configured. Rather than change the bony components, autoimmune and inflammatory diseases affect the tunnel's soft tissues and decrease the tunnel's volume. Because the tunnel's neural components remain most sensitive to increased pressure, changes in sensory and motor function are among the first symptoms of tunnel damage. The upper section of the tunnel, containing the medial plantar neurovascular structures, remains more sensitive to volume changes than the lower section, which contains the lateral plantar neurovascular structures.

The tibial nerve, like the median nerve, has a rich vascularity, but it is sensitive to ischemia. Compression of the vasa vasorum, which surrounds the nerve, will lead to ischemia and neurologic symptoms. Increased vascular compromise during standing and walking accounts for the crises that appreciate in patients with tarsal tunnel syndrome. In several idiopathic cases that have been relieved by surgery, the nerves were normal in appearance. These cases have been proposed to be vascular in nature.

Procedure

Tapping the area over the posterior tibial nerve (medial plantar nerve) with a reflex hammer produces tingling distal to the percussion. The paresthesia that radiates into the foot indicates tarsal tunnel syndrome.

Confirmation Procedures

Duchenne's sign, electrodiagnosis

Reporting Statement

Tinel's foot sign is positive. The presence of this sign indicates tarsal tunnel syndrome that involves the medial plantar nerve.

~ Clinical Pearl ~

The medial plantar nerve enters the foot after passing beneath the medial ligament of the ankle, which it shares with the posterior tibial and flexor tendons. The structure of this feature is comparable to the carpal tunnel of the wrist. The medial plantar nerve is vulnerable to compression by swelling of the tendons or by space-occupying lesions, such as ganglia. Tarsal tunnel syndrome is not common, but it should be considered for patients who have neurologic symptoms in the hindfoot.

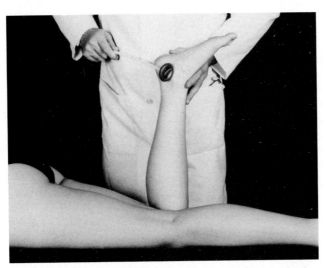

Fig. 12–36 The patient is lying prone on the examination table. The leg may be extended at the knee or flexed. The examiner percusses the posterior tibial nerve (medial plantar nerve) with a reflex hammer. Paresthesia that is elicited distal to the percussion indicates tarsal tunnel syndrome.

Bibliography

American Academy of Orthopaedic Surgeons: *Joint motion: Method of measuring and recording,* Edinburgh, 1965, British Orthopaedic Association.

American Medical Association: *Guides to the evaluation of permanent impairment,* ed 3, Chicago, 1990, The Association.

Apley AG, Solomon L: *Concise system of orthopaedics and fractures,* London, 1988, Butterworth-Heinemann.

Barton NJ: Arthroplasty of the forefoot in rheumatoid arthritis, *J Bone Joint Surg,* 55B:126, 1973.

Beeson PB, McDermott W: *Textbook of medicine* ed 13, Philadelphia, 1971, WB Saunders.

Binak K, Regan TJ, Christensen RC, Hellems HK: Arteriovenous fistula: Hemodynamic effect of occlusion and exercise, *Am Heart J,* 60:495, 1960.

Brahms MA: Common foot problems, *J Bone Joint Surg,* 49A:1653, 1967.

Cahill DR: The anatomy and function of the contents of the human tarsal sinus and canal, *Anat Rec,* 153:1, 1965.

Cailiet R: Foot and ankle pain, Philadelphia, 1979, FA Davis.

Cipriano JJ: *Photographic manual of regional orthopaedic and neurological tests,* ed. 2, Baltimore, 1991, Williams and Wilkins.

Coffman JD: Peripheral collateral blood flow and vascular reactivity in the dog, *J Clin Invest,* 45:923, 1966.

Coffman JD, Mannick JA: An objective test to demonstrate the circulatory abnormality in intermittent claudication, *Circulation,* 33:177, 1966.

Cohen HL, Brumlik J: *A manual of electroneuromyography,* New York, 1968, Harper and Row.

Colter JM: Lateral ligamentous injuries of the ankle, In Hamilton WC (editor): *Traumatic disorder of the ankle,* New York, 1984, Springer-Verlag.

Cooke TDV, Lehmann PO: Intermittent claudication of neurogenic origin, *Can J Surg,* 11:151, 1968.

Cox JM: *Low back pain, mechanism, diagnosis, and treatment,* ed. 5, Baltimore, 1990, Williams and Wilkins.

D'Ambrosia RD: *Musculoskeletal disorders regional examination and differential diagnosis,* Philadelphia, 1977, JB Lippincott.

Dandy DJ: *Essential orthopaedics and trauma,* Edinburgh, 1989, Churchill Livingstone.

Dejong RN: *The neurological examination incorporating the fundamentals of neuroanatomy and neurophysiology,* ed 3, New York, 1967, Harper and Row.

Doherty M, Doherty J: *Clinical examination in rheumatology,* London, 1992, Wolfe Publishing.

DuVries HL: Five myths about your feet, *Today's health,* 45:49-51, Aug. 1967.

DuVries HL: *Surgery of the foot,* ed 2, St. Louis, 1965, Mosby.

Fegan WG, Fitzgerald DE, Beesley WH: A modern approach to the injection treatment of varicose veins and its applications in pregnant patients, *Am Heart J,* 68:757, 1964.

Friedman SA, Holling HE, Roberts B: Etiologic factors in aorto-iliac and femoro-popliteal vascular disease, *N Engl J Med,* 271:1382, 1964.

Gampstorp I: Normal conduction velocity of ulnar, median, and peroneal nerves in infancy, childhood and adolescence, *Acta Paediatrica Scand Suppl,* 146:68, 1963.

Gardner E, Gray DJ: The innervation of the joints of the foot, *Anat Rec,* 161:141, 1968.

Gardner E, Gray DJ, O'Rahilly R: *Anatomy: A regional study of human structure,* ed 4, Philadelphia, 1975, WB Saunders.

Gilliatt RW: Normal conduction in human and experimental neuropathies, *Proc R Soc Lond (Biol),* 59:989, 1966.

Gray H: *Anatomy of the human body,* (Edited by CM Goss) ed 28, Philadelphia, 1966, Lea and Febiger.

Hamilton WC: Anatomy, In Hamilton WC (editor): *Traumatic disorder of the ankle,* New York, 1984, Springer-Verlag.

Hart FD: *French's index of differential diagnosis,* ed. 10, Baltimore, 1973, Williams and Wilkins.

Inman VT: *The joints of the ankle,* Baltimore, 1976, Williams and Wilkins.

Inman VT: DuVries' *Surgery of the foot,* ed. 3, St. Louis, 1973, Mosby.

Jahss MH: *Disorders of the foot,* Philadelphia, 1982, WB Saunders.

Katz WA: *Rheumatic diseases diagnosis and management,* Philadelphia, 1977, JB Lippincott.

Kelikian H, Kelikian AS: *Disorders of the ankle,* Philadelphia, 1985, WB Saunders.

Kendall HO, Kendall FP, Wadsworth GE: *Muscles testing and function,* ed. 2, Baltimore, 1971, Williams and Wilkins.

Kleiger B: Mechanisms of ankle injury, *Orthop Clin North Am,* 5:127, 1974.

Klenerman L: *The foot and its disorders,* ed. 2, Boston, 1982, Blackwell Scientific Publications.

Kouchoukos NT, Levy JF, Balfour JF, Butcher HR: Operative therapy for femoral-popliteal arterial occlusive disease, *Circulation,* 35 (suppl 1):174, 1967.

Lloyd-Roberts GC, Clark RC: Ball and socket ankle joint in metatarsus adductus varus (S-shaped or serpentine foot), *J Bone Joint Surg,* 55B:193, 1973.

Magee DJ: *Orthopedic physical assessment,* Philadelphia, 1987, WB Saunders.

Mann RA: *Surgery of the foot,* St. Louis, 1986, Mosby.

Mannick JA, Nabseth DC: Axillofemoral bypass graft, *N Engl J Med,* 278:461, 1988.

Mazion JM: *Illustrated manual of neurological reflexes/signs/tests, part I, orthopedic signs/tests/maneuvers for office procedure, part II,* Orlando, 1980, Daniels Publishing.

McRae R: *Clinical orthopaedic examination,* ed. 3, Edinburgh, 1990, Churchill Livingstone.

Medical Economics Books: *Patient care flow chart manual,* ed. 3, Oradell, NJ, 1982, Medical Economics Books.

Mennell JM: *Foot pain,* Boston, 1969, Little, Brown.

Milgram JE: Office measures for relief of painful foot, *J Bone Joint Surg,* 46A:1095, 1964.

Morton DJ: Biomechanics of the human foot, *In American Academy of Orthopaedic Surgeons Instructional Course Lectures,* vol 2, Ann Arbor, Mich, 1944, J W Edwards.

Mubarak SJ, Hargens AR: *Compartment syndromes and Volkmann's contracture,* vol 3, Philadelphia, 1981, WB Saunders.

Mullark RE: *The anatomy of varicose veins,* Springfield, IL, 1965, Charles C Thomas.

O'Donoghue DH: *Treatment of injuries to athletes,* ed. 3, Philadelphia, 1976, WB Saunders.

Omer GE, Spinner M: *Management of peripheral nerve problems,* Philadelphia, 1980, WB Saunders.

Pecina NM, Krmpotic-Nemanic J, Markiewitz AD: *Tunnel syndromes,* Boston, 1991, CRC Press.

Post M: *Physical examination of the musculoskeletal system,* Chicago, 1987, Mosby.

Rasmussen O, Tovberg-Jansen I: Anterolateral rotational instability in the ankle joint, *Acta Orthop Scand,* 52:99, 1981.

Salter RB, Harris WR: Injuries involving the epiphyseal plate, *J Bone Joint Surg,* 45A:587, 1963.

Schadt DC, Hines EA Jr., Juergens JL, Barker NW: Chronic atherosclerotic occlusion of the femoral artery, *JAMA,* 175:937, 1961.

Seymour N, Evans DK: A modification of the Grice subtalar arthrodesis, *J Bone Joint Surg,* 50B:372, 1968.

Smorto MP, Basmajian JV: *Clinical electroneurography: An introduction to nerve conduction tests,* Baltimore, 1972, William & Wilkins.

Spittell JA Jr, Palumbo PJ, Love JG, Ellis FH Jr.: Arteriovenous fistula complicating lumbar disk surgery, *N Engl J Med,* 268:1162, 1963.

Tachdjian MO: *The child's foot,* Philadelphia, 1985, WB Saunders.

Thompson T, Doherty J: Spontaneous rupture of the tendon of achilles: A new clinical diagnostic test, *Anat Rec,* 158:126, 1967.

Thurston SE: *The little black book of neurology,* Chicago, 1987, Mosby.

Turek SL: *Orthopaedics principles and their application,* ed. 3, Philadelphia, 1977, JB Lippincott.

Waddell G, McCulloch JA, Kummel E, Venner RM: Nonorganic physical signs in low back pain, *Spine,* 5(1):65, 1980.

Wagner FW Jr: The dysvascular foot: A system for diagnosis and treatment, *Foot Ankle,* 2:64, 1981.

Wilkins RW, Coffman JD: Tests of peripheral vascular efficiency, *Practitioner,* 188:346, 1962.

Wood JE: *The veins,* Boston, 1965, Little, Brown.

Zsoter T, Cronin RFP: Venous distensibility in patients with varicose veins, *Can Med Assoc J,* 94:1293, 1966.

CHAPTER

~ *13* ~

Malingering

*F*eigned illness, or malingering, is a sensitive medicolegal issue. Illness or injury that cannot be supported by medical fact not only confounds the physician's diagnostic procedures and health care delivery, but also serves as an element of fraud in the third-party payer system. Patients participating in this behavior are a bane.

Not all patients who feign an illness are completely aware of their actions. Some patients embellish symptoms and physical signs as learned responses or traits, while others present physical problems with hysterical emotional overlays. The latter group occurs mostly because of fear of the unknown.

Two major categories of hysterical disorders are identified: (1) patients with a fictitious illness, such as in malingering or Munchausen's syndrome, and (2) patients with signs and symptoms that have no organic basis, but who are not deliberately attempting to mislead the physician.

Frequently trivial physical trauma or disease is at the root of a portrayed illness or injury. Often by the time symptom embellishment is clinically recognized, the complaints are of such a magnitude that they are completely incongruous with the original illness or injury. A patient who originally experienced a minor, clinically documented upper respiratory infection now presents with symptoms and subjective complaints that resemble those for histoplasmosis or black-lung disease. Yet another patient may present with total leg disability following a minor thigh contusion. Both patients have in common the total lack of clinical findings to support the complaints, and some type of secondary gain serves as a driving force behind the medical charade.

Individuals may feign physical symptoms to continue in a less strenuous job at work, or they may receive a parking space closer to their place of employment. These individuals may also fake symptoms to gain control over family members or fellow workers. The injured party may also allow others to do work the patient would ordinarily do.

The diagnosis of hysteria should be established only on the basis of positive evidence. Even if the patient has an obvious hysterical disorder, a serious organic illness may still be present.

Conversion symptoms have a physiologic or pathologic substrate. A *conversion disorder* denotes a process in which a patient's emotions become transformed into physical (motor or sensory) manifestations. These patients are asking for help but in an inappropriate way. Conversion symptoms often occur in mentally defective individuals or in adolescents, as a way of coping (albeit inadequately) with the environment. Common presentations include blindness, deafness, paresis, sensory disturbances, ataxia, seizures, and unconsciousness.

Malingering is defined as the conscious misrepresentation of thoughts, feelings, and facts, and it is a condition in which symptoms and signs associated with pain or dysfunction are either partially or entirely feigned for secondary gain. Most commonly, malingering occurs in the setting of the workplace, where worker's compensation is an issue.

It is difficult to label patients as hysterics, frauds, or malingerers. This is rarely accomplished without reaping the wrath of the patient or substantial legal repercussions.

The actual percentage of patients who are malingerers is undetermined. However, it has been estimated that 2% of all patients seeking health care are malingering. Obviously, the ascertainment of the inaccuracy of a patient's report of pain and disability is a difficult process, but the possibility of malingering should be raised in the mind of the treating physician when major discrepancies or inconsistencies appear in the patient's medical situation.

Armed with Borg pain scales, Oswestry disability indices, symptom magnification indexing, and neuroorthopedic malingering tests, the physician is able to substantiate or refute the existence of malingering in any given case. These tests and indices are usually employed with the more traditional neuroorthopedic physical examinations. A singular positive finding or test does not indicate that the patient is magnifying or faking symptoms. Rather, the malingering diagnosis is based on the preponderance of positive malingering-test findings *and* the absence of findings from traditional neuroorthopedic tests. Any positive findings must be further correlated with the medical history of the patient. It is the constellation of positive malingering tests, normal findings in traditional tests, and medical history discrepancies that form the malingering diagnosis. Malingering and psychogenic rheumatism patients primarily complain of pain, sensory losses, or paralysis in any combination.

Index of Tests

Pain qualification and quantification

    Axial trunk-loading test

    Burn's bench test

    Flexed-hip test

    Flip sign

    Libman test

    Magnuson's test

    Mannkopf's sign

    Marked part pain-suggestibility test

    Plantar flexion test

    Related joint motion test

    Seeligmüller's sign

    Trunk rotational test

Sensory deficit qualification and quantification

    Anosmia testing

    Coordination-disturbance testing

    Cuignet's test

    Facial anesthesia testing

    Gault test

    Janet's test

    Limb-dropping test (upper extremities)

    Lombard's test

    Marcus Gunn's sign

    Midline tuning-fork test

    Optokinetic nystagmus test

    Position-sense testing

    Regional anesthesia testing

    Romberg's sign

    Snellen's test

    Stoicism indexing

Paralysis qualification and quantification

    Bilateral leg-dropping test

    Hemiplegic posturing

    Hoover's sign

    Simulated foot-drop testing

    Simulated forearm-and-wrist-weakness testing

    Simulated grip-strength-loss testing

    Tripod test (bilateral leg-fluttering test)

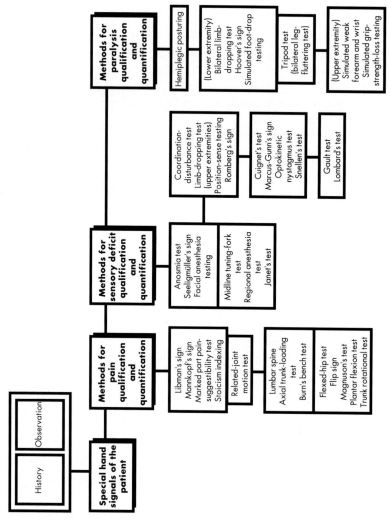

Fig.13–1 Malingering Assessment.

GENERAL PROCEDURES

General Patient Observation

There is consensus among physicians that malingering is readily detected with appropriate medical and psychologic tests. Most patients who have remained conscious during an injury can give an adequate description of what happened. A malingerer is vague and on guard while describing the incidents of an injury or accident. However, some patients, who also remain conscious at the time of injury, are not as observant as others, and these patients will be somewhat vague. There are also patients whose personalities are characterized by a complete lack of definitiveness about everything.

A malingerer often appears quarrelsome, nervous, and ill at ease. General observation of the patient before and after the physical examination may reveal that the patient is fully capable of movements or activities that were claimed to be impossible in the physical examination.

Note how the patient enters and behaves in the reception room. It is helpful if a nonprofessional staff person takes the patient's history and engages the claimant in conversation. Many remarks that will help place the examining physician on guard can be elicited.

When hearing loss is the complaint, speak to the patient calmly and in a very low tone of voice to test the patient's response. With visual-disturbance complaints, give the patient a magazine with fine print to read while waiting, and later ask something about the subject matter.

Ask the patient to describe the accident in detail. Encourage the patient to go through as many of the painful motions as possible. Often, the extreme interest of the examiner in the patient's story will cause the patient to move the arms, legs, or back in a normal manner.

Try to observe the patient tying the shoes, walking down a hallway, bending at the waist, drinking at a fountain, pulling or pushing a door, or many other unguarded activities of daily living.

Detailed History

Occasionally, the physician is called upon to distinguish fraud or exaggeration from organic injury. As should be apparent by now, this is not an easy task. An examination, when deception or exaggeration is suspected, should be completed with a strictly impartial attitude on the part of the examiner. The patient must be accorded all the tact and courtesy that is ordinarily extended to any other patient. If the doctor-patient rapport is compromised, confidence is destroyed and questions and tests, which are constructed to evoke sincerity on the part of the patient, become unreliable.

In many instances the patient grudgingly gives the history. The malingering patient may remark "I've told this to the last doctor, and I don't see any reason to repeat it." The patient also may deny permission to review previous x-ray findings or case histories, stating that the attorney can only grant such permission. The genuine patient usually will not hesitate in this regard.

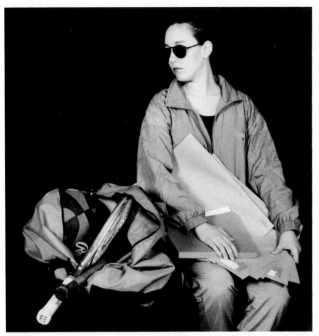

Fig. 13–2 When observing a malingering patient, the examiner will note the following: (1) the patient will fail to make consistent eye contact and may obscure eye contact with sunglasses; (2) the patient may be dressed in clothing that indicates athletic involvement, which is inappropriate for an injury, of a supposedly disabled patient; (3) the patient usually carries a voluminous medical file and an aggregation of radiographs from doctor to doctor; (4) the patient may be impatient; (5) the patient may be unwilling to participate in a full examination, not wanting to risk exposure of the feigned illness. Other subtle signs to watch for are appointments—such as a tennis match immediately following the examination of the disabled lower back—that are inappropriate for the disability.

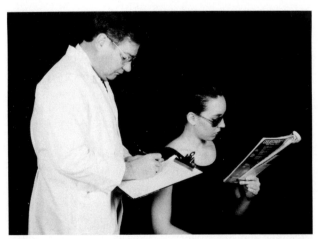

Fig. 13–3 A detailed history from a malingering patient is difficult to acquire and assess. The patient may relate queer and exaggerated stories of the injurious event, or the patient may act disinterested and distant in the history interview. The patient avoids eye contact.

Malingerers will give an involved and long history, most of which is often discovered to be false.

When the patient's history, actions, and examination findings suggest that symptoms are exaggerated, it is the duty of the physician to make the examination so complete that there will be no question as to the actual extent of any organic disease or injury.

The physician's next duty is to decide whether the patient is a malingerer attempting to defraud and deceive, or whether hysteria or neurasthenia exists, in which the patient benignly imagines the disability. Many patients become convinced that a certain type of disability is due to a specific injury. If the physician can establish sufficient confidence with the patient to explain and treat the condition effectively, often the exaggerated symptoms will disappear. However, with malingering, any attempt on the part of the physician to confront the patient results in further exaggeration.

To achieve a secondary gain, the malingerer must use subterfuge. Exaggeration usually is obvious no matter how cleverly it is performed. The malingerer exhibits slyness of expression and watches the examiner carefully during the various procedures. The patient may try to impress the examiner with the importance of the case and frequently reiterates a great degree of personal honesty. The patient appears to be constantly suspicious that detection is likely and attempts to avoid disclosure.

A detailed history is the first essential, and many times the answers to questions must be requested repeatedly. The patient may give strange stories about the exact nature of an accident or the treatment that was previously administered for the condition.

Psychogenic Rheumatism Profile

Patients with psychiatric disorders may develop pain as part of the symptoms associated with mental illness. Patients with pain also may develop psychiatric disorders as part of the symptoms associated with the physical illness. Pain associated with neurosis is more common than pain associated with schizophrenia or endogenous depression. There are four reasons for psychologic illness that cause the appearance or exacerbation of pain: (1) patient anxiety, (2) psychiatric hallucination, (3) increased tension in the muscles, with associated inadequate circulation and the accumulation of metabolic byproducts (lactic acid), and (4) hysteria with conversion reactions.

Psychogenic rheumatism is a term used to describe patients who have musculoskeletal psychiatric disorders. An example of psychogenic rheumatism that is associated with back pain is camptocormia, which is a special form of conversion hysteria that occurs mainly in military service personnel and industrial workers. The disease is characterized by the patient's assumption of a posture in which the back is flexed acutely, the arms hang loosely, and the patient's eyes are directed downward. The posture disappears when the patient assumes a recumbent position. Many of the

---

Symptoms and Signs of Psychogenic Rheumatism★

1. Dramatic urgency for an appointment that is not justified by the severity of the disease.
2. A list (in writing), of complaints so long and detailed that no fact is left out.
3. Multiple test results, including EKG, EMG, EEG, barium enema, upper GI, CT scans, myelograms, and MRI, with no positive findings.
4. The patient demands to review the laboratory data first, to determine the cause of the symptoms. Any minor abnormalities are highlighted by the patient.
5. Preoccupation with future disability from minor physical changes.
6. Those who accompany the patient may be entirely separated from the patient's condition or intensely supportive. The companion may be highlighting every abnormality, frequently using the pronoun "we" during the description of tests or treatments.
7. Inability of the patient to relax during the examination.
8. Marked theatrical responses to questions concerning pain.
9. The patient frequently holds onto the physician during the examination, as a gesture of seeking support.

★From *Clinics in Rheumatic Diseases,* 5:797 Philadelphia, 1979, WB Saunders.

---

afflicted individuals are males, whose parents have had back disorders. Therapy for the condition involves separation of the individual from the source of stress. Patients who have this condition and are in the military have had quick recoveries within days of receiving the news that they have been discharged from the armed forces.

Symptoms and signs found in patients with psychogenic rheumatism are listed in the box above.

The malingerer exaggerates or fakes a condition or injury. It is important to believe the history the patient relates even though malingering is suspected.

In many instances a malingerer can be extremely convincing during the examination. The malingering patient usually complains of sensory loss, paralysis, pain, or a combination of these symptoms. A hysterical patient will claim similar problems. Unlike the hysterical patient, the malingerer consciously attempts to deceive the doctor.

Two separate sets of criteria have been developed to document the likelihood of malingering, the Emory Pain Control Center inconsistency profile and Ellard's profile of inconsistency. Although these inconsistency profiles were developed independently, they are similar.

Combined Emory and Ellard Inconsistency Profiles*

1. Discrepancies become apparent between a patient's complaints of terrible pain and an attitude of calmness and well-being.

2. A complete workup for organic disease by two or more physicians is negative.

3. The patient makes dramatized complaints that are vague or have global implications. "It just hurts," or "I hurt bad." This may be further attested by malingering hand signals.

4. The patient exaggerates a trivial pathologic condition (such as a *mild* strain, muscular cramp or contusion) and embellishes it with medical terms learned from previous contact with physicians. "My back spasms paralyze my legs."

5. The patient overemphasizes gait or posture abnormalities that develop suddenly, persist, and cannot be substantiated objectively. For example, the patient complains of a limp that is not confirmed by a specific pattern of wear on old shoes or the patient reports daily use of a cane or back brace, but these items show little wear.

6. The patient resists evaluation or rehabilitation when the stated goal of therapy is a return to gainful employment.

7. The patient exhibits a lack of motivation to learn new coping skills, despite verbal reports of compliance with treatment. (For instance, the patient will show no increase in back motion despite claims of completing range-of-motion exercise daily).

8. The patient misses appointments for objective studies that measure function, motion, or vocational capabilities.

9. The patient has an unconventional response to treatment, such as reports of increased symptoms following therapy, that follows no anatomic or physiologic pattern. For example, the patient may respond to tranquilizers as if they are stimulants and vice versa.

10. The patient shows resistance to treatment procedures, especially in the presence of intense complaints of pain.

11. Psychologic or emotional disturbances are absent.

12. Psychologic tests are inconsistent and without clinical presentations. For example, the MMPI profile indicates a psychotic disorder, but no clinical signs of psychosis are present.

13. Discrepancies arise between reports by the patient and spouse or other close relatives.

14. Personal and occupational history appears unstable.

15. The patient's personal history reflects a character disorder that might include drug or alcohol abuse, criminal or compulsive behavior, erratic personal relationships, and violence.

*From Evans RC: Malingering/symptoms exaggeration, In Sweere JJ (ed): *Chiropractic Family Practice,* Gaithersburg, 1992, Aspen Publishers.

Special Hand Signals by the Patient

How a patient uses the hands to describe the area of pain is useful in determining the validity of the complaints. Patients with organic, pain-producing lesions are concerned that the source of the pain might be missed. When directed to point to the pain, this type of patient will touch the part with one or two fingers, which is representative of a more focal appreciation of the discomfort. In severe expression of the symptoms, this patient also may place the examiner's hand on the exact location of the pain. These patients do not want to risk having the source missed and not treated.

The psychogenic rheumatic patient uses the whole hand to paint the area of involvement with pain. Because this type of patient perceives the lesion abnormally, the distribution is painted to cover a whole body part. More than one dermatome boundary is crossed by this pain, and this patient's discomfort is real. The discomfort may have origin in an organic lesion but, because of learned responses or fear, the patient rubs the whole part with the hand to indicate its extent. Careful questioning and guidance will help this patient better define the most focal trigger areas.

At first malingering patients take care not to touch the area they claim experiences pain. Because the complaint is a sham, touching of the part abets the lie. The examiner often inadvertently aids this process by physically touching the area of complaint, before the patient has. The patient now only has to agree with the frustrated examiner, concerning the exact location of the pain.

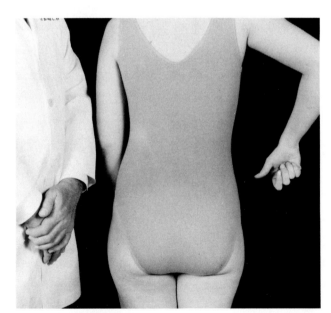

Fig. 13–4 At first the malingering patient takes care not to touch the area of claimed pain. The complaint is a sham, so the patient allows the examiner to touch the part first, and then the patient simply agrees with the suggested origin of pain.

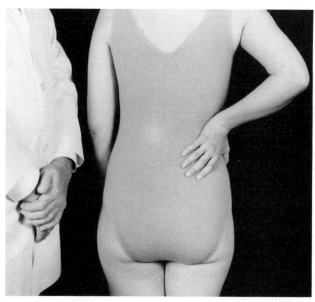

Fig. 13–5 The hysteric patient, or the patient with psychogenic rheumatism, paints the area of complaint with the whole hand. The discomfort is real, but the borders of the complaint exceed the known anatomic distributions. Careful investigation will define the focal triggers.

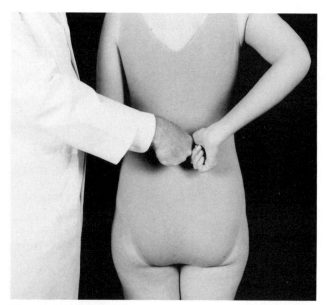

Fig. 13–6 Patients experiencing organic pain for the first time are concerned that the lesion will be missed. This patient will touch the part, precisely locating it with one or two fingers. The patient also may hold the examiner's finger on the spot of worst complaint.

PAIN QUALIFICATION AND QUANTIFICATION

Overview

Pain is an image that becomes perfected in the sensorium of the cerebral cortex. This pain image is created by stimuli that have passed through a chain of lower centers, in which they are modified and refined. Even at the cortical level, the pain image is subject to changes by associated constitutional and emotional factors. Stimuli coming from the same source and passing through the same modifications by the lower centers, will produce in one patient a pain image of bright and burning colors, and in another, a faded out, unimpressive design. The patient's constitution is mirrored in this difference.

The three main relay stations for sensory stimuli wandering from the periphery to the sensory cortex are (1) the peripheral sensory nervous system, with its cell station in the spinal ganglia, (2) the pathways and centers in the spinal cord and medulla, and (3) the sensory centers of the diencephalon, especially the thalamus. Each of the latter two have intermediate, subsidiary relay stations.

In general, the closer to the axis of the body, the more scant is the distribution of sensory end organs in the tissues and the less precise the allocation of the pain source. There are some exceptions. Some deep-lying structures are intensely sensitive because of their rich endowment with pain-conducting terminal fibers, in contrast to other structures occupying the same anatomic plane. An example is sacrolumbalgia with characteristic trigger points from injured ligamentous structures that lie beneath the covering musculature. The periosteum is another highly sensitive structure. Sensory nerves are obvious exceptions from the rule because they are the conductors of pain.

The differential diagnosis and evaluation of pain depend on a description of the intensity of the unpleasant sensation, a comparison by the patient to other known sensations, and an attempted designation of the severity of the pain based on a number system.

The spectrum of pain awareness and severity varies from a minimal pain response that is tolerated and easily overlooked to an unbearable sensation that interferes with the individual's productive activities.

There are physiologic variations of the pain threshold from one person to another. There is an inherent, definable difference in the pain level that varies from congenital insensitivity to pain or to a state of hypersensitivity to almost any external stimulus.

Congenital insensitivity to pain is recognized as a true syndrome in which the person does not respond to epicritic stimuli, or even fractures of the extremities, by anything other than a descriptive comment concerning the injury. These patients do not complain of pain.

A high threshold of pain is recognized in many individuals who tolerate painful stimuli—such as heat, cold, sharp, or heavy pressure—and recognize the abnormal sensation

---

Borg-Type Pain Scale★

On a scale of 1–10, place an X at your current pain level.

Normal	Low pain	Moderate pain	Intense pain	Emergency
( ) 0	( ) 1	( ) 4	( ) 7	( ) 10
	( ) 2	( ) 5	( ) 8	
	( ) 3	( ) 6	( ) 9	

Scoring: (0–3) Patients at this level may be able to return to work depending on many factors. (4–5) The transitional zone may indicate a significant degree of impairment for a nonsymptom magnifying patient or a low level of impairment for a patient who has a low pain threshold. (6–10) This level indicates a severe pathologic condition or symptom magnification behavior. Above (10) indicates symptom magnification.

★From Borg G: Psychophysical bases of perceived exertion, *Med Sci Sports Exerc* 14(5):377, 1982.

---

and the kind of sensation but who are able to accept the stimulus with minimal response.

A temporary, limited awareness of pain occurs immediately after certain severe injuries, such as a tear of major ligaments around the knee during a football game or a severe inversion injury to the ankle resulting in massive ligamentous tear. The individual experiences sudden, exquisite pain at the time of the injury and may become hypotensive, nauseated, and faint. During the recovery phase the injured part may be manipulated with little or no discomfort in certain instances. However, within several minutes after injury the pain pattern associated with periosteal injury, distended synovium and capsule, and pressure from hematoma, becomes severe.

An average reaction to pain stimuli characterizes that which most individuals have to a sudden sharp point, to excessive heat, or to a severe rotary injury to a joint. The individual with an average pain tolerance will describe pain in the shoulder as dull and aching but compatible with moderate limitation of the activities of daily living. If the pain is more severe, the condition will be described as sharp, lancinating, and intermittently severe. The circadian cycle affects the intensity of the pain. Complaints of pain are usually greater at night and may increase as barometric pressure increases. External modalities—such as excessive heat or cold, or an unusual degree of compression or forcible rotation—cause pain to increase.

The individual's personality affects the average reaction to pain. Those with hysterical personalities or with a tendency for hypochondriasis or those who are anxious and depressed respond with more frequent and intense complaints concerning pain, and they overreact to the severity of the stimulus. Pain is affected by sleep deprivation and an unnaturally high anxiety level. Individuals with a labile personality who have acute pain, may overreact to painful stimulus. The same individuals may become dependent and passive and accept chronic pain, although they frequently complain about the effect of the pain on their personality. For example, they state that the pain lessens their sex drive and performance and alters their disposition. The emotional aspects of pain cannot be separated from the physical aspects. A severe toothache that interferes with sleeping, eating, and working is represented by a much higher degree of pain and responds less readily to medications and external applications than does the acute form of pain that is present for only a short period and does not affect rest and nutrition.

A patient who actually is in pain, demonstrates a definite pallor or change in the facial features. Pain often will produce positive evidence, through involuntary muscle spasm and contractures, leading to postural attitudes for relief. The patient who is in genuine pain will perspire freely and flinch consistently. Also, the pulse will increase suddenly, the blood pressure may rise, and the pupils will dilate. In a malingerer, the pulse does not change, the pupils do not dilate abnormally and the complaints of pain will usually be greater than the clinical findings can support.

Anesthesia denotes a state in which a patient gives no demonstrable recognition of external stimuli except for stimuli that involves movement of the part with extreme pressure that causes tendon or bone stimulation.

Hypesthesia (hypoesthesia) is the diminution of the ability to recognize cutaneous stimulation caused by pressure made with a sharp point or a dull object. This description usually designates alteration of a dermatome.

Dysesthesia is an uncomfortable, unpleasant sensation that results from stimulation of a cutaneous region, caused or affected by peripheral nerve trauma or regeneration. Stimulation of one side of a digit may actually be felt in an adjacent digit.

Paresthesia is painful tingling, aching, and/or burning along the course of a peripheral nerve that results from percussion of the involved nerve or stimulation of the skin in the autonomous zone of the involved nerve.

Hyperesthesia is the unpleasant feeling of excessive sensation that results from cutaneous stimulation. Hair follicles in the geographic dermatome are excessively sensitive to touch, as are the skin and cuticle, of that digit.

Cold intolerance is the dull, deep, aching sensation in a segment of the extremity that occurs as the environmental temperature is lowered. The more rapidly the temperature drops the greater is the pain. The pain distribution is not well localized and is not relieved immediately by warming the part. The pain associated with cold intolerance may be minimal if the temperature is dropped slowly but may be severe if warm-up is accomplished too rapidly.

Burning, searing, cutting, and hot are terms commonly used by individuals with peripheral dysfunction lesions that result from complete or partial nerve trauma.

Pain problems can be categorized as (1) pure nerve pain, (2) pain associated with nerve and vascular insufficiency, or (3) pain related to numerous local alterations, such as inadequate skin coverage, fibrosis, bone pressure, tendon irritation, and collagen fibrosis.

Determining the most relevant factors, whether biologic or psychologic, should be incorporated into a prospective assessment of each patient. The goal is the identification of individuals who will and will not benefit from medical and surgical management of pain.

Oswestry-Type Pain-Disability Questionnaire*

This questionnaire has been designed to give the examiner information about pain and how it affects your ability to manage in everyday life. Please circle, in each section, only *one* statement that most closely applies to you.

Section 1: Pain intensity
1. I can tolerate the pain I have without having to use painkillers.
2. The pain is bad, but I manage without taking painkillers.
3. Painkillers give complete relief from pain.
4. Painkillers give moderate relief from pain.
5. Painkillers give very little relief from pain.
6. Painkillers have no affect on the pain, and I do not use them.

Section 2: Personal care (washing, dressing, etc.)
1. I can look after myself normally, without causing extra pain.
2. I can look after myself normally, but it causes extra pain.
3. It is painful to look after myself, and I am slow and careful.
4. I need some help, but I manage most of my personal care.
5. I need help everyday in most aspects of self care.
6. I do not get dressed. I wash with difficulty and stay in bed.

Section 3: Lifting
1. I can lift heavy weights without increased pain.
2. I can lift heavy weights, but it gives added pain.
3. Pain prevents me from lifting heavy weights off the floor, but I can manage if they are conveniently positioned, such as on a table.
4. Pain prevents me from lifting heavy weights, but I can manage light to medium weights if they are conveniently positioned.
5. I can lift only very light weights.
6. I cannot lift or carry anything at all.

Section 4: Walking

1. Pain does not prevent me from walking any distance.
2. Pain prevents me from walking more than 1 mile.
3. Pain prevents me from walking more than 1/2 mile.
4. Pain prevents me from walking more than 1/4 mile.
5. I can only walk using a cane or crutches.
6. I am in bed most of the time and have to crawl to the toilet.

Section 5: Sitting

1. I can sit in any chair as long as I like.
2. I can only sit in my favorite chair as long as I like.
3. Pain prevents me from sitting more than 1 hour.
4. Pain prevents me from sitting for more than 1/2 hour.
5. Pain prevents me from sitting more than 10 minutes.
6. Pain prevents me from sitting at all.

Section 6: Standing

1. I can stand as long as I want without added pain.
2. I can stand as long as I want, but it gives me added pain.
3. Pain prevents me from standing for more than 1 hour.
4. Pain prevents me from standing for more than 30 minutes.
5. Pain prevents me from standing for more than 10 minutes.
6. Pain prevents me from standing at all.

Section 7: Sleeping

1. Pain does not prevent me from sleeping well.
2. I can sleep well only by using sleeping tablets.
3. Even when I take sleeping tablets, I have less than 6 hours of sleep.
4. Even when I take sleeping tablets, I have less than 4 hours of sleep.
5. Even when I take sleeping tablets, I have less than 2 hours of sleep.
6. Pain prevents me from sleeping at all.

Section 8: Sexual activity

1. My sexual activity is normal and causes no extra pain.
2. My sexual activity is normal but causes some extra pain.
3. My sexual activity is nearly normal but is very painful.
4. My sexual activity is severely restricted by pain.
5. My sexual activity is nearly absent because of pain.
6. Pain prevents any sexual activity at all.

Section 9: Social life

1. My social life is normal and gives me no extra pain.
2. My social life is normal but increases the degree of pain.
3. Pain has no significant effect on my social life, other than limiting my more energetic interests, such as dancing.
4. Pain restricts my social life, and I do not go out often.
5. Pain has restricted by social life to my home.
6. I have no social life because of pain.

Section 10: Traveling

1. I can travel anywhere without added pain.
2. I can travel anywhere, but it gives me added pain.
3. Pain is bad, but I manage journeys of more than 2 hours.
4. Pain restricts me to a journey of less than 1 hour.
5. Pain restricts me to short, necessary journeys that take no longer than 30 minutes.
6. Pain prevents me from traveling, except to the doctor or hospital.

Scoring

Each item is given a point value ranging from 0–5, from top to bottom, for a potential total score of 0–50. The score is doubled for a total percentage score. If an item is not answered, [or an answer is made up by the patient] it is dropped from the total potential score and the total percentage is calculated using the remaining answers. The percentages are interpreted as follows: 0%–20% indicates minimal disability in the activities of daily living (ADL), 20%–40% moderate ADL disability, 40%–60% severe ADL disability, 60%–80% crippled ADL disability, 80%–100% symptom magnification or bed bound.

*From Fairbank JTC: The Oswestry low back disability questionnaire, *Physiotherapy*, 66:271, 1980, Chartered Society of Physiotherapy.

Pure malingering is suggested by the following characteristics: (1) the simulation of a nonexisting illness or injury, (2) the voluntary provocation, aggravation, and protraction of disease by artificial means, and (3) false allegations about the existence of some malady, such as epilepsy

---

∿ Tips for Assessment of Pain ∿

Feigning or pretense of nonexisting symptoms by word, gesture, action, or behavior is *simulation* (positive malingering) or *dissimulation* (negative malingering). The deliberate and designed feigning of disease or disability, or the intentional concealment of disease, if it exists, is *pure malingering*. The magnification or intensification of symptoms that already exist is *partial malingering* or *exaggeration*. Ascribing morbid phenomena or symptoms to a definite cause, although the cause may be recognized or ascertained to have no relationship to the symptoms, is *false imputation*.

Comment

In the valid patient, any antalgic position can be taken as a sign that pain can be alleviated or abolished. An antalgic position, which is assumed automatically, cannot easily be simulated, and it is a protective measure. With uncomplicated lumbosacral strain, the typical antalgic position when standing is slight forward flexion. When maintaining this position, it is not only the abdominal muscles, as forward flexors of the trunk, that are under tension but also the long back muscles, even though they are extensors. The antalgic position does not merely block extension, but it also prevents an excess of forward flexion.

Procedure

The examiner presses the patient's cranium in a downward direction. The existing antalgic positioning must not be disturbed during the axial loading. The axial loading may elicit pain in the neck, but it should not elicit pain in the lower back. Suspect malingering if the patient indicates that pain is felt in the lower back.

Confirmation Procedures

Burn's bench test, flexed-hip test, flip sign, Magnuson's test, plantar flexion test, trunk rotational test

> **Reporting Statement**
>
> The axial trunk-loading test is positive and elicits a complaint of pain in the lumbar spine. This result suggests a lack of organic basis for the lower back complaint.

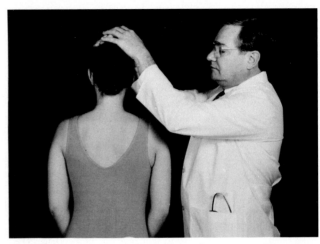

Fig. 13–7 The patient is in the standing position. The examiner presses downward on the patient's head with both hands carefully and not disturbing the existing antalgic posture. The axial loading may elicit pain in the neck, but should not elicit pain in the lower back. Lower back pain is a positive finding and indicates a lack of organic basis for the lower back complaint.

∼ Burn's Bench Test ∼

Comment

A herniated disc can be defined as the herniation of the nucleus pulposus through the fibers of the annulus fibrosus.

The patient's major complaint is a sharp lancinating pain. Often there is a prior history of intermittent episodes of localized back pain. The pain also radiates down the leg in the anatomic distribution of the affected nerve root, and it is usually described as deep and sharp, progressing from above downward. The onset of pain may be insidious or sudden and may be associated with a tearing or snapping sensation in the spine. Occasionally, when sciatica develops, the back pain resolves. Once the annulus is ruptured, it may no longer be under tension. Disc herniation occurs with sudden physical effort when the trunk is flexed or rotated. The sciatica may vary in intensity, and it may be so severe that a patient is unable to ambulate and feels as if the back is locked.

Procedure

The patient is instructed to kneel on a stool and bend the trunk forward, far enough to allow touching of the floor with fingertips or hands. Patients who may be expected to perform this test successfully include those afflicted with sciatica, sacralization, spondylolisthesis, compression fractures of vertebra, etc. A malingerer will fail to perform the maneuver and usually states "I can't do it," or words to that effect, even before attempting the move.

Confirmation Procedures

Axial trunk-loading test, flexed-hip test, flip sign, Magnuson's test, plantar flexion test, trunk rotational test

---

Reporting Statement

Burn's bench test cannot be accomplished. This result suggests a lack of organic basis for the patient's lower back complaint.

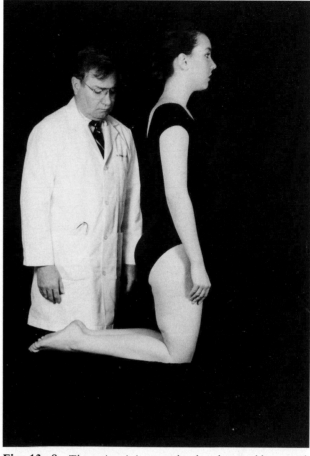

Fig. 13–8 The patient is instructed to kneel on a table or stool, approximately 18 inches from the floor.

Continued.

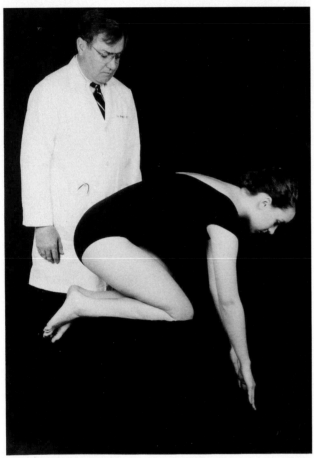

Fig. 13-9 The patient is then instructed to flex the trunk forward.

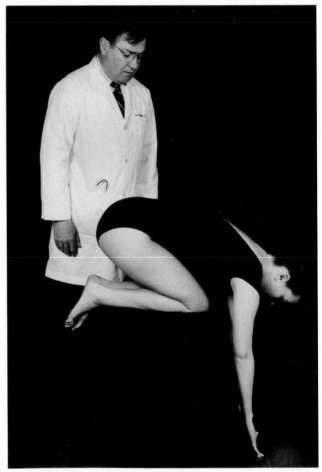

Fig. 13-10 This flexion should be far enough to allow the patient to touch the floor. This maneuver does not affect the lumbar tissues to any significant degree. A malingering patient will fail to perform the maneuver, stating "I can't do it," or words to that effect.

Comment

Acute pain in the back that radiates down to the knee but will not radiate beyond this point without neurologic abnormality, is usually due to an acute muscle or ligament injury in the lumbar spine. The symptoms can be precipitated by a sudden violent movement or by a comparatively trivial movement following a period of hard work.

Tall, slim patients with willowy backs and weak muscles are especially prone to acute back strains, as are those in sedentary occupations. Those who sit for a long time and then have to lift heavy weights without an adequate warm-up are very vulnerable. Such occupations include a delivery person, who may drive in a vehicle over bumpy surfaces for more than an hour with the spine flexed and then leap out of the seat to lift a heavy weight from the vehicle.

The sacroiliac joints are also subject to acute strains. Although the joints have a large surface area, they have poor mechanical cohesion and violent twisting strains can cause severe pain around the joints.

Procedure

Place one hand under the patient's lumbar spine and the other hand under the patient's knee. Lift the knee while flexing the hip. If the patient indicates that lower back and/or leg pain is felt in the lower back, before the lumbar spine moves, suspect malingering.

Confirmation Procedures

Axial trunk-loading test, Burn's bench test, flip sign, Magnuson's test, plantar flexion test, trunk rotational test

Reporting Statement

The flexed hip test elicits pain before movement at the lumbosacral spine occurs. This test demonstrates a lack of organic basis for the patient's complaint.

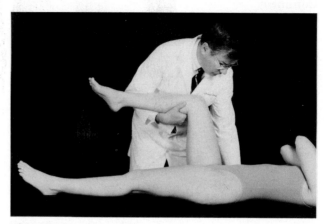

Fig. 13–11 The patient is supine on the examination table. The examiner places one hand under the patient's lumbar spine, palpating the bony landmarks of the L5 and S1 spinous processes. The examiner maintains contact with these landmarks. While the knee is passively held in 90 degrees of flexion, the examiner flexes the hip to 90 degrees. If lower back and/or leg pain is experienced before the L5 and S1 spinouses separate, malingering is suspected.

Comment

With the patient who has a valid lower back injury, a full neurologic examination is warranted for the patient if there are continued root symptoms. Enhanced imaging (CT, MRI) is indicated if there is continued disabling pain, despite a period of absolute rest, and if the distribution of the pain does not give a clear indication of which root is involved. Enhanced studies are required if there is paralysis of any muscle that does not recover within a few days. Further investigation is required if there is any disturbance of micturition. If the pain is clearly in the distribution of a lumbar root but is not accompanied by any stiffness of the back, enhanced studies are warranted. This situation may be observed in spinal neurofibromata.

Procedure

While the patient is lying in a supine position on the examining table, the examiner raises the patient's affected leg, keeping the knee straight. If this movement is limited by pain or muscle resistance, the examiner then directs the patient to sit up, making sure the legs are kept flat on the table. If the patient can sit in this manner without pain, the test is positive. Sitting with the legs straight out reproduces the same maneuver as a straight leg-raising test.

Confirmation Procedures

Axial trunk-loading test, Burn's bench test, flexed-hip test, Magnuson's test, plantar flexion test, trunk rotational test.

> ### Reporting Statement
>
> Flip sign is present and indicates a lack of organic basis for the patient's complaint.

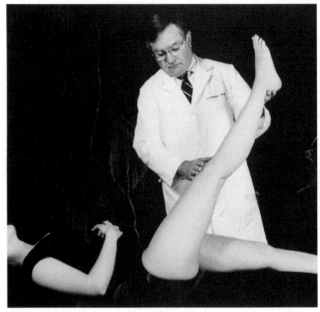

Fig. 13–12 The patient is lying supine on the examination table. The examiner performs a straight-leg raising test on the affected side, noting the limitation of movement because of pain or muscle spasm.

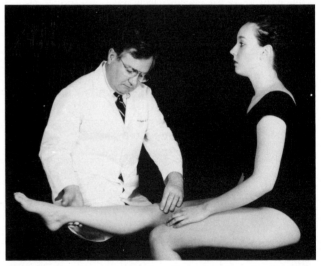

Fig. 13–13 The patient is then directed to sit at the side of the examination table, with the legs dangling over the edge. On pretext of examining an uninvolved joint of the leg, the examiner fully extends the knee of the affected leg, effecting a straight-leg raising sciatic stretch maneuver. If the maneuver does not elicit pain, the test is positive and malingering should be suspected. In a modification of this test, the patient is directed to sit up from the position in Fig. 13–12, with the legs extended and flat on the examination table. If the patient can sit up in this manner, the test is positive.

Comment

Central pain is usually characterized by spontaneous pain, hyperpathia, and hyperalgesia. The term *spontaneous pain* is used to denote the absence of extrinsic stimuli, which ordinarily produce pain. Spontaneous pain is frequently differentiated from evoked pain in which the stimuli are obvious. Hyperpathia designates a painful overreaction to different stimuli and is associated with diminished sensibility to the form of stimulation that excites such a reaction. Hyperalgesia is an overreaction without diminished sensibility or sensory loss. In the last two, regardless of the threshold value, the sensation evoked is abnormal. These painful sensations always develop in an explosive manner, are of an excessive, compelling, diffuse, and complex nature, and they continue unduly after stimulation has ceased.

Procedure

The examiner applies finger pressure to the mastoid process. The pressure is gradually increased until the patient states that it is becoming noticeably uncomfortable. This point is an indication of that patient's pain threshold, which varies from patient to patient. The threshold gives the examiner an idea if this patient has a low, high, or moderate pain threshold. The threshold is not to be used specifically as a criteria for malingering. Identifying a patient's pain threshold will quantify discomfort in this patient and applies to this patient only. This testing procedure will be useful during interpretation of palpation findings or subjective statements concerning pain or discomfort.

Confirmation Procedures

Mannkopf's sign, marked part pain-suggestibility test, related joint motion test.

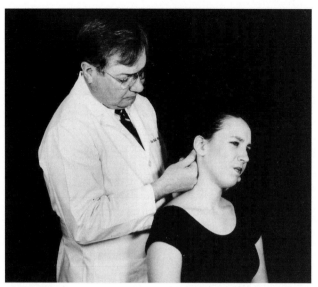

Fig. 13–14 The patient is seated, and the examiner is positioned behind the patient. The examiner applies thumb pressure to the mastoid process and gradually increases the pressure until the patient states that it is becoming noticeably uncomfortable. The test may be repeated for comparison on the opposite mastoid process. This test provides an indication of the patient's pain threshold and is a useful index for interpretation of palpation findings in later examination procedures.

Reporting Statement

Libman's sign demonstrates an unusually low threshold for pain in the patient.

Libman's sign demonstrates a normal threshold for pain in this patient.

Comment

Cutaneous tenderness is present when pain and discomfort are elicited by a normally innocuous amount of pressure. This tenderness may be related to, but is slightly different from, hyperalgesia. Pain may or may not be concomitantly present. The tenderness may be due to a direct, underlying pathologic condition, such as occurs with inflammatory lesions or after trauma to the skin, subcutaneous, and muscular tissue. The tenderness may occur as a result of peripheral nerve lesions, or it may occur as a result of a visceral or deep, somatic pathologic condition at some distance from the tenderness. The tenderness may be present over the area where pain is felt, or it may be absent entirely from that area and found at some distant point. The latter condition exists in visceral disease, for example in cholecystitis, in which the pain is felt in the back at the angle of the scapula, while the tenderness is felt in the skin of the upper right quadrant. Cutaneous tenderness may be elicited by pinching the skin or pressing on it, and it should always be compared with a symmetrically identical area on the opposite side.

Procedure

The patient with lower back pain is directed to point to the site of the pain. The examiner marks that site. The examiner then distracts the patient by performing an examination away from the marked site of pain and later resumes the examination of the lower back. The test is positive with any significant change in the location of the pain. The test is significant as evidence of simulated pain, hysteria, or malingering.

Confirmation Procedures

Axial trunk-loading test, Burn's bench test, flexed-hip test, flip sign, plantar flexion test, trunk rotational test

---

Reporting Statement

Magnuson's test is positive with significant changes between the location of the sites of pain during testing. This result indicates a lack of organic basis for the patient's lower back complaint.

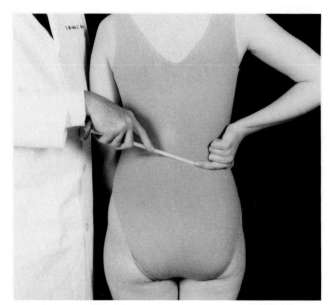

Fig. 13–15 The patient may be standing or seated for this test. The patient is directed to point to the site of lower back pain. The examiner marks the site.

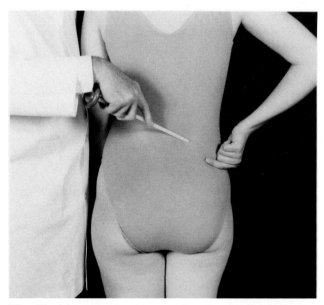

Fig. 13–16 Following distraction by other examination procedures, the patient is instructed to once again point to the location of the lower back pain. The test is positive when the patient identifies any site other than the original. The test is significant for simulated lower back pain, hysteria, or malingering.

Comment

The autonomic nervous system is a division of the peripheral nervous system that distributes to smooth muscle and glands throughout the body. By definition the autonomic nervous system is entirely a motor (efferent) system and is automatic in the sense that most of its functions are carried out below the conscious level.

The sympathetic division of the autonomic nervous system is thrown into activity in preparing the organism for fight or flight, and it causes a mass response because of the existence of sympathetic ganglion chains or plexuses where the preganglionic synapse occurs. In action the sympathetic nervous system produces vasoconstriction of the skin and viscera, shifting more blood to the brain, skeletal muscles, and heart.

Procedure

The examiner establishes the patient's resting pulse rate, and the patient is made as comfortable as possible. Then, without changing the patient's position, the examiner applies mechanical pressure or electrical stimulation over the painful area, while monitoring the pulse rate. An increase in pulse rate of 10 or more beats per minute constitutes a positive sign. The sign is absent in simulated pain.

Confirmation Procedures

Libman's sign, marked part pain-suggestibility test, related joint motion test

---

Reporting Statement

Mannkopf's sign is present on the right, with an increase in the patient's baseline pulse rate by a factor of 10 bpm. This increase indicates that an organic basis exists for the patient's musculoskeletal complaint.

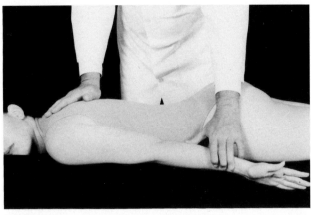

Fig. 13–17 The test may be applied for any area of musculoskeletal pain. The examiner palpates the patient's resting radial pulse and establishes a baseline index.

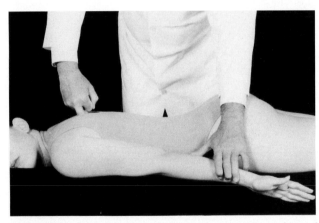

Fig. 13–18 The examiner applies firm pressure, or any form of noxious stimulation, over the area of the pain. The examiner again palpates the patient's radial pulse. An increase of 10 or more beats per minute in the pulse rate is a positive sign. The sign is absent in simulated pain.

Comment

Hypochondriacal neurosis denotes a preoccupation with bodily processes, in which the individual becomes unduly concerned about possible dysfunctions that are largely imagined or exaggerated. The patient's thoughts are occupied by health issues, and there is concern that one or more illnesses exist. Contrary facts are not reassuring. The symptoms chosen for expression are frequently those experienced by close associates. In psychodynamic terms, the hypochondriacal person is immature and never achieved an external object relationship, focusing instead on the body for the major and often sole means of communicating with others. Underlying these complaints is the need for continual reassurance that an illness does not exist and that someone cares and is willing to listen.

Procedure

The examiner applies pressure to the described painful point and marks it. The patient is distracted by examination of some other part of the body and pressing on new, tender areas. The examiner returns to the area of original complaint and asks the patient to close the eyes and then locate the tender points. If the patient cannot place the points of pain/tenderness closer than 2 inches from the marked area, exaggeration is suspected.

Confirmation Procedures

Libman's sign, Mannkopf's sign, related joint motion test

Reporting Statement

The marked part pain-suggestibility test is positive and indicates a lack of organic basis for the patient's pain.

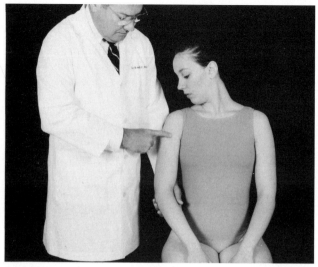

Fig. 13–19 The patient is seated. The examiner instructs the patient to identify the area of pain. The examiner applies pressure to the site, confirming the pain reaction. The site is marked or noted by some non stimulating method. The patient is distracted with other examination procedures.

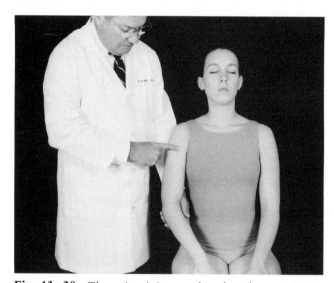

Fig. 13–20 The patient is instructed to close the eyes.

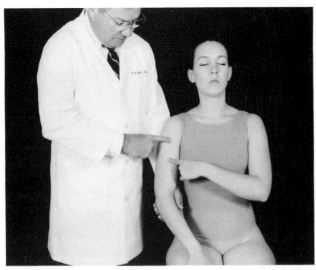

Fig. 13–21 With the eyes closed the patient is asked to once again identify the site of pain. If the patient cannot place the point of pain within 2 inches of the original site, exaggeration is suspected. It is important that the examiner *not* remind the patient of the original location, especially by touch.

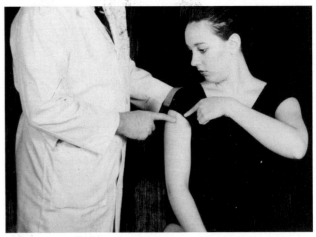

Fig 13–22 In an alternative method of determining pain suggestibility the examiner first suggests a certain point as the source of pain and marks it.

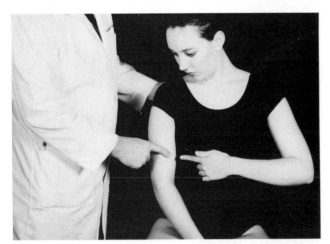

Fig. 13–23 By distracting the patient with different testing procedures the examiner suggests a nearby, but new point of discomfort and notes whether the pain shifts with the suggestion.

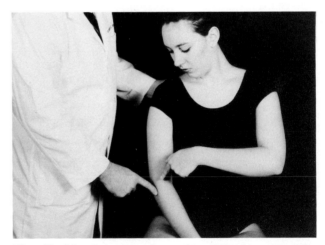

Fig. 13–24 If the site of pain does shift, this suggestibility indicates exaggeration of pain. It is important that the examiner *not* remind the patient of the original location, especially by touch.

Comment

There are several maneuvers that tighten the sciatic nerve and, in doing so, further compress an inflamed nerve root against a herniated disc. With the straight-leg raising maneuver, the L5 and S1 nerve roots move 2 to 6 mm at the level of the foramen. The L4 nerve root moves a shorter distance, and the more proximal nerve roots show little motion. Thus the straight-leg raising test is important and has value in detecting lesions of the fifth lumbar and first sacral nerve root.

Procedure

The patient is instructed to raise the legs, one at a time, until pain is felt in the lower back or the leg. The angle at which the pain occurs is noted, and the patient lowers the leg. The examiner places one hand under the patient's knee and one hand under the patient's foot and raises the lower extremity, keeping the knee slightly flexed. The leg is raised to one half of the height at which the pain was originally elicited. The foot is plantar flexed at this point. If the patient indicates that this move causes lower back pain, suspect malingering.

Confirmation Procedures

Axial trunk-loading test, Burn's bench test, flexed-hip test, flip sign, Magnuson's test, trunk rotational test

---

Reporting Statement

The plantar flexion test is positive on the right and indicates a lack of organic basis for the patient's sciatic pain.

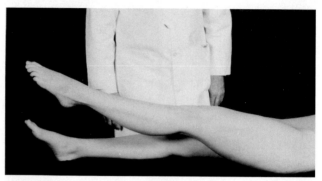

Fig. 13–25 The patient is lying supine on the examination table. The patient is instructed to raise the extended, affected leg, until pain is felt in the lower back or in the leg. The examiner notes the angle at which pain occurs. The patient lowers the leg to the table.

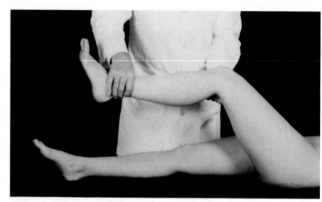

Fig. 13–26 The examiner places one hand under the patient's knee and one hand under the ankle and elevates the leg, keeping the knee slightly flexed. The leg is elevated to a point below the production of the original pain.

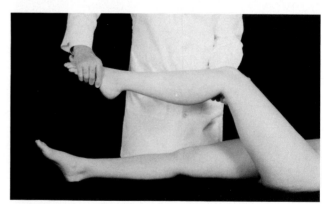

Fig. 13–27 The examiner plantar flexes the foot. If the patient indicates that the final maneuver caused lower back pain, malingering is suspected.

Comment

Most but not all orthopedic conditions are associated with some restriction of movement in the related joint. Complete loss of movement follows surgical ablation of a joint (arthrodesis) or may occur during some pathologic process, such as infection, where fibrous or bony tissue binds the articular surfaces together. The joint then cannot be moved, either actively or passively. In many conditions there is a loss of that part of the range of motion that allows the joint to be brought into its neutral position. The common loss of movement usually prevents the joint from being fully extended. This is known as a fixed flexion deformity.

Procedure

The painful part is either actively or passively moved. This move is performed with isometric resistance of a muscle group that is nearby but is in no way associated with the pain. If the patient complains of pain, the examiner moves the muscle group or related joint later, judging the inaccuracy of the statements and the correlated reactions. This assessment is accomplished by using a flexor group where an extensor group may produce pain in the joint. Where the same muscle serves more than one movement, test all movements.

Confirmation Procedures

Libman's sign, Mannkopf's sign, marked part pain-suggestibility test

> ### Reporting Statement
>
> The related joint motion test is positive on the right. This result indicates embellished pain.

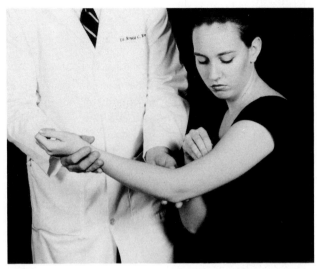

Fig. 13−28 The patient identifies the area of musculoskeletal complaint, especially the point at which motion of the affected joint is uncomfortable. The examiner confirms this reported site of pain with the patient. For example, the patient identifies that flexion of the elbow hurts the biceps musculature.

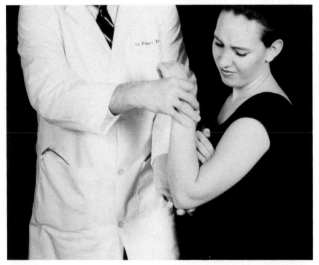

Fig. 13−29 The examiner places the painful joint or part into isometric testing, of a muscle group that is nearby, but unrelated to the primary injury group. For example, the examiner isometrically tests the triceps muscle group. If the patient complains of the original pain, the examiner moves the primary muscle group later in the examination, noting the accuracy of statements and reactions to the original findings. Discrepancies suggest exaggeration of symptoms or malingering.

Comment

Trigeminal neuralgia is characterized by a sudden attack of excruciating pain of short duration and along the distribution of the fifth cranial nerve. The attack is normally precipitated by mild stimulation of a trigger zone in the area of the pain, and is characterized by recurrent paroxysms of sharp, stabbing pains in the distribution of one or more branches of the nerve. The onset is usually in middle or late life, and the incidence is higher in females. The pain may be described as a burning or searing pain that occurs in lightning-like jabs, lasting only 1–2 minutes or as long as 15 minutes. The frequency of attacks varies from many times a day to several times a month or a year. The patient often tries to immobilize the face during conversation or attempts to swallow food without chewing in order to avoid irritating the trigger zone.

Procedure

Mydriasis (dilated pupil) is present on the side of the face that is afflicted with neuralgia. The sign is present as long as pain is present. The sign is absent in cases of hysteria or malingering.

Confirmation Procedures

Anosmia testing, facial anesthesia testing

Reporting Statement

Seeligmüller's sign is absent on the right and indicates hysterical face pain.

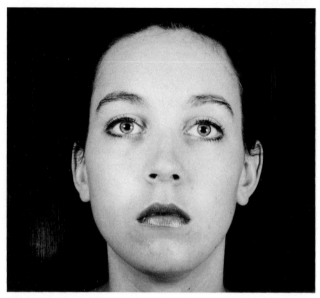

Fig. 13–30 In the patient complaining of facial neuralgia the examiner observes the pupils for mydriasis. A dilated pupil is a usual finding with facial neuralgia and is absent in cases of hysteria or malingering.

Comment

During flexion of the trunk the strain falls first on the iliolumbar ligament. Next strain is transmitted to the interspinous ligaments, from the fifth lumbar vertebra upward, then to the dorsolumbar fascia, particularly to the sacral triangle. During extension the impingement signs prevail over the tension effects. The articulation comes first and the interspinous ligaments follow. The ligamentum flavum escapes impingement. During axial rotation the iliolumbar ligament becomes strained first, then the intertransverse. During lateral flexion the sequence on the convex side is (1) quadratus, (2) ligamentum flavum, and (3) the interspinous ligament.

The legs transmit their effect through the pelvis. Single-leg raising causes no pelvic movement, although it does cause contraction of the contralateral gluteus maximus. Double-leg raising tilts the pelvis into extension. The ischial tuberosities serve as fulcrums.

Procedure

The patient rotates the trunk. The examiner ensures that the pelvis rotates as well. If the patient indicates that this causes lower back pain, suspect malingering. The lumbar spine is not moving. Instead the whole spine is rotated from the hips and thighs.

Confirmation Procedures

Axial trunk-loading test, Burn's bench test, flexed-hip test, flip sign, Magnuson's test, plantar flexion test

Reporting Statement
The trunk rotational test is positive and elicits pain in the lumbar spine on the right. This result indicates a lack of organic basis for the patient's lumbar spine complaint.

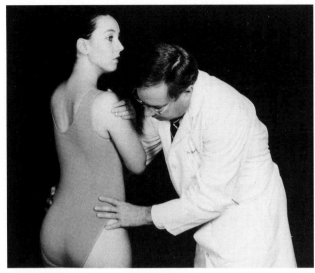

Fig. 13-31 The patient is in the standing position with the arms folded across the chest. The examiner instructs the patient to rotate the trunk, while making sure that the pelvis is rotated simultaneously. If the patient indicates that this move causes pain in the lower back, the test is positive and indicates malingering.

SENSORY DEFICIT QUALIFICATION AND QUANTIFICATION

Overview

The nervous system does not perceive external events directly. Instead, the brain receives an abstract picture that is a composite of nerve impulses that originate at the periphery. The transformation of external stimuli into conductible impulses is called transduction. Sensibility is the reception or encoding of external stimuli and the transmission of impulses along nerve fibers. In broad terms, sensibility encompasses sight, smell, sound, taste, temperature change, pain, touch-pressure, and movement or change in position. Sensibility is the modality of prime importance. Touch-pressure is the ability to recognize touch, whether moving across the surface or continually applied to a single spot.

In contrast to sensibility, which is primarily a peripheral phenomenon, sensation is the central reception and conscious recognition of external stimuli. Sensation involves several facets of central nervous system function. Some of these facets are voluntary, and some are involuntary. Among these facets are the orderly reception and integration of impulses from several sources, association with other information (either current or from memory storage), assimilation and interpretation of such data, and finally, elevation to the conscious level. All of these facets may result, at the patient's discretion, in an appropriate response.

The transmission of impulses from skin surface to cerebral cortex requires a chain of three afferent neurons. The cell body of the first-order afferent neuron lies in the dorsal ganglion, and the other two are in the spinal cord and brain. From a practical standpoint the examiner has access only to the axon of the first order afferent neuron, its receptors, and the skin that contains them.

Sensation may be divided into three groups: superficial, deep, and combined. Superficial sensation is concerned with touch, pain, temperature, and two-point discrimination; deep sensation is concerned with muscle and joint position sense (proprioception) and deep muscle pain and vibration sense (pallesthesia). The combination of superficial and deep sensory mechanisms is involved in stereognosis, the recognition and naming of familiar objects placed in the hand; and topognosis, the ability to localize cutaneous stimuli. Stereognosis depends on the integrity of the cerebral cortex.

Cutaneous sensibility is divided into two groups, epicritic and protopathic, each served by a different neuron. Epicritic senses are concerned with perception of light touch, two-point discrimination, and small differences in temperature; the protopathic senses are concerned with pain and more marked changes of temperature.

∼ Tips for Assessment of a Sensory Deficit ∼

In the evaluation of what appears to be psychogenic changes in sensation, it is always essential to recall that there is some variation in the nerve supply in normal individuals. Furthermore, hysterical or malingered changes may be superimposed on organic anesthesia in peripheral nerve lesions and other neurologic disorders. Hysterical (or malingered) hemianesthesia, which almost invariably occurs on the left side, may occasionally be accompanied by an ipsilateral decrease or loss of the senses of vision, hearing, smell, and taste.

Comment

The central connections of the olfactory nerve are complex. Association fibers to the tegmentum and pons pass directly as third-order neurons from the anterior perforated substance, and indirectly from the hippocampus, via the fornix and olfactory projection tracts, through the mamillary bodies and anterior nuclei of the thalamus. Reflex connections, thus established within the nuclei of the other cranial and spinal nerves, may be functionally significant during swallowing and digestion.

The olfactory nerve may serve as a portal of entry for cryptogenic infections of the brain and meninges (poliomyelitis, epidemic meningitis, and encephalitis).

Disorders of the sense of smell may be caused be inflammatory and other lesions of the nasal cavity, fracture of the anterior fossa of the skull, tumors of the frontal lobe and pituitary region, meningitis, hydrocephalus, posttraumatic cerebral syndrome, arteriosclerosis, cerebrovascular accidents, certain drug intoxications, psychoses, neuroses, and congenital defects.

Special syndromes involving the olfactory nerve include the Foster-Kennedy syndrome (unilateral optic atrophy, with or without anosmia, and contralateral papilledema) and the aura of epilepsy.

Anosmia may be of significance. Bilateral anosmia commonly occurs with colds, rhinitis, etc. Unilateral anosmia may be of diagnostic significance in locating brain lesions, such as tumors, at the base of the frontal lobe.

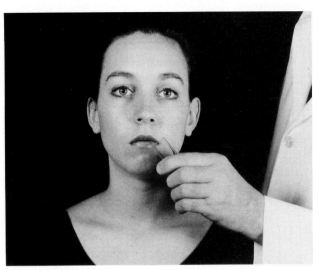

Fig. 13–32 In complaints of loss of smell, the patient is instructed to index various odors by smelling aromatics, such as peppermint, clove, vanilla, coffee grounds, and finally spirit of ammonia. An individual with feigned anosmia will claim the inability to smell any of the substances. Using spirit of ammonia directly irritates the trigeminal nerve endings in the nose. A damaged olfactory nerve does not impair the patient's ability to notice (smell) pungent ammonia. Anosmia to ammonia suggests a psychogenic or manufactured complaint.

Procedure

With complaints involving the loss of the sense of smell, the patient is directed to index various odors by smelling aromatics such as peppermint, clove, vanilla, coffee grounds (uncooked), and then finally, spirit of ammonia. An individual with psychogenic loss of smell frequently claims the inability to smell any of these substances. Ammonia is extremely pungent and actually irritates the trigeminal nerve endings in the nose, rather than being smelled by the olfactory nerve proper. Hence, a damaged olfactory nerve does not impair a patient's ability to notice (smell) the pungent ammonia fumes.

Confirmation Procedures

Seeligmüller's sign, facial anesthesia testing

Reporting Statement

Anosmia testing demonstrates normal function of the olfactory nerve. This result suggests feigned anosmia.

Comment

Tremors are involuntary movements in one or more parts of the body, produced by rhythmical alternate contractions of opposing muscle groups. Tremors are symptoms of constitutional diseases or disorders rather than clinical entities.

In differentiating tremors the examiner should note their rate, rhythm, and distribution and the effect of movement or rest. A rapid tremor oscillates 8 to 10 times per second, a slow tremor 3 to 5 times per second. Tremors may be fine or coarse. Intention tremor appears during, or is accentuated by, volitional movements of the affected part. Resting tremors are present when the involved part is at rest, but they diminish or disappear during active movements.

Transient tremors, without particular significance, may occur in healthy individuals during hunger, chilling, excitement, or after physical exertion.

Procedure

With coordination disturbances the patient is instructed to touch tip of the nose while the eyes are open. The patient is then instructed to close the eyes and again touch the tip of the nose. With organic cerebellar lesions an intention crescendo tremor manifests as the finger approaches the nose. The malingerer will move the finger in a guided but devious course toward the nose, without exhibiting the intention tremor.

Confirmation Procedures

Limb-dropping test (upper extremities), position-sense testing, Romberg test

---

Reporting Statement

Coordination-disturbance testing does not demonstrate involuntary intention crescendo tremors. This result indicates a lack of organic basis for the patient's complaint of a loss of coordination.

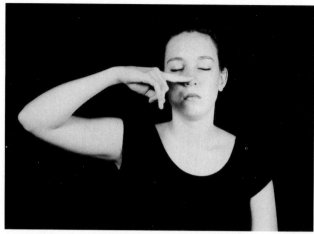

Fig. 13–33 The seated patient is instructed to touch the tip of the nose while the eyes are open. The patient is then instructed to close the eyes and again touch the tip of the nose. With organic cerebellar lesions an intention crescendo tremor manifests as the finger approaches the nose.

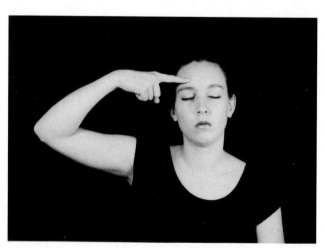

Fig. 13–34 The malingering patient will move the finger toward the nose in a guided, but devious course, without the intention tremor.

Comment

Optic atrophy is commonly divided into primary and secondary (or postneuritic) categories. Primary optic atrophy results from a degeneration of the nerve fibers following retrobulbar neuritis that results from syphilis, central retinal artery occlusion, glaucoma, trauma, or any condition or drug that causes injury to the optic nerve along its intracanalicular or intracranial course. With secondary optic atrophy, degeneration of the nerve fibers is accompanied by glial formation on the nerve head and is caused by optic neuritis or severe and prolonged papilledema.

Visual loss is directly proportional to the degree of nerve atrophy. Total blindness and a dilated, fixed pupil may result. In primary optic atrophy, the disc is white or grayish with sharp edges and a saucer-shaped excavation. The lamina cribrosa is clearly visible. The retina is usually normal. In secondary optic atrophy, the disc is dirty white with irregular and indistinct margins and is covered by glial tissue that conceals the lamina cribrosa. Evidence of previous inflammation, such as sheathed vessels, may be seen in the retina.

Procedure

Without a positive Marcus Gunn's sign but with continued complaint of unilateral blindness, the examiner places a refractive lens over the "good eye," ostensibly to test it. The lens actually deprives the eye of any effective vision. The malingering patient is directed to read a Snellen chart. This is accomplished perfectly with the blind eye.

Confirmation Procedures

Marcus Gunn's sign, optokinetic nystagmus test, Snellen's test

---

Reporting Statement

Cuignet's test is positive for simulated blindness in the right eye.

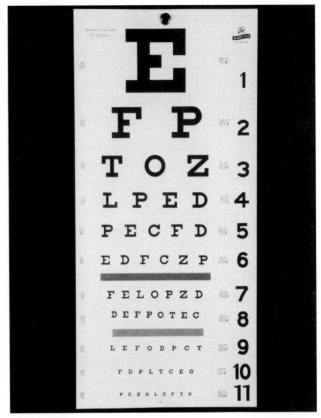

Fig. 13−35 The seated patient is placed at an appropriate distance from a Snellen eye chart. The patient is instructed to read the chart with one eye at a time. With simulated unilateral blindness, the patient will claim that the blind eye cannot read the chart.

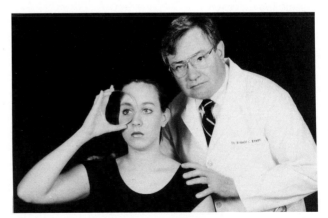

Fig. 13−36 The examiner places a refractive, but myopic lens over the good eye, ostensibly to aid its vision and test it. The patient is again instructed to read the Snellen chart. The lens deprives the eye of any effective vision. If the chart is read, it was done so with the blind eye. If the chart can be read, the test is positive and indicates simulated unilateral blindness.

Comment

Neuritis is a disease of a nerve. As an affectation of a single nerve, it is called mononeuritis. Of two or more nerves in separate areas, the disease is called mononeuritis multiplex, and if it affects many nerves simultaneously, it is called polyneuritis. The term implies a syndrome of sensory, motor, reflex, and vasomotor symptoms, singly or in combination, produced by lesions of the nerve roots or peripheral nerves.

Sensory symptoms may be prominent. Descriptive terms—such as tingling, pins-and-needles sensation, burning, boring, and stabbing—are used by the patient. Pain, often worse at night, may be aggravated by touching the affected area or by temperature changes. Numbness and objective loss of sensation occur, in severe cases, in stocking-and-glove distributions. The nerve trunks may be tender. When sensory loss is profound, painless ulcers may appear on the digits or joints may be painlessly enlarged (Charcot joints).

Procedure

With symptoms of facial anesthesia the examiner applies a vibrating tuning fork to the numb side of the patient's forehead, near the midline. The malingerer or hysteric will state that there is no sensation. When the examiner moves the application of the tuning fork just across the midline, the patient now reports sensing the vibrations immediately. The lack of vibration sense on the "numb" side is an impossibility because the bone tissue conducts vibration, which is applied to the area of claimed anesthesia, to the normal side. This test is valid even for a pathologic bone condition or an organic bone disease.

Confirmation Procedures

Seeligmüller's sign, anosmia testing

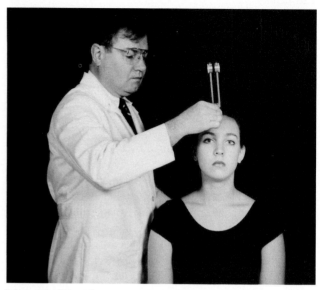

Fig. 13–37 The patient is seated. The examiner applies a vibrating tuning fork to the numb side of the forehead, near the midline of the forehead. The patient is asked to identify sensations of vibration across the forehead. If the patient denies feeling the vibration on the numb side of the forehead, the test is repeated just across the midline, on the normal side of the forehead. If the patient feels the vibration only on the normal side, hysteria or malingering is suspected.

Reporting Statement

Facial anesthesia testing is positive on the right for hysterical or simulated facial anesthesia.

Comment

Perceptive deafness is impaired hearing caused by disorders of the inner ear, the eighth (auditory) nerve, cerebral pathways, or the auditory center.

Causes include involvement of these structures in infectious diseases—such as meningitis, syphilis, typhoid, mumps, measles, and hemolytic streptococcal infection; tumors of the cerebellopontine angle, temporal lobe, eighth nerve, or cochlea; trauma to these organs, such as from skull fracture; injury by such toxic substances as quinine, arsenic, alcohol, salicylates, mercury, or aminoglycoside antibiotics (kanamycin); psychogenic disturbances; or physiologic dysfunction that may occur in senility and from excessive noise.

Excessive noise is a common cause of hearing loss. The loss is more pronounced in the high frequencies and traditionally has been caused by industrial noise and exposure to heavy gunfire. Recently, the condition has appeared in adolescents, caused by excessive electronic amplification of music.

Procedure

Deafness is a form of sensory deprivation easily feigned and as easily tested. Although the complaint is the inability to hear any sound, the patient with such a conversion reaction may startle to a loud noise and can be awakened from a sound sleep by the same.

A startled response to sound is an important finding when testing a noncooperative, hysterical, or malingering patient. The examiner can gain a crude estimate of the patient's hearing ability by using the auditory-palpebral reflex.

When a patient hears a loud sound, an involuntary blink is the response. With the patient's normal ear covered, an assistant standing behind the patient (out of the patient's line of sight) can clap the hands or pop a bag. The examiner observes the patient for blinking or a startled response. If the patient has a response, the examiner can be certain that the patient heard something. If the patient does not respond, the significance of the test is doubtful.

Confirmation Procedure

Lombard's test

Reporting Statement

Gault's test is positive and elicits an auditory-palpebral reflex. This result indicates simulated deafness.

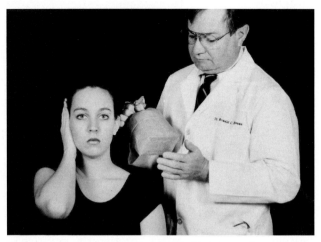

Fig. 13–38 The patient is seated and is instructed to cover the normal ear. The examiner or an assistant is positioned behind the patient, out of the patient's peripheral vision.

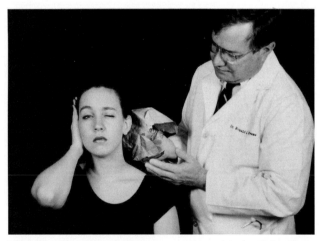

Fig. 13–39 The examiner or an assistant claps hands loudly or pops a bag. The examiner observes the patient for involuntary blinking or a startle response (auditory-palpebral reflex). If the response is present, the test is positive and indicates that the deaf ear heard something. This result suggests malingering.

Comment

Hysterical paralysis of one limb usually provides little difficulty during diagnosis. The affected limb may be either rigid or flaccid, and there is no true muscular atrophy and no alteration in the muscular response to electrical stimulation. The reflexes provide the most information. With hysterical paralysis the reflexes may be exaggerated, but they are never lost.

More often than not, a limb that is the seat of hysterical paralysis also presents complete insensibility to all forms of stimulation, and the upper limit of such anesthesia may end abruptly at a level for which there is no anatomic basis.

Procedure

If anesthesia is the complaint, the patient is instructed to close the eyes. The patient is then directed to answer "yes" if a pinprick is felt on the skin or "no" if not. Obviously the only appropriate answer is silence when the supposedly anesthetic area is touched.

Confirmation Procedures

Facial anesthesia testing, midline tuning-fork test, regional anesthesia testing

---

Reporting Statement

Janet's test indicates simulated anesthesia on the right.

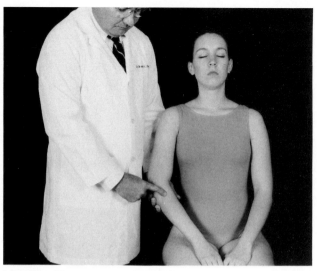

Fig. 13–40 In this test for anesthesia the patient may be seated or recumbent. The patient is instructed to close the eyes.

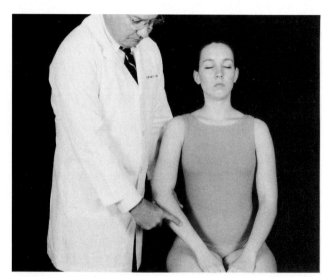

Fig. 13–41 As the examiner touches the involved part, either with a finger or sharp object, the patient is directed to indicate feeling the touch by saying "yes" and not feeling the touch by saying "no." The only appropriate answer, when the anesthetic area is touched, is silence. The test is positive when the patient identifies with the answer "no." The test indicates hysteria or malingering.

Comment

Level of consciousness is a phrase that refers to certain processes that provide awareness of one's self and the environment. Terms used to describe pathologic alterations in the level of consciousness are determined, largely, by the degree of patient arousal. These alterations range from confusion to somnolence, stupor, and coma.

The examiner should be familiar with conditions that, in some respects, resemble stupor or coma. Akinetic mutism is a state of wakeful unresponsiveness in which the patient has no meaningful mental content or purposeful movement but seems to be awake. This condition may follow bilateral cerebral damage (the apallic state), lesions of the upper midbrain or diencephalon, and, rarely, hydrocephalus. The locked-in syndrome is a condition in which the patient is conscious and aware, but paralyzed and anarthric. Eye movements are preserved and may be of use for communication. The condition is due to a lesion of the ventral portion of the pons.

Disease processes involving two general areas of the central nervous system can alter consciousness. These are lesions, either in both cerebral hemispheres or in the deep midline structures, in the upper brainstem near the central core of the gray matter. Diseases producing disturbances of the level of consciousness fall into four main categories: (1) supratentorial mass lesions that secondarily compress deep midline structures, (2) infratentorial lesions that directly damage the central brainstem core, (3) metabolic disorders that widely depress or interrupt cortical function, and (4) psychiatric disorders resembling coma.

Procedure

Reduced awareness or faked stoicism is attempted to portray a reduced level of consciousness. In a conversion reaction or malingering, the pupillary and corneal reflexes and plantar responses will be normal, although reduced awareness or increased pain tolerance is exhibited.

Often when a patient feigning reduced consciousness has a hand held up by the examiner, and then dropped over the patient's face, it is consciously swerved to keep the hand from striking the face. A patient with an organically reduced level of consciousness will not make this movement of avoidance and will usually have pupillary abnormalities and other positive neurologic signs.

Confirmation Procedures

Coordination-disturbance testing, position-sense testing, Romberg test

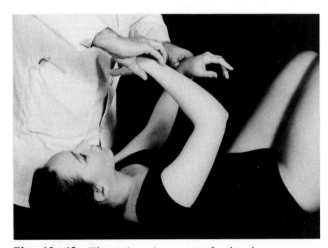

Fig. 13–42 The patient, in a state of reduced awareness or consciousness, is recumbent on the examination table. The examiner elevates the patient's arms by the wrists.

Continued.

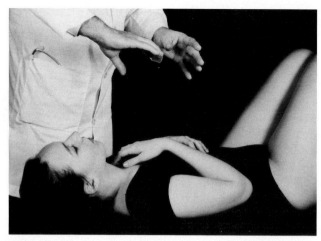

Fig. 13–43 The arms are allowed to drop over the patient's chest.

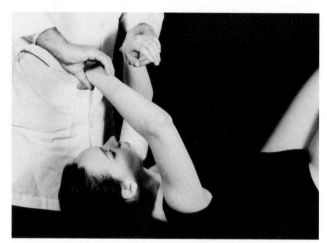

Fig. 13–44 The test is repeated, this time with the examiner holding the arms over the patient's head and face.

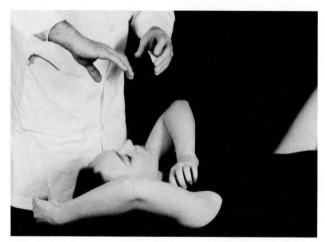

Fig. 13–45 The arms are allowed to drop. The test is positive when the arms are swerved to avoid striking the face. A positive test indicates a lack of organic basis for the reduced level of awareness or consciousness.

Comment

Anomalies of the external auditory canal, eardrum, middle ear, or eustachian tube that interfere with the conduction of sound waves to the inner ear may be responsible for conductive deafness. In this category are mechanical obstructions of the external auditory canal for a foreign object, cerumen, furuncle, osteoma, or stenosis. Perforation, scarring, or inflammation of the tympanic membrane also restrict sound-wave movement in the ear. Ankylosis of the ossicles, middle ear inflammation (acute or chronic) or tumor, osteosclerotic involvement of the oval window margin restrict the vibration of the footplate of the stapes. Obstruction of the eustachian tube by inflammation, stenosis, tumor, or lymphoid hypertrophy at the ostium also diminishes conductive hearing.

Procedure

Lombard's auditory test is a test of hearing that relies on the effect of induced noise on a subject's hearing responses. The test is used in the investigation of nonorganic hearing loss. The patient with hearing loss is seated for this examination. The examiner engages the patient in conversation or has the patient read aloud from a page. As the reading progresses or the conversation continues, background noise is induced and amplified. If the patient's voice grows louder with the background noise, the testing is positive and indicates nonorganic hearing loss.

Confirmation Procedure

Gault test

Reporting Statement
Lombard's test is positive. This result indicates simulated deafness.

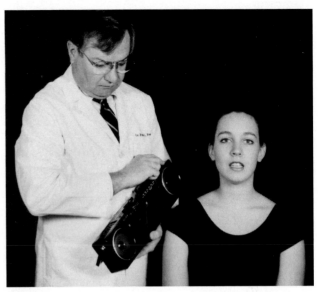

Fig. 13–46 The patient with hearing loss is seated for this examination. The examiner engages the patient in conversation or has the patient read aloud from a page. As the reading progresses or the conversation continues, background noise is induced and amplified. If the patient's voice grows louder with the background noise, the testing is positive and indicates nonorganic hearing loss.

Comment

Optic neuritis is inflammation of that portion of the optic nerve that is ophthalmoscopically visible. This inflammation occurs with meningitis, encephalitis, syphilis, acute febrile diseases, foci of infection, and multiple sclerosis and with poisoning by methyl alcohol, carbon tetrachloride, lead, and thallium. Optic neuritis is almost always unilateral. Disturbances of vision are the only symptoms, which vary from minimal contraction of the visual field with enlargement of the blind spot to complete blindness and pain during motion of the globe. The maximum reduction of vision is frequently reached within 1 or 2 days. The disease can last for months. Ophthalmoscopic examination discloses hyperemia and minimal edema of the disc in the early stages, with more noticeable changes in advanced cases.

The Marcus Gunn's sign represents an afferent pupillary defect due to a lesion of the optic nerve. Resting pupil sizes are normal. Both direct and consensual pupillary responses are decreased (reduced constriction) with bright illumination of the involved side. Both responses are normal with illumination of the normal side. When moving the light back to the involved eye, both pupils dilate, and both constrict with stimulation on the normal side.

Procedure

If there is an organic basis for unilateral blindness, the lesion must be situated anteriorly to the optic chiasm and the pupillary reaction is usually abnormal. Marcus Gunn's sign is especially useful for evaluating the existence of unilateral blindness.

To elicit the Marcus Gunn's sign the patient's eyes are fixed at a distant point and a strong light shines on the intact eye. A crisp, bilateral contraction of the pupils is noted. Upon moving the light to the affected eye, both pupils dilate for a brief period. When the light is returned to the intact eye, both pupils contract promptly and remain contracted. This response indicates damage to the optic nerve, on the affected side.

Confirmation Procedures

Cuignet's test, optokinetic nystagmus testing, Snellen's test

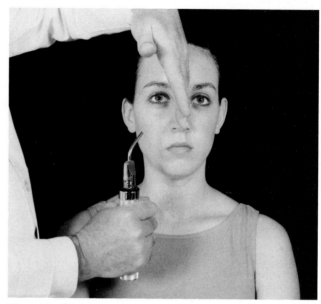

Fig. 13–47 To elicit the Marcus Gunn's sign, the seated patient's eyes are fixed at a distant point. The examination room is dimmed and a strong light is shone on the normal eye. The examiner notes a crisp bilateral contraction of the pupils.

> ### Reporting Statement
>
> Marcus Gunn's sign cannot be demonstrated. The absence of this sign indicates normal optic nerve functioning bilaterally.

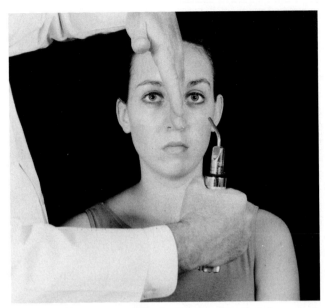

Fig. 13–48 Upon moving the light to the affected eye, both pupils dilate for a brief period.

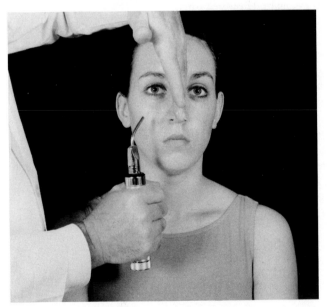

Fig. 13–49 On return of the light to the intact eye, both pupils contract promptly and remain contracted. This response indicates damage to the optic nerve on the affected side. The absence of Marcus Gunn's sign in unilateral blindness indicates a nonorganic basis for the complaint.

Comment

Fibers conveying touch, superficial pain, and temperature pass via cutaneous nerves to mixed nerves, where they are joined by fibers carrying impulses from joints, ligaments, and muscles. Lesions of cutaneous nerves will not cause proprioceptive sensory loss, but interruption of mixed nerves and pure motor nerves will. All sensory fibers have their cell station in the ganglia of the cranial nerves or the posterior spinal roots. The spinal roots enter the posterolateral aspect of the cord in the root entry zone. Fibers conveying touch and postural sensibility pass upward in the posterior columns to the nuclei gracilis and cuneatus in the medulla. Those from the lower half of the body lie medially and those from the upper half of the body occupy the lateral portion of the posterior column. These fibers cross the midline of the CNS as sensory decussation and form the medial lemniscus, then pass upward through the brainstem to the thalamus.

Procedure

Many feigned complaints fall in the category of sensory loss. Complaints of this kind usually manifest as numbness or anesthesia of a body part. The major distinguishing factor between feigned numbness and organic anesthesia is the disregard of the former for anatomic continuity. Indeed feigned numbness includes all levels of sense (light touch, heat, cold, position, deep pressure, etc.) However, such instances of sensory loss are physically impossible without spinal cord transection.

Conversion reactions that involve only the sensory systems are difficult to prove. Organic sensory losses follow known anatomic distributions, but conversion reaction sensory disturbances follow the patient's perception of human anatomy.

Patients with organic sensory disturbances are able to perceive a vibrating tuning fork placed on either side of the head or on either side of the sternum because the conduction vibrates through the bone. In a conversion reaction the sternum or head is split. For example, vibration is perceived on one side of the midline of the forehead or sternum but not on the other.

Confirmation Procedures

Janet's test, regional anesthesia testing

Reporting Statement

The midline tuning-fork test is positive. This test indicates simulated anesthesia on the right.

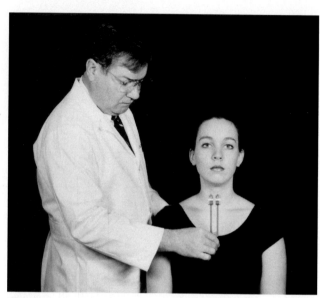

Fig. 13–50 The patient may be seated or recumbent. The examiner places a vibrating tuning fork on the affected side of the sternum, near the midline. The patient is instructed to identify areas of perceived vibration. If the patient does not feel the vibration, the tuning fork is moved across the midline, to the normal side. The test is positive if the patient identifies that vibration is only felt on the normal half of the body and not on the affected side. The positive test indicates hysteria, conversion reaction, or malingering.

Comment

Nystagmus is a rhythmic horizontal or vertical oscillation of the eyeballs. This oscillation is more pronounced when the patient is looking in certain directions. Nystagmus is often a sign of cerebellar, vestibular, or labyrinthine disease, and it is a common sign in certain systemic diseases, such as multiple sclerosis. Prolonged use of the eyes with insufficient illumination and in strained positions, such as that maintained by miners, and fatigue of the eye muscles, especially when due to errors of refraction, also may be causative. Vestibular stimulation causes nystagmus.

Procedure

With faked blindness the patient will often avoid personal injury when walking and will blink to unexpected physical threats. Pupillary reactions are normal and optokinetic nystagmus is normal.

To demonstrate optokinetic nystagmus the examiner instructs the patient to keep the eyes open. The examiner holds a ruler or a tape measure 10 inches in front of the patient's face, ostensibly to measure pupillary distances. As the pupils constrict, which demonstrates attempted focusing, the ruler is moved from left to right across the patient's field of vision. A patient who can see the ruler will fix the vision on the vertical markings and develop an involuntary eye movement called optokinetic nystagmus. This is a similar phenomenon to a person riding in a vehicle and looking out the window watching telephone poles go by. This test is used when routine eye examination reveals a normal fundus and intact pupillary reactions to light.

With organic blindness, pupillary reflexes are abnormal and optokinetic nystagmus is absent. Hysterical field defects, when plotted out on a tangent screen, will not change with the varying distance between the patient and the screen.

Confirmation Procedures

Cuignet's test, Marcus Gunn's sign, Snellen's test

Reporting Statement

Optokinetic nystagmus is present and does not support the patient's complaint of blindness.

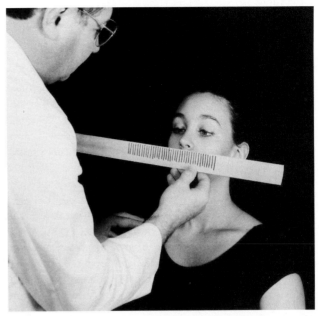

Fig. 13–51 The patient is seated. The examiner instructs the patient to keep the eyes open. A ruler or a tape measure is held approximately 10 inches in front of the patient's face. The examiner holds the ruler still and observes the patient's eyes for slight pupil constriction, indicating the attempt of the eyes to focus on the ruler markings.

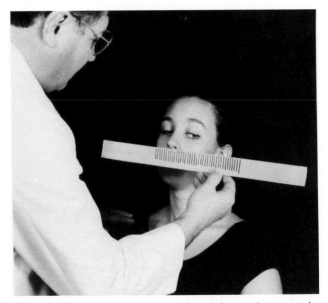

Fig. 13–52 The ruler is moved from left to right, across the patient's field of vision. A patient who can see the ruler, will fix the vision on the vertical markings, and develop an involuntary eye movement, called optokinetic nystagmus. This test is used when routine eye examination reveals a normal fundus and intact pupillary reactions to light. Optokinetic nystagmus suggests a lack of organic basis for the blindness.

Comment

Hereditary spastic paraplegia is familial, but it may be present without a history of cases in previous generations because sporadic cases do occur. The symptoms are those of a slowly progressive degeneration of the pyramidal tracts, starting between 3 and 15 years of age but rarely at older ages. For a time there is only a spastic paraplegia, but gradually spastic weakness spreads to the upper limbs and ultimately to the bulbar muscles. There is no sensory loss, but optic atrophy may occur. The disease takes many years to run its course and is one of the heredofamilial group, of which Friedreich's ataxia is the best known. With the latter disease, symptoms usually come on in childhood or adolescence and the earliest complaints are of weakness and clumsiness of the legs. Ataxia of gait is apt to obscure the presence of weakness because of pyramidal degeneration. This is more so as tendon reflexes are diminished or absent and tone is reduced. The ataxia is partly due to degeneration of the spinocerebellar tracts and partly due to loss of position sense.

Procedure

If a patient claims that the position of a body part cannot be differentiated, the patient is directed to close the eyes, and the examiner bends the patient's fingers or toes up or down. The patient is instructed to state what direction the examiner is bending the digit. A patient may report contrary findings by saying "up" when the examiner is bringing the digit down, and vice versa. With organic sensory loss, the patient has a 50% chance of correctly guessing the digit position. The malingerer's reporting average is always contrary to the actual digit position and therefore incorrect a majority of the time.

Confirmation Procedures

Coordination-disturbance testing, limb dropping test (upper extremities), Romberg test

---

Reporting Statement

Position-sense testing is positive on the right. This result indicates feigned loss of position sense.

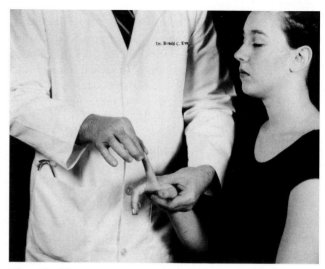

Fig. 13–53 The patient may be seated or recumbent. The patient is instructed to close the eyes. The examiner bends the patient's finger (or toe) up.

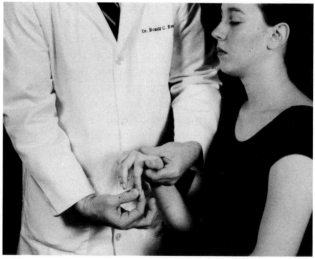

Fig. 13–54 The finger or toe is then bent down. The patient is instructed to identify the direction of the digit movement. The patient may report contrary findings to the actual position of the digit. In organic sensory loss the patient has a 50% chance of success rate at guessing the digit position. The test is positive when the patient is consistently wrong. This result suggests malingering.

Comment

Conversion of anxiety into symptoms of dysfunction of various organs or parts of the body is a common characteristic of conversion hysteria. The emotional conflict, instead of being experienced consciously, is converted into physical symptoms involving voluntary muscles or special sense organs. The patient often appears unconcerned about the sensory or motor paralysis (la belle indifference). The reaction not only serves to allay anxiety, but also may provide some secondary gain. The conversion symptom does not always follow the anatomic distribution of the sensorimotor nerves, but it is determined symbolically (glove or stocking anesthesia, tunnel vision). These reactions help in understanding the nature of the unconscious conflict.

Procedure

To define a regional complaint of numbness, the examiner uses a straight pin or a Wartenberg pinwheel and delineates the areas where the claimed numbness ceases. The usual organic cause of anesthesia or paresthesia is peripheral neuritis. With peripheral neuritis the upper border of the anesthesia is blurry and usually different for each different sensation tested, such as pain, touch, heat, and vibration. In the hysterical or malingering patient, the border of anesthesia is extremely abrupt, stopping at a wrist crease, or some other external anatomic area that is unrelated to the dermatome pattern. This numbness landmark may even vary from examination to examination.

Most malingerers claim a simultaneous loss of all forms of sensation, including touch, pain, temperature, and vibratory sensation. All losses are identical as to extent and accurate neural distribution or dermatome patterns are not present.

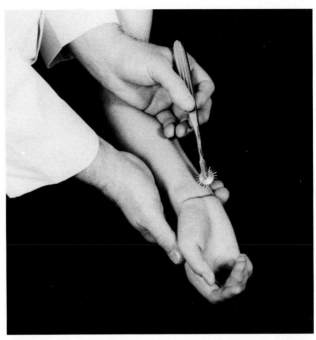

Fig. 13–55 The patient may be seated or recumbent for this test. The patient identifies the area of numbness. The examiner, using a pin or Wartenberg pinwheel, delineates the boundaries of the numbness. The test is positive when the borders of the anesthesia are extremely abrupt, stopping at some anatomic landmark unrelated to the dermatome involved. Such a sensory deficit distribution suggests malingering or hysteria.

Confirmation Procedures

Janet's test, midline tuning-fork test

Reporting Statement

Regional anesthesia testing indicates a loss of all sensory modalities that do not follow known anatomic distributions. This loss indicates a lack of organic basis for the patient's complaint of anesthesia.

～ Romberg's Sign ～
STATION TEST

Comment

Tabetic or ataxic gait is characteristic of posterior column disease and results from the loss of proprioceptive sense in the extremities. The patient walks on a wide base, slapping the feet, and usually watches the legs to know where they are. When the eyes are closed or the patient is in the dark, the ataxia is much worse. Clumsiness and uncertainty are characteristic. The feet are placed too widely apart and in taking a step the patient lifts the advancing leg abruptly and too high and then stamps or slaps the foot solidly to the ground. Uneven spacing of steps, tottering, and swaying occur, usually with deviation to one side or the other.

Procedure

With this disorder of balance loss, the patient is instructed to stand with the feet together, first with the eyes open, then with the eyes closed. With organic sensory ataxia, the patient will sway the body from the ankles. Swaying from the hips, toward a wall to catch one's self in the nick of time, suggests malingering.

Confirmation Procedures

Coordination-disturbance testing, limb-dropping test (upper extremities), position-sense testing

Reporting Statement

Romberg's sign is absent. The patient sways from the hips. The absence of this sign indicates a lack of organic basis for the patient's ataxia.

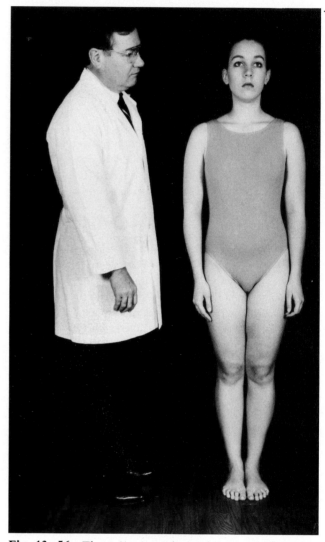

Fig. 13–56 The patient is standing and instructed to place the feet close together. The patient's eyes are open.

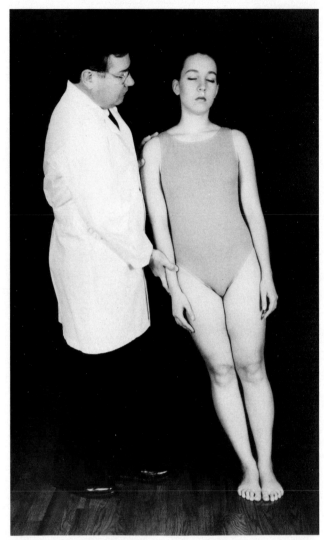

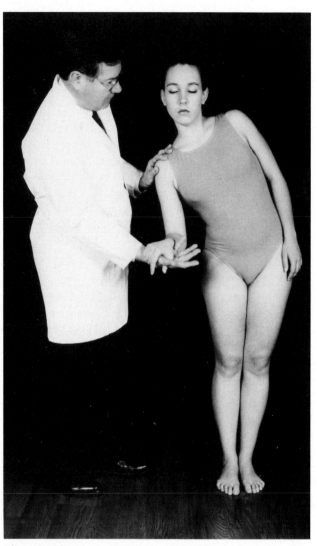

Fig. 13–57 While maintaining this narrowed base, the patient is instructed to close the eyes. In organic ataxia the patient will lose balance, usually by falling from the ankles toward the side of the cerebellar lesion. The examiner maintains proximity to the patient for safety.

Fig. 13–58 The malingering patient will sway from the pelvis, usually toward a wall, catching the fall in the nick of time. In this instance, the sign is absent and indicates a lack of organic basis for the patient's loss of balance.

Comment

Color blindness may be hereditary or acquired. Hereditary types are transmitted as recessive characteristics, sometimes X-linked. These include achromatopsia (total color blindness), monochromatism (partial color blindness, with ability to recognize one of the three basic colors remaining), and dichromatism (ability to recognize two of the three basic colors).

In normal (trichromatic) vision, the eye can perceive three light primaries (red, blue, green) and can mix these in suitable portions, so white or any color of the spectrum can be matched. Color blindness can result from a lessened capacity to match three primary colors. It can be dichromatic vision, in which only one pair of the primary colors is perceived, the two colors being complimentary to each other. Most dichromats are red-green blind and confuse red, yellow, and green.

Procedure

For pretended color blindness in one eye, the patient is requested to look at alternate red and green letters. The admittedly good eye is covered with a red glass. If the green letters are read, evidence of fraud is present.

Confirmation Procedures

Cuignet's test, Marcus Gunn's sign, optokinetic nystagmus testing

Reporting Statement
Snellen's test is positive on the right. This result indicates feigned color blindness on that side.

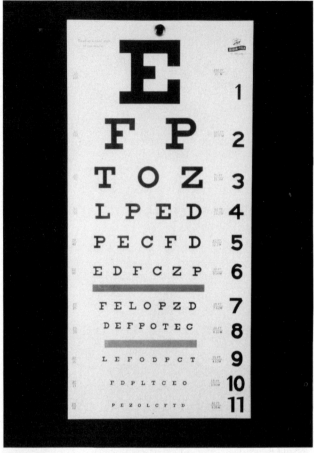

Fig. 13–59 The seated patient is placed an appropriate distance from a Snellen eye chart. The patient is instructed to read the red and green letters, using one eye at a time. The patient will state that the color blind eye can not read the chart.

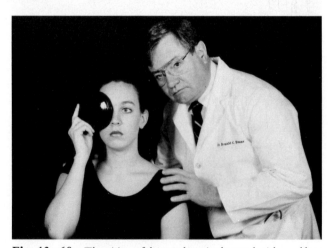

Fig. 13–60 The vision of the good eye is obscured with a red lens and the patient is instructed to reread the chart. If the green letters are read, the test is positive. A positive test indicates that the vision of the alleged blind eye is preserved. This suggests malingering.

Comment

Although it is rare, some patients are born with a lack of any pain appreciation. This is a congenital indifference to pain or an inability to perceive it at all. Whether the patient feels the pain but is indifferent to it, or whether the patient lacks any pain sensation is difficult to determine. The patient does not suffer. The cause of this congenital absence of pain perception is unknown. As children, these patients undergo falls and bumps but never cry. The defect is central rather than peripheral because the child recognizes the stimulus without exhibiting signs of pain. Normal nerve endings, which subserve pain sensibilities, are found in the skin and periosteum. Free nerve endings are also found in the glandular tissue. Progressive degenerative changes of the Charcot type are observed in the adult joints of these patients.

Procedure

The interval between eye blinks in the average patient is 25 to 30 seconds. A 60-second lapse between blinks, while staring straight ahead, indicates a patient who is stoic.

A stoic patient can be described as impassive and calm in the face of pain and discomfort. They may also be cool and indifferent to the sensations elicited in testing.

Confirmation Procedures

Libman's sign, Mannkopf's sign, marked part pain-suggestibility test, related joint motion test

---

Reporting Statement

The stoicism index for this patient is greater than 60 seconds. This result indicates a congenital insensitivity to pain.

The stoicism index for the patient is 10. This result indicates hypersensitivity to pain.

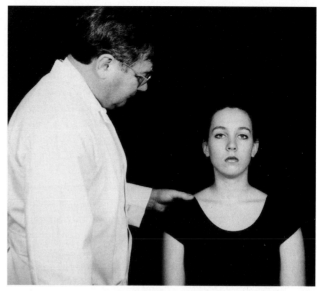

Fig. 13–61 The patient is seated, and the examiner observes the interval between blinks, as the patient stares straight ahead.

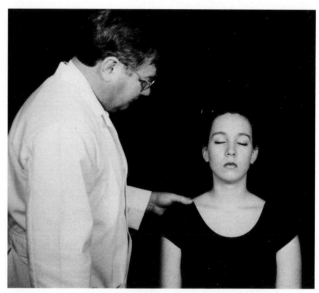

Fig. 13–62 A lapse of 60 seconds or more between blinks indicates decreased sensitivity to pain. A lapse of less than 20 seconds indicates a patient hypersensitive to pain.

PARALYSIS QUALIFICATION AND QUANTIFICATION

Overview

Motion is a fundamental property of most animal life. In the simple unicellular animals, motion and locomotion depend upon the contractility of protoplasm and the action of accessory organs, such as cilia or flagella. The lowest multicellular animals possess rudimentary neuromuscular mechanisms. In higher forms, motion is based on the transmission of impulses from a receptor through an afferent neuron and ganglion cell to muscle. This same principle is found in the reflex arc of higher animals, including humans, in whom the anterior spinal cord has developed into a central regulating mechanism. This central regulating mechanism is concerned with initiating and integrating movements.

Motor disturbances include weakness and paralysis, which may result from lesions of the voluntary motor pathways or of the muscles themselves. Impaired motor functioning may result from involvement of muscle, myoneural junction, peripheral nerve, or the CNS.

The types of paralysis or paresis are based on the location. Hemiplegia is a spastic or flaccid paralysis of one side of the body and extremities, limited by the median line sagittally. Monoplegia is a paralysis of one extremity only. Diplegia is a paralysis of any two corresponding extremities, both of which are usually lower extremities but may be upper extremities. Paraplegia is a symmetric paralysis of both lower extremities. Quadriplegia, or tetraplegia, is a paralysis of all four extremities. Hemiplegia alternans (crossed paralysis) is a paralysis of one or more ipsilateral cranial nerves and contralateral paralysis of the arm and leg.

Paralyses occur in many patients with hysteria, and they may be spastic or flaccid. With hysterical contracture the affected muscles are not atrophied, except in severe cases of long duration. The deep tendon reflexes are increased, and a spurious ankle-clonus may be present, but Babinski's sign is not observed. The limbs are most affected as is the case with hemiplegia, monoplegia, or paraplegia. Less often the muscles of the face are affected. Certain attitudes are characteristic of hysterical paralyses. The elbows, wrists, and fingers are kept flexed, and the arms are adducted. The hip and knee are extended, and the foot is held in a position of talipes equinovarus. Ptosis of the face may be simulated by spasm of the orbicularis palpebrarum, torticollis by contracture of the sternomastoid. In the less severe cases the stiffness and paresis are neither complete nor marked enough for the condition to be called a contracture. The deformity produced is the result of active muscular spasm. In severe and longstanding cases a true contracture results and the limb cannot be straightened by ordinary mechanical means. Highly characteristic of hysterical contracture is the patient's use of antagonistic muscles to prevent passive or active correction of the deformity exhibited.

∾ Tips for Assessment of Paralysis ∾

Abnormalities of the motor system, which may be manifestations of both hysteria and malingering, include disturbances of muscle strength and power; disorders of tone; dyskinesia; and abnormalities of corrdination, station, and gait. There are rarely changes in volume or contour (except for wasting from disuse) and no abnormalities on electromyography. These motor changes of psychic etiology may resemble almost any type of motor disturbance that is brought about by organic disease of the nervous system.

In both hysterical and malingered paralyses the patient makes little effort to contract the muscles necessary for executing the desired movement. The patient may remain calm and indifferent while demonstrating the lack of strength. The patient may also show little sign of alarm at the presence of complete paralysis and may smile cheerfully during the examination. Reliable evidence that the patient is not exerting all available power in an attempt to carry out a voluntary movement can be elicited by watching and palpating the contraction of the antagonists as well as the agonists.

Comment

Muscle imbalance at the hip encourages subluxation and dislocation. When the equilibrium between the flexor-adductor group and the abductor-extensor group is altered so the former overpowers the latter, the femoral neck is pulled medially to a more vertical position.

Disproportionate muscle forces necessary for producing subluxation and dislocation occur most often in children with myelomeningocele. Paralysis or paresis in one or both lower extremities is present at birth in more than 90% of the infants with thoracolumbar or lumbar myelomeningocele, and in more than 50% with lumbosacral or sacral myelomeningocele. The peculiar muscle imbalance is also found, but this is uncommon in cerebral palsy, poliomyelitis, and diseases and injuries of the cauda equina.

Procedure

Lower extremities are usually portrayed to be either weak or completely paralyzed. To determine a weak hip or leg, the patient is placed on the examination table in a supine position. The examiner flexes the legs at the hip, keeping the knees straight. The examiner holds the legs in an elevated position by cradling the patient's feet in a hand and instructs the patient to push the legs downward and hard against the examiner's hand. The examiner suddenly pulls the hand away. If leg weakness is of an organic origin, the affected leg will fall to the examining table. If the weakness is faked, the leg may move up or hang in midair for a moment before falling, because of hip muscle flexor actuation.

Confirmation Procedures

Hoover's sign, simulated foot-drop testing, tripod test (bilateral leg-fluttering test)

> ### Reporting Statement
>
> Lower extremity limb-dropping test indicates feigned paresis of the right leg.

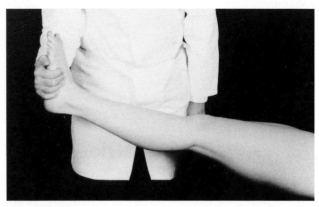

Fig. 13–63 The patient is lying supine on the examination table. The examiner performs a bilateral straight-leg raising test. As the legs are in the elevated position, the examiner instructs the patient to push the heel of the legs downward, against the examiner's resistance.

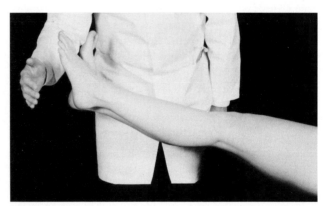

Fig. 13–64 The examiner unexpectedly pulls the supporting hand away from the legs. The leg affected with simulated paralysis will hang in the air momentarily before falling to the table. This result represents a positive test and indicates hysteria or malingering.

Comment

Intracerebral hemorrhage destroys the parenchyma. Cerebral thrombosis or embolism causes necrosis of the parenchyma (infarction, encephalomalacia) in the area supplied by the occluded vessel. If the embolus is septic and infection spreads beyond the vessel wall, encephalitis, brain abscess, or meningitis may result.

Specific symptoms are determined by the site of the lesion. Cerebral hemorrhage is most common in the region of the thalamus and internal capsule and is usually accompanied by severe hemiplegia, hemianesthesia, speech disturbance and sometimes hemianopsia. Because the middle cerebral artery or its branches are frequently the site of thrombosis or embolism, common symptoms are hemiplegia (affecting the arm more than the leg) and cortical sensory loss in the affected limbs. Various disturbances (aphasia and apraxia) may follow damage to the dominant hemisphere.

Procedure

Paralysis is yet another symptom presentation from the repertoire of the hysteric, psychogenic, rheumatic, or malingering patient.

A patient with a feigned paralyzed leg and arm may incorrectly assume there also will be difficulty in turning the head toward the paralyzed side. Pronation drift (the inability to hold the pronated arms still) is absent on station and gait.

Reporting Statement

Hemiplegic posturing is present and is inconsistent with organic hemiplegia.

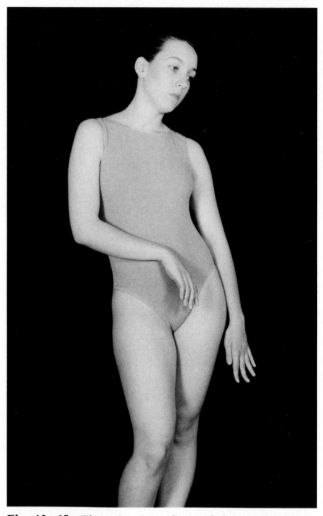

Fig. 13–65 The patient is standing, and the examiner assesses the patient's posture. In feigned paralysis, the paralyzed arm and leg are held in typical flexion contractures. The patient incorrectly assumes that the head cannot be turned toward the paralyzed side. Pronation drift is absent. This behavior indicates malingering or hysteria.

Comment

Neurologic loss is usually described as a sensory or motor deficit. The sensory loss may produce hypoesthesia, paresthesia, or hyperesthesia and may manifest as pain or numbness over a specific area. The motor deficits may be described as a weakness, stiffness, or more commonly as difficulty in walking far, running, or jumping. If there is outright paralysis, the onset may have been sudden or insidious. The paralysis may be flaccid or spastic. Flaccidity is associated with lower motor neuron disorders and spasticity with upper motor neuron disorders. The examiner must determine if the symptoms have increased or decreased and to what degree the patient is disabled. The examiner must also determine if there has been a loss of sphincter control of the bladder and rectum.

Procedure

Hoover's sign is helpful in differentiating between organic and hysterical paralysis. When a supine patient is directed to lift the paralyzed or affected one leg, it is normal for the patient to unconsciously press the heel of the unaffected leg against the examination table. In organic hemiplegia, this downward pressure is accentuated on the healthy side, as the patient attempts to raise the paretic leg. If the examiner places a hand under the heel, this pressure can be felt. In malingering there will be no, or very little, pressure on the opposite side of the affection as the patient attempts to raise the involved extremity.

Confirmation Procedures

Bilateral limb-dropping test (lower extremities), simulated foot-drop testing, tripod test (bilateral leg-fluttering test)

> ### Reporting Statement
>
> Hoover's sign is present on the right. The presence of this sign indicates feigned leg paresis.

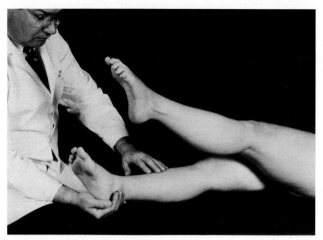

Fig. 13–66 The patient is lying supine on the examination table. The examiner places one hand under the heel of the unaffected leg. The patient attempts to lift the paralyzed leg off the table. The organically paralyzed patient presses the unaffected leg firmly downward, when attempting to flex the paralyzed hip. Because the malingerer is not trying, this synergistic action does not occur. The sign is present when the counterpressure is absent on the unaffected side. The sign indicates malingering or hysteria.

Comment

Complicated, coordinated movements are examined by observing the patient's manner of walking. Paresis will produce a slow, guarded, short-stepped, and shuffling gait. Paralysis of the anterior tibial muscles, especially by anterior horn or peripheral nerve lesion, causes a drop foot and produces a steppage gait. To avoid tripping over the plantar flexed foot, the extremity is advanced with the knee and hip flexed. With spasticity the legs are advanced slowly with shortened steps, and the toes scrape the ground. Adductor tightness produces a scissors gait, by which the legs are alternately crossed. With the ataxic, or tabetic, gait the patient must constantly observe the placement of the feet because of the absence of deep position sense. The hip is flexed and externally rotated and the forefoot is strongly dorsiflexed before being thrown down with the heel striking first. The patient is unable to stand with the eyes closed. In contrast, cerebellar ataxia is not aided by visual assistance. The gait appears stumbling and drunken, as the patient sways from side to side, and there is a tendency to fall toward the side of the lesion.

Procedure

With feigned total leg weakness/paralysis a patient may pretend to be unable to raise the forefoot while walking. This complaint must be separated from organic foot drop. The patient is standing and the examiner is positioned behind the patient. The patient is instructed to maintain a rigid and narrow-based posture, with the feet close together. In a surprise move the examiner grasps the shoulders of the patient and pulls the patient's body backward. The examiner notes the movement of the toes and forefoot. If the forefoot rises, the test is positive. A positive test indicates feigned foot drop.

Confirmation Procedures

Bilateral limb-dropping test (lower extremities), Hoover's sign, tripod test (bilateral leg-fluttering test)

> ### Reporting Statement
>
> Simulated foot-drop testing is positive. This result indicates a feigned steppage gait or foot drop.

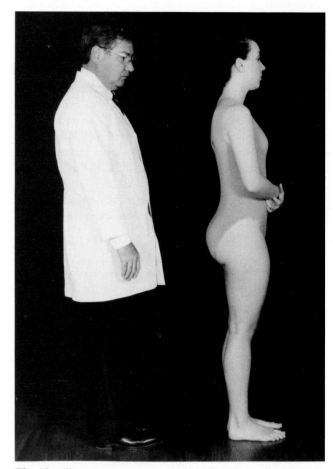

Fig.13–67 The patient is standing, and the examiner is positioned behind the patient. The patient is instructed to maintain a rigid and narrow-based posture with the feet close together.

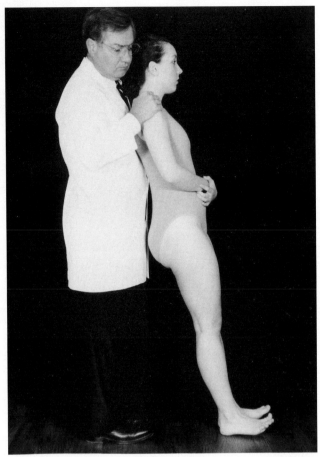

Fig. 13–68 In a surprise move, the examiner grasps the shoulders of the patient and pulls the patient's body backward. The examiner notes the movement of the toes and forefoot. If the forefoot rises, the test is positive. The positive test indicates feigned foot drop.

Comment

Although the function of one hand may be assessed, the impairment of function in one hand may clearly affect many activities that normally involve both hands performing together. The degree of overall functional impairment may be investigated by inquiring about or testing the patient's ability to perform certain tasks. This can be assessed efficiently with the Lamb Bilateral Hand Activity Index illustrated in the box below. When progress is being measured, each of these items listed in the box below may be scored on a scale of 0-5, or 0-10, and added. A total score of 80 or 160, respectively, represents a return to normal bilateral hand functions.

Activities Performed with Both Hands Acting Together★

1) Unscrew the top from a bottle.
2) Fill a cup and drink.
3) Open a can with a can-opener.
4) Remove a match from a box and light it.
5) Use a knife and fork for eating.
6) Apply toothpaste to a toothbrush and clean teeth.
7) Put on a jacket.
8) Close buttons on clothing.
9) Fasten a belt around the waist.
10) Tie shoe laces.
11) Sharpen a pencil.
12) Write messages.
13) Use a dial telephone.
14) Staple papers together.
15) Wrap string around a package.
16) Use playing cards.

★Modified from McRae R: *Clinical orthopaedic examination*, ed 3, Edinburgh, 1990, Churchill, Livingstone.

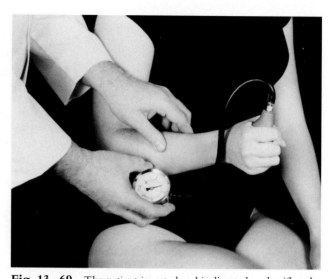

Fig. 13–69 The patient is seated and is directed to dorsiflex the wrist. If this move cannot be accomplished, the examiner instructs the patient to grip and squeeze a dynamometer. As the patient squeezes, the examiner palpates the forearm musculature. The test is positive when the examiner notes synergistic contraction of the forearm extensors and observes slight wrist dorsiflexion. The test is significant for feigned muscular weakness.

Procedure

If the complaint is persisting forearm or wrist weakness that is not associated with grip-strength loss, the patient is directed to dorsiflex the wrist. If this cannot be done, the patient is then asked to squeeze a dynamometer while the examiner palpates the patient's forearm. In functional or feigned weakness the examiner will feel the patient's forearm extensors contract synergistically and will see the wrist extend when the patient squeezes.

Confirmation Procedures

Simulated grip-strength-loss testing

Reporting Statement

Testing for simulated weakness of the forearm and wrist is positive on the right. This result indicates feigned muscular weakness.

Comment

When a patient presents with weakness, the physician must consider many possible causes. There is such a wide range of differential diagnosis that an evaluation for all the possible causes of weakness not only would be cumbersome but also costly for the patient and time consuming for the examiner. Perhaps even more important, the patient is exposed to potentially hazardous and painful tests that might be unnecessary. It is desirable, therefore, to ascertain the anatomic locus of the patient's weakness.

When a weak patient presents with evidence of motor unit disease and the cause is not myopathic, then the patient is probably suffering from a neuropathy. The differential diagnosis of neuropathy includes many diseases that present with similar symptoms (symmetric distal sensory losses). However, occasionally patients with neuropathy may present with the following symptoms: (1) thickened nerves (hypertrophic neuropathy), (2) mononeuritis, (3) radiculopathy, (4) cranial nerve involvement, (5) autonomic disturbances, (6) ascending neuritis, and (7) weakness without sensory findings.

Procedure

When grip-strength loss is the complaint, the patient is directed to squeeze the examiner's fingers with the paralyzed hand as hard as possible. While the patient does this, the examiner suddenly tears the fingers away. If grip weakness is due to organic disease, a sudden tug will break the grasp easily. If the weakness is being faked, strong resistance is likely to be encountered before the malingerer realizes the error or contradiction and releases the grip.

Confirmation Procedures

Simulated forearm-and-wrist-weakness testing

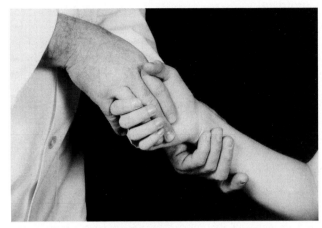

Fig. 13–70   The seated patient is instructed to grip and squeeze the examiner's fingers with the paralyzed hand as hard as possible.

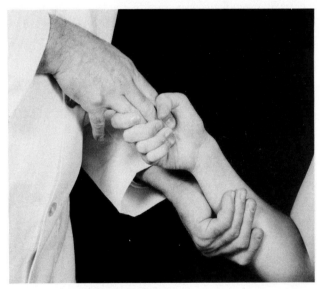

Fig. 13–71   As the patient continues the grip, the examiner unexpectedly tears the fingers from the grip. Strong resistance is likely to be encountered before the patient realizes the error and releases the grip. In organic disease, the sudden tug will break the grasp easily. The test is positive for feigned loss of grip.

Reporting Statement
Simulated grip-strength-loss testing is positive on the right. This result indicates feigned loss of strength.

～ Tripod Test (Bilateral Leg-Fluttering Test) ～

Comment

Lesions of the lower motor neurons may be located in the ventral gray column of the spinal cord or brainstem or in their axons, which constitute the ventral roots of the spinal nerves or the cranial nerves. Lesions may result from trauma, toxins, infections, and vascular disorders or congenital malformations, degenerative processes, or neoplasms. Signs of lower motor neuron lesions include flaccid paralysis of the involved muscles, muscle atrophy, and a degeneration reaction. Reflexes of the involved muscle are diminished or absent and no pathologic reflexes are obtainable.

Procedure

A patient may attempt to fake a leg paralysis as the result of a further faked lumbar intervertebral disc syndrome. In this instance the patient is instructed to sit on the examination table with the knees flexed at 90 degrees and the legs hanging dependent. The patient is directed to rapidly and repeatedly extend and relax, or flex, the legs. If lumbar disc involvement exists, the patient will need to lean backward to perform this maneuver, if able to do it at all. The patient feigning disc involvement can accomplish the maneuver without assuming such a tripod posture.

Confirmation Procedures

Bilateral limb-dropping test (lower extremities), Hoover's sign, simulated foot-drop testing

---

Reporting Statement

Tripod testing is negative, and simulated lumbar pain is indicated.

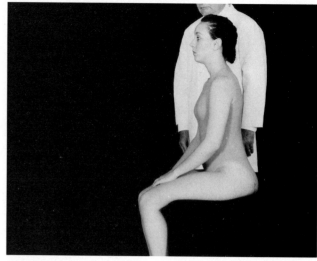

Fig. 13–72 The patient is instructed to sit on the examining table with the knees flexed at 90 degrees and the legs hanging dependent.

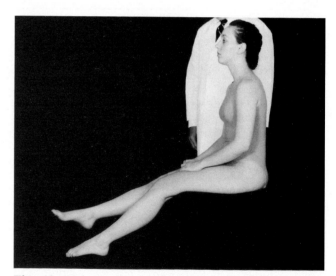

Fig. 13–73 The patient is directed to rapidly and repeatedly extend the legs, in a flutter maneuver.

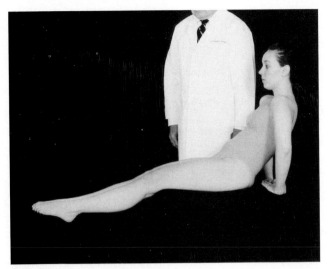

Fig. 13–74   If a lumbar disc involvement exists, the patient will need to lean backward to perform this maneuver, if the patient is even able to perform the maneuver at all.

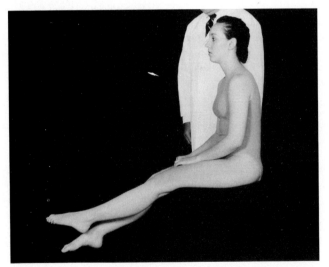

Fig. 13–75   The patient who is feigning disc involvement can accomplish the maneuver without assuming such a tripod posture.

Bibliography

American Medical Association: *Guides to the evaluation of permanent impairment,* ed 3, Chicago, 1990, The Association.

Apley AG, Solomon L: *Concise system of orthopaedics and fractures,* London, 1988, Butterworth-Heinemann.

Aronoff GM: *Evaluation and treatment of chronic pain,* Baltimore, 1985, Urban and Schwartzenberg.

Aronoff GM, McAlary PW, Witkower A, Berdell MS: Pain treatment programs: Do they run workers to the workplace? *Spine,* 2: 123, 1987.

Benson DF, Blumer D: *Psychiatric aspect of neurologic disease,* New York, 1975, Grune and Stratton.

Borenstein DG, Wiesel SW: *Low back pain, medical diagnosis and comprehensive management,* Philadelphia, 1987, WB Saunders.

Borg G: Psychophysical bases of perceived exertion, *Med and Science in Sport and Exercise,* 14:(5):377, 1982.

Bradley LA: Multivariate analysis of the MMPI profiles of low back pain patients, *J Behav Med,* 1:253, 1978.

Brena SF, Chapman SL: Pain and litigation, Textbook of pain, Edinburgh, 1984, Churchill Livingstone.

Cipriano JJ: *Photographic manual of regional orthopaedic and neurological tests,* ed 2, Baltimore, 1991, Williams and Wilkins.

Cousins MJ, Phillips GD: *Acute pain management,* New York, 1986, Churchill Livingston.

D'Ambrosia RD: *Musculoskeletal disorders regional examination and differential diagnosis,* Philadelphia, 1977, JB Lippincott.

Dandy DJ: *Essential orthopaedics and trauma,* Edinburgh, 1989, Churchill Livingstone.

DeMeyer W: Technique of the neurologic examination: A programmed text, New York, 1969, McGraw-Hill.

American Psychiatric Association: *Diagnostic and statistical manual of mental disorders* ed 3, Washington, 1980, The Association.

Doherty M, Doherty J: *Clinical examination in rheumatology,* London, 1992, Wolfe Publishing.

Dorland's Illustrated medical dictionary, ed 27, Agnew LRC (editor), Philadelphia, 1988, WB Saunders.

Ellard J: Psychological reactions to Compensable Injury, *Med J Aust,* 8:349, 1970.

Evans RC: Malingering/symptoms exaggeration, In Sweere JJ (editor): *Chiropractic family practice, a clinical manual,* Gaithersburg, 1992, Aspen Publication.

Evans RC: *Overview of orthopedic malingering, capit homecoming and educational symposium,* Rotorura, 1986, Phillip Institute of Science and Technology.

Fairbank JTC: The Oswestry low back pain disability questionnaire, *Physiotherapy,* 8:66, 271, 1980.

Finneson BE: Low back pain, ed 2, Philadelphia, 1981, JB Lippincott.

Gentry WD, Newman MC, Goldner JL, Baeyer CV: Relation between graduated spinal block technique and MMPI for diagnosis and prognosis of chronic low back pain, *Spine* 2(3), 1977.

Goldner JL, Jones WB: Anomalous innervation of the forearm and hand, *J Bone Joint Surg,* 48(A):604, 1966.

Goldner JL, Fisher G: Index ray deletion-complication and sequelae, *J Bone Joint Surg* 54(A):898, 1972.

Goldner JL, and others: Upper limb pain, proceedings ASSH, *J Bone Joint Surg* 54(A):899, 1972.

Goldner JL: Volkman's ischemia contracture, In Flynn JE (editor) *Hand surgery,* ed 2, Baltimore, 1975, Williams and Wilkins.

Goldner JL: Musculoskeletal aspects of emotional problems, editorial, *South Med J,* 69:1, 1976.

Goldner JL, Bright DS: The effect of extremity blood flow on pain and cold tolerance, In Omer G, Spinner M: *Peripheral nerve injuries,* Philadelphia, 1979, WB Saunders.

Gunn CC, Bilbrandt WE: Early and subtle signs in low back sprain, *Spine,* 3:267, 1978.

Guyton AC: *Structure and function of the nervous system,* Philadelphia, 1972, WB Saunders.

Hart FD: *French's index of differential diagnosis,* ed 10, Baltimore, 1973, Williams and Wilkins.

Heilman KM, Watson RT, Greer M: *Handbook for differential diagnosis of neurologic signs and symptoms,* New York, 1977, Appleton-Century-Crofts.

Holvey DN, Talbott JH: *The Merck manual of diagnosis and therapy,* ed 12, New Jersey, 1972, Merck.

Jabaley ME, Burns JE, Orcutt BA, Bryant WM: Comparison of histologic and functional recovery after peripheral nerve repair, *J Hand Surg* [AM], 1:119, 1976.

Jacobs JW: Screening for organic mental syndromes in the medically ill, *Ann Intern Med,* 86:40, 1977.

Katz WA: *Rheumatic diseases diagnosis and management,* Philadelphia, 1977, JB Lippincott.

Keefe FJ: Behavioral assessment and treatment of chronic pain: Current status and future directions, *J Consult Clin Psychol,* 50: 896, 1982.

Kelsey JL: An epidemiological study of acute herniated lumbar intervertebral disc, *Rheum Rehab,* 14:144, 1975.

Kendall HO, Kendall FP, Wadsworth GE: *Muscles testing and function,* ed 2, Baltimore, 1971, Williams and Wilkins.

Levin H, Conley CL: Thrombocytosis associated with malignant disease, *Arch Intern Med,* 114:497, 1964.

Loewebstein WR: Biological transducers, *Scientific American,* 203: 98, 1960.

Magee DJ: *Orthopedic physical assessment,* Philadelphia, 1987, WB Saunders.

Mayer TG: A prospective two year study of functional restoration in industrial low back injury: An objective assessment procedure, *JAMA,* 258: 1763, 1987.

Mayo Clinic and Mayo Foundation: *Clinical examinations in neurology,* ed 5, Philadelphia, 1981, WB Saunders.

Mazion JM: *Illustrated manual of neurological/reflexes/signs/tests, Part I, Orthopedic signs/tests/maneuvers for office procedure, Part II,* Orlando, 1980, Daniels Publishing.

McBride ED: Disability evaluation and principles of treatment of compensable injuries, ed 6, Philadelphia, 1963, JB Lippincott.

McRae R: *Clinical orthopaedic examination,* ed 3, Edinburgh, 1990, Churchill Livingstone.

Medical Economics Books: *Patient care flow chart manual,* ed 3, Oradell, NJ, 1982, Medical Economics Books.

Melzack R: *The McGill pain questionnaire: Pain measurement and assessment,* New York, 1983, Raven Press.

Merskey H: *Pain and psychological medicine, textbook of pain,* Edinburgh, 1984, Churchill Livingstone.

Million T, Green CJ, Meagher RB: *Million behavioral health inventory,* ed 3, Minneapolis, 1982, Interpretive Scoring System.

Mountcastle VB: Sensory receptors and neural encoding: Introduction to sensory processes, In Mountcastle VB (editor): *Medical physiology,* St. Louis, 1974, Mosby.

Mountcastle VB: The view from within: Pathways to the study of perception, *Johns Hopkins Med J,* 136:109, 1975.

Nachemson AL: The lumbar spine: an orthopaedic challenge, *Spine,* 1:59, 1976.

O'Donoghue DH: Treatment of injuries to athletes, ed 3, Philadelphia, 1976, WB Saunders.

Olson WH, Brumback RA: *Handbook of symptom-oriented neurology,* Chicago, 1989, Mosby.

Omer GE, Spinner M: Management of peripheral nerve problems, Philadelphia, 1980, WB Saunders.

Osterweis M, Kleinman A, Mechanic D: *Pain and disability: Clinical, behavioral and public policy perspectives, report of the institute of medicine committee on pain, disability and chronic illness behavior,* Washington, DC, 1987, National Academy Press.

Pilling LF, Brannick TL, Swenson WM: Psychological characteristics of patients having pain as a presenting symptom, *Can Med Assoc J,* 97:287, 1967.

Reed R: *Malingering, symposium papers,* Los Angeles, 1986, American College of Chiropractic Orthopedists.

Rockwood CA Jr, Eilbert RE: Camptocormia, *J Bone Joint Surg,* 51(A):533, 1969.

Rotes-Querol J: The syndrome of psychogenic rheumatism, *Clin Rheum Dis,* 5:797, 1979.

Schram S, Taylor T: Tension signs in lumber disc prolapse, *Clin Orthop,* 75:195, 1971.

Sherman MS: The nerves of bones, *J Bone Joint Surg,* 45(A):522, 1963.

Thurston SE: *The little black book of neurology,* Chicago, 1987, Mosby.

Truex RC, Carpenter MB: Human neuroanatomy, ed 6, Baltimore, 1969, Williams and Wilkins.

Turek SL: Orthopaedics principles and their application, ed 3, Philadelphia, 1977, JB Lippincott.

Waddell G: An approach to backache, *Br J Hosp Med,* 28:187, 1982.

Waddell G: A new clinical model for the treatment of low back pain, *Spine,* 12:632, 1987.

Walshe FMR: Diseases of the nervous system, ed 11, Baltimore, 1970, Williams and Wilkins.

Walters A: Psychogenic regional pain alias hysterical pain, *Brain,* 84:1, 1961.

Wing PC, Wilfling FJ, Kokan PJ: *Comprehensive analysis of disability following lumbar intervertebral fusion: Medical diagnosis and management,* Philadelphia, 1987, WB Saunders.

Listing of Tests, Alphabetically and Anatomically

CERVICAL SPINE

Bakody sign
Barre-Lieou sign
Bikele's sign
Brachial plexus tension test
Dejerine's sign
DeKleyn's test
Distraction test
Foraminal compression test
Hallpike maneuver
Hautant's test
Jackson cervical compression test
Lhermitte's sign
Maximum cervical compression test
Naffziger's test
O'Donoghue maneuver
Rust's sign
Shoulder depression test
Soto-Hall sign
Spinal percussion test
Spurling's test
Swallowing test
Underburg's test
Valsalva maneuver
Vertebrobasilar artery functional maneuver

SHOULDER

Abbott-Saunders test
Adson's test
Allen maneuver
Apley's test
Apprehension test
Bryant's sign
Calloway's test
Codman's sign
Costoclavicular maneuver
Dawbarn's sign
Dugas' sign

George's screening procedure
Halstead maneuver
Hamilton's test
Impingement sign
Ludington's test
Mazion's shoulder maneuver
Reverse Bakody maneuver
Roos' test
Shoulder compression test
Speed's test
Subacromial push button sign
Supraspinatus press test
Transverse humeral ligament test
Wright's test
Yergason's test

ELBOW

Cozen's test
Elbow flexion test
Golfer's elbow test
Kaplan's sign
Ligamentous instability test
Mills's test
Tinel's sign at the elbow

FOREARM, WRIST, AND HAND

Allen's test
Bracelet test
Bunnell-Littler test
Carpal lift sign
Cascade sign
Dellon's moving two-point discrimination test
Finkelstein's test
Finsterer's sign
Froment's paper sign
Interphalangeal neuroma test
Maisonneuve's sign

Phalen's sign
Pinch grip test
Shrivel test
Test for tight retinacular ligaments
Tinel's sign at the wrist
Tourniquet test
Wartenberg's sign
Weber's two-point discrimination test
Wringing test

THORACIC SPINE

Adam's positions
Amoss's sign
Anghelescu's sign
Beevor's sign
Chest expansion test
First thoracic nerve root test
Forestier's bowstring sign
Passive scapular approximation test
Rib motion test
Schepelmann's sign
Spinal percussion test
Sponge test
Sternal compression test

LUMBAR SPINE

Antalgia sign
Bechterew's sitting test
Bilateral leg-lowering test
Bowstring sign
Bragard's sign
Cox sign
Demianoff's sign
Deyerle's sign
Double leg-raise test
Ely's sign
Fajersztajn's test
Femoral nerve traction test
Heel/toe walk test
Hyperextension test
Kemp's test
Kernig/Brudzinski sign
Lasègue differential sign
Lasègue rebound test
Lasègue sitting test
Lasègue test
Lewin punch test
Lewin snuff test
Lewin standing test
Lewin supine test
Lindner's sign
Match stick test
Mennell's sign
Milgram's test

Minor's sign
Nachlas test
Néri's sign
Prone knee-bending test
Quick test
Schober's test
Sicard's sign
Sign of the buttock
Skin pinch test
Spinal percussion test
Straight-leg raising test
Turyn's sign
Vanzetti's sign

PELVIS AND SACROILIAC JOINT

Anterior innominate test
Belt test
Erichsen's sign
Gaenslen's test
Gapping test
Goldthwait's sign
Hibb's test
Iliac compression test
Knee-to-shoulder test
Laguerre's test
Lewin-Gaenslen's test
Piedallu's sign
Sacral apex test
Sacroiliac resisted-abduction test
Smith-Petersen test
Squish test
Yeoman's test

HIP

Actual leg length test
Allis' sign
Anvil test
Apparent leg-length test
Chiene's test
Gauvain's sign
Guilland's sign
Hip telescoping test
Jansen's test
Ludloff's sign
Ober's test
Patrick's test
Phelp's test
Thomas test
Trendelenburg's test

KNEE

Abduction stress test
Adduction stress test
Apley's compression test

Apprehension test for the patella
Bounce home test
Childress duck waddle test
Clarke's sign
Drawer test
Dreyer's sign
Fouchet's sign
Lachman test
Lateral pivot shift maneuver
Losee test
McMurray sign
Noble compression test
Patella ballottement test
Payr's sign
Q-angle test
Slocum's test
Steinmann's sign
Thigh circumference test
Wilson's sign

LEG, ANKLE, AND FOOT

Anterior drawer sign of the ankle
Buerger's test
Claudication test
Duchenne's sign
Foot tourniquet test
Helbings' sign
Hoffa's test
Homans' sign
Keen's sign
Morton's test
Moszkowicz' test
Moses' test
Perthes' test
Strunsky's sign
Thompson's test
Tinel's foot sign

MALINGERING AND PSYCHOGENIC RHEUMATISM

Special hand signals by the patient
Axial trunk-loading test
Burn's bench test
Flexed-hip test
Flip sign
Libman test
Magnuson's test
Mannkopf's sign
Marked part pain-suggestibility test
Plantar flexion test
Related joint motion test
Seeligmüller's sign
Trunk rotational test
Anosmia testing
Coordination-disturbance test
Cuignet's test
Facial anesthesia test
Gault test
Janet's test
Limb-dropping test (upper extremities)
Lombard's test
Marcus Gunn's sign
Midline tuning-fork test
Optokinetic nystagmus test
Position-sense testing
Regional anesthesia testing
Romberg's sign
Snellen's test
Stoicism indexing
Bilateral limb-dropping test (lower extremities)
Hemiplegic posturing
Hoover's sign
Simulated foot-drop testing
Simulated forearm-and-wrist-weakness testing
Simulated grip-strength-loss test
Tripod test (bilateral leg-fluttering test)

Listing of Tests According to the Position of the Patient

THE STANDING EXAMINATION

Adam's positions
Antalgia sign
Anterior innominate test
Axial trunk-loading test
Belt test
Burn's bench test
Chest expansion test
Childress duck waddle test
Claudication test
Dejerine's sign
Forestier's bowstring sign
Heel/toe walk test
Helbings' sign
Hemiplegic posturing
Kemp's test
Lewin punch test
Lewin snuff test
Lewin standing test
Magnuson's test
Mazion's shoulder maneuver
Mennell's sign
Néri's bowing sign
Passive scapular approximation test
Perthes' test
Quick test
Romberg's sign
Schepelmann's sign
Schober's test
Simulated foot-drop testing
Spinal percussion test
Trendelenburg's test
Underburg's test
Valsalva maneuver
Vanzetti's sign

THE SITTING EXAMINATION

Abbott-Saunders test
Adson's test

Allen's test
Anosmia testing
Apley's compression test
Apprehension test
Apprehension test for the patella
Bakody sign
Barre-Lieou sign
Bechterew's sitting test
Bikele's sign
Bracelet test
Brachial plexus tension test
Bryant's sign
Bunnell-Littler test
Calloway's test
Carpal lift sign
Cascade sign
Codman's sign
Coordination-disturbance testing
Costoclavicular maneuver
Cozen's test
Cuignet's test
Dawbarn's sign
Dellon's moving two-point discrimination test
Deyerle's sign
Distraction test
Dugas' test
Elbow flexion test
Facial anesthesia test
Finkelstein's test
Finsterer's sign
First thoracic nerve root test
Flip sign
Foraminal compression test
Froment's paper sign
Gault test
George's screening procedure
Golfer's elbow test
Halstead maneuver

Hamilton's test
Hautant's test
Impingement sign
Interphalangeal neuroma test
Jackson cervical compression test
Janet's test
Kaplan's sign
Lasègue sitting test
Libman test
Ligamentous instability test
Lindner's sign
Lombard's test
Ludington's test
Ludloff's sign
Lhermitte's sign
Maisonneuve's sign
Marcus Gunn's sign
Marked part pain suggestibility test
Maximum cervical compression test
Midline tuning-fork test
Mills's test
Minor's sign
Naffziger's test
Optokinetic nystagmus test
O'Donoghue maneuver
Payr's sign
Phalen's sign
Piedallu's sign
Pinch grip test
Regional anesthesia test
Reverse Bakody maneuver
Roos' test
Rust's sign
Seeligmüller's sign
Shoulder compression test
Shoulder depression test
Shrivel test
Simulated forearm-and-wrist-weakness testing
Simulated grip-strength-loss testing
Slocum's test
Snellen's test
Speed's test
Spurling's test
Stoicism indexing
Subacromial push button sign
Supraspinatus press test
Swallowing test
Test for tight retinacular ligaments
Tinel's sign at the elbow
Tinel's sign at the wrist
Tourniquet test
Transverse humeral ligament test
Tripod test (bilateral leg-fluttering test)
Vertebrobasilar artery functional maneuver

Wartenberg's sign
Weber's two-point discrimination test
Wright's test
Wringing test
Yergason's test

THE SUPINE EXAMINATION

Abduction stress test
Actual leg length test
Adduction stress test
Allis' sign
Amoss's sign
Anghelescu's sign
Anterior drawer sign of the ankle
Anvil test
Apparent leg-length test
Beevor's sign
Bilateral limb-dropping test (lower extremities)
Bilateral leg-lowering test
Bounce home test
Bowstring sign
Bragard's sign
Buerger's test
Calf circumference test
Chiene's test
Clarke's sign
Cox sign
DeKleyn's test
Demianoff's sign
Deyerle's sign
Double leg-raise test
Drawer test
Dreyer's sign
Duchenne's sign
Fajersztajn's test
Flexed-hip test
Tourniquet test
Fouchet's sign
Gapping test
Goldthwait's sign
Guilland's sign
Hallpike maneuver
Hip telescoping test
Homans' sign
Hoover's sign
Jansen's test
Keen's sign
Kernig/Brudzinski sign
Knee-to-shoulder test
Lachman test
Laguerre's test
Lasègue differential test
Lasègue rebound test
Lasègue test

Lateral pivot shift maneuver
Lewin supine test
Limb-dropping test (upper limbs)
Losee test
McMurray sign
Milgram's test
Morton's test
Moszkowicz' test
Noble compression test
Patella ballottement test
Patrick's test
Plantar flexion test
Rib motion test
Sicard's sign
Sign of the buttock
Smith-Petersen test
Soto-Hall sign
Squish test
Steinmann's sign
Sternal compression test
Straight-leg raising test
Strunsky's sign
Thigh circumference test
Thomas test
Turyn's sign
Wilson's sign

SIDE-LYING EXAMINATION

Femoral nerve traction test
Gaenslen's test
Gauvain's sign
Iliac compression test
Lewin-Gaenslen's test
Match stick test
Ober's test
Sacroiliac resisted-abduction test
Skin pinch test

PRONE EXAMINATION

Apley's compression test
Ely's sign
Erichsen's sign
Hibb's test
Hoffa's test
Hyperextension test
Mannkopf's sign
Moses' test
Nachlas test
Phelp's test
Prone knee-bending test
Sacral apex test
Sponge test
Thompson's test
Tinel's foot sign
Yeoman's test

APPENDIX C

Glossary of Abbreviations

A	Assessment
Abd. hall.	Abductor hallucis
Abd. dig. V	Abductor digiti five
Abd. poll. brev.	Abductor pollicis brevis
Abd. poll. long.	Abductor pollicis longus
abnl	Abnormal
AC	Acrocyanosis
ACJ	Acromioclavicular joint
A & D	Amplitude & Duration
Abd. long.	Abductor longus
ADL	Activities of daily living
AE	Above elbow
AJ	Ankle jerk
AK	Above knee
AKA	Above-knee amputation
ALS	Amyotrophic lateral sclerosis
amb	Ambulate
AMP	Amputation
Amp. sl	Amplitude slightly increased
Ampl, dur&#	Amplitude, duration & number
ANA	Antinuclear antibody
Anc	Anconeus
ANF	Antinuclear factor
ant	Anterior
Ant. tib.	Anterior tibialis
AP and lat.	Anterior-posterior and lateral
ARM	Active range of motion
AS	Left ear
AU	Both ears
A&W	Alive and Well
ax	Axillary
B	Brisk
Bic	Biceps
Biceps fem.	Biceps femoris
BJ	Biceps jerk
BJM	Bones, joints, & muscles
BK	Below knee
BKA	Below-knee amputation
BP	Blood pressure
Brachionad	Brachionadialis
Bru	Bruised
C/O	Complaint of
c/o	Complaining of

C1–C8	Cervical 1st root through cervical 8th root
C1–C2	1st cervical vertebrae 2nd cervical vertebrae
Ca	Carcinoma
CAT	Computerized axial tomography
CC	Chief complaint
cm	Centimeter, centimeters
CM	Costal margin
CMC	Carpometacarpal
CNS	Central nervous system
cond	Condition
cont	Continue
Dr.	Doctor
DRG	Diagnosis Related Groups
DTR	Deep tendon reflexes
dur	duration
Dx	Diagnosis
e.r.	Evoked response
EBV	Epstein–Barr virus
ECU	Extensor carpi ulnaris
edx	Electrodiagnosis
EEG	Electroencephalogram
EJ	Elbow jerk
EKG	Electrocardiogram
EMG	Electromyogram
Enc	Encourage
EPS	Extraparametal symptoms
ESR	Erythrocyte sedimation rate
eval	Evaluation
Evoked pot.	Evoked potential
Exam	Examination
ext	External
Ext. ind	Extensor indices
Ext. c. rad. B	Extensor carpi radialis brevis
Ext. c. rad. L	Extensor carpi radialis longus
Ext. dig. brev.	Extensor digitorum brevis
Ext. dig. comm.	Extensor digitorum communis
Ext. dig. long.	Extensor digitorum longus
Ext. hall. long.	Extensor hallucis longus
Ext. poll. brev.	Extensor pollicis brevis
Ext. poll. long.	Extensor pollicus longus
extr	Extremity
FB	Foreign body
FHx	Family history
FLEX	Flexion
Flex. c. rad.	Flexor carpi radialis
Flex. c. uln.	Flexor carpi ulnaris
Flex. dig. prof.	Flexor digitorum profundus
Flex. dig. subl.	Flexor digitorum sublimis
ft	Foot
FUO	Fever of undetermined origin
FWB	Full weight bearing
FX	Fracture
Gastroc	Gastrocnemius

Glut. max.	Gluteus maximus
Glut. med.	Gluteus medius
GP	General practitioner
GSW	Gunshot wound
H&P	History and physical
Ha	Headache
HBP	High blood pressure
HEENT	Head, eyes, ears, nose & throat
ht	Height
Hx	History
ICS	Intercostal space
IM	Intramuscular
Inf. glut.	Inferior gluteal
Infraspin.	Infraspinatus
Instr	Instruction
IP	Interphalangeal
IPJ	Interphalangeal joint
JRA	Juvenile rheumatoid arthritis
jt	Joint
KJ	Knee jerk
Lab	Laboratory
LBP	Low blood pressure
LMN	Lower motor neuron
LMP	Last menstrual period
LOA	Left occiput anterior
LOC	Loss of consciousness
LOM	Limitation of motion
LOP	Left occiput posterior
med	Median
ML	Midline
mp	Metacarpophalyngeal
MPJ	Metacarpophalangeal joint
MRI	Magnetic resonance imaging
MS	Multiple sclerosis
MTP	Metatarsophalangeal
MUAP's	Motor unit action potentials
N	Nerve
N&V	Nausea and vomiting
N/A	Not applicable
NAD	No acute distress
NCV	Nerve conduction velocity
NKA	No known allergies
NR	Normal range
NRC	Nerve root compression
N/V	Nausea/vomiting
NVD	Nausea, vomiting, and diarrhea
NWB	Nonweight bearing
OA	Osteoarthritis
obt	Obturator
Ortho	Orthopedic
O.T.	Occupational therapy
OTC	Over the counter
PA	Posteroanterior
palp	Palpate, palpated, palpable
PE	Physical examination

pect. maj.	Pectoralis major
pect. min.	Pectoralis minor
Periph	Peripheral
Peron. brevis	Peroneus brevis
Peron. long.	Peroneus longus
PERRLA	Pupils equal, round, reactive to light and accommodation
PH	Past history, personal history
PI	Present illness
PID	Pelvic inflammatory disease
PIP	Proximal interphalangeal
PIPJ	Proximal interphalangeal joint
PM&R	Physical medicine and rehabilitation
po	Phone order
pos	Positive
post	Posterior
post	After
PP	Proximal phalanx
PR	Pulse rate
PRIND	Partial Residual Ischemic Neurovascular Deficit
prn	As the occasion arises (pro re nata)
prod	Productive
Pron. quad.	Pronator quadratus
Pron. ter.	Pronator teres
prox	Proximal
P.T.	Physical Therapy
pt	Patient
PVD	Peripheral vascular disease
PWB	Partial weight-bearing
RA	Rheumatoid arthritis
Rehab	Rehabilitation
RF	Rheumatic fever
Rhomb	Rhomboids
RIND	Reversible Ischemic Neurologic Deficit
RLE	Right lower extremity
R/O	Rule out
ROM	Range of motion
ROS	Review of systems
rp	Radial pulse
RPO	Right posterior oblique
R.T.	Recreation Therapy
RTO	Return to office
RUE	Right upper extremity
S&S	Signs and symptoms
S1–S5	Sacral 1st root through sacral 5th root
S1–S2	First, second heart sounds
Sciat	Sciatic
SCM	Sternocleidomastoid
SD	Standard deviation
Sed. rate	Sedimentation rate
Semi. memb.	Semimembranosis
Sens	Sensory
Ser. ant.	Serratus anterior
SF	Spinal fluid
SHx	Social history

SI	Sacroiliac
SIJ	Sacroiliac joint
SLE	Systemic lupus erythematosis
SLR	Straight leg raises
SMA-12	Sequential multiple analysis (12-channel biochemical profile)
SOAP	Subjective, Objective, Assessment, Plan
SOB	Short of breath
sol.	Soleus
St	Strong
Strep	Streptococcus
Sup. glut.	Superior gluteal
Suprascap	Suprascapular
Supraspin	Supraspinatus
Sx	Symptoms
T	Temperature
T1-T12	1st thoracic root through 12th thoracic root
Tc	Transcutaneous
thor	Thoracic
Ther	Therapy
THR	Total hip replacement
TIA	Transient ischemic attack
tib	Tibial
ting	Tingling
TJ	Triceps jerk
TMJ	Temporomandibular joint
tol	Tolerated
tp	Treatment plan
TPR	Temperature, pulse, and respiration
Trap	Trapezius
Tric	Triceps
Tx	Treatment
UMN	Upper motor neuron
UA	Urinalysis
vib	Vibration
Vig	Vigorous

Cross-Reference Tables for Tissue or Area Examined

	Nerve root	VBA Syndrome	Brachial plexus	Meningitis	IVD syndrome	Tumor	Fracture	Dural irritation	Sprain	Facet	Myospasm	Subluxation	Arthritis
Bakody sign	●												
Barre-Lieou sign		●											
Bikele's sign			●	●									
Brachial plexus tension test	●		●		●	●	●						
Dejerine's sign	●												
DeKleyn's test		●											
Distraction test	●									●	●		
Foraminal compression test	●												
Hallpike maneuver		●											
Hautant's test		●											
Jackson cervical compression test					●	●				●		●	●
L'hermitte's sign								●					
Maximum cervical compression test	●									●	●		
Naffziger's test	●					●			●		●		
O'Donoghue maneuver									●		●		
Rust's sign							●		●			●	●
Shoulder depression test	●							●		●			
Soto-Hall sign				●	●		●			●		●	●
Spinal percussion test					●		●					●	
Spurling's test	●												
Swallowing test					●	●							●
Underburg's test		●											
Valsalva maneuver					●	●							
Vertebrobasilar artery functional maneuver		●											

Fig. D–1   Cervical spine cross-reference table for tissue or area being examined.

	Biceps tendon	Scalenus anticus syndrome	Thoracic outlet syndrome	Rotator cuff	Anterior dislocation	Posterior dislocation	Supraspinatus tendon	Subacromial bursa	Subclavian arterial stenosis	Adhesive capsulitis	Transverse humeral ligament
Abbott-Saunders test	●										
Adson's test		●	●								
Allen maneuver			●								
Apley's test				●							
Apprehension test					●	●					
Bryant's sign					●	●					
Calloway's test					●	●					
Codman's sign					●		●				
Costoclavicular maneuver			●								
Dawbarn's sign								●			
Dugas test					●	●					
George's screening procedure									●		
Halstead maneuver			●								
Hamilton's test					●	●					
Impingement sign	●						●				
Ludington's test	●										
Mazion's shoulder maneuver				●	●	●				●	
Reverse Bakody maneuver		●	●								
Roos' test			●								
Shoulder compression test			●						●		
Speed's test	●										
Subacromial push button sign					●		●				
Supraspinatus press test							●				
Transverse humeral ligament test	●										●
Wright's test			●								
Yergason's test	●										●

Fig. D–2 Shoulder joint cross-reference table for tissue or are examined.

	Lateral epicondylitis	Radiohumeral bursitis	Cubital tunnel syndrome	Medial epicondylitis	Neuropathy	Sprain
Cozen's test	●	●				
Elbow flexion test			●			
Golfer's elbow test				●		
Kaplan's sign	●					
Ligamentous instability test						●
Mills's test	●					
Tinel's sign at the elbow					●	

Fig. D–3 Elbow joint cross-reference table for tissue or area examined.

Diagnosis	Allen's test	Bracelet test	Bunnell-Littler test	Carpal lift sign	Cascade sign	Dellon's moving two-point discrimination test	Finkelstein's test	Finsterer's sign	Froment's paper sign	Interphalangeal neuroma test	Maisonneuve's sign	Phalen's sign	Pinch grip test	Shrivel test	Test for tight retinacular ligaments	Tinel's sign at the wrist	Tourniquet test	Wartenberg's sign	Weber's two-point discrimination test	Wringing test
Anterior interosseous syndrome													●							
Carpal tunnel syndrome												●				●	●			●
Colles' fracture											●									
Neuroma										●										
Ulnar neuropathy						●			●							●	●	●	●	
Aseptic necrosis								●												
Tenosynovitis							●													
Denervation						●								●				●		
Sprain				●																
Carpal fracture				●	●			●												
Digit contractures			●											●						
Rheumatoid arthritis		●			●															
Arterial stenosis	●																●			

Fig. D-4 Forearm, wrist, and hand cross-reference table for tissue or area examined.

	Adam's positions	Amoss's sign	Anghelescu's sign	Beevor's sign	Chest expansion test	First thoracic nerve root test	Forestier's bowstring sign	Passive scapular approximation test	Rib motion test	Schepelmann's sign	Spinal percussion test	Sponge test	Sternal compression test
Fibrositis												●	
Strain											●		
Fracture											●		
Intercostal syndrome									●	●			
Rib injury									●	●			●
T1-T2 nerve root						●		●					
Myelopathy				●									
Tuberculosis			●										
Sprain		●									●		
IVD syndrome		●									●		
Anklylosing spondylitis		●			●		●		●				
Scoliosis	●												

Fig. D-5   Thoracic spine cross-reference table for tissue or area examined.

Condition	Antalgia sign	Bechterew's sitting test	Bilateral leg-lowering test	Bowstring sign	Bragard's sign	Cox sign	Demianoff's sign	Deyerle's sign	Double leg-raise test	Ely's sign	Fajersztajn's test	Femoral nerve traction test	Heel/toe walk test	Hyperextension test	Kemp's test	Kernig/Brudzinski sign	Lasègue differential sign	Lasègue rebound test
Lower extremity joints																		
Fracture																		
Denervation																		
Myofascitis																		
Hamstring spasm																		
Sacroiliac lesion																		
Meningitis																●		
L2-L3-L4												●		●				
Femoral nerve										●		●		●				
Hip lesion										●							●	
Sprain								●							●			
Spinal neuropathy				●	●					●			●	●	●		●	
Cord tumor					●													
Mechanical lower back			●				●		●						●			
Subluxation		●																
Dural adhesions		●									●							
IVF encroachment		●	●															
Sciatica		●		●				●			●		●					
IVD syndrome	●	●	●		●	●			●		●		●		●			●

Fig. D-6 Lumbar spine cross-reference table for tissue or area examined.

	Lasègue sitting test	Lasègue test	Lewin punch test	Lewin snuff test	Lewin standing test	Lewin supine test	Lindner's sign	Match stick test	Mennell's sign	Milgram's test	Minor's sign	Nachlas test	Néri's sign	Prone knee-bending test	Quick test	Schober's test	Sicard's sign	Sign of the buttock	Skin pinch test	Spinal percussion test	Straight-leg raising test	Turyn's sign	Vanzetti's sign
Lower extremity joints															●								
Fracture											●									●			
Denervation								●											●				
Myofascitis					●														●				
Hamstring spasm				●																			
Sacroiliac lesion		●				●			●		●	●	●										
Meningitis																							
L2-L3-L4														●									
Femoral nerve														●									
Hip lesion																		●					
Sprain									●		●									●			
Spinal neuropathy	●						●										●						
Cord tumor		●								●											●		
Mechanical lower back		●										●	●			●		●	●	●			
Subluxation													●										
Dural adhesions		●																			●		
IVF encroachment		●																					
Sciatica	●	●			●	●	●										●					●	●
IVD syndrome		●	●	●		●		●		●	●		●						●	●	●		

	Anterior innominate test	Belt test	Erichsen's sign	Gaenslen's test	Gapping test	Goldthwait's sign	Hibb's test	Iliac compression test	Knee-to-shoulder test	Laguerre's test	Lewin-Gaenslen's test	Piedallu's sign	Sacral apex test	Sacroiliac resisted-abduction test	Smith-Petersen test	Squish test	Yeoman's test
Pyogenic sacroilitis									●								
Fracture								●									
Subluxation							●	●	●	●	●	●	●				●
Sprain					●		●	●	●	●	●	●	●			●	●
Lumbosacral syndrome		●		●		●									●		
Sacroiliac pathology	●	●	●	●	●	●	●	●	●	●	●	●	●		●		●

Fig. D–7 Pelvis cross-reference table for tissue or area examined.

	Actual leg-length test	Allis' sign	Anvil test	Apparent leg-length test	Chiene's test	Gauvain's sign	Guilland's sign	Hip telescoping test	Jansen's test	Ludloff's sign	Ober's test	Patrick's test	Phelp's test	Thomas test	Trendelenburg's test
Subluxation															●
Coxa vara															●
Poliomyelitis															●
Legg-Calvé-Perthes disease															●
Hip flexion contracture														●	
Gracillis contracture													●		
Iliotibial band											●				
Osteoarthritis									●						●
Meningeal irritation							●								
Pelvic obliquity	●			●											
Calcaneal fracture			●												
Tibial/fibular fracture			●												
Coxa p athology			●			●			●			●	●	●	
Fracture			●		●					●					●
Tibial dysplasia		●													
Hip dislocation		●						●							●
Leg Length	●			●											

Fig. D–8 Hip joint cross-reference table for tissue or area examined.

	Abduction stress test	Adduction stress test	Apley's compression/distraction test	Apprehension test for the patella	Bounce home test	Childress duck waddle test	Clarke's test	Drawer test	Dreyer's sign	Fouchet's sign	Lachman test	Lateral pivot shift maneuver	Losee test	McMurray sign	Noble compression test	Patella ballottement test	Payr's sign	Q-angle test	Slocum's test	Steinmann's sign	Thigh circumference test	Wilson's sign
Osteochondritis																						●
Quadriceps																					●	
Valgus deformity																		●				
Effusion																●						
Anterolateral rotary syndrome													●					●				
Patellar syndromes							●			●								●				
Patellar fracture									●													
Posterior oblique ligament								●			●								●			
Arcuate-popliteus complex								●			●	●							●			
Posterior cruciate ligament								●											●			
Iliotibial band								●				●			●				●			
Posterior capsule								●				●							●			
Anterior cruciate ligament								●			●	●							●			
Chondromalacia patellae							●			●								●				
Patellar dislocation				●														●				
Lateral meniscus			●			●	●							●						●		
Medial meniscus			●			●	●							●			●			●		
Lateral collateral ligament		●										●							●			
Medial collateral ligament	●							●											●			

Fig. D–9 Knee joint cross-reference table for tissue or area examined.

	Talofibular ligament	Vascular	Atrophy	Peroneal nerve paralysis	Foot pronation	Calcaneus fracture	Thrombophlebitis	Fibular fracture	Neuroma	Metatarsalgia	Achilles tendon	Tarsal tunnel syndrome
Anterior drawer sign of the ankle	●											
Buerger's test		●										
Calf circumference test			●									
Claudication test		●										
Duchenne's sign				●								
Foot tourniquet test		●										
Helbings' test					●							
Hoffa's test						●						
Homans' sign		●					●					
Keen's sign								●				
Morton's test									●	●		
Moszkowicz' test		●										
Moses' test		●					●					
Perthes' test		●										
Strunsky's sign										●		
Thompson's test						●					●	
Tinel's foot sign												●

Fig. D–10   Lower leg, ankle, and foot cross-reference table for
tissue or area examined.

	Axial trunk-loading test	Burn's bench test	Flexed-hip test	Flip sign	Libman's sign	Magnuson's test	Mannkopf's sign	Marked part pain-suggestibility test	Plantar flexion test	Related joint motion test	Seeligmüller's sign	Trunk rotational test	Anosmia testing	Coordination-disturbance test	Cuignet's test
Paresis															
Stoicism															
Consciousness															
Anesthesia															
Deafness															
Facial anesthesia															
Blindness															●
Cerebellar lesions														●	
Trigeminal nerve													●		
Olfactory nerve													●		
Facial pain											●				
General pain					●		●	●		●					
Sciatica				●					●						
Lower back	●	●	●			●			●			●			

PAIN   **SENSORY**

Cond'd.	SENSORY													MOTOR						
	Facial anesthesia testing	Gault test	Janet's test	Limb-dropping test (upper extremities)	Lombard's test	Marcus Gunn's sign	Midline tuning-fork test	Optokinetic nystagmus test	Position-sense testing	Regional anesthesia testing	Romberg's sign	Snellen's test	Stoicism indexing	Bilateral limb-dropping test (lower extremities)	Hemiplegic posturing	Hoover's sign	Simulated foot-drop testing	Simulated forearm-and-wrist-weakness testing	Simulated grip-strength-loss test	Tripod test (bilateral leg-fluttering test)
Paresis														●	●	●	●	●	●	
Stoicism													●							
Consciousness				●									●							
Anesthesia			●				●			●										
Deafness		●			●															
Facial anesthesia	●									●										
Blindness						●		●				●								
Cerebellar lesions									●		●				●	●				
Trigeminal nerve																				
Olfactory nerve																				
Facial pain																				
General pain																				
Sciatica																				
Lower back																				●

Fig. D–11 Malingering cross-reference table for tissues or area examined.

Index